Progress in Allergy and Clinical Immunology
Volume 3, Stockholm

Progress in Allergy and Clinical Immunology Volume 3, Stockholm

Proceedings of the XVth International Congress of Allergology and Clinical Immunology
and the 1994 Annual Meeting of the European Academy of Allergology and Clinical Immunology
Stockholm, June 26–July 1, 1994

Edited by
S. G. O. Johansson
Department of Clinical Immunology, Karolinska Hospital, Stockholm, Sweden

Associate Editors
J. Björkander (Sweden), B. Björkstén (Sweden), S.-E. Dahlén (Sweden), F.B. Michel (France), T. Miyamoto (Japan), T. Söderström (Sweden)

Hogrefe & Huber Publishers
Seattle · Toronto · Bern · Göttingen

Library of Congress Cataloging-in-Publication Data

is available via the Library of Congress Marc Database under the
LC Catalog Card Number 94-074177.

Canadian Cataloguing in Publication Data

International Congress of Allergology and Clinical Immunology (15th : 1994 : Stockholm, Sweden)
Progress in allergy and clinical immunology, volume 3, Stockholm : proceedings of the XVth International Congress of Allergology and Clinical Immunology and the European Academy of Allergology and Clinical Immunology 1994 annual meeting, Stockholm, June 26–July 1, 1994
Includes bibliographical references and index
1. Allergy – Congresses. 2. Immunopathology – Congresses. I. Johansson, S. G. O. (Stig Gunnar Olof), 1938–   . II. European Academy of Allergology and Clinical Immunology. Meeting (1994: Stockholm, Sweden). III. Title.

RC583.2.I57   1995   616.97   C95-930181-X

USA: P.O. Box 2487, Kirkland, WA 98083-2487
                    Phone (206) 820-1500, Fax (206) 823-8324
CANADA: 12 Bruce Park Avenue, Toronto, Ontario M4P 2S3
                    Phone (416) 482-6339
SWITZERLAND: Länggass-Strasse 76, CH-3000 Bern 9
                    Phone (031) 300-4500, Fax (031) 300-4590
GERMANY: Rohnsweg 25, D-37085 Göttingen
                    Phone (0551) 49609-0, Fax (0551) 49609-88

Printed and bound in Germany

ISBN 0-88937-122-9

Contents

Contents

Preface

For the first time, the International Association of Allergology and Clinical Immunology (IAACI) and the European Academy of Allergology and Clinical Immunology (EAACI) have joined together for a collaborative congress: the XVth ICACI and EAACI '94. The joint efforts of the societies resulted in a scientific program that included 60 symposia, with invited speakers covering allergological and immunological aspects of most diseases. The response to the Congress was tremendous! More than 6000 participants from 80 countries attended what became one of our largest meetings ever.

This volume, the third in the series on *Progress in Allergy and Clinical Immunology*, presents the main papers from the plenary symposia, main symposia, and joint symposia – all in all 14 of the most prestigious sessions held during the Congress. It is our belief that the book will not only be useful as a position report on the state of the art of allergology and clinical immunology in 1994. It should also serve as an important tool in the process of continuing education and provision of information to physicians and scientists in these fields. On behalf of the Editors, I would like to express our sincere appreciation to the contributors and to the Publishers, Hogrefe & Huber, for their cooperation in producing this important volume.

S. G. O. Johansson
Stockholm, Fall 1994

Allergen Presentation in the Airways

Patrick G Holt, Delia J Nelson, Andrew S McWilliam, Christine McMenamin, Natalie Bilyk, Deborah H Strickland*

Keywords: Antigen presentation, respiratory tract, dendritic cells, MHC class II, alveolar macrophages, T-helper cells, CD8+ T cells

Primary immune responses to inhaled allergen are initiated in the regional lymph nodes (RLN) by allergen-bearing dendritic cells (DC) which migrate from the airway wall. They normally perform a "sentinel" role in surveillance for antigen, which they process and store for future presentation to T cells after migration to RLN; the latter requires a GM-CSF-dependent maturational step, which is actively inhibited while they are *in situ* by cytokine signals from alveolar macrophages (AM). The turnover time of the DC is less than 72 h in the steady state, and is markedly accelerated during inflammation, where their density can transiently increase by up to 300%. They are highly sensitive to steroids, in both normal and inflamed airway tissue. Secondary immune responses to inhaled antigens occur throughout lung and airway tissues, and can potentially be triggered by any cells bearing MHC class II, although the available evidence suggests that DC and monocytes are probably the only functionally significant populations present. Resident AM strongly inhibit local T-memory cell (especially Th2) proliferation in the lung, but permit activation of individual T cells to the stage of IL-2R expression and cytokine secretion, thus limiting the magnitude of the local secondary T-effector cell response to a "single hit."

Regulation of Primary Immunity to Inhaled Antigen/Allergen

Inhalation of protein antigens triggers an initial Th2-dependent IgE plasma cell response in the regional lymph nodes (RLN) draining the upper respiratory tract. In immunologically normal disease-free animals undergoing continuous inhalation exposure, this IgE response is short lived, and is terminated by the onset of a state of "tolerance" or "immune deviation" involving selective suppression of IgE/delayed-type hypersensitivity (DTH) reactivity, with the concomitant preservation of low grade antigen-specific IgG, IgA, and Th1-like T-helper cell activity (1–3). If inhalation exposure occurs during periods of hormonal imbalance, immunological dysfunction (in particular "immaturity"), or exposure to agents causing inflammation at the level of the airway mucosa, the IgE response may instead persist, producing a state of clinical hypersensitivity to the allergen (1–3). An identical series of mechanisms are operative during the primary response to dietary allergens, which ideally leads to a state of host-protective "oral tolerance" (4).

Regardless of whether allergen inhalation results in a state of unresponsiveness ("tolerance") or hypersensitivity, the key cellular events which determine the outcome of the overall response occur in the paracortical regions of the RLN draining the nasopharynx and the major conducting airways. The antigen presenting cell (APC) which controls this response must accordingly have the following characteristics: (i) it must be capable of efficiently sampling extracellular fluids within the airway epithelium; (ii) it must be capable of directed migration to paracortical zones in RLN; and (iii) it must be highly efficient in activating *naive* T cells. The only cell population which meets these criteria are dendritic cells (DC; 5), in particular the DC population recently described in our laboratory as resident within the epithelium of the conducting airways and the alveolar wall (6).

* Division of Cell Biology, Institute for Child Health Research, PO Box 855, West Perth, Western Australia 6872.

DC Population in the Respiratory Tract Tissues

Since the original description of the DC network within the alveolar septa and airway epithelium in humans (7) and experimental animals (8, 9), considerable progress has been made in characterization of these cells, as summarized below.

Density, Distribution, and Surface Phenotype in the Steady State

In healthy adult animals, DC are distributed throughout the respiratory tract, from the nasal mucosa to the alveolar septa, their overall density at individual sites reflecting intensity of local stimulation by inhaled particulates, namely, highest in the nasal turbinates and the epithelium of the large airways (10, 11).

The majority of the DC constitutively express high levels of MHC class II (Ia), but a subset has recently been identified which is Ia⁻ (9–11). These DC express CD4, together with some (but not all) of the surface markers characteristic of macrophages; additionally, the DC populations in the airway epithelium can be distinguished from those of the conducting airways on the basis of differential expression of these latter markers (9, 10). A distinguishing feature of human respiratory tract DC is surface expression of variable levels of CD1 a or CD1 c; Birbeck granule expression is also highly variable (12).

Function

Analogous to epidermal Langerhans cells (ELC; 5), airway and lung DC are restricted to antigen acquisition/processing while *in situ*, and only develop the capacity to present antigen to T cells after migration to RLN, where they mature under stimulation from GM-CSF (13, 14). While *in situ*, they are prevented from responding to GM-CSF by signals derived from endogenous tissue macrophages, particularly the resident AM population (13, 14).

Population Dynamics

Recent studies employing a radiation chimera model indicate that 85% of the airway DC population is renewed every 48–72 h, with net migration to RLN being matched by net recruitment of bone-marrow derived precursors (15). This is a much more rapid turnover than typical DC populations such as ELC, and is matched only by gut wall DCs (15).

Response to Inflammation

The density of airway DC has been shown to increase in chronic inflammation in animals employing a model of cedar workers asthma (10), and also in the nasal mucosa of human rhinitics in the pollen season (16). More dramatic changes occur during acute inflammation to inhaled bacterial products, where airway intraepithelial DC density can increase by up to 300% within 2 h of exposure (10, 17); unlike PMN which migrate into the epithelium and continue through to the airway surface, the freshly recruited DC remain within the inflamed epithelium (presumably sampling the antigenic environment) for several hours, and then home selectively to RLN (7).

Ontogeny

The airway DC population is initially "seeded" in fetal life, but at birth the cells of the network (approx. one third as dense as in adults) do not express Ia; the latter is progressively upregulated between birth and weaning in response to inhaled inflammatory stimuli, and during this period the overall DC density increases towards adult levels (11).

Steroid Sensitivity

Administration of topical (inhaled) or systemic steroids markedly reduces the density and also decreases the surface Ia expression of airway DC. These effects have been documented in adult animals in the steady state and during acute inflammation (18), and also in newborn animals where the kinetics of postnatal development is reduced (11). One locus of action of steroids in this system is at the level of migration of bone-marrow derived DC precursors from the blood into the airway mucosa (15).

Regulation of Secondary Immune Responses to Inhaled Allergen in Sensitized Animals

Unlike naive T cells, which require inductive signals from DC, sensitized T-memory cells can theoretically respond to processed antigen presented in conjunction with class II MHC molecules on the surface of virtually any cell type, including epithelial cells, fibroblasts, B cells, monocytes/macrophages, and even eosinophils (19).

In the context of the respiratory tract, there is little direct evidence to suggest a significant local role in this process for cells other than DC and monocytes. While B cells function effectively as APC *in vitro*, B-cell infiltration into lung tissues is not a feature of immunoinflammatory diseases such as asthma, and Ia^+ epithelial cells appear more likely to deliver an anergizing as opposed to activating signal, as shown for type II alveolar epithelial cells (reviewed in 19).

Cells of the mononuclear phagocytic lineage appear to play a major, and dualistic role. On the one hand, monocytes are acknowledged as excellent APC for T-memory cells, but as noted above mature resident AM (into which the monocytes develop after migration into lung) suppress the APC function(s) of DC (9, 13, 14), and inhibit the capacity of primed T cells to respond to antigen or mitogen (19). The acquisition of this T-cell-suppressive phenotype occurs relatively slowly over a period of several days after monocytes enter the lung, and is inhibited/reversed by a combination of GM-CSF and TNF-α (20).

The mechanism(s) by which mature AM suppress T-cell activation are only partly understood, and the process appears to be multifactorial (reviewed in 21). However, recent studies indicate that AM regulation in this context does not equate to simple inhibition of T-cell function, but instead involves limitation of the expression of effector function(s) by individual T cells to a "single hit," i.e., they display normal Ca^{2+} flux, TcR down-modulation, cytokine secretion (including IL-2), and expression of IL-2R, but are prevented from responding to the IL-2 signal, and are consequently unable to progress beyond the G_0/G_1 phases of the cell cycle (21). This appears to be a mechanism to limit local T-cell activation to the minimum required for host protection, thus minimizing immunoinflammatory damage to the delicate tissues involved in gas exchange. There are intriguing suggestions in the literature that this mechanism may be less effective in diseases such as chronic asthma, but convincing proof is lacking.

Recent evidence in support of the operation of this overall mechanism *in vivo* has been provided by experiments in rats and mice involving the *in situ* depletion of AM via intratracheal administration of a liposome-encapsulated selective macrophage toxin. These studies demonstrated that AM-depleted animals displayed markedly enhanced secondary immune responses to inhaled allergen, characterized by large infiltrates of activated T and B cells into lung and airway tissue (21, 22). The AM-deficient animals additionally showed preferential amplification of secondary IgE responses indicating selectivity of this control mechanism towards Th2 regulation (23), possibly via the IFN-α/IL-12 pathways.

Acknowledgments

This work is supported by the National Health and Medical Research Council of Australia and Glaxo Australia

Address for correspondence:

Patrick G Holt
Division of Cell Biology
Institute for Child Health Research
PO Box 855, West Perth
Western Australia 6872

References

1. Holt PG, Sedgwick JD. Suppression of IgE responses following antigen inhalation: A natural homeostatic mechanism which limits sensitization to aeroallergens. *Immunol Today* 1987; 8:14.

2. Holt PG, McMenamin C. Defence against allergic sensitization in the healthy lung: The role of inhalation tolerance. *Clin Exp Allergy* 1989; 19:255.

3. McMenamin C, Holt PG. The natural immune response to inhaled soluble protein antigens involves major histocompatibility complex (MHC) class I-restricted $CD8^+$ T cell-mediated but MHC class II-restricted $CD4^+$ T cell-dependent immune deviation resulting in selective suppression of IgE production. *J Exp Med* 1993; 178:889.

4. Mowat AM. The regulation of immune responses to dietary protein antigens. *Immunol Today* 1987; 8:93.

5. Steinman RM. The dendritic cell system and its role in immunogenicity. *Annu Rev Immunol* 1991; 9:271.

6. Holt PG, Schon-Hegrad MA, McMenamin PG. Dendritic cells in the respiratory tract. *Int Rev Immunol* 1990; 6:139.

7. Holt PG, Schon-Hegrad MA, Phillips MJ, McMenamin PG. Ia-positive dendritic cells form a tightly meshed network within the human airway epithelium. *Clin Exp Allergy* 1989; 19:597.

8. Holt PG, Schon-Hegrad MA, Oliver J, Holt BJ, McMenamin PG. A contiguous network of dendritic antigen-presenting cells within the respiratory epithelium. *Int Arch Allergy Appl Immunol* 1990; 91:155.

9. Holt PG, Schon-Hegrad MA, Oliver J. MHC class II antigen-bearing dendritic cells in pulmonary tissues of the rat. Regulation of antigen presentation activity by endogenous macrophage populations. *J Exp Med* 1988; 167:262.

10. Schon-Hegrad MA, Oliver J, McMenamin PG, Holt PG. Studies on the density, distribution, and surface phenotype of intraepithelial class II major histocompatibility complex antigen (Ia)-bearing dendritic cells (DC) in the conducting airways. *J Exp Med* 1991; 173:1345.

11. Nelson DJ, McMenamin C, McWilliam AS, Brenan M, Holt PG. Development of the airway intraepithelial Dendritic Cell network in the rat from class II MHC (Ia) negative precursors: Differential regulation of Ia expression at different levels of the respiratory tract. *J Exp Med* 1994; 179:203.

12. Soler P, Moreau A, Basset F, Hance AJ. Cigarette smoking-induced changes in the number and differentiated state of pulmonary dendritic cells/Langerhans cells. *Am Rev Respir Dis* 1989; 139:1112.

13. Holt PG, Oliver J, McMenamin C, Schon-Hegrad MA. Studies on the surface phenotype and functions of dendritic cells in parenchymal lung tissue of the rat. *Immunology* 1992; 75:582.

14. Holt PG, Oliver J, Bilyk N, McMenamin C, McMenamin PG, Kraal G, Thepen T. Downregulation of the antigen presenting cell function(s) of pulmonary dendritic cells *in vivo* by resident alveolar macrophages. *J Exp Med* 1993; 177:397.

15. Holt PG, Haining S, Nelson DJ, Sedgwick JD. Origin and steady-state of class II MHC-bearing dendritic cells in the epithelium of the conducting airways. *J Immunol* 1994; 153: 256.

16. Fokkens WJ, Vroom TM, Rijntjes E, Mulder PG. Fluctuation of the number of CD1(T6)-positive dendritic cells, presumably Langerhans cells, in the nasal mucosa of patients with an isolated grass-pollen allergy before, during, and after the grasspollen season. *J Allergy Clin Immunol* 1989; 84:39.

17. McWilliam AS, Nelson DJ, Holt PG. Rapid dendritic cell recruitment is a hallmark of the acute inflammatory response at mucosal surfaces. *J Exp Med* 1994; 179:1331.

18. Nelson DJ, McWilliam AS, Haining S, Holt PG. Downmodulation of airway intraepithelial Dendritic Cell populations following local and systemic exposure to steroids. *Am J Resp Crit Care Med* (in press).

19. Holt PG. Regulation of antigen-presenting function(s) in lung and airway tissues. *Eur Respir J* 1993; 6:120.

20. Bilyk N, Holt PG. Inhibition of the immunosuppressive activity of resident pulmonary alveolar macrophages by granulocyte/macrophage colony-stimulating factor. *J Exp Med* 1993; 177:1773.

21. Strickland DH, Kees UR, Holt PG. Suppression of T-cell activation by pulmonary alveolar macrophages: Dissociation of effects on TcR, IL-2R expression, and proliferation (submitted).

22. Thepen T, McMenamin C, Oliver J, Kraal G, Holt PG. Regulation of immune response to inhaled antigen by alveolar macrophages: differential effects of *in vivo* alveolar macrophage elimination on the induction of tolerance vs. immunity. *Eur J Immunol* 1991; 21:2845.

23. Thepen T, McMenamin C, Girn B, Kraal G, Holt PG. Regulation of IgE production in presensitised animals: In vivo elimination of alveolar macrophages preferentially increases IgE responses to inhaled allergen. *Clin Exp Allergy* 1992; 22:1107.

T Cells, Cytokines, and IgE Regulation in Allergic Disease

Sergio Romagnani*

Keywords: IgE, Th1, Th2

In the last few years, a great deal of progress has been made in understanding the mechanisms underlying human allergic disorders. Activation by allergens of type 2 helper T cells (Th2) in genetically predisposed individuals is responsible for both the production of IgE antibodies (via IL-4 and IL-13) and eosinophilia (via IL-5), which represent the hallmarks of allergic disorders. The mechanisms responsible for Th2-type responses against allergens or helminths and for Th1-type responses against intracellular bacteria have also been at least partially clarified. Early production of IL-12 and interferons promotes Th1-type responses, whereas early production of IL-4 favors Th2-type responses. More recently, we have shown that Th2, but not Th1, cells express the CD30 molecule. CD30 might be a distinctive marker of T cells producing Th2-type cytokines which is involved in the differentiation/activation pathway of these cells.

Introduction

In the last few years, the mechanisms that regulate the synthesis of human IgE have been widely investigated (reviewed in 1 and 2). Human IgE synthesis results from the collaboration between a subset of CD4+ helper T (Th) cells, and B cells. CD4+ Th cells provide B cells with at least two signals: one signal is delivered by T cell-derived interleukin (IL)-4 (3, 4) which induces germ-line ε expression (5). Another T cell-derived cytokine, IL-13, can also induce germ-line ε expression in B cells, but it seems to be two- to five-fold less potent than IL-4 in inducing IgE production (6). The other signal, which is required for the expression of a productive mRNA and for the synthesis of IgE protein, is represented by a Th-B cell-to-cell physical interaction (7, 8). This interaction occurs between the CD40L expressed on the activated Th cell and the CD40 molecule constitutively expressed on the B cell (9–11). In contrast, CD4+ Th cells that do not produce IL-4 or produce high concentrations of IFN-γ do not support IgE synthesis, and IFN-γ can suppress the IL-4-dependent IgE synthesis (3, 4). Other soluble factors have been shown, at least *in vitro*, to have some negative or positive regulatory effects on human IgE synthesis (Figure 1).

Th Cells Involved in the Human IgE Synthesis Belong to the Th2 Subset

Altered proportions of IL-4- and/or IFN-γ-producing phytohemagglutinin (PHA)-induced T-cell clones were found in the peripheral blood (PB) of patients with the hyper-IgE syndrome (12), severe atopic disorders, or helminthic infestations (13). Subsequently, it was shown that most T cells infiltrating the conjunctiva of patients with vernal conjunctivitis developed into T-cell clones that appeared to be very similar to the Th2 cells already described in mouse (14) because of their ability to produce large amounts of IL-4 but no, or limited amounts of, IFN-γ (15). Likewise, high proportions of T-cell clones with similar cytokine profile were derived from the skin of patients with atopic dermatitis (16, 17). By using a different experimental approach, i.e., *in situ* hybridization, cells exhibiting specific signals for IL-5 mRNA, but not for IFN-γ, were found at the site of the 24-h late phase reactions in skin biopsies from atopic patients (18). Similar cells were also located beneath the epithelial basement membrane in endobronchial mucosal biopsies (19) and in the bronchoalveolar fluid from patients with extrinsic asthma (20).

* Division of Clinical Immunology and Allergy, University of Florence, Italy.

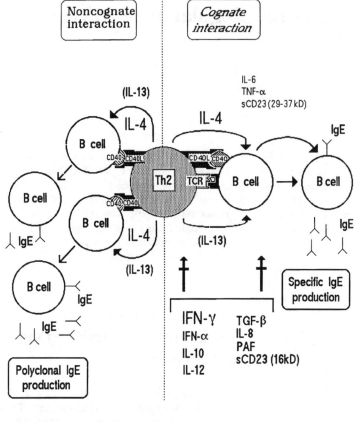

Figure 1. Role of T cells and cytokines in the regulation of human IgE synthesis. At least two signals are required by B cells to synthesize IgE. The first signal is provided by Th2 cell-derived IL-4 or IL-13, which promote the isotype switching to IgE; the second signal is provided by the interaction between CD40L on the activated T cell and CD40 on the B cell.

To investigate whether the Th2-like cells present in the airway mucosa of patients with allergic respiratory disorders actually reflected a T-cell response to inhaled allergens, biopsy specimens were obtained from the bronchial or nasal mucosa of patients with grass pollen-induced bronchial asthma or rhinitis 48 h after positive bronchial or nasal provocation test with grass pollen extract. T-cell clones derived from these and control specimens were then assessed for their phenotype, allergen-specificity, profile of cytokine secretion and ability to provide B cell help for IgE synthesis. Proportions ranging from 14 to 22% of CD4[+] T-cell clones derived from stimulated mucosa were specific for grass allergens; most of them exhibited a clear-cut Th2 profile and induced IgE synthesis in autologous PB B cells. In contrast, none of T-cell clones derived from control tissues was specific for grass allergens, and only a minority of them showed the Th2 phenotype (21). These findings provide convincing evidence that Th2 cells specific for the relevant allergen appear in the mucosa soon after allergen inhalation. These cells, because of their

cytokine profile, might well play a triggering role in the initiation of the allergic cascade.

Main Properties of Human Th2 Cells

To provide additional information on both the nature and function of Th cells responsible for the human IgE synthesis in allergic patients and in individuals infested by helminth parasites, our strategy has been to establish T-cell clones specific for allergens (*Dermatophagoides pteronyssinus* group I, *Der p* I; *Lolium perenne* group I, *Lol p* I; and *Poa pratensis* group IX, *Poa p* IX), helminthic components (excretory/secretory antigen of *Toxocara canis,* TES), bacterial components (protein purified derivative, PPD, of *Mycobacterium tuberculosis,* tetanus toxoid, TT, and streptokinase, SK) and viruses (influenza virus).

When large series of PPD- or TES-specific T-cell clones derived from two healthy individuals were compared, a clear cut dichotomy in the profile of cytokine secretion was observed. Virtually all PPD-specific clones produced IL-2 and IFN-γ, but not IL-4 and IL-5 (Th2), whereas the great majority of TES-specific clones produced IL-4 and IL-5, but not IL-2 and IFN-γ (Th1). PPD-specific T-cell clones that failed to secrete IL-4 and IL-5, and TES-specific T-cell clones that failed to secrete IL-2 and IFN-γ, were found to lack transcripts for IL-4 and IL-5 or for IL-2 and IFN-γ, respectively (22). High numbers of Der p I-, *Lol p* I-, or *Poa p* IX-specific T-cell clones were obtained from mite- or grass-sensitive atopic individuals and compared for their phenotype of cytokine secretion with PPD- or TT-specific T-cell clones derived from the same donors. Virtually all the allergen-specific T-cell clones produced IL-4 (and IL-5) in response to stimulation with PMA plus anti-CD3 antibody, and a proportion of them failed to produce IFN-γ. When assessed with the specific antigen under MHC-restricted conditions, the great majority of allergen-

specific T-cell clones behave as Th2-like helper T cells. While most T-cell clones specific for TT produced both IL-4 and IFN-γ (particularly in response to PMA plus anti-CD3 antibody), all T-cell clones specific for PPD produced high amounts of IFN-γ, but most of them did not produce IL-4 and IL-5 (23).

Interestingly, PPD-specific (Th1) and TES- or allergen-specific (Th2) clones showed other distinctive functional properties. The majority of Th1, but only a minority of Th2, clones were cytolytic (24). Only Th2 clones provided help for B-cell IgE synthesis, whereas both Th1 and Th2 clones at low T-B cell-to-cell ratios provided helper functions for other immunoglobulin classes. At high T-B ratios, however, the helper function of Th1 clones was limited by their cytolytic activity towards the antigen-presenting cell (APC), including B cells (24, 25). Finally, Th1, but not Th2, clones induced procoagulant activity and tissue factor production in human monocytes, and these activities were suppressed by both IL-4 and IL-10 produced by Th2 cells (Del Prete et al., submitted for publication). The main functional properties of human Th1 and Th2 clones are summarized in Table 1.

Table 1. Main functional properties of human Th1 and Th2 clones.

Functions	Th1	Th2
Cytokine secretion		
IFN-γ	+++	−
TNF-β	+++	−
IL-2	+++	+
TNF-α	+++	+
GM-CSF	++	++
IL-3	++	+++
IL-6	+	+++
IL-10	+	+++
IL-13	+	+++
IL-4	−	+++
IL-5	−	+++
Regulation by cytokines		
IL-2	up	up
IL-4		up
IFN-γ		down
IL-10	down	down
Cytolytic potential	+++	−
IgE	−	+++
IgM, IgG, IgA		
At low T: B cell ratios	+++	++
At high T: B cell ratios	−	+++
Macrophage activation		
Induction of PCA	+++	−
TF production	+++	−

Abnormal IL-4 Production by Th Cells from Atopic Subjects

Additional elements of complexity emerged when the phenotype of cytokine secretion of PPD-, TT-, or SK-specific T-cell lines and clones obtained from the PB of atopic and nonatopic donors was compared. Even if all clones specific for bacterial constituents from both atopic and nonatopic donors were able to produce elevated concentrations of IFN-γ, a clear difference emerged with regard to their ability to produce IL-4. PPD-, TT-, and SK-specific T-cell lines derived from atopic donors but not from nonatopics were able to produce high amounts of IL-4 and IL-5. More importantly, 37% of PPD-specific TCC derived from atopic patients, but only 4% of those obtained from nonatopic individuals, produced IL-4 in response to stimulation with the specific antigen (26). Similar results were obtained when T-cell clones were generated from cord blood lymphocytes of newborns from atopic parents (Piccinni et al., manuscript in preparation). These data suggest that atopic patients have an enhanced ability to produce IL-4, even in response

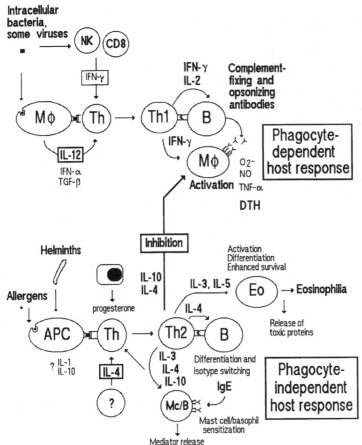

Figure 2. The two main pathways of specific immunity based on their dependence or independence of phagocyte recruitment in the effector response.

Th2 = type 2 helper T lymphocyte; TCR = T cell receptor; - = stimulatory effect; - = inhibitory effect.

From reference (33).

Mø = macrophage; Th = CD4[+] helper T lymphocyte; CD8[+] = CD8[+] T lymphocyte; NK = natural killer cell; B = B lymphocyte; DTH = delayed-type hypersensitivity; Eo = eosinophil; APC = antigen presenting cell; Mc/B = cell of the mast cell/basophil lineage; ? = the nature of the cell(s) providing IL-4 at the triad (APC/Ag/Th) recognition level is still unclear.

to antigens other than common environmental allergens or helminthic components. This aberrant IL-4 production by Th cells may represent one of the immune alterations encoded by non-MHC genes that control basal IgE levels (27). However, the molecular alteration(s) responsible for the enhanced ability of Th cells from atopic patients to produce IL-4 are at present unknown.

Mechanisms Involved in the Development of Th1 or Th2 Cells

Factors that regulate the development of human Th1 and Th2 clones have been investigated using PB lymphocytes cultured with PPD, TES, or allergens in the presence or in the absence of cytokines

and/or anti-cytokine antibodies. The presence of IL-4 in bulk cultures before cloning shifted the differentiation of PPD-specific T cells from the Th1 to the Th0, or even to the Th2 phenotype. In contrast, the addition of both IFN-γ and anti-IL-4 antibody induced allergen- as well as TES-specific T cells to differentiate into Th0, or even Th1, instead of Th2 clones (28). IFN-α, TGF-β, NKSF (IL-12), poly-I-C, and influenza virus also promoted the differentiation of allergen- or TES-specific T cells into Th0 or Th1, instead of Th2 clones (28–31). In contrast, anti-IL-12 antibody favored the differentiation of PPD-specific T cells into Th0 or Th2, instead of Th1 clones (30). IFN-α and IL-12 are produced predominantly by macrophages, cells that have an important role in the presentation of corpuscolate antigens to Th cells. Therefore, it is reasonable to suggest that, given the capacity of viruses and intracellular bacteria to stimulate macrophage production of IFN-α and IL-12 (which induce IFN-γ production by both T cells and NK cells), Th cells may be simultaneously presented with processed antigen plus cytokines that induce them to differentiate towards a Th1 phenotype (32).

Taken together, these data suggest that intracellular bacteria and some viruses induce specific immune responses of the Th1 type at least partly because they either directly stimulate NK cells to produce IFN-γ, or because they induce macrophage production of IFN-α and IL-12, which in turn stimulate NK cell growth and IFN-γ production. The production of high concentrations of IFN-γ by NK cells, although important, does not appear to be sufficient for the induction of Th1 responses. Indeed, the addition of anti-IFN-γ antibody to bulk cultures does not prevent or reverse the inhibitory effect of poly-I-C on the differentiation of allergen-specific T cells into Th2 clones. In contrast, the poly-I-C-induced Th0/Th1 differentiation of allergen-specific T cells could be driven to the Th0/Th2 profile by the simultaneous addition of antibodies reactive with IFN-γ, IFN-α, and IL-12 (32; Manetti et al., manuscript in preparation) . It can be concluded, therefore, that intracellular bacteria and some viruses induce Th1 responses because the profile of the "natural" immune response they evoke provides optimum conditions (high concentrations of IL-12 and IFN-γ in absence of IL-4) for the development of Th1 cells (Figure 2) (33).

The reason why soluble allergens and some helminth components promote the differentiation of Th cells into the Th2 phenotype is less clear. The presence in the microenvironment of IL-4 in concomitance with no, or low concentrations of, IFN-γ seems to represent a favorable condition for the development of Th2 cells. The other component necessary for the development of Th2 cells – the presence of IL-4 – raises the important question of the cellular source of IL-4. Since T cells seem to be unable to differentiate into IL-4-producing cells in the absence of IL-4, IL-4 production by a non-T cell must be involved. Non-T cells from mouse spleen and human bone marrow, probably belonging to the mast cell/basophil lineage, as well as mature basophils and mast cells, can release IL-4 (34–37). Thus, IL-4 production by cells of the mast cell/basophil lineage might very well reflect a means through which Th2 cells can be strikingly amplified *in vivo* during allergic reactions and parasitic infestations. Whether these cells also play a role in the primary Th2 responses remains to be established.

More recently, we have shown that other soluble factors may favor the development of Th2 cells. Addition in bulk culture before cloning of an IL-1 receptor antagonist (IL-1ra) inhibited the development of Der p I-specific T cells into Th2 cells, suggesting that the presence of endogenously produced IL-1 may be important for the development of Th2 cells (38). Likewise, progesterone present in bulk culture before cloning appeared to shift the differentiation of PPD- or SK-specific T cells from the Th1 to the Th0 phenotype. More importantly, stimulation of established Th1 clones with progesterone in combination with insoluble anti-CD3 antibody induced mRNA expression and production of small but significant amounts of IL-4 (Piccinni et al., manuscript in preparation). These findings are consistent with the recent demonstration of increased IL-4 expression at the placental level during murine pregnancy (39). It has been indeed suggested that Th2 cytokines produced at the maternal-fetal interface may contribute to successful pregnancy by inhibiting the fetus-rejecting activity of Th1 responses (40). Thus, IL-4 appears to be the critical factor for the development of Th2 responses, but IL-1, IL-10, and progesterone itself may play an ancillary role in favoring such a type of development (Figure 2).

CD30 is a Distinctive Marker for Activated Th2 Cells

One of the main problems in studying the role of Th1 and Th2 subsets in different disease states is the lack of reliable markers capable of identifying these cell subsets. To overcome this problem, in a recent study we have assessed a large panel of human CD4[+] T-cell clones with established Th1, Th2, or Th0 profiles of cytokine secretion for the expression of different CD antigens. By using a monoclonal antibody specific for CD30, a member of the so-called TNF receptor superfamily (41) already known for its presence on the surface membrane of Hodgkin and Reed-Sternberg cells (42), we found that Th1 clones showed low or undetectable expression of CD30 protein, whereas Th2 clones expressed high levels of surface CD30 and released detectable amounts of soluble CD30. Th0 clones showed an intermediate pattern of CD30 expression and release (43, 44). Furthermore, CD4[+] CD30[+] T cells specific for *Lol p* I grass pollen allergen and inducible to the production of

Th2-type cytokines were sorted out from the circulation of grass-sensitive patients in concomitance with seasonal exposure to grass pollen and the appearance of allergic symptomatology (43). Finally, elevated concentrations of the soluble form of CD30 were found in the serum of high proportions of HIV-infected individuals (45) and of allergic patients showing high IgE serum levels (Giannarini et al., manuscript in preparation). Thus, CD30 appears to be involved in the differentiation/activation pathway of Th2 cells and may represent a marker for activated human T cells producing Th2-type cytokines (43, 44).

Concluding Remarks

In the last few years, the mechanisms responsible for the triggering and maintenance of allergic disorders have been extensively clarified. There is no longer any doubt that hyperproduction of IgE in allergic people results from the helper activity on B cells of Th cells able to produce IL-4, but not IFN-γ (Th2 cells). These Th2 cells, because of their ability to produce IL-5, are also responsible for the eosinophilia that is often associated with hyperproduction of IgE in both allergic subjects and helminth-infested patients. The mechanisms by which helminths preferentially activate Th2 cells are still obscure. Likewise, the reason why environmental allergens promote a prevalent Th2 response only in a minority of human beings (so-called atopics) is unclear.

The results of several studies suggest that a better knowledge of factors that modulate the activation of Th2 cells may provide a means for therapeutic interventions in IgE-mediated disorders through successful transformation of a Th2-like into a Th1- or Th0-like response. For instance, a bias toward Th1 activation could be achieved in vitro either by addition of IL-12 or IFNs, and/or neutralization of IL-4 in the microenvironment where the Th cell-allergen interaction occurs. A further characterization of the events required for selective activation of Th1 or Th2 cells might offer potential sites for pharmacological manipulation of Th1 and Th2 activation, leading to the development of drugs that selectively activate or inhibit specific Th subsets in vivo.

Acknowledgments

This work was supported by funds provided by CNR (ACRO Project) and European Community Biotechnology network.

Address for correspondence:

Sergio Romagnani
Istituto di Clinica medica 3
Viale Morgagni, 85
I-50134 Florence
Italy

References

1. Romagnani S. Regulation and deregulation of human IgE synthesis. *Immunol Today* 1990; 11:316.

2. Vercelli D, Geha RS. Regulation of IgE synthesis in humans: a tale of two signals. *J Allergy Clin Immunol* 1991; 88:285.

3. Del Prete GF, Maggi E, Parronchi P, Chretien I, Tiri A, Macchia D, Ricci M, Banchhereau J, de Vries J, Romagnani S. IL-4 is an essential factor for the IgE synthesis induced in vitro by human T cell clones and their supernatants *J Immunol* 1988; 140:4193.

4. Pene JF, Rousset F, Briere F, Chretien I, Bonnefoy JY, Spits H, Yokota T, Arai N, Arai K-I, Banchereau J, de Vries J. IgE production by normal human lymphocytes is induced by interleukin 4 and suppressed by interferons g and a and prostaglandin E2. *Proc Natl Acad Sci USA* 1988; 85:6880.

5. Gauchat J-F, Lebman DA, Coffman RL, Gascan H, de Vries JE. Structure and expression of germline trasncripts in human B cells induced by interleukin-4 to switch to IgE production. *J Exp Med* 1990; 172:463.

6. Punnonen J, Aversa G, Cocks BG, McKenzie ANJ, Menon S, Zurawski G, de Waal Malefyt R, de Vries JE. Interleukin 13 induces interleukin 4-independent IgG4 adn IgE synthesis and CD23 expression by human B cells. *Proc Natl Acad Sci USA* 1993; 90:3730.

7. Parronchi P, Tiri A, Macchia D, De Carli M, Biswas P, Simonelli C, Maggi E, Del Prete GF, Ricci M, Romagnani S. Noncognate contact-dependent B cell activation can promote IL-4-dependent *in vitro* human IgE synthesis. *J Immunol* 1990; 144:2102.

8. Vercelli D, Jabara HH, Arai K, Geha RS. Induction of human IgE synthesis requires interleukin 4 and T/B cell interactions involving the T cell receptor/CD3

complex and MHC class II antigens. *J Exp Med* 1989; 169:1295.

9. Jabara HH, Fu SM, Geha RS, Vercelli D. CD40 and IgE: synergism between anti-CD40 monoclonal antibody and interleukin 4 in the induction of IgE synthesis by highly purified human B cells. *J Exp Med* 1990; 172:1861.

10. Spriggs MK, Armitage RJ, Strockbine L, Clifford L, Macduff BM, Sato TA, Maliszewski CR, Fanslow WC. Recombinant human CD40 ligand stimulates B cell proliferation and immunoglobulin E secretion. *J Exp Med* 1992; 176:1543.

11. Fuleihan R, Ramesh N, Loh R, Jabara HH, Rosen FS, Chatila T, Fu SM, Stamenkovic I, Geha RS. Defective expression of the CD40 ligand in X chromosome-linked immunoglobulin deficiency with normal or elevated IgM. *Proc Natl Acad Sci USA* 1993; 90:2170.

12. Del Prete GF, Tiri A, De Carli M, Macchia D, Parronchi P, Rossi ME, Pietrogrande MC, Ricci M, Romagnani S. Defective in vitro production of interferon-gamma and tumor necrosis factor-alpha by circulating T cells from patients with the Hyper-IgE syndrome. *J Clin Invest* 1989; 84:1830.

13. Romagnani S, Del Prete GF, Maggi E, Parronchi P, Tiri A, Macchia D, Giudizi MG, Almerigogna F, Ricci M. Role of interleukins in induction and regulation of human IgE synthesis. *Clin Immunol Immunopathol* 1989; 50:13.

14. Mosmann TR, Cherwinski H, Bond MW, Giedlin MA, Coffman RL. Two types of murine helper T cell clone. I. Definition according to profiles of lymphokine activities and secreted proteins. *J Immunol* 1986; 136:2348.

15. Maggi E, Biswas P, Del Prete GF, Parronchi P, Macchia D, Simonelli C, Emmi L, De Carli M, Tiri A, Ricci M, Romagnani S. Accumulation of Th2-like helper T cells in the conjunctiva of patients with vernal conjunctivitis. *J Immunol* 1991; 146:1169.

16. van der Heijden FL, Wierenga EA, Bos JD, Kapsenberg ML. High frequency of IL-4-producing CD4+ allergen-specific T lymphocytes in atopic dermatitis lesional skin. *J Invest Dermatol* 1991; 97:389.

17. van Reijsen FC, Bruijnzeel-Koomen CAFM, Kalthoff FS, Maggi E, Romagnani S, Westland JKT, Mudde GC. Skin-derived aero-allergen specific T cell clones of TH2 phenotype in patients with atopic dermatitis. *J Allergy Clin Immunol* 1992; 90:184.

18. Kay AB, Yin, S, Varney V, Gaga M, Durham SR, Moqbel R, Wardlaw AJ, Hamid Q. Messenger RNA expression of the cytokine gene cluster, interleukin 3 (IL-3, IL-4, IL-5, and granulocyte/macrophage colony-stimulating factor, in allergen-induced late-phase cutaneous reactions in atopic subjects. *J Exp Med* 1991; 173:775.

19. Hamid Q, Azzawi M, Ying S, Moqbel R, Wardlaw

AJ, Corrigan CJ, Bradley B, Durham SR, Collins JV, Jeffery PK, Quint DJ, Kay AB. Expression of mRNA for interleukin-5 in mucosal bronchial biopsies from asthma. *J Clin Invest* 1991; 87:1541.

20. Robinson DS, Hamid Q, Ying S, Tsicopoulos A, Barkan J, Bentley AM, Corrigan C, Durham SR, Kay AB. Predominant Th2-like bronchoalveolar T-lymphocyte population in atopic asthma. *N Engl J Med* 1992; 326:298.

21. Del Prete GF, De Carli M, D'Elios MM, Maestrelli P, Ricci M, Fabbri L, Romagnani S. Allergen exposure induces the activation of allergen-specific Th2 cells in the airway mucosa of patients with allergic respiratory disorders. *Eur J Immunol* 1993; 23:1445.

22. Del Prete G.F, De Carli M, Mastromauro C, Macchia D, Biagiotti R, Ricci M, Romagnani S. Purified protein derivative of Mycobacterium tuberculosis and excretory-secretory antigen(s) pf Toxocara canis expand in vitro human T cells with stable and opposite (type 1 T helper or type 2 T helper) profile of cytokine production. *J Clin Invest* 1991; 88:346.

23. Parronchi P, Macchia D, Piccinni M-P, Biswas P, Simonelli C, Maggi E, Ricci M, Ansari A.A, Romagnani S. Allergen- and bacterial antigen-specific T-cell clones established from atopic donors show a different profile of cytokine production. *Proc Natl Acad Sci USA* 1991; 88:4538.

24. Del Prete G.F, De Carli M, Ricci M, Romagnani S. Helper activity for immunoglobulin synthesis of T_H1 and T_H2 human T cell clones: the help of Th1 clones is limited by their cytolytic capacity. *J Exp Med* 1991; 174:809.

25. Romagnani S. Human TH1 and TH2: Doubt no more. *Immunol Today* 1991; 12:256.

26. Parronchi P, De Carli M, Manetti R, Simonelli C, Piccinni M-P, Macchia D, Maggi E, Del Prete GF, Ricci M, Romagnani S. Aberrant interleukin (IL)-4 and IL-5 production in vitro by CD4+ helper T cells from atopic subjects. *Eur J Immunol* 1992; 22:1615.

27. Marsh DG, Neely JD, Breazeale DR, Ghosh B, Freidhoff LR, Ehrich-Kautzky E, Schou C, Krishnaswamy G, Beaty TH. Linkage analysis of IL4 and other chromosome 5q31.1 markers and total serum immunoglobulin E concentrations. *Science* 1994; 264:1152.

28. Maggi E, Parronchi P, Manetti R, Simonelli C, Piccinni MP, Santoni Rugiu F, De Carli M, Ricci M, Romagnani S. Reciprocal regulatory role of IFN-γ and IL-4 on the in vitro development of human T_H1 and Th2 clones. *J Immunol* 1992; 148:2142.

29. Parronchi P, De Carli M, Manetti R, Simonelli C, Sampognaro S, Piccinni M-P, Macchia D, Maggi E, Del Prete GF, Romagnani S. IL-4 and IFNs exert opposite regulatory effects on the development of cytolytic potential by TH1 or TH2 human T cell clones. *J Immunol* 1992; 149:2977.

30. Manetti R, Parronchi P, Giudizi, MG, Piccinni MP, Maggi E, Trinchieri G, Romagnani S. Natural killer stimulatory factor (NKSF/IL-12) induces Th1-type specific immune responses and inhibits the development of IL-4 producing Th cells. *J Exp Med* 1993; 177:1199.

31. Manetti R, Gerosa F, Giudizi MG, Biagiotti R, Parronchi P, Piccinni MP, Sampognaro S, Maggi E, Romagnani S, Trinchieri G. Interleukin-12 induces stable priming for interferon-g (IFN-γ) production during differentiation of human T helper (Th) cells and transient IFN-γ production in established Th2 cell clones. *J Exp Med* 1994; 179:1273.

32. Romagnani S. Induction of T_H1 and T_H2 response: A key role for the 'natural' immune response? *Immunol Today* 1992; 13:379.

33. Romagnani S, Maggi E. TH1 vs TH2 responses in HIV infection. *Curr Opin Immunol* 1994; (in press)

34. Ben Sasson SZ, LeGros G, Conrad DH, Finkelman FD, Paul WE. Cross-linking Fc receptors stimulate splenic non-B, non-T cells to secrete IL-4 and other lymphokines. *Proc Natl Acad Sci USA* 1990; 87:1421–1425.

35. Piccinni MP, Macchia D, Parronchi P, Giudizi MG, Bani D, Alterini R, Grossi A, Ricci M, Maggi E, Romagnani S. Human bone marrow non-B, non-T cells produce interleukin 4 in response to cross-linkage of Fce and Fcg receptors. *Proc Natl Acad Sci USA* 1991; 88:8656–8660.

36. Bradding P, Feather IH, Howarth PH, Mueller R, Roberts JA, Britten K, Bews JPA, Hunt TC, Okayama Y, Heusser CH, Bullock GR, Church MK, Hogate ST. Interleukin 4 is localized to and released by human mast cells. *J Exp Med* 1993; 176:1381.

37. Brunner T, Heusser CI, Dahinden CA. Human peripheral blood basophils primed by interleukin 3 (IL-3) produce IL-4 in response to immunoglobulin E receptor stimualtion. *J Exp Med* 1993; 177:605.

38. Manetti R, Barak V, Piccinni MP, Sampognaro S, Parronchi P, Maggi E, Dinarello CA, Romagnani S. Interleukin 1 favors the in vitro development of type 2 T helper (Th2) human T cell clones. *Res Immunol* 1994; 145:93.

39. Delassus S, Coutinho GC, Saucier C, Darche S, Kourilsky P. Differential cytokine expression in maternal blood and placenta during murine gestation. *J Immunol* 1994; 152:2412.

40. Wegmann TG, Lin H, Guilbert L, Mosmann TR. Bidirectional cytokine interactions in the maternal-fetal relationship: Is successful pregnancy a Th2 phenomenon? *Immunol Today* 1993; 14:353.

41. Durkop H, Latza U, Hummel M, Eitelbach F, Seed B, Stein H. Molecular cloning and expression of a new member of the nerve growth factor receptor family which is characteristic for Hodgkin's disease. *Cell* 1992; 68:1.

42. Stein H, Mason DY, Gerdes J, O'Connor N, Wainscoat J, Pallesen G, Gatter K, Falini B, Delsol G, Lemke H, Schwarting R, Lennert K. The expression of the Hodgkin's disease-associated antigen Ki-1 in reactive and neoplastic lymphoid tissue. Evidence that Reed-Sternberg cells and hysticocytic malignancies are derived from activated lymphoid cells. *Blood* 1985; 66:848.

43. Del Prete GF, De Carli M, Almerigogna F, Daniel CK, D'Elios MM, Zancuoghi G, Vinante F, Pizzolo G, Romagnani S. Preferential expression of CD30 by human CD4+ T cells producing Th2-type cytokines. *FASEB J* 1995 (in press).

44. Manetti R, Annunziato F, Biagiotti R, Giudizi MG, Piccinni M-P, Giannarini L, Sampognaro S, Parronchi P, Vinante F, Pizzolo G, Maggi E, Romagnani S. CD30 expression by CD8 + CD30+ T cell clones in human immunodeficiency virus (HIV) infection, *J Exp Med* 1994 (1n press).

45. Pizzolo G, Vinante F, Morosato L, Nadali G, Chilosi M, Gandini G, Sinicco A, Raiteri R, Semenzato G, Stein H, Perona G. High serum levels of the soluble form of CD30 molecule in the early phase of HIV-1 infection as an independent predictor of progression to AIDS. *AIDS* 1994; 8:741.

Adhesion Molecules in Allergy

Craig D Wegner*

Keywords: Adhesion molecules, asthma, respiratory viral infection, eosinophil, lymphocyte, respiratory syncytial virus

Cell surface adhesive glycoproteins are the principal regulators of nearly all aspects of immune/inflammatory responses. The upregulated expression of intercellular adhesion molecule-1 (ICAM-1) on endothelium and epithelium at sites of allergic and asthmatic inflammation is supported by animal experiments demonstrating that antagonism of ICAM-1 attenuates allergen-induced airway eosinophilia and hyperresponsiveness in primates, as well as respiratory syncytial virus-induced lymphocyte infiltration and impaired alveolar gas exchange in mice. In allergy and asthma, the selective upregulation of vascular cell adhesion molecule-1 (VCAM-1) on the endothelium by the Th2 lymphocyte (or mast cell) derived cytokine IL-4 has been hypothesized to mediated the specific and characteristic eosinophilic and lymphocytic infiltrate found in these diseases. *In vitro* as well as *in vivo* data both support and contradict this hypothesis.

Introduction

To properly defend the host against foreign invaders such as bacteria or viruses, leukocytes must come into intimate contact or "adhesion" with cellular and noncellular substrates. Leukocytes attach to endothelial cells so that they can migrate from the circulation to sites of ongoing inflammation. They attach to antigen-presenting cells, such as alveolar macrophages and epithelial dendritic cells, so that a normal antigen specific immune response can occur. Finally, leukocytes attach to appropriate target cells so that lysis of virally infected or tumor cells can occur.

Beyond simply providing the traction for leukocyte trafficking and the mooring for their docking, the cell surface adhesive glycoproteins that consummate cell-cell and cell-matrix attachments perform an active "regulatory" role in directing and managing inflammatory responses. The basal or enhanced of expression of adhesion molecules on inflamed endothelium and epithelium supports the focal accumulation and retention of leukocytes at sites of inflammation (1). On leukocyte activation, some adhesion molecules increase their binding avidity and/or expression while others are shed presumably to accommodate anchoring and migration, respectively (2). Finally, adhesion itself, under appropriate costimulatory/cooperative conditions, causes the signaling, priming or activation of leukocytes (3, 4).

Thus, it is obvious that adhesion molecules play a critical role in allergic responses. In the sections below, both *in vitro* and *in vivo* evidence for the contribution of specific adhesion glycoproteins in allergic, asthmatic and respiratory viral responses are reviewed.

Endothelial Adhesion Molecule Expression

At inflammatory foci, mediators generated as part of the inflammatory response such as cytokines, thrombin, vasoactive peptides, etc., cause the upregulated expression of at least two families of adhesion molecules on the surface of endothelial cells. P-selectin and E-selectin are members of the selectin family so named because of their lectin or carbohydrate binding domains. These molecules are relatively rapidly as well as transiently expressed after endothelial stimulation and contribute to the initial attachment (rolling) of circulating leukocytes to the endothelium presumably because of the rapid but weak carbohydrate-carbohydrate interactions (5). Intercellular adhesion molecule-1 (ICAM-1) and vascular cell adhesion molecule-1 (VCAM-1) are members of the immunoglobulin supergene family with five and six or seven, respectively, C-like domains. The upregulated expression

* Department of Immunological Diseases, Boehringer Ingelheim Pharmaceuticals, Inc., Ridgefield, CT, USA.

of these molecules is slower in onset and more prolonged than the selectins, hence the apparent important role of these molecules in chronic inflammatory/allergic responses (asthma, rhinitis). In addition, the interaction of these molecules with their respective leukocyte integrin receptors (CD11a and CD11b for ICAM-1; VLA-4 for VCAM-1) while slower in onset is stronger than that for the selectins. Hence these endothelial adhesion ligands contribute importantly to firm adhesion require for leukocyte migration and transendothelial migration (5).

VLA-4/VCAM-1, IL-4, Th2 Lymphocyte Hypothesis

The selective accumulation of eosinophils and lymphocytes in allergic responses has been hypothesized to be generated by a VLA-4/VCAM-1 pathway induced by the release of IL-4 and IL-5 from Th2 lymphocytes (6). This hypothesis is based on the following observations: (i) the marked expression of VLA-4 on basophils, eosinophils and lymphocytes, but not neutrophils and only minimally on monocytes, (ii) the selective upregulation of VCAM-1 on endothelial cells by singular or costimulation with IL-4, (iii) the principal source of IL-4 is the Th2 lymphocyte (IL-5 is also released by mast cells), (iv) IL-4 enhances, and induces class switching to, IgE production by B lymphocytes, and (v) Th2 lymphocytes are also the major source of IL-5, a selective stimulator of eosinophil differentiation, adhesion and activation. Support of this hypothesis is found in two animal models. In guinea pigs, the eosinophil accumulation induced in a passive cutaneous anaphylaxis (PCA) reaction or by the intradermal injections of platelet-activating factor (PAF), leukotriene B$_4$, or C5a-des-Arg was in all cases inhibited by an anti-VLA-4 monoclonal antibody (mAb) (7). In inhaled allergen challenged sheep, treatment with an anti-VLA-4 mAb prevented the late-phase broncho-obstruction and subsequent increase in airway responsiveness (8).

However, the following additional observations do not support this hypothesis: (i) In conditions where ICAM-1 is expressed (i.e., most, since there is a small constitutive expression of ICAM-1 on most endothelial cells in vivo), the VLA-4/VCAM-1 mediated adhesion to, and migration through, endothelial monolayers by eosinophils and lymphocytes is dominated by the CD18/ICAM-1 pathway (9, 10). (ii) In contrast to ICAM-1, VCAM-1 expression is not enhanced in the bronchial biopsies of asthmatics, even during acute exacerbations requiring emergency room attention (S. Montefort and S. T. Holgate, personal communication). (iii) In the sheep allergen challenge model, despite efficacy on function parameters (see above), the anti-VLA4 mAb did not attenuate eosinophil or total leukocyte influx (8). Therefore, the positive effects of anti-VLA-4 mAbs in the above mentioned animal models may be the consequence of a VLA-4/fibronectin mediated migration and/or activation of eosinophils within the interstitium rather than an attenuation of a VLA-4/VCAM-1 transendothelial diapedesis pathway.

Epithelial Adhesion Molecule Expression

Of the endothelial adhesion molecules mentioned above, only ICAM-1 is found on the surface of lung epithelial cells. Constitutive ICAM-1 expression is low on airway epithelial cells cultured to confluent monolayers in vitro, but can be impressively enhanced by cytokine stimulation (Figure 1). IFN-γ is the strongest cytokine enhancer of epithelial ICAM-1 expression with IL-1β, TNF-α, and IL-4 (but not LPS) also effective. The time course of enhanced ICAM-1 expression [onset at ≥2 h and peak at 12–16 h (11)] is similar to that reported for endothelial cells in vitro and human skin keratinocytes in vivo (12) and indicative of the required de novo protein synthesis. It has been argued that the adhesion of leukocytes to epithelium plays an important role in their retention, activation and cell mediated cytotoxicity at that site (1, 13). This is portrayed in Figure 2.

Primate Model of Allergen-Induced Airway Hyperresponsiveness

Airway hyperresponsiveness is the most characteristic an important feature of bronchial asthma. Its severity correlates with the intensity of symptoms, diurnal variations in airway caliber and therapy required (14). Once established, airway

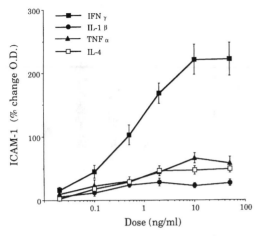

Figure 1. Dose response effects of 16 h of stimulation with inflammatory cytokines on ICAM-1 expression on confluent monolayers of the rhesus monkey bronchus epithelial cell line 4MBr-5. ICAM-1 is plotted as percentage change above basal expression (n ≥ 5). From (29) with permission.

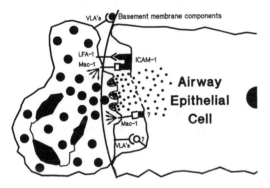

Figure 2. Cartoon depicting possible adhesion molecules and interactions involved in the retention, activation and tissue mediated injury proximal to the airway epithelium.

hyperresponsiveness can remain stable for years, persist apparently in the absence of allergen inhalation, airway inflammation and epithelial desquamation, and thus, possibly become permanent due to irreversible (or at least slowly reversible) alterations in airway ultrastructure (15, 16). However, results from several studies indicate that the onset or development of airway hyperresponsiveness is induced by repeated allergen inhalation and linked to the activation of lymphocytes, the infiltration of eosinophils, and their damage and/or desquamation of airway epithelium (6, 17, 18). Consequently, understanding of the molecular

basis for the development of airway hyperresponsiveness is critical to the clinical management of asthma early in its history (i. e., before airway hyperresponsiveness becomes persistent).

In adult male cynomolgus monkeys with a naturally occurring hypersensitivity to *Ascaris suum* extract, we have reported that *Ascaris* inhalation induces an activation of airway lymphocytes as well as a prolonged airway eosinophilia and that chronic airway eosinophilia is associated with marked airway hyperresponsiveness (11). Multiple (three or more alternate day), but not a single, inhalations of antigen were found to produce an increase (usually more than eight-fold) in airway responsiveness to inhaled methacholine of severity correlated to the degree of epithelial desquamation (11, 19). To explore the role of specific adhesion glycoproteins in this model, mouse anti-human mAbs to ICAM-1, E-selectin or Mac-1 (CD11b), that showed functional cross-reactivity in cynomolgus monkeys, were administered intravenously, daily beginning one day prior to three alternate day *Ascaris* inhalations. The monkeys were rested five or more weeks between each study, to allow the induced airway inflammation and hyperresponsiveness to resolve, and the mAb treatment study was compared to bracketing control studies in each animal. Allergen inhalation was found to increase ICAM-1 expression on airway and alveolar endothelium and epithelial as well as inducing E-selectin expression only on airway endothelium (1, 20). Treatment with the anti-ICAM-1 mAb R6.5 attenuated both the eosinophil infiltration and increase in airway responsiveness (60 ± 8% and 92 ± 34%, respectively) (1). In contrast, administration of the anti-E-selectin mAb CL2 did not significantly inhibit the eosinophil infiltration (×10³/ml BAL: 507 ± 118 in control vs. 430 ± 114 in CL2 treated) or the increase in airway responsiveness (change in log PC_{100}: −1.16 ± 0.27 in control vs. −1.24 ± 0.29 in CL2 treated) (11). Finally, the anti-Mac-1 mAb LM2, while not reducing the eosinophil infiltration, significantly inhibited the activation of airway eosinophils (BAL supernatant eosinophil peroxidase (EPO) activity in O. D. units: 618 ± 210 in control vs. 185 ± 41 in LM2 treated) as well as the increase in airway responsiveness (change in log. PC_{100}: −0.99 ± 0.16 in control vs. −0.14 ± 0.15 in LM2 treated) (12).

Results with the anti-Mac-1 mAb indicate that the inhibition of induced airway hyperresponsiveness by treatment with the anti-ICAM-1 mAb may have been due to an attenuation of an epithelial

ICAM-1 binding eosinophil Mac-1 costimulatory, eosinophil activation signal in addition to its attenuation of eosinophil infiltration via blocking endothelial ICAM-1. To investigate this possibility further, a placebo controlled crossover study design was used to evaluate the effects of daily inhalation administration of the anti-ICAM-1 mAb R6.5 to selectively target epithelial ICAM-1. In animals who experienced greater than a half-log increase in airway responsiveness during either arm of the study, inhaled R6.5 treatment completely blocked the induced airway hyperresponsiveness in two animals, blocked by ~50% in two additional animals, and was ineffective in two others. However, serum levels of IgM anti-R6.5 antibodies (possibly neutralizing the administered R6.5) were detected in both animals in which R6.5 was ineffective and in one of the two in which it inhibited only 50%. Inhaled R6.5 also attenuated eosinophil activation (BAL supernatant EPO activity) in most animals consistent with the antagonism of a costimulatory activation of eosinophils via their adhesion to epithelial ICAM-1 (22).

Murine Model of Respiratory Viral Infection

Respiratory viral infections are a major cause of hospitalization in infants, the elderly and patients with cardiopulmonary restrictions (23). In addition, respiratory infections are the most common cause of the onset or exacerbation of airway hyperresponsiveness and asthma symptoms (24). Several lines of evidence suggest that the morbidity of these infections is a consequence of the immune/inflammatory response rather than the cytopathic effects of the virus (25). To investigate further the role of the inflammatory response as well as the specific adhesion molecules involved, we have developed a murine model of respiratory syncytial virus (RSV) infection.

In mice, as in humans, RSV infection causes a bronchiolitis and/or pneumonia with perivascular and bronchiolar lymphocytic cuffing as well as occasional foci of alveolar lymphocytic infiltration. This is associated with an impairment of alveolar gas exchange as well as in increase in airway responsiveness (26). The role of ICAM-1 was evaluated since ICAM-1 is heavily, constitutively expressed on alveolar epithelium (27) and it is (see

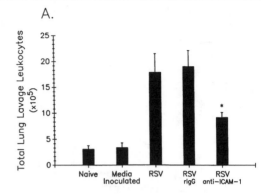

A.

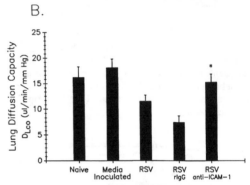

B.

Figure 3. Effects of anti-ICAM-1 (YN1/1.7: 3 mg/kg, i.p., b.i.d.) versus control rat IgG on the increase in lung lavage (airspace lumen) leukocytes (A) and impairment in alveolar gas exchange (B) 6 days after inoculation with RSV or control HEp-2 media in mice. Bars represent the mean ± SE (n = 4–6). Asterisk (*) signifies significant protection by anti-ICAM-1 compared to RSV alone as well as RSV plus rIgG treatment (p<0.05 by Student's *t* test).

above) an important contributor to lymphocyte recruitment, antigen presentation and lymphocyte activation or cell mediated cytotoxicity. Female Balb/c mice (≥15 weeks of age) were inoculated intranasally with RSV A2 stain or control HEp-2 media and treated with a rat mAb to murine ICAM-1 (YN1/1.7) or control rat IgG (3 mg/kg, i.p., b.i.d.). Six days later [peak of the inflammatory response (26)] the mice were anaesthetized and their tracheas cannulated. Respiratory system resistance (Rrs) and dynamic compliance (Crs) were measured by forced oscillations (4–40 Hz) (28). Diffusion capacity of the lungs for carbon monoxide (D_{Lco}) was determined by the single breath method (28). Airway responsiveness was assessed by determining the concentration of nebulized and inhaled methacholine to produce a 100% increase in Rrs

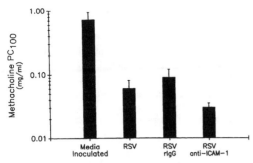

Figure 4. Effects of anti-ICAM-1 (YN1/1.7: 3 mg/kg, i. p., b.i.d.) versus control rIgG on the increase in airway responsiveness to inhaled methacholine (decrease in the PC_{100}) 6 days after inoculation with RSV in mice. Bars represent the mean ± SE (n = 8–9).

(PC_{100}). Lung lavage was performed to assess leukocyte influx. RSV infection induced a 4-fold increase in lung lavage leukocytes, 15% decrease in D_{Lco}, and 10-fold increase in airway responsiveness (decrease in PC_{100}) without significantly altering Rrs or Crs (26). YN1/1.7 (anti-ICAM-1) treatment significant attenuated the leukocyte infiltration (Figure 3A) as well as completely inhibiting the impairment in gas exchange (Figure 3B). Interestingly, despite this marked effect on the inflammation response, the RSV-induced airway hyperresponsiveness was not attenuated (Figure 4).

These results suggest that the morbidity of impaired gas exchange caused a by a respiratory viral infection may be largely due to the intensity of the inflammatory response and thus reversed by anti-inflammatories. In contrast, the more chronic morbidity of increase in airway responsiveness (increase in asthma symptoms?) seems to be independent of the inflammatory response and may be more associated with the cytopathic effects of the virus.

Summary

It is now clear that adhesion molecules play a critical regulatory role in all aspects of an allergic inflammatory response including leukocyte trafficking, antigen presentation, leukocyte activation, and cell mediated cytotoxicity. In addition, several studies including those described above indicate that antagonism of but a single adhesion molecule (e. g., ICAM-1) may provide a novel mechanistic approach to the attenuation of allergic inflammatory responses, and, more importantly, their associated organ dysfunctions.

Address for correspondence:

Craig D Wegner
Abbott Laboratories
Dept. 46R Bldg. AP9
100 Abbott Park Road
Abbott Park, IL 60064-3500
USA

References

1. Wegner CD, Gundel RH, Reilly P, Haynes N, Letts LG, Rothlein R. Intercellular adhesion molecule-1 (ICAM-1) in the pathogenesis of asthma. *Science* 1990; 247:456–459.

2. Kishimoto TK, Jutila MA, Berg EL, Butcher EC. Neutrophil Mac-1 and MEL-14 adhesion proteins inversely regulated by chemotactic factors. *Science* 1989; 245:1238–1241.

3. van Seventer GA, Newman W, Shimizu Y, Nutman TB, Tanaka Y, Horgan KJ, Gopal TV, Ennis E, O'-Sullivan D, Grey H, Shaw S. Analysis of T cell stimulation by superantigen plus major histocompatibility complex class II molecules or by CD3 monoclonal antibody: Costimulation by purified adhesion ligands VCAM-1, ICAM-1, but not ELAM-1. *J Exp Med* 1991; 174:901–913.

4. Wegner CD, Wallace RW. Adhesion molecules that regulate inflammatory cell interactions. In Chung FK, Barnes PJ (Eds.). *Pharmacology of the respiratory tract: Clinical and experimental.* New York: Marcel Dekker, 1992, pp. 223–252.

5. von Andrian UH, Berger EM, Ramezani L, Chambers JD, Ochs HD, Harlan JM, Paulson JC, Etzioni A, Arfors KE. *In vivo* behavior of neutrophils from two patients with distinct inherited leukocyte adhesion deficiency syndromes. *J Clin Invest* 1993; 91:2893–2897.

6. Kay AB. T lymphocytes and their products in atopic allergy and asthma. *Int Arch Allergy Appl Immunol* 1991; 94:189–193.

7. Weg VB, Williams TJ, Lobb RR, Nourshargh S. A monoclonal antibody recognizing very late activation antigen-4 inhibits eosinophil accumulation *in vivo. J Exp Med* 1993; 177:56–566.

8. Abraham WM, Sielczak MW, Ahmed A. Cortes A, Lauredo IT, Kim J, Pepinsky B, Benjamin CD, Leone D, Lobb RR, Weller PF. a_4-Integrins mediate antigen-

induced late bronchial responses and prolonged airway hyperresponsiveness in sheep. *J Clin Invest* 1994; 93:776–787.

9. Vachula M, Vanepps DE. *In vitro* models of lymphocyte transendothelial migration. *Invasion Metastasis* 1992; 12:66–81.

10. Ebisawa M, Bochner BS, Georas SN, Schleimer RP. Eosinophil transendothelial migration induced by cytokines: Role of endothelial and eosinophil adhesion molecules in IL-1 beta-induced transendothelial migration. *J Immunol* 1992; 149:4021–4028.

11. Wegner CD, Rothlein R, Gundel RH. Adhesion molecules in the pathogenesis of asthma. *Agents Actions Suppl* 1991; 34:529–544.

12. Vejlsgaard GL, Ralfkiaer E, Avnstrop C, Czajkowski M, Marlin SD, Rothlein R. Kinetics and characterization of intercellular adhesion molecule-1 (ICAM-1) expression on keratinocytes in various inflammatory skin lesions and malignant cutaneous lymphomas. *J Am Acad Dermatol* 1989; 20:782–790.

13. Simon RH, DeHart PD, Todd III RF. Neutrophil-induced injury of rat pulmonary alveolar epithelial cells. *J Clin Invest* 1986; 78:1375–1386.

14. Hargreave FE, Ryan G, Thomson NC, O'Byrne PM, Latimer K, Juniper EF, Dolovich J. Bronchial responsiveness to histamine or methacholine in asthma: Measurement and clinical significance. *J Allergy Clin Immunol* 1981; 68:347–355.

15. Lundgren R, Soderberg M, Horstedt P. Stenling R. Morphological studies of bronchial mucosal biopsis from asthmatics before and after ten years of treatment with inhaled steroids. *Eur Respir J* 1988; 1:883–889.

16. Brewster CE, Howarth PH, Djukanovic R, Wilson J, Holgate ST, Roche WR. Myofibroblasts and subepithelial fibrosis in bronchial asthma. *Am J Respir Cell Mol Biol* 1990; 3:507–511.

17. Boulet L-P, Cartier A, Thomson NC, Roberts RS, Dolovich J, Hargreave FE. Asthma and increases in nonallergic bronchial responsiveness from seasonal pollen exposure. *J Allergy Clin Immunol* 1983; 71:399–406.

18. Gleich GJ, Flavanhan NA, Fujisawa T, VanHoutte PM. The eosinophil as a mediator of damage to respiratory epithelium: A model for bronchial hyperreactivity. *J Allergy Clin Immunol* 1988: 81:776–781.

19. Wegner CD, Torcellini CA, Clarke CC, Letts LG, Gundel RH. Effects of single and multiple inhalations of antigen on airway responsiveness in monkeys. *J Allergy Clin Immunol* 1991; 87:835–841.

20. Wegner CD, Gundel RH, Rothlein R, Letts LG. Expression and probable roles of cell adhesion molecules in lung inflammation. *Chest* 1992; 101:34S-39S.

21. Wegner CD, Gundel RH, Letts LG. Efficacy of monoclonal antibodies against adhesion molecules in animal models of asthma. *Agents Actions Suppl* 1993; 43:151–162.

22. Wegner CD, Gundel RH, Churchill L, Letts LG. Adhesion glycoproteins as regulators of airway inflammation: Emphasis in the role of ICAM-1. In Holgate ST, Austen KF, Lichtenstein LM, Kay AB (Eds) *Asthma: Physiology, immunopharmacology, and treatment*, 4th edn. London: Academic Press, 1993, pp. 227–241.

23. Dolin R. Common viral respiratory infections. In *Harrison's Principles of internal medicine*, 11th edn. New York: McGraw-Hill, 1987, pp. 700–705.

24. Busse WW. Respiratory infections and bronchial hyperreactivity. *J Allergy Clin Immunol* 1988; 81:770–775.

25. Murphy BR, Sotnidov AV, Lawrence LA, Banks SM, Prince GA. Enhanced pulmonary histopathology os observed in cotton rats immunized with formulin-inactivated syncytical virus or purified F glycoprotein and challenged with RSV 3–6 months after immunization. *Vaccine* 1990; 8:497–502.

26. Raymond EL, McFarland ML, Van GY, Wolyniec WW, Churchill L, Letts LG, Wegner CD. Characterization of the lung inflammation and dysfunction induced by respiratory syncytical virus (RSV) infection in mice. *J Respir Crit Care Med* 1994; 149:A48 (Abstract).

27. Kang B-H, Crapo JD, Wegner CD, Letts LG, Chang L-Y. Intercellular adhesion molecule-1 expression on the alveolar epithelium and its modification by hyperoxia. *Am J Respir Cell Mol Biol* 1993; 9:350–355.

28. Wegner CD, Wolyniec WW, LaPlante AM, Marschman K, Lubbe K, Haynes N, Rothlein R, Letts LG. Intercellular adhesion molecule-1 (ICAM-) contributes to pulmonary oxygen toxicity in mice: Role of leukocytes revised. *Lung* 1992; 170:267–279.

29. Churchill L, Gundel RH, Letts LG, Wegner CD. Contribution of specific cell-adhesive glycoproteins to airway and alveolar inflammation and dysfunction. *Am Rev Respir Dis* 1993; 148:S83–S87.

Regulation of Human Mast Cell and Basophil Function

Gianni Marone, Giuseppe Spadaro, Arturo Genovese*

Keywords: Basophils, cyclosporin A, histamine, leukotriene C$_4$, mast cells

Human basophils and mast cells play a fundamental role in the pathogenesis of allergic disorders through the elaboration of proinflammatory mediators and immunoregulatory cytokines. Altered basophil/mast cell releasability has been documented in patients with allergic disorders (bronchial asthma, allergic rhinitis, atopic dermatitis, and chronic urticaria). Basophil and mast cell releasability can be modulated *in vitro* by nimesulide, a recently identified nonsteroidal anti-inflammatory drug, corticosteroids, type IV cyclic AMP phosphodiesterase inhibitors, protein kinase inhibitors, and immunophillin ligands (cyclosporins and FK-506). The latter group of agents are of particular interest since they exert immunosuppressive and anti-inflammatory effects on human basophils and mast cells *in vitro* as well *in vivo*.

Anatomical, immunological, and pharmacological observations indicate that human basophils and mast cells play a role in allergic disorders by elaborating proinflammatory mediators (1) and various cytokines (2–5). It has been shown, for instance, that basophils in sputum from asthmatics increase before an asthmatic attack (6) and after allergen-induced asthmatic responses (7). Mast cells have been identified in the bronchoalveolar lavage (BAL) fluid (8) and in the bronchial mucosa and submucosa of asthmatic patients (9). Post-mortem examinations have revealed basophils in the airway lumen, in the bronchial epithelium, and in the submucosa of fatal asthma cases (10). Basophil and/or mast cell releasability is known to be altered in patients with atopic dermatitis (11), chronic urticaria (12), and bronchial asthma (8).

An interesting finding was that human basophils (5) and mast cells (2–4) generate cytokines after immunological activation. Moreover, activated basophils and mast cells express the ligand for CD40 (CD40L), thereby providing the cell contact signal required for IgE synthesis by human B cells (13). Thus, taken together these observations suggest that basophils and mast cells play a crucial role in allergic disorders, not only by producing inflammatory mediators, but also by regulating IgE synthesis independently of T cells.

Basophils, like other granulocytes, differentiate and mature in the bone marrow, and circulate in the blood; they are not under normal conditions found in connective tissue. Human mast cell progenitors (CD34$^+$ cells), on the contrary, are present in bone marrow, in cord blood, and in fetal liver cells; they complete their differentiation in connective tissue, where they are often adjacent to blood and lymph vessels, near or within nerves, and beneath epithelial surfaces (14). It may be assumed that basophils and mast cells play distinct roles in various types and phases of allergic reactions involving the respiratory tract (15) and skin (16).

Basophils can migrate into certain inflamed tissues. One example of this is that they are recruited to the site of late-phase reactions and synthesize most of the mediators recovered in nasal lavage and skin blister models during late-phase reactions (15, 16). Mast cells seem to be involved predominantly in immediate reactions.

In this article we will focus on agents modulating human basophil and mast cell functions that appear to hold promise for the treatment of inflammatory diseases.

Nonsteroidal Anti-Inflammatory Drugs

The recent identification of two isoenzymes of cyclo-oxygenase (type I and type II) has generated

---

*   Division of Clinical Immunology and Allergy, University of Naples Federico II, School of Medicine, Naples, Italy.

new impetus in this area (17). Aspirin and other nonsteroidal anti-inflammatory drugs (NSAID) exacerbate asthma in about 20% of patients (18), a finding that has been ascribed to their ability to potentiate the release of basophil and mast cell mediators (19). Indomethacin (INDO), meclofenamic acid (MCA), and acetylsalicylic acid (ASA) increase IgE-mediated histamine release (20, 21) and the *de novo* synthesis of LTC_4 from basophils (21). The potency of NSAID in enhancing IgE-mediated histamine release was significantly correlated with their capacity to inhibit the cyclooxygenase pathway (22).

The NSAID nimesulide (4-nitro-2-phenoxymethane sulfonanilide; NIM) is chemically unrelated to other compounds of the same class. Indeed, its functional acid group is sulfonanilide (23). NIM and its active metabolite 4-hydroxy-nimesulide (OH-NIM) inhibited the release of histamine and leukotriene C_4 (LTC_4) from basophils activated by antigen and anti-IgE (24). NIM also inhibited histamine, LTC_4, and prostaglandin D_2 (PGD_2) release from lung parenchymal and skin mast cells (25). In addition, NIM and OH-NIM increased, whereas ASA and INDO reversed, the inhibitory effect of the adenylate cyclase agonists PGE_1 and forskolin (25). NIM appears to be the only NSAID that possesses such properties. The latter observation might explain why it is well tolerated in most patients with ASA idiosyncrasy (26). Studies are under way to characterize its biochemical mechanism of action in the light of the two isozymes of cyclooxygenase (17).

Corticosteroids

Glucocorticoids are one of the therapeutic mainstays in most allergic disorders. Even patients with mild asthma are affected by inflammation of the bronchial mucosa (27, 28), and so the use of inhaled and systemic corticosteroids is increasing worldwide. Intravenous corticosteroids cause rapid basopenia, whereas skin tissue histamine remains unchanged (29). It has been found that only prolonged treatment with topical corticosteroids can reduce skin mast cell number and inhibit the allergen-induced wheal-and-flare response (30). Similarly, short-term *in vitro* incubation with corticosteroids did not alter mediator release from basophils, but prolonged (12–24 h) incubation with prednisolone,

dexamethasone, or deflazacort inhibited IgE-mediated histamine secretion from these cells (31, 32). Interestingly, even when human lung and skin mast cells were incubated for lengthy periods with dexamethasone, their ability to release mediators after anti-IgE challenge remained unchanged (33). This series of studies provides a clear example of the pharmacological heterogeneity of human $Fc\epsilon RI^+$.

The fact that human basophils (5) and mast cells (2–4) are a major source of cytokines leads to the question: Can corticosteroids modulate the synthesis of cytokines in immunologically activated $Fc\epsilon RI^+$ cells?

Phosphodiesterase Inhibitors and Adenylate Cyclase Activators

Cyclic AMP (cAMP) is an important second messenger in most inflammatory cells, and it can exert an inhibitory effect on these cells (19). Leukocytes from patients with atopic dermatitis were found to have increased levels of cAMP phosphodiesterase (PDE) activity (34), an abnormality that can be reversed by inhibition of cAMP PDE. Also, the increased IL-4 production by atopic mononuclear cells correlated with enhanced PDE activity and was reversed by a selective type IV PDE inhibitor (34). This suggests the PDE isozyme is a therapeutic target for the control of atopic skin disease.

There are at least five classes of cAMP PDE, each being the product of a distinct gene or of a family of genes (35). These PDE isozymes differ in: (1) kinetic characteristics; (2) physical characteristics; (3) tissue distribution; (4) endogenous activators and inhibitors (e. g., Ca^{2+}/calmodulin, cGMP); and (5) subcellular distribution (35). Several PDE inhibitors can be used as pharmacological probes. These fall into two main categories: (1) nonspecific inhibitors of PDE activity such as theophylline and 3-isobutyl-1-methylxanthine; and (2) selective inhibitors of individual PDE isozymes. The latter comprises compounds such as rolipram, a selective inhibitor of the cAMP-specific PDE (PDE IV), and zaprinast, a selective inhibitor of the cGMP-specific PDE (PDE V) (35). Both cAMP PDE III and PDE IV are found in purified basophils (36).

Rolipram dose-dependently inhibited IgE- and PAF-induced histamine release from basophils, whereas the type III PDE inhibitor SK&F 95654 and zaprinast, the PDE V inhibitor, had no effect (36, 37). Consequently PDE IV seems to be the prime isozyme in the regulation of cAMP content in basophils and mast cells.

Isoproterenol and other catecholamines inhibit antigen-induced histamine secretion from basophils and mast cells, presumably by binding to β-adrenergic receptors (19). The β_2-agonist fenoterol inhibited IgE-mediated histamine release from both human basophils and mast cells, and the dose-response inhibition curve was paralleled by a fenoterol-induced increase in cAMP levels in leukocytes (38). Unfortunately, fenoterol cannot be included among the therapeutic agents, because it has been reported to be associated with an increased risk of death or near death from asthma (39). Newer β_2-adrenergic agonists with interesting pharmacokinetic properties, such as salmeterol and formoterol, might also inhibit the release of mediators from lung mast cells (40).

Protein Kinase and Tyrosine Kinase Inhibitors

Protein Kinase C (PKC) is known to play a major role in signal transduction by phosphorylating such diverse proteins as channels, receptors, other kinases, and cytoskeletal proteins (41). Phorbol esters (TPA) and bryostatins can activate human basophils, but not mast cells, to release histamine (42, 43). Anti-IgE- and TPA-induced activation of basophils is paralleled by a rapid rise in membrane-associated PKC, which is correlated with the amount of histamine released (44). Appropriate concentrations of staurosporine, a PKC inhibitor, inhibit TPA-induced mediator release from basophils (44). Interestingly, both TPA and bryostatins inhibit anti-IgE-induced mediator release from skin and lung mast cells (43, 45). The identification of several isoforms of PKC (46) may help in identifying novel molecular targets for therapeutic agents useful in the management of basophil- and mast cell-mediated inflammatory diseases.

In rodent mast cells and mast cell lines, IgE cross-linking causes tyrosine phosphorylation to increase (47). This suggests that a tyrosine kinase may be involved in either the activation of phos-

pholipase C or in the regulation of long-term responses. Four different inhibitors of tyrosine kinases were tested on IgE-dependent histamine release from human lung mast cells and basophils, and the inhibitory profiles were strikingly different, possibly reflecting differences in IgE-dependent signal transduction mechanisms (48).

Immunophilin Ligands

Cyclosporin A (CsA), a cyclic undecapeptide that inhibits T-cell responses (49), has recently offered some insight into the mechanisms of signal transduction in immune cells. Cyclophilin A (CyP) is the first of a family of proteins with high affinity for CsA and low affinity for inactive analogs such as CsH (50). CyP is an immunophilin, a class of intracellular proteins that is emerging as a new pathway of intracellular signaling in immune and inflammatory cells. Two major classes of immunophilins, the CyP and FK-binding proteins (FKBP), have been identified, purified, and cloned (51). There are at least four human isoforms of CyP (52). Two natural macrolides, FK-506 and rapamycin (RAP), bind with high affinity to FKBP (53).

Binding of CsA to CyP and of FK-506 to FKBP is essential to their immunosuppressive activity (49). The CsA-CyP complexes, as well as the FK-506-FKBP complexes, bind to calcineurin (Cn) (54), which has a catalytic A subunit (CnA) and a regulatory B subunit (CnB); the CnA subunit has a binding site for calmodulin (CaM) and for the CnB subunit. Cn has the biochemical requirements of the common target of immunophilin-drug complexes and is thus a potential component of the signaling pathways involved in the activation of immune cells. Complexes of CsA or FK-506 and their respective intracellular binding proteins inhibit the CaM-dependent protein phosphatase 2B, which is essential in the signal transduction pathway for lymphocytes (55), basophils (56–59, 62) and mast cells (58, 60, 61) (Table 1).

RAP exerts distinct immunosuppressive activities, presumably by binding to FKBP, but its molecular mechanism of action is different from that of FK-506 (63). The third component to which the RAP-FKBP complex binds has been recently identified, and is not Cn (64).

CsA inhibited histamine and eicosanoid release from human basophils and mast cells challenged

21

Table 1. The immunological relevance of calcineurin (Cn)/phosphatase 2B activity.

- Cn is a key rate-limiting enzyme in T-cell signal transduction and in basophil/mast cell mediator release
- IL-2 production by T cells activated through the TCR/CD3 complex is correlated with the level of phosphatase 2B activity
- Cells expressing low levels of Cn (e. g., T cells) are more sensitive to CsA/FK-506
- Overexpression of Cn overcomes the CsA/FK-506-mediated inhibition of NF-AT-dependent cytokine gene transcription
- Immunosuppressive activity of cyclosporin analogs correlates with inhibition of Cn phosphatase 2B activity
- Cn is involved in signalling events that lead to degranulation of basophils, mast cells, and cytotoxic T cells
- Cn activity plays a role in TCR/CD3-mediated induction of apoptosis in T cell hybridomas

with antigen or anti-IgE (56, 59). Inhibition occurred even when the drug was added during release. CsH, which has extremely low affinity for CyP, did not affect IgE-mediated activation of these cells. CsA and its analogs (CsG, CsC, and CsD) inhibit the release of mediators from basophils and mast cells, presumably by interacting with CyP (59).

In vivo administration of a single oral dose of CsA (7 mg/kg) in normal volunteers caused a rapid and significant inhibition of histamine release from basophils obtained *ex vivo* and challenged *in vitro* with anti-IgE, f-Met-Leu-Phe (FMLP), and compound A23187 (62). The inhibitory effect of CsA was extremely rapid. It peaked at 1–5 h, then slowly declined up to 13 h. In a second series of experiments, healthy volunteers were given oral CsA (5 mg/kg twice a day) or placebo for 5 days. Basophil releasability in response to anti-IgE, FMLP, and A23187 was inhibited 30–60% throughout the course of CsA treatment. Placebo had no such effect. These experiments provide a rare example of how an *in vivo* administered drug can modulate basophil releasability *ex vivo*. These results might explain, at least in part, the efficacy of CsA in some patients with severe asthma and atopic dermatitis (49).

Compound FK-506, but not RAP, also inhibits histamine and LTC_4 release from basophils and mast cells challenged with antigen and anti-IgE. Interestingly, RAP acts as a competitive antagonist of

FK-506, presumably at the level of FKBP (56, 57, 61). It thus appears that binding to FKBP is necessary, but not sufficient to deliver the inhibitory signal for the release of proinflammatory mediators from basophils and mast cells.

Immunophilin ligands such as CsA and FK-506 might also affect the release of cytokines from mast cells (63). Preliminary observations suggest that this new class of drugs, with anti-inflammatory and immunosuppressive properties, has similar effects on human $Fc\epsilon RI^+$ cells. Therefore, these compounds might play a dual role in the control of immune disorders by inhibiting the release of proinflammatory mediators and the *de novo* synthesis of immunoregulatory cytokines.

Acknowledgments

The original work presented in this article was supported in part by grants from the CNR (Project FATMA: Subproject Prevention and Control of Disease Factors; Project No. 94.00607.PF41) and the MURST (Rome, Italy).

Address for correspondence:

Prof. Gianni Marone
Cattedra di Immunologia Clinica e Allergologia
Facoltà di Medicina
Via S. Pansini, 5
I-80131 Napoli
Italy

References

1. Marone G, Casolaro V, Cirillo R, Stellato C, Genovese A. Pathophysiology of human basophils and mast cells in allergic disorders. *Clin Immunol Immunopathol* 1989; 50:S24-S40.
2. Walsh LJ, Trinchieri G, Waldorf HA, Whitaker D. Human dermal mast cells contain and release tumor necrosis factor a, which induces endothelial leukocyte adhesion molecule 1. *Proc Natl Acad Sci USA* 1991; 88:4220–4224.
3. Bradding P, Feather IH, Howarth PH, Mueller R, Roberts JA, Britten K, Bews JPA, Hunt TC, Okayama Y, Heusser CH, Bullock GR, Church MK, Holgate ST. Interleukin 4 is localized to and released by human mast cells. *J Exp Med* 1992; 176:1381–1386.
4. Möller A, Lippert U, Lessmann D, Kolde G, Hamann K, Welker P, Schadendorf D, Rosenbach, Luger T,

Czarnetzki BM. Human mast cells produce IL-8. *J Immunol* 1993; 151:3261–3266.

5. MacGlashan DW Jr, White JM, Huang S-K, Ono SJ, Schroeder JT, Lichtenstein LM. Secretion of IL-4 from human basophils. The relationship between IL-4 mRNA and protein in resting and stimulated basophils. *J Immunol* 1994; 152:3006–3016.

6. Kimura I, Tanizaki Y, Saito K, Takahashi K, Ueda N, Sato S. Appearance of basophils in the sputum of patients with bronchial asthma. *Clin Allergy* 1975; 5:95–98.

7. Pin I, Freitag AP, O'Byrne PM, Girgis-Gabardo A, Watson RM, Dolovich J, Denburg JA, Hargreave FE. Changes in the cellular profile of induced sputum after allergen-induced asthmatic responses. *Am Rev Respir Dis* 1992; 145:1265–1269.

8. Casolaro V, Galeone D, Giacummo A, Sanduzzi A, Melillo G, Marone G. Human basophil/mast cell releasability. V. Functional comparisons of cells obtained from peripheral blood, lung parenchyma and bronchoalveolar lavage in asthmatics. *Am Rev Respir Dis* 1989; 139:1375–1382.

9. Crimi E, Chiaramondia M, Milanese M, Rossi GA, Brusasco V. Increase of mast cell numbers in bronchial mucosa after the late-phase asthmatic response to allergen. *Am Rev Respir Dis* 1991; 144:1282–1286.

10. Koshino T, Teshima S, Fukushima N, Takaishi T, Hirai K, Miyamoto Y, Arai Y, Sano Y, Ito K, Morita Y. Identification of basophils by immunohistochemistry in the airways of post-mortem cases of fatal asthma. *Clin Exp Allergy* 1993; 23:919–925.

11. Marone G, Giugliano R, Lembo G, Ayala F. Human basophil releasability.II. Changes in basophil releasability in patients with atopic dermatitis. *J Invest Dermatol* 1986; 87:19–23.

12. Casolaro V, Cirillo R, Genovese A, Formisano S, Ayala F, Marone G. Human basophil releasability. IV. Changes in basophil releasability in patients with chronic urticaria. *J Immunol Res* 1989; 1:67–73.

13. Gauchat JF, Henchoz S, Mazzei G, Aubry JP, Brunner T, Blasei H, Life P, Talabot D, Flores-Romo L, Thompson J, Kishi K, Butterfield J, Dahinden C, Bonnefoy JY. Induction of human IgE synthesis in B cells by mast cells and basophils. *Nature* 1993; 365:340–343.

14. Galli SJ. New concepts about the mast cell. *N Engl J Med* 1993; 328:257–265.

15. Bascom R, Pipkorn U, Lichtenstein LM, Naclerio RM. The influx of inflammatory cells into nasal washings during the late response to antigen challenge. Effect of systemic steroid pretreatment. *Am Rev Respir Dis* 1988; 138:406–412.

16. Charlesworth EN, Hood AF, Soter NA, Kagey-Sobotka A, Norman PS, Lichtenstein LM. Cutaneous late-phase response to allergen: mediator release and inflammatory cell infiltration. *J Clin Invest* 1989; 83:1519–1526.

17. Meade EA, Smith WL, DeWitt DL. Differential inhibition of prostaglandin endoperoxide synthase (cyclooxygenase) isozymes by aspirin and other nonsteroidal anti-inflammatory drugs. *J Biol Chem* 1993; 268:6610–6614.

18. Stevenson DD. Cross-reactivity between aspirin and other drugs/dietary chemicals. A critical review. In Pichler WJ, Stadler BM, Dahinden C, Pécoud AR, Frei PC, Schneider C, de Weck AL (Eds) *Progress in allergy and clinical immunology.* Toronto: Hogrefe & Huber Publishers, 1989, pp. 462–466.

19. Marone G, Kagey-Sobotka A, Lichtenstein LM. Effects of arachidonic acid and its metabolites on antigen-induced histamine release from human basophils in vitro. *J Immunol* 1979; 123:1669–1677.

20. Marone G, Kagey-Sobotka A, Lichtenstein LM. IgE-mediated histamine release from human basophils: differences between antigen E- and anti-IgE-induced secretion. *Int Arch Allergy Appl Immunol* 1981; 65:339–348.

21. Marone G, Columbo M, Cirillo A, Condorelli M. Studies on the pathophysiology of aspirin idiosyncrasy. In Bonomo L, Tursi A (Eds) *Recent advances in allergology.* Florence: OIC Medical Press, 1986, pp. 77–97.

22. Wojnar RJ, Hearn T, Starkweather S. Augmentation of allergic histamine release from human leukocytes by nonsteroidal anti-inflammatory analgesic agents. *J Allergy Clin Immunol* 1980; 66:37–45.

23. Swingle KF, Moore GGI, Grant TJ. 4-nitro-2-phenoxymethanesulfonanilide (R-805): A chemically novel anti-inflammatory agent. *Arch Int Pharmacodyn* 1976; 221:132–139.

24. Marino O, Casolaro V, Meliota S, Stellato C, Guidi G, Marone G. Inhibition of histamine release from human FcεRI$^+$ cells by nimesulide. *Agents Actions* 1992; 32:C311-C314.

25. Casolaro V, Meliota S, Marino O, Patella V, de Paulis A, Guidi G, Marone G. Nimesulide, a sulfonanilide non-steroidal antiinflammatory drug, inhibits mediator release from human basophils and mast cells. *J Pharmacol Exp Ther* 1993; 267:1375–1385.

26. Andri L, Senna G, Betteli C, Givanni S, Scaricabarozzi I, Mezzelani P, Andri G. Tolerability of nimesulide in aspirin-sensitive patients. *Ann Allergy* 1994; 72:29–32.

27. Beasley R, Roche WR, Roberts JA, Holgate ST. Cellular events in the bronchi in mild asthma and after bronchial provocation. *Am Rev Respir Dis* 1989; 139.806–17.

28. Marone G, Casolaro V, Spadaro G, Genovese A. Bronchoalveolar lavage. In Weiss EB, Stein M (Eds) *Bronchial asthma. Mechanisms and therapeutics.*

Boston: Little Brown and Company, 1993, pp. 309–313.

29. Dunsky EH, Zweiman B, Fischler E, Levy DA. Early effects of corticosteroids on basophils, leukocyte histamine, and tissue histamine. *J Allergy Clin Immunol* 1979; 63:426–432.

30. Lavker RM, Schechter NM. Cutaneous mast cell depletion results from topical corticosteroid usage. *J Immunol* 1985; 135:2368–2373.

31. Stellato C, Casolaro V, Renda A, Genovese A, Marone G. Anti-inflammatory effect of deflazacort. *Int Arch Allergy Immunol* 1992; 99:340–342.

32. Marone G, Stellato C, Renda A, Genovese A. Anti-inflammatory effects of glucocorticoids and cyclosporin A on human basophils. *Eur J Clin Pharmacol* 1993; 45 (Suppl 1):S17-S20.

33. Schleimer RP, Schulman ES, MacGlashan DW Jr, Peters SP, Hayes EC, Adams GK III, Lichtenstein LM, Adkinson NF Jr. Effects of dexamethasone on mediator release from human lung fragments and purified human lung mast cells. *J Clin Invest* 1983; 71:1830–1835.

34. Chan SC, Li S-H, Hanifin JM. Increased interleukin-4 production by atopic mononuclear leukocytes correlates with increased cyclic adenosine monophosphate-phosphodiesterase activity and is reversible by phosphodiesterase inhibition. *J Invest Dermatol* 1993; 100:681–684.

35. Beavo JA, Reifsnyder DH. Primary sequence of cyclic nucleotide phosphodiesterase isozymes and the design of selective inhibitors. *Trends Pharmacol Sci* 1990; 11:150–155.

36. Peachell PT, Undem BJ, Schleimer RP, MacGlashan DWJr, Lichtenstein LM, Cieslinski LB, Torphy TJ. Preliminary identification and role of phosphodiesterase isozymes in human basophils. *J Immunol* 1992; 148:2503–2510.

37. Columbo M, Horowitz E, McKenzie-White J, Kagey-Sobotka A, Lichtenstein LM. Pharmacologic control of histamine release from human basophils induced by platelet activating factor. *Int Arch Allergy Immunol* 1993; 102:383–390.

38. Marone G, Ambrosio G, Bonaduce D, Genovese A, Triggiani M, Condorelli M. Inhibition of IgE-mediated histamine release from human basophils and mast cells by fenoterol. *Int Arch Allergy Appl Immunol* 1984; 74:356–361.

39. Spitzer WO, Suissa S, Ernst P, Horwitz RI, Habbick B, Cockroft D, Boivin J-F, McNutt M, Buist AS, Rebuck AS. The use of β-agonists and the risk of death and near death from asthma. *N Engl J Med* 1992; 326:501–506.

40. Nials AT, Ball DI, Butchers PR, Coleman RA, Humbles AA, Johonson M, Vardey CJ. Formoterol on airway smooth muscle and human lung mast cells:

A comparison with salbutamol and salmeterol. *Eur J Pharmacol* 1994; 251:127–135.

41. Beaven MA, Rogers J, Moore JP, Hesketh TR, Smith GA, Metcalfe JC. The calcium signal and correlation with histamine release in 2H3 cells. *J Biol Chem* 1984; 259:7129–7136.

42. Schleimer RP, Gillespie E, Lichtenstein LM. Release of histamine from human leukocytes stimulated with the tumor-promoting phorbol diesters. I. Characterization of the response. *J Immunol* 1981; 126:570–574.

43. Patella V, Casolaro V, Ciccarelli A, Pettit GR, Columbo M, Marone G. The antineoplastic bryostatins affect differently human basophils and mast cells. *Blood* 1994, in press.

44. Warner JA, MacGlashan DW Jr. Signal transduction events in human basophils: a comparative study of the role of protein kinase C in basophils activated by anti-IgE antibody and formyl-methionyl-leucyl-phenylalanine. *J Immunol* 1990; 145:1897–905.

45. Massey WA, Cohan VL, MacGlashan DWJr, Gittlen SW, Kagey-Sobotka A, Lichtenstein LM, Warner JA. Protein kinase C modulates immunoglobulin E-mediated activation of human mast cells from lung and skin. I. Pharmacologic inhibition. *J Pharmacol Exp Ther* 1991; 258:824–829.

46. Coussens L, Parker PJ, Rhee L, Yang-Feng TL, Chen E, Waterfield MD, Francke U, Ullrich A. Multiple, distinct forms of bovine and human protein kinase C suggest diversity in cellular signaling pathways. *Science* 1986; 233:859–866.

47. Benhamou M, Gutkind JS, Robbins KC, Siraganian RP. Tyrosine phoshorylation coupled to IgE receptor mediated signal transduction and histamine release. *Proc Natl Acad Sci USA* 1990; 87:5327–5330.

48. Lavens SE, Peachell PT, Warner JA. Role of tyrosine kinases in IgE-mediated signal transduction in human lung mast cells and basophils. *Am J Respir Cell Mol Biol* 1992; 7:637–644.

49. Marone G, de Paulis A, Casolaro V, Ciccarelli A, Spadaro G, Patella V, Stellato C, Cirillo R, Genovese A. Are the anti-inflammatory properties of cyclosporin A useful in the treatment of chronic asthma? In Melillo G, O'Byrne PM, Marone G (Eds) *Respiratory allergy. Advances in clinical immunology and pulmonary medicine.* Amsterdam: Elsevier, 1993, pp. 251–260.

50. Marone G, de Paulis A, Ciccarelli A, Casolaro V, Cirillo R. Mechanism(s) of action of cyclosporin A. *Seminars Clin Immunol* 1991; 2:11–6.

51. Standaert RF, Galat A, Verdine GL, Schreiber SL. Molecular cloning and overexpression of the human FK506-binding protein FKBP. *Nature* 1990; 346:671–674.

52. Bergsma DJ, Eder C, Gross M, Kersten H, Sylvester D, Appelbaum E, Cusimano D, Livi GP, McLaughlin

MM, Kasyan K, Porter TG, Silverman C, Dunnington D, Hand A, Prichett WP, Bossard MJ, Brandt M, Levy MA. The cyclophilin multigene family of peptidyl-prolyl isomerases. Characterization of three separate human isoforms. *J Biol Chem* 1991; 266:23204–23214.

53. Jin Y-J, Albers MW, Lane WS, Bierer BE, Schreiber SL, Burakoff SJ. Molecular cloning of a membrane-associated human FK506- and rapamycin-binding protein, FKBP-13. *Proc Natl Acad Sci USA* 1991; 88:6677–6681.

54. Liu J, Farmer JDJr, Lane WS, Friedman J, Weissman I, Schreiber SL. Calcineurin is a common target of cyclophilin-cyclosporin A and FKBP-FK506 complexes. *Cell* 1991; 66:807–815.

55. O'Keefe SJ, Tamura J, Kincaid RL, Tocci MJ, O'Neil EA. FK-506- and CsA-sensitive activation of the interleukin-2 promoter by calcineurin. *Nature* 1992; 357:692–694.

56. de Paulis A, Cirillo R, Ciccarelli A, Condorelli M, Marone G. FK-506, a potent novel inhibitor of the release of proinflammatory mediators from human FcεRI+ cells. *J Immunol* 1991; 146; 2374–2381.

57. de Paulis A, Cirillo R, Ciccarelli A, de Crescenzo G, Oriente A, Marone G. Characterization of the anti-inflammatory effect of FK-506 on human mast cells. *J Immunol* 1991; 147:4278–4285.

58. Marone G, Triggiani M, Cirillo R, Giacummo A, Siri L, Condorelli M. Cyclosporin A (CsA) inhibits the release of histamine and peptide leukotriene C$_4$ from human lung mast cells. *Ricerca Clin Lab* 1988; 18:53–9.

59. Cirillo R, Triggiani M, Siri L, Ciccarelli A, Pettit GR, Condorelli M, Marone G. Cyclosporin A rapidly inhibits mediator release from human basophils presumably by interacting with cyclophilin. *J Immunol* 1990; 144:3891–3897.

60. Stellato C, de Paulis A, Ciccarelli A, Cirillo R, Patella V, Casolaro V, Marone G. Anti-inflammatory effect of cyclosporin A on human skin mast cells. *J Invest Dermatol* 1992; 98:800–804.

61. de Paulis A, Stellato C, Cirillo R, Ciccarelli A, Oriente A, Marone G. Anti-inflammatory effect of FK-506 on human skin mast cells. *J Invest Dermatol* 1992; 99:723–728.

62. Casolaro V, Spadaro G, Patella V, Marone G. *In vivo* characterization of the anti-inflammatory effect of cyclosporin A on human basophils. *J Immunol* 1993; 151:5563–5573.

63. Hatfield SM, Mynderse JS, Roehm NW. Rapamycin and FK-506 differentially inhibit mast cell cytokine production and cytokine-induced proliferation and act as reciprocal antagonists. *J Pharmacol Exp Ther* 1992; 261:970–976.

64. Brown EJ, Albers MW, Shin TB, Ichikawa K, Keith CT, Lane WS, Schreiber SL. A mammalian protein targeted by G1-arresting rapamycin-receptor complex. *Nature* 1994; 369:756–758.

Eosinophils: Functional Aspects

Monique Capron*, Bouchaïb Lamkhioued*, Delphine Aldebert*, Abdelilah Soussi Gounni*, Ariane Dubost*,**, Emmanuel Delaporte**, André Capron*

Keywords: Eosinophils, IgE receptors, granule proteins, cytokines, Th1, Th2, bullous pemphigoid

Eosinophils exhibit numerous membrane receptors, including members of the immunoglobulin family (FcγR, FcαR), members of the integrin family (β$_1$ and β$_2$ integrins), as well as members of the cytokine receptor family. Lectin-type molecules have also been demonstrated recently. Eosinophils are not only the source of cytotoxic or proinflammatory mediators, but also of cytokines and growth factors, among which are their own factors of differentiation. The aim of the present review is to illustrate recent aspects of eosinophil functions, with a particular emphasis on FcεRI and IgE-dependent degranulation in an autoimmune disease, bullous pemphigoid, as well as on the synthesis of different cytokines by distinct subsets of eosinophils. Taken together, these results allow us to reconsider the role of eosinophils in immune response.

Introduction

Over the past 20 years, several lines of evidence have raised the interest in the effector function of eosinophils in a variety of clinical states associated with hypereosinophilia, including parasitic and allergic diseases (1). The cytolytic potential of eosinophils has been extensively studied in cytotoxicity assays against parasite larvae. These mechanisms are strictly dependent on antibodies and/or complement, which interact with specific receptors on the eosinophil membrane. Adhesion molecules allowing cellular interactions and tissue migration have also been described on eosinophils. The differentiation and activation of eosinophils are controlled by hemopoietic growth factors, namely IL-3, GM-CSF, and specifically IL-5, which bind to the corresponding membrane receptors. Indeed, eosinophils possess a large variety of membrane receptors, which belong to different gene super-families, including members of the immunoglobulin family (such as FcγR or FcαR), members of the integrin family (VLA4 as a β1 integrin or LFA1/CD11a, CR3/Mac1/CD11b, CR4/p150,95/CD11c, and CD18 as β2 integrins), and members of the cytokine receptor family (IL-3, GM-CSF, or IL-5 receptor). Eosinophils also show molecules with a lectin domain such as FcεRII/CD23 (C-type lectin) or, more recently discovered, Mac2/ε binding protein (S-type lectin).

Studies on eosinophil mediators have revealed that eosinophils are not only the source of cytotoxic (granule basic proteins, major basic protein or MBP, eosinophil cationic protein or ECP, eosinophil derived neurotoxin or EDN, and eosinophil peroxidase or EPO) and proinflammatory mediators (leukotriene C$_4$ or LTC$_4$, prostaglandin E$_2$ or PGE$_2$, and neuropeptides), but can also release various cytokines and growth factors (the interleukins IL-1, IL-6, IL-8, transforming growth factors TGF-α, TGF-β, and the tumor necrosis factor TNF-α), including their own factors of differentiation (IL-3, GM-CSF, and IL-5).

The aim of the present review is to highlight some recent aspects of eosinophil functions, with particular emphasis on IgE-dependent release of granule proteins and on the synthesis of Th1 versus Th2 cytokines by distinct subpopulations of eosinophils.

Expression of the High Affinity IgE Receptor (FcεRI) by Human Eosinophils

Several IgE binding molecules have been identified on eosinophils. The low affinity FcεRII/CD23 and

---

*   Centre d'Immunologie et de Biologie Parasitaire, Institut Pasteur, Lille, France.
** Service de Dermatologie A, Centre Hospitalier Régional Universitaire, Lille, France.

Mac2/ε binding proteins are expressed by sub-populations of human eosinophils and participate in IgE binding and IgE-mediated cytotoxicity towards parasitic targets (2, 3). The demonstration that the high affinity IgE receptor (FcεRI) could be detected on Langerhans cells in the skin led us to investigate its expression by eosinophils (4).

FcεRI is a tetrameric structure composed of one IgE-binding α chain, one β chain, and two disulfide-linked γ chains. Anti-FcεRI α chain mAb (15–1) used in flow cytometry analysis bound to 13–73% of eosinophils from patients with hyper-eosinophilic syndromes. Immunostaining experiments performed on cytocentrifuged preparations of purified blood eosinophils or tissue sections from patients with atopic dermatitis revealed that some eosinophils were positively stained with anti-FcεRI α chain mAb. These results indicate that the α chain of FcεRI can be detected in a subpopulation of eosinophils which varies between patients, in contrast to mast cells which constitutively express FcεRI (4).

The expression of mRNA encoding the α chain of FcεRI was detected by Northern hybridization, using the corresponding cDNA probe (4). Again, the intensity of signal varied between individual patients. The β and γ chain mRNAs were detected by a more sensitive RT-PCR technique. These results clearly showed that eosinophils, and not the contaminating cells, lymphocytes or neutrophils, expressed the three components of FcεRI (4).

The involvement of FcεRI in IgE-mediated functions of eosinophils was next investigated. First, anti-FcεRI α chain mAb significantly inhibited, in a dose-dependent manner, the binding of radio-labeled human myeloma IgE to eosinophils (4). We could also demonstrate that mAb to FcεRI chain, but not isotypic control mAb, inhibited the IgE-dependent cytotoxicity mediated by eosinophils against parasitic targets (4). These results provide the first evidence that, in addition to its role in mediating allergic responses, FcεRI may participate in a physiologic protective immune response. They lead to the concept that not only IgE and its low-affinity IgE receptor (5), but also the high affinity IgE receptor, probably arose during evolution to protect organisms against pathogens, rather than to induce pathological allergic reactions.

Release of Granule Proteins after IgE-Dependent Activation

Effector functions of eosinophils against parasites, as well as against mammalian cells, appear to be mainly mediated by the release of cationic proteins such as MBP, ECP, EDN, and EPO (1). Moreover, it has been recently shown that EPO, but not ECP, could be released by purified eosinophils from patients with a parasitic infection or with allergic diseases, after addition of the specific antigen or anti-IgE antibodies, suggesting that IgE-dependent activation could lead to a differential release of granule proteins (6). Experiments were then performed in order to determine whether cross-linking of FcεRI could induce EPO release from eosinophils. Highly significant levels of EPO (index of release >15) could be detected after stimulation of purified eosinophils with the anti-FcεRI α chain mAb 15–1, and anti-mouse IgG antibodies as cross-linking reagent (4). In contrast, no significant EPO release was obtained in the presence of unrelated isotype control mAb, or with the various controls. These results suggest that EPO could be released through engagement of FcεRI, and they also indicate that IgE bound to FcεRI expressed by eosinophils could trigger their degranulation. The selectivity of EPO release through FcεRI was investigated by using a radioimmunoassay to evaluate the exocytosis of ECP in aliquots of the same supernatants in which EPO was detected. No significant release of ECP was detected after stimulation of eosinophils with the anti-FcεRI α chain mAb 15–1 and further incubation with anti-mouse IgG antibodies. In contrast, elevated levels of ECP were obtained in supernatants of the same eosinophil preparations after activation with secretory IgA. These results confirm our previous reports showing that EPO but not ECP was released after IgE-dependent activation, whereas ECP was released after IgG– or IgA-dependent activation (6). The reasons for differential exocytosis of eosinophil granule proteins are not clear. However, our findings are consistent with the hypothesis that engagement of FcεRI drives the same signal-inducing eosinophil degranulation as IgE immune complexes.

The possible interactions between IgE and eosinophils have been recently investigated in *bullous pemphigoid* (BP), a subepidermal blistering disease. This disease is characterized by circulating autoantibodies reactive with antigenic components of hemidesmosomes, including a major autoantigen named BP230. Increased IgE levels associated with tissue and blood eosinophilia are often observed, but without any precise function. In addition, the detection of eosinophil granule proteins in tissue lesions or in bullous fluids as well in the blood allowed us to investigate whether IgE-mediated activation of eosinophils could lead to degranulation and mediator release. Specific IgE antibodies to the recombinant BP230 autoantigen were detected in the blood and in bullous fluids from patients with BP. Moreover, surface IgE was observed by immunostaining on blood and tissue eosinophils. Interestingly, addition of either the recombinant antigen or anti-IgE, but not anti-IgG, induced the release of eosinophil peroxidase (EPO).

These results suggest that, similarly to the situation observed in parasitic infections or in allergic diseases, eosinophils with surface IgE can respond to a major autoantigen by releasing pharmacologically active mediators which may contribute to the damage in this autoimmune disease.

Synthesis of Cytokines by Eosinophils

Human eosinophils were shown to synthesize IL-5 in a variety of diseases, such as celiac disease (7), asthma (8), hypereosinophilic syndromes (9), eosinophilic cystitis (10), and, more recently, atopic dermatitis, herpetiform dermatitis, and bullous pemphigoid, but not in Crohn's disease, for instance (11). These findings, as well as the detection of IL-5 protein in a restricted proportion of eosinophils, led us to suggest the existence of IL-5 positive and IL-5 negative eosinophils. The existence in mice and men of distinct subpopulations of CD4 positive T helper cells producing either IL-2 and IFN-γ (Th1 subset), or IL-4, IL-5, and IL-10 (Th2 subset), led us to investigate the synthesis of IFN-γ, as a prototype for the Th1 cytokines. Using in situ hybridization with an anti-sense probe coding for human IFN-γ, or immunostaining with mAb to IFN-γ, we showed that human eosinophils could express IFN-γ mRNA and protein. To further investigate the expression of Th1 versus Th2 cytokines by eosinophils, we next looked at IL-10. The same experimental approaches revealed the expression of IL-10 mRNA and protein by eosinophils. Finally, results of double in situ hybridization or double immunostaining indicated the existence of subpopulations of eosinophils which coexpress either IL-5 and IL-10 or IFN-γ. Obviously, much additional work will be required to identify the particular patterns of eosinophil cytokine expression and secretion in the various diseases associated with hypereosinophilia. However, it is reasonable to suspect that eosinophils will turn out to be particularly important sources of cytokines, especially in allergic diseases and parasitic infections.

Finally, we recently showed that IFN-α, widely used for the treatment of hypereosinophilic syndromes (9), is able to inhibit eosinophil release of granule proteins and IL-5, suggesting that it has a direct effect on eosinophils.

Conclusion

In conclusion, eosinophils, which were for a long time a poorly characterized cell population, now seem to participate in all steps of the immune response, not only as a source of cytotoxic and proinflammatory mediators, but also as cells that are capable of elaborating a number of cytokines that might contribute to inflammation, chemotaxis, activation, and cell growth, as well as to the regulation of the immune response.

Address for correspondence:

Dr Monique Capron
Centre d'Immunologie et de Biologie Parasitaire
Unité INSERM U167
Institut Pasteur
1 rue du Pr A Calmette, B.P. 245
F-59019 Lille Cédex
France

References

1. Spry CJF. Eosinophils. *A comprehensive review and guide to the scientific and medical literature.* Oxford: Oxford Medical Publications, 1988.

2. Capron M, Truong MJ, Aldebert D, Gruart V, Suemura H, Delespesse G, Tourvieille B, Capron A.

Heterogeneous expression of CD23 epitopes by eosinophils from patients. Relationships with IgE-mediated functions. *Eur J Immunol* 1991; 21:2423.

3. Truong MJ, Gruart V, Liu FT, Prin L, Capron A, Capron M. IgE-binding molecules (Mac-2/εBP) expressed by human eosinophils. Implication in IgE-dependent eosinophil cytotoxicity. *Eur J Immunol* 1993; 23:3230.

4. Soussi Gounni A, Lamkhioued B, Ochiai K, Tanaka Y, Capron A, Kinet JP, Capron M. High affinity IgE receptor on eosinophils is involved in defence against parasites. *Nature* 1994; 367:183.

5. Capron A, Dessaint JP, Capron M, Joseph M, Ameisen JC, Tonnel AB. From parasites to allergy: A second receptor for IgE. *Immunol Today* 1986; 7:15.

6. Tomassini M, Tsicopoulos A, Tai PC, Gruart V, Tonnel AB, Prin L, Capron A, Capron M. Release of granule proteins by eosinophils from allergic and other hypereosinophilic patients upon immunoglobulin dependent activation. *J Allergy Clin Immunol* 1991; 88:365.

7. Desreumaux P, Janin A, Colombel JF, Prin L, Plumas J, Emilie D, Torpier G, Capron A, Capron M. Interleukin-5 messenger RNA expression by eosinophils in the intestinal mucosa of patients with coeliac disease. *J Exp Med* 1992; 175:293.

8. Broide DH, Paine MM, Firestein GS. Eosinophils express interleukin-5 and granulocyte macrophage-colony-stimulating factor mRNA at sites of allergic inflammation in asthmatics. *J Clin Invest* 1992; 90:1414.

9. Desreumaux P, Janin A, Dubucquoi S, Copin MC, Torpier G, Capron A, Capron M, Prin L. Synthesis of interleukin-5 by eosinophils in patients with eosinophilic heart diseases. *Blood* 1993; 82:1553.

10. Dubucquoi S, Janin A, Desreumaux P, Rigot JM, Copin MC, François M, Torpier G, Capron M, Gosselin B. Evidence for eosinophil activation in eosinophilic cystitis. *Eur Urol* 1994; 25:254.

11. Dubucquoi S, Desreumaux P, Janin A, Klein O, Goldman M, Tavernier J, Capron A, Capron M. Interleukin-5 synthesis by eosinophils: Association with granules and immunoglobulin-dependent secretion. *J Exp Med* 1994; 179:183.

Chemokines: Chemotactic Factors that Activate Basophils (Histamine-Releasing Factors) and Eosinophils

Allen P Kaplan, Piotr Kuna, Sesha R Reddigari*

Keywords: Basophils, chemokines, MCAF/MCP-1, RANTES, interleukins, eosinophils

Chemokines are cytokines possessing chemotactic activity for neutrophils, eosinophils, basophils, lymphocytes, and monocytes. Many of these also activate such cells to induce secretion of a wide variety of inflammatory substances. Histamine-releasing factors are basophil activators, most of which reside in the β chemokine subgroup. MCAF/MCP-1 is the most potent, followed by RANTES and MIP Iα/β. Basophils can be "primed" for histamine release due to these chemokines by prior stimulation with IL-3, IL-5, or GM-CSF, while inhibition of histamine release is seen with a wide variety of α or β chemokines typified by IL-8. This phenomenon may represent "receptor class desensitization" in which agonists act on different receptors coupled to the same or similar G proteins. RANTES is also a potent chemotactic factor and secretagogue for eosinophils. Chemokines such as MCAF/MCP-1 and RANTES may have an important role in the development of the late-phase reaction. Finally, the ratio of IL-8/MCAF determined in nasal washings of ragweed sufferers is markedly diminished during their symptomatic session due to decreased IL-8 and augmented MCAF. Thus, the ratio of inhibitors or agonists for cells such as basophils may determine symptoms during allergy season.

Introduction

The term "chemokines" describes a series of structurally related cytokines that function as chemotactic factors and therefore recruit inflammatory cells into an area of tissue injury. These cells are also activated. There are two subgroups of chemokines, shown in Table 1, termed α and β. All chemokines have a molecular weight of approximately 8 kDa

Table 1. The chemokine family.

Subfamily α	Subfamily β
Platelet factor 4	MCAF/MCP-1
β-thromboglobulin	MCP-2
CTAC III/NAP-2	MCP-3
Interleukin-8 (NAP-1)	RANTES
Melanoma growth factor (GRO/MGSA)	MIP-1α
Macrophage inflammatory peptide (MIP-2)	MIP-1β
IP-10	I-309
	HC-11, 14

and have four critical cysteine residues positioned similarly. The first two cysteines may have a single amino acid between them (C-X-C) characteristic of the α subgroup, or these two cysteines may be adjacent (C-C) as is seen in the β subgroup. These cytokine-like molecules bind to heparin, although their relative affinities vary, and the α and β subgroups are encoded on different chromosomes, i. e., chromosomes 4 and 17, respectively. Cytokine-like molecules inducing basophil secretion (histamine-releasing factors or HRF) thus far identified are members of the β chemokine family although both α and β chemokines may have a role in the recruitment and activation of basophils, eosinophils, monocytes, and lymphocytes. A partial chemotactic profile of these factors is given in Table 2.

* Division of Allergy, Rheumatology, and Clinical Immunology, Department of Medicine, SUNY – Stony Brook, Health Sciences Center, Stony Brook, NY, USA.

30

Table 2. Chemotactic factors.

	Neutrophils	Monocytes	T Cells	Basophils	Eosinophils
α-Chemokines					
PF4	+	+			
IL-8	++		+		
NAP-2	+				
β-Chemokines					
MCP-1		++		++	
MCP-2		++		+	
MCP-3		++		++	+
RANTES		+	+	+	++
MIP-1α	+	+	+ (CD8)	+	+
MIP-1β	+	+	+ (CD4)	+	

Histamine-Releasing Factors/Basophil Activation

A variety of reports confirmed the original observation that mononuclear cells or platelets are capable of producing cytokines that cause basophil degranulation and histamine release, although there was little progress in isolating and characterizing such factors on a molecular basis until the chromatographic separation reported by Baeza et al. (1). A combination of ion exchange chromatography and gel filtration separated HRF into at least three fractions, each of which released histamine upon incubation with human basophils. Thus, HRF appeared to be the result of a single factor with multiple molecular forms or multiple gene products with overlapping functions. The latter proved to be correct. Application of HPLC methodology and preparative elution from SDS gels led to purification of an 8–10 kDa protein (2), and amino-acid sequence analysis revealed it to be CTAP III/NAP-2, an α chemokine. Microheterogeneity was evident since the gel band appeared broad and the amino-acid sequence of the upper half of the band corresponded to CTAP III, while the amino-acid sequence of the lower half was identical, though the sequence began with amino acid no. 16. Enzymatic cleavage of purified CTAP III (produced from platelets) with purified elastase or supernatants from activated monocytes removes the N-terminal 15 residues and converts it to NAP-2 (Figure 1). These proved to be plentiful chemokines, each of which was active on basophils in the 0.5–10.0 µg/ml range and were therefore relatively weak on a molar basis. CTAP III was originally

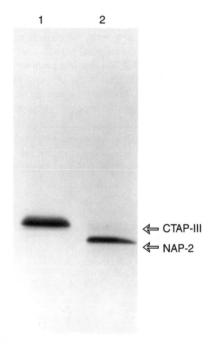

Figure 1. SDS gel electrophoresis of CTAP III (left) and NAP-2 (right). CTAP III was purified by affinity chromatography of platelet supernatants and NAP-2 isolated by elastase digestion of CTAP III and reisolation by affinity chromatography.

described as an activator of fibroblasts (connective tissue activating protein) to stimulate cell synthesis of DNA, sulfated glycosaminoglycans, hyaluronic acid, and PGE$_2$. NAP-2 retains these activities of CTAP III but acquires the capacity to attract neutrophils and to activate them (neutrophil activating protein-2). CTAP III and NAP-2 are equipotent with respect to their capacity for basophil histamine release (3). NAP-1, described earlier, is identical to IL-8 (Table 1), a potent chemotactic factor and activator of neutrophils (4).

Subsequent studies proceeded either by further purification and characterization of HRF using HPLC methodology or by assaying all of the described α or β chemokines for activity on human basophils or mast cells. Kuna et al. (5) and Alam et al. (6) demonstrated that MCAF or MCP-1, a β chemokine, is a potent HRF (Figure 2). MCAF/MCP-1 accounts for 50–60% of the total histamine-releasing capability of mononuclear cell supernatants and about 90% of the activity of the initial chromatographic peak, which also contains CTAP III/NAP-2 and IL-8. For example, immunoabsorption of peak I using monoclonal antibodies to CTAP III leaves a faint band in the same position upon SDS gel electrophoresis, which retains approximately 90% of the original activity and corresponds to MCAF/MCP-1 by immunoblotting. This protein was discovered by two groups, hence the two designations: "monocyte chemotactic and activating protein" or "monocyte chemotactic

protein-1" (4, 7). It is produced by monocytes (and other cells) and attracts monocytes and activates them. It is also chemotactic for basophils and, as HRF, activates them to release histamine. Histamine release is G-protein dependent, is exceedingly rapid with a $t_{1/2}$ of approximately 30 seconds (5), and its potency is equal to that of IgE plus antigen (8) (Table 2). Since the late-phase allergic reaction is characterized by basophil infiltration and protracted histamine release, MCAF/MCP-1 production must be considered to be one of the contributing factors. Soon thereafter, Bischoff et al. (9) confirmed the activity of MCAF/MCP-1 upon basophils. MCP-2 and MCP-3 are closely homologous to MCP-1, but can be separated from it by ion exchange chromatography (10). MCP-2 is a trace protein possessing about half the HRF activity of MCP-1 (unpublished observations), though its contribution to the total activity of mononuclear cells or platelet supernatants is not known. MCP-3, on the other hand, has similar activity to MCP-1 on basophils, but is far less plentiful (11).

Another β chemokine with basophil chemotactic activity and HRF activity is RANTES (12). This

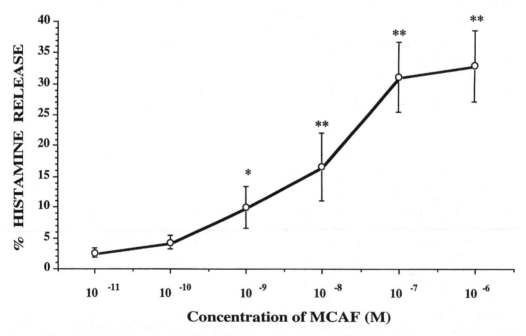

Figure 2. Dose-dependent histamine release by MCAF. Basophils of six individuals were challenged with MCAF from 10^{-11} to 10^{-6} M, and the percentage histamine release was determined. Results are expressed as a mean percentage of histamine release ± SEM. *p ≤ 0.022; **p ≤ 0.014 vs. histamine release induced by 10^{-11} M MCAF (Wilcoxon's rank sum test).

chemokine was first described as a product of T lymphocytes, which is chemotactic for monocytes and a subpopulation of "memory" lymphocytes (13). Since it is a β chemokine like MCAF/MCP-1, we tested recombinant material for HRF activity and found it to be half as potent as MCAF/MCP-1. It had the same dose response (10^{-9}–10^{-7}M) range with equally rapid histamine release, but on average, the percent histamine release was half of that seen with MCAF/MCP-1. Whereas virtually all subjects tested were responsive to MCAF/MCP-1 – whether atopic or not – 80% of subjects' basophils responded to RANTES, atopic subjects' cells being more responsive (8).

MIP Iα and MIP Iβ are closely related molecules originally described in rodents as macrophage inflammatory factors (14). Both are β-type chemokines that are chemotactic for activated human lymphocytes. MIP Iβ recruited primarily CD4+ T cells, while MIP Iβ recruited CD8+ T cells (15). MIP Iα has been reported to have HRF activity on the basophils of atopic subjects (14 of 20 responded at 10^{-9}–10^{-7}M) (15) which is similar to the activity of RANTES. Our own studies of both MIP Iα and MIP Iβ found only 6 of 20 responders, the potency being 30–40% of that of RANTES (8). MIP Iα is chemotactic for basophils, and that activity is comparable to MCAF/MCP-1 (16).

IL-8 (NAP-1) is an α chemokine reported to possess histamine-releasing activity upon basophils; however, its contribution to the activity seen in mononuclear cell/platelet supernatants is uncertain.

No significant histamine release is seen unless basophils are first primed (pretreated) with IL-3, IL-5, or GM-CSF. Release of both histamine and LTC$_4$ has been reported (17, 18, 19), though the priming effect is more pronounced on leukotriene secretion. We have found that only an occasional subject has significant histamine release to IL-3 plus IL-8, and that our data are, in general, negative (8). Further, IL-8 is contained in the peak I of fractionated supernatants and accounts for less than 5% of the activity present. Thus, we do not feel IL-8 to be a major contributor to HRF activity on basophils. The most potent factors thus far reported are MCAF/MCP-1, MCP-3, and RANTES, with lesser contributions by MIP Iα,β and CTAP III/NAP-2 (8). The relative potency of these agents relative to anti-IgE is shown in Figure 3.

Priming Basophils for HRF-Induced Secretion

The responsiveness of basophils to HRF can be modulated by preincubation with low concentrations of cytokines which, themselves, are unable to induce secretion. Thus, preincubation of basophils with (10^{-9}–10^{-8} M) IL-3 or IL-5 or GM-CSF can augment the release of histamine by a subsequent exposure to 10^{-7} M MCAF/MCP-1 or 10^{-7} M RANTES. The overlapping activities (in this in-

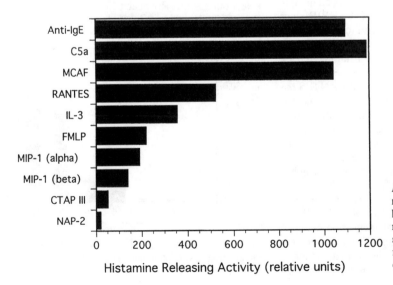

Figure 3. Figure depicting the relative potency of the various histamine releasing chemokines relative to other secretagogues such as C5a, anti-IgE$_4$, and f-met-leu-phe as well as the non-chemokine cytokine, IL-3.

33

stance priming) by this group of cytokines may be related to the fact that the receptors for these cytokines share a subunit, i.e., they consist of an α chain that is specific for each, and a common β chain. Higher concentrations of IL-3, and to a lesser degree GM-CSF, can directly induce histamine release from basophils (20, 8). In general, the responsive subjects are atopic individuals whose cells are likely primed *in vivo*. Immunoabsorption of IL-3 from cell supernatants depletes HRF activity by about 15–20%. This is likely due to the priming effect of IL-3 rather than its ability to induce secretion directly based on the relative concentrations required. IL-3 is, therefore, unusual in that it is the only cytokine that is not a chemokine that can cause basophil secretion and contributes significantly to HRF activity (Figure 3). Immunoabsorption of MCAF/MCP-1, RANTES, and IL-3 accounts for a 75–80% reduction in the total HRF activity of mononuclear cells/platelet derived supernatants.

active process that inhibits secretion. This phenomenon is referred to as homologous "desensitization" as is seen with ligand-receptor interactions that are coupled to G proteins as described for chemotactic factors. Preincubation with RANTES similarly desensitizes itself.

However, we have found that preincubation of basophils with a wide variety of α or β chemokines tested at 5×10^{-9} M inhibit subsequent secretion by optimal MCAF/MCP-1 (10^{-7} M). Washing the cells after the initial incubation reverses the inhibition. Inhibition by RANTES was 69%, by MIP Iα 49%, by MIP Iβ 43%, by PF4 57%, by IL-8 41%, by CTAP III 27%, and by IP10 15% (24). This may reflect "receptor class desensitization," in which the agonists act on different receptors which couple to the same or very similar G proteins. The kinase that phosphorylates the occupied receptor to uncouple it from the G protein acts also on other non-occupied receptors to uncouple them also and diminish the response.

Chemokine-Dependent Inhibition of Basophil Histamine Release

Soon after the concept of HRF evolved, mononuclear cell supernatants were found to contain an inhibitor of HRF-dependent histamine release, and the activity was designated histamine release inhibitory factor or HRIF (21). IL-8 has been thought to fulfill the function attributed to HRIF since preincubation of basophils with concentrations ranging from 10^{-11} to 10^{-8} M inhibit HRF-induced histamine release (22) as well as histamine release due to recombinant MCAF. Subsequently, preincubation with low concentrations of RANTES has been shown to inhibit HRF or MCAF-induced histamine release (23), suggesting that inhibition may be a more general phenomenon. However, the mechanism is unclear since there are little data available regarding chemokine receptors.

It is of interest that preincubation of basophils with concentrations of MCAF that are insufficient to cause histamine secretion prevents secretion by a subsequent challenge with 10^{-7} M MCAF. Washing the cells after the initial incubation does not reverse the process, suggesting either receptor blockade by a high-affinity ligand that cannot be removed by simple washing or induction of some

Activation of Eosinophils

Since eosinophils are major effector cells of allergic inflammation and may be derived from the same precursor cell as the basophil, it is of interest to test the various chemokines for eosinophil chemotactic activity and/or eosinophil activation and degranulation. Recently, Kameyoshi et al. (25) demonstrated that RANTES is chemotactic for eosinophils, while Rot et al. (26) demonstrated that RANTES also degranulates them. However, the

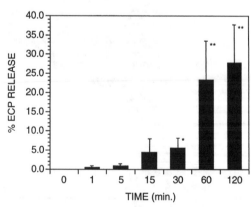

Figure 4. Time course of release of eosinophil cationic protein from eosinophils upon stimulation with 10^{-7} M RANTES.

concentration necessary and the time course of activation were not specified and cytochalasin B-treated cells were utilized in studies of secretion. A later report by Alam et al. (27) confirmed that RANTES is chemotactic for purified eosinophils between 10^{-8} M and 10^{-9} M, and demonstrated that it upregulated the expression of CD11b/CD18, caused release of eosinophil cationic protein, and rendered the cells "hypodense," suggesting an activated phenotype. Figure 4 shows a time-course of release of eosinophil cationic protein upon incubation of purified human eosinophils with recombinant RANTES. In contrast to basophils, secretion is a slow process increasing over hours. Other β chemokines with eosinophilotactic activity are MCP-3 (11) and MIP Iα (Table 2).

Concluding Comments

Chemokines, HRF, and Allergic Diseases

One of the areas of particular relevance to these data is the potential contribution of chemokines to the late-phase allergic response. There are some data to suggest that HRF is functionally present in cutaneous late-phase reactions (28), and that injection of chemokines in rodents (29) can elicit a response that resembles the late phase. Data in human diseases are only preliminary; however, identification of the specific proteins involved and development of specific reagents for their quantitation and detection in body fluids and within tissues will allow such studies to be completed. HRF activity has been found in nasal washings of allergic subjects which decreases with topical steroid therapy (30, 31) or immunotherapy (32). It is also found in bronchoalveolar lavage fluids (33). Preseasonal immunotherapy also modulates HRF production in seasonal asthmatics (34).

There are considerable data to indicate that basophils infiltrate tissues during the late phase, and that there is protracted histamine release in the absence of tryptase secretion suggesting basophil degranulation. It is unclear whether persisting antigen is a prerequisite for a late-phase reaction, but there is certainly a ready mechanism by which such histamine release can occur in the absence of antigen or IgE antibody. Quantitatively, the most striking change during the late phase is the infiltration and activation of eosinophils. RANTES and MIP Iα and β may be key factors involved in the recruit-ment and activation of such cells. The increment in T_4^+ helper cells and monocytes is small, but such cells are activated and may provide a ready source of chemokines. The possibility that mast cells, basophils, and/or eosinophils produce chemokines as well must also be examined since they secrete a variety of cytokines that were heretofore unsuspected.

Address for correspondence:

Allen P Kaplan
Division of Allergy, Rheumatology
and Clinical Immunology
Department of Medicine
SUNY – Stony Brook
Health Sciences Center
Stony Brook, NY 11794
USA

References

1. Baeza ML, Reddigari SR, Haak-Frendscho M, Kaplan AP. Purification and further characterization of human mononuclear cell histamine releasing factor. *J Clin Invest* 1988; 83:1204.

2. Baeza ML, Reddigari SR, Kornfeld D, Ramani N, Smith EM, Hossler PA, Fischer T, Castor CW, Gorevic PG, Kaplan AP. Relationship of one form of human histamine releasing factor to connective tissue activating peptide-III. *J Clin Invest* 1990; 85:1516.

3. Reddigari SR, Kuna P, Miragliotta GF, Kornfeld D, Baeza ML, Castor CW, Kaplan AP. Connective tissue-activating peptide III and its derivative, neutrophil-activating peptide-2, release histamine from human neutrophils. *J Allergy Clin Immunol* 1992; 89:666.

4. Yoshimura T, Matsushima Y, Tanaka S, Robinson EA, Appella E, Oppenheim JJ, Leonard EJ. Purification of a human monocyte-derived neutrophil chemotactic factor that has peptide sequence similarity to other host defense cytokines. *Proc Natl Acad Sci USA* 1987; 84:9233.

5. Kuna P, Reddigari SR, Rucinski D, Oppenheim JJ, Kaplan AP. Monocyte chemotactic and activating factor is a potent histamine-releasing factor for human basophils. *J Exp Med* 1992; 175:489.

6. Alam R, Lett-Brown MA, Forsythe PA, Anderson-Walters DJ, Kenamore C, Kormoo C, Grant JA. Monocyte chemotactic and activating factor is a potent histamine-releasing factor for basophils. *J Clin Invest* 1992; 89:723.

7. Matsushima K, Morishita K, Yoshimura T, Lavu S, Kobayashi Y, Lew W, Appella E, Kung HF, Leonard EJ, Oppenheim JJ. Molecular cloning of a human monocyte-derived neutrophil chemotactic factor (MDNCF) and the induction of MDNCF mRNA by IL-1 and tumor necrosis factor. *J Exp Med* 1988; 167:1883.

8. Kuna P, Reddigari SR, Schall TJ, Rucinski D, Sadick M, Kaplan AP. Characterization of the human response to cytokines, growth factors, and histamine releasing factor of the intercrine/chemokine family. *J Immunol* 1993; 150:1932.

9. Bischoff SC, Krieger M, Brunner T, Dahinden CA. Monocyte chemotactic protein 1 is a potent activator of human basophils. *J Exp Med* 1992; 175(5):1271.

10. Van Damme J, Proost P, Lenaerts J-P, Opdenakker G. Structure and functional identification of two human, tumor-derived monocyte chemotactic proteins (MCP-2 and MCP-3) belonging to the chemokine family. *J Exp Med* 1992; 176:59.

11. Dahinden CA, Geiser T, Brunner T, von Tscharner V, Caput D, Ferrara P, Minty A, Baggiolini M. Monocyte chemotactic protein 3 is a most selective basophil and eosinophil chemokine. *J Exp Med* 1994; 179:751.

12. Kuna P, Reddigari SR, Schall TJ, Rucinski D, Viksman MY, Kaplan AP. RANTES, A monocyte and T lymphocyte chemotactic cytokine releases histamine from human basophils. *J Immunol* 1992; 149:636.

13. Schall T, Bacon K, Toy K, Goeddel D. Selective attraction of monocytes and T lymphocytes of the memory phenotype by cytokine RANTES. *Nature* 1990; 347:669.

14. Davatelis G, Tekamp-Olson P, Wolpe SD, Hermsenk K, Luedke K, Gallegos C, Coit D, Merryweather J, Cerami A. Cloning and characterization of a c-DNA for murine macrophage inflammatory protein (MIP), a novel monokine with inflammatory and chemokinetic properties. *J Exp Med* 1988; 117:1939.

15. Taub DD, Conlon K, Lloyd AR, Oppenheim JJ, Kelvin DJ. Preferential migration of activated CD4+ and CD8+ T cells in response to MIP Iα and MIP Iβ. *Science* 1993; 260:355.

16. Alam R, Forsythe PA, Stafford S, Lett-Brown MA, Grant JA. Macrophage inflammatory protein Iα activates basophils and mast cells. *J Exp Med* 1992; 176:781.

17. Bischoff SC, Brunner T, De Weck AL, Dahinden CA. IL-5 modifies histamine release and leukotriene generation by human basophils in response to diverse agonists. *J Exp Med* 1990; 172:1577.

18. Bischoff SC, De Weck AL, Dahinden CA. IL-3 and granulocyte/macrophage-colony-stimulating factor render human basophil responsive to low concentration of complement component C3 a. *Proc Natl Acad Sci USA* 1990; 87:6813.

19. Dahinden CA, Kurimoto Y, De Weck AL, Lindley I, Dewald B, Baggiolini M. The neutrophil-activating peptide NAF/NAP-1 induces histamine release and leukotriene release by IL-3-primed basophils. *J Exp Med* 1989; 170:1787.

20. Haak-Frendscho M, Arai N, Arai K-I, Baeza ML, Finn A, Kaplan AP. Human recombinant granulocyte-macrophage colony-stimulating factor and IL-3 cause basophil histamine release. *J Clin Invest* 1988; 82:17.

21. Alam R, Grant JA, Lett-Brown MA. Identification of a histamine releasing inhibitory factor produced by human mononuclear cells *in vitro*. *J Clin Invest* 1988; 82:2056.

22. Kuna P, Reddigari SR, Kornfeld D, Kaplan AP. IL-8 inhibits histamine release from human basophils induced by histamine releasing factors, connective tissue activating peptide III, and IL-3. *J Immunol* 1991; 147:1920.

23. Alam R, Forsythe PA, Lett-Brown MA, Grant JA. IL-8 and RANTES inhibit basophil histamine release induced with monocyte chemotactic and activating factor/monocyte chemotactic protein-1 and histamine releasing factor. *Am J Respir Cell Mol Biol* 1992; 7:427.

24. Kuna P, Reddigari SR, Rucinski D, Schall TJ, Kaplan AP. Chemokines of the α and β subclass inhibit human basophil responsiveness to monocyte chemotactic and activating factor/monocyte chemoattractant protein I. *J Allergy Clin Immunol*, in press.

25. Kameyoshi Y, Dörschner A, Mallet AI, Christophers E, Schröder J-M. Cytokine RANTES released by thrombin-stimulated platelets is a potent attractant for human eosinophils. *J Exp Med* 1992; 176:587.

26. Rot A, Krieger M, Brunner T, Bischoff SC, Schall TJ, Dahinden CA. RANTES and macrophage inflammatory protein Iα induce the migration and activation of human eosinophil granulocytes. *J Exp Med* 1992; 176:1489.

27. Alam R, Stafford S, Forsythe PA. RANTES is a chemotactic and activating factor for human eosinophils. *J Immunol* 1993; 150:3442.

28. Warner JA, Pienkowski MM, Plaut M, Norman PS, Lichtenstein LM. Identification of histamine releasing factor(s) in the late phase of cutaneous IgE-mediated reactions. *J Immunol* 1986; 136:2583.

29. Anderson-Walters D, Kumar D, Grant JA, Alam R. Monocyte chemoattractant peptide-1 (MCP-1) and macrophage inflammatory peptide-1 (MIP-1), the two major histamine releasing factors, induce immediate and late foot pad swelling reactions in mice *in vivo*. *J Allergy Clin Immunol* 1993; 91:313.

30. Sim TC, Alam R, Forsythe PA, Welter JB, Lett-Brown MA, Grant JA. Measurement of histamine-releasing factor activity in individual nasal washings: relationship with atopy, basophil response, and mem-

brane-bound IgE. *J Allergy Clin Immunol* 1992; 89:1157.

31. Sim TC, Hilsmeier RA, Alam R, Allen RK, Lett-Brown MA, Grant JA. Effect of topical corticosteroids on the recovery of histamine releasing factors in nasal washings of patients with allergic rhinitis. *Am Rev Resp Dis* 1992; 145:1316.

32. Brunet C, Bedard P-M, Lavoie A, Jobin M, Hebert J. Allergic rhinitis to ragweed pollen II. Modulation of histamine releasing factor production by specific immunotherapy. *J Allergy Clin Immunol* 1992; 89:87.

33. Alam R, Welter JB, Forsythe PA, Lett-Brown MA, Rankin JA, Boyars M, Grant JA. Detection of histamine release inhibitory factor- and histamine releasing factor-like activities in bronchoalveolar lavage fluids. *Am Rev Respir Dis* 1990; 141:666.

34. Kuna P, Alam R, Kuzminska B, Rozniecki J. The effect of preseasonal immunotherapy on the production of histamine releasing factor (HRF) by mononuclear cells from patients with seasonal asthma: results of a double blind placebo-controlled, randomized study. *J Allergy Clin Immunol* 1989; 83:816.

New Concepts in the Understanding of Asthma: Introductory Remarks

Mario Ricci*

Keywords: Th2-like cells, mast cells, cytokines, IL-4 gene promoter

As is well known, Th2-like cells are required for IgE production by B cells. They accumulate in the target tissues of allergic inflammation and seem to be involved, together with mast cells, in the induction and maintenance of allergic bronchial asthma. Undoubtedly, knowledge of the importance of cytokines in the airway allergic inflammation has made possible further advances in understanding the pathogenesis of bronchial asthma. Mediators and cytokines produced by mast cells and Th2-like cells are involved in the induction of microvascular changes, upregulation of particular adhesion molecules in endothelial and epithelial cells, migration, and activation of inflammatory cells, mainly eosinophils. Macrophages may also be considered as cells potentially involved in allergic inflammation. Certainly, in the open disease, multidirectional cellular and molecular interactions occur. Strong evidence has been provided for the dominant role of IL-4 in the Th2-like cell development in atopics. Consequently, as is extensively discussed in this review, attention has recently been centered on understanding the molecular mechanisms regulating IL-4 gene expression on T cells and other cells and their possible deregulation in atopics.

Introduction

According to the traditional view, in allergic respiratory disorders the inhaled allergens react with specific IgE bound to FcεRI receptors on the surface of the mast cells (and basophils) and induce, by cross-linking of receptors, the release of cellular mediators responsible for acute phase reactions and allergic inflammation.

A more complex integrative view of how the pathophysiological alterations responsible for allergic diseases come about has been recently ad-vanced (1, 2). This view will be susceptible to better definition in the future.

There is no doubt that knowledge of the involvement of cytokines and chemokines in allergic inflammation has made possible considerable advances. Cytokines are able to consistently influence the functions of a variety of cell types in a marked and persistent way, particularly by inducing "de novo" expression of multiple genes. The cytokine network provides the most appropriate and convincing basis for intercellular communications and control.

In these introductory remarks, first the advances concerning the role of Th2-like cells in the induction and maintenance of airway allergic inflammation will be briefly reviewed, and then the factors that may favor the development of allergen-specific Th2-like cells in atopics will be discussed.

Th2-Like Cells and Airway Allergic Inflammation

Th2-Like Cells in Humans and Their Role in Inducing IgE Synthesis by B Cells

As was previously demonstrated in mice, it has been possible to show the existence in humans of Th1-and Th2-like cells by studying the profile of cytokine production by T cell clones (TCC) from peripheral blood (PB) specific for *Toxocara* parasitic antigens (TPA) and TCC specific for endocellular bacterial antigens (3). Moreover, at the same time it has been shown that bone marrow cells belonging to mast cell/basophil lineages produced IL-4 when activated by anti-IgE antibodies (4). According to our present knowledge, IL-4 as well as some cytokines of the same family are produced by mucosal mast cells and basophils.

* Institute of Clinica Medica III, University of Florence, Italy.

It is known that Th2-like cells are required for IgE production. Resting B cells require signals delivered by a physical interaction with activated Th2-like cells at the level of the paracortical area of lymph nodes and at the level of different zones of germinal centers. Close physical interactions between T and B cells are necessary to induce B cell IgE synthesis. Different signals are required. One signal is represented by the release of IL-4 and/or IL-13 by activated Th2-like cells; other signals are dependent on the interactions occurring between costimulatory molecules, such as CD40 on the surface of B cells and CD40 L on the surface of T cells. IL-4 and IL-13 provide important switching signals. Other complementary signals provided by IL-5, IL-6, IL-9 and sCD23 can potentiate the IgE synthesis. An inhibitory activity on IgE production is exerted by IFN-γ, IFN-α, IL-8, IL-10, IL-12 and TGF-β (2). It has been recently shown that mast cells and basophils express the ligand for CD40 and can induce IgE production in the presence of IL-4; basophils can do this even in the absence of IL-4 (5).

Allergen-Specific Th2-Like Cells are Expanded in Atopic Subjects, Particularly at Level of Target Tissues

The phenotype of cytokine production by T cells from peripheral blood (PB) and target tissues of atopic subjects has been extensively investigated. The results of these investigations can be summarized as follows:

1. In atopic subjects allergens preferentially expand T cell clones (TCC) with the Th2 phenotype of cytokine secretion (6).
2. CD4+ TCC from atopics display an aberrant *in vitro* production of IL-4 and IL-5, even in response to antigens other than allergens.
3. TCC established from PB of atopics can produce concordant concentrations of IL-3, IL-4, IL-5, and GM-CSF (7).
4. TCC derived from umbilical cord blood of newborns from atopic parents consistently proliferate *in vitro* in response to allergens (8); according to preliminary results, a significant percentage show the Th2-like profile of cytokine production.
5. Late-phase cutaneous reactions to allergens, allergen-induced rhinitis, and asthma are associated with the activation of the IL-3, IL-4, IL-5, and GM-CSF gene cluster (2, 8, 10).
6. Allergen exposure induces the activation of al-

lergen-specific Th2 cells in the airway mucosa of patients with allergic respiratory disorders, increased Th2-type cytokine mRNA expression, and eosinophil recruitment in bronchoalveolar lavage (BAL) (10, 11).

These data, taken together, suggest that Th2-like cells are expanded mainly at the level of target tissues of atopic subjects. Aeroallergen sensitization can occur during fetal life; in fact, allergen-specific Th2-like cells can be already expanded at birth. Thus, in atopics, overexpression not only of the IL-4 gene, but also of other genes of IL-4 gene family members, namely IL-3, IL-5, and GM-CSF genes, appears to be present.

Th2-Like Cells and Effector Mechanisms of Airway Allergic Inflammation

The traditional view of the pathogenesis of airway allergic inflammation cannot explain a number of observations related to pathological findings (persistence, even in the mildest asthmatics, of a unique form of inflammation), to clinical and pathophysiological findings (persistence of some alterations, such as bronchial hyperreactivity, even in the mildest forms and between attacks), and to the beneficial effects of some therapeutic interventions such as steroids and cromolyn sodium.

At present it is possible to propose that at least two principal types of cells, mast cells and T cells, can be involved in the initiation of the effector mechanisms of tissue allergic inflammation, namely in bronchial asthma.

Mast cells present in the airway mucosa are stimulated by inhaled allergens and release mediators responsible for the acute phase reactions. Some mediators produced by these cells, such as LTs and PAF, also possess chemotactic activity. Furthermore, as previously reported, mast cells (and basophils) produce IL-4 and some cytokines of the same family when activated. Human mucosal mast cells also produce TNF-α, IL-6, and IL-8.

Even T cells appear to play a central role in the pathogenesis of allergic inflammation (12). At the level of the respiratory mucosa these cells can be activated by allergen molecules presented by antigen-presenting cells (APC) such as dendritic cells.

Mediators and cytokines produced by mast cells and T cells are both involved in the induction of microvascular changes, upregulation of particular adhesion molecules on endothelial and epithelial cells, and migration and activation of inflammatory cells, mainly eosinophils. Thus, multidirectional cellular and molecular interactions can occur.

Monocytes-macrophages may also be considered as cells potentially involved in the initiation and in the maintenance of allergic inflammation. These cells express low affinity FcεRII receptors and could be stimulated by allergen molecules, as well as by different mediators and cytokines, to release in turn mediators and cytokines.

As is well known, there is a strong evidence for the central proinflammatory role of eosinophils in allergic, intrinsic, and occupational asthma. Eosinophils can injure the respiratory mucosa fundamentally by releasing their basic proteins, oxygen free radicals, and lipid mediators such as LTC$_4$ and PAF. The latter can contribute to microvascular leakage, bronchoconstriction, and mucus secretion. Moreover, activated eosinophils have been recently shown to be able to elaborate diverse cytokines such as IL-3, TGF-α, TGF-β_1, GM-CSF, IL-1, IL-6, and IL-5. The ability to elaborate cytokines represents a new way in which eosinophils may contribute to the regulation of diverse inflammatory alterations in airway mucosal tissues. Thus, it is reasonable to suggest that a cascade of different cell types, cytokines, and mediators actively participates in self-strengthening "circular" mechanisms supporting airway allergic inflammation.

Development of Th2-Like cells in Atopic Patients

To study the predisposing factors that favor the development of Th2-like cells, a great deal of attention has been focused on the interactions between allergen peptides, APC, and T cells. An understanding of these factors is obviously of a great importance to better clarify the genesis of the atopic state and to plan new approaches to the problems of prevention and therapy.

Role of Particular Antigen Presenting Cells (APC), HLA Class II Molecules, TCR Repertoire, Costimulatory Molecules, and Microenviromental Cytokines in the Development of Th2-Like Cells

That dendritic cells (DC) of respiratory mucosa play a special role in driving the primary and secon-

dary responses to allergens has been supported by some data. However, further work is still necessary to definitely clarify the actual importance of DC in driving the development of allergen-specific Th2-like cells.

Genetic data available suggest that class II molecules on the APC play a permissive role in the binding with allergen peptides, but that they are not the sole determinants of the responses to allergens. At present, no clear results are available about the possible role of particular structures of TCR chains or of the costimulatory molecules in the induction of Th2 cell development. According to results obtained in humans *in vitro* and in animal models *in vitro* and *in vivo*, IL-4 favors the differentiation of Th2 cells, whereas IFN-γ, IL-12, IFN-α, and TGF-β inhibit the development of Th2 cells (13, 14). All the studies provide strong evidence for a dominant role of IL-4 in the differentiation of naive and memory T cells into Th2 cells (15). Recently, it has also emerged that IL-13 is important in the regulation of IgE production by B cells. However, whereas both IL-4 and IL-13 represent switching signals for B cells for IgE production, the positive activity of IL-4 on Th2 cell development has not been shown to be shared by any other cytokines.

The question of the nature of the cells that can provide IL-4 in the endogenous microenvironment of lymphoid tissues, particularly in the primary responses to allergens, remains to be solved. IL-4 could be provided by cells other than T cells. However, even though these cells can be important during ongoing IgE responses, it is difficult to imagine that at the beginning of the primary responses mast cells and basophils may be activated through crosslinking of surface IgE molecules. In these conditions the relevance of IgE-independent stimulation has to be definitely proved.

Molecular Mechanisms Able to Govern the Expression of IL-4 Gene and of Other Genes of the Same Cytokine Family

In humans, the genes coding for the "Th2 cytokines" map on the long arm of chromosome 5 q 31.1. The transcription of the IL-4 gene has been shown to be regulated by multiple promoter elements acting together. Recent reports have confirmed that the P sequence is one of the most important regulatory elements in human IL-4 gene expression (16, 17). Another four P sites have been identified in the murine IL-4 gene promoter, suggesting the existence of more complex mechanisms involved in the regulation of IL-4 gene expression (16).

A new positive regulatory element I (PRE-I) with strong basal enhancing activity has been identified in the distal promoter of the human IL-4 gene. Its enhancer function is strongly suppressed by a negative regulatory element (NRE) (18). The usual function of IL-4 NRE seems to be a safeguard against IL-4 gene overexpression.

Very recently, other studies have been carried out by molecular dissection of the murine IL-4 gene promoter. All the P sites identified in the regulatory region of mouse IL-4 gene promoter interact with a family of transcription factors (nuclear factors P, NF(P)) specific for T cells, but not for the different T cell subsets. NF(P) have some characteristics similar to those of the cytoplasmic component of the nuclear factor of activated T cells (NF-ATc), which is a transcription factor involved in the transcription of IL-2 gene.

The molecular dissection of the murine IL-4 gene promoter has made it possible to identify two sequences, termed consensus sequences 1 (CS1) and CS2. CS1 appears to be more important for the inducibility of the IL-4 promoter and to have Th2-specific functions. CS2 shows some resemblance to the·CLEO element (19).

Undoubtedly, evidence for a common regulation of the cytokine genes of the IL-4 family is of a great interest. The so-called CLE0 (consensus lymphokine element 0) is shared by the promoters of the GM-CSF, IL-4, IL-3, and IL-5 genes (20). This element seems to play an important role in the coordinate induction of IL-4, IL-3, IL-5, and GM-CSF genes (16). Moreover, the P sequence of human IL-4 gene promoter has homology with the corresponding regulatory region of IL-5 gene (17). An intergenic enhancer, located between the IL-3 and GM-CSF loci, is required for the regulated activation of IL-3 and GM-CSF gene expression in T cells.

Concluding Remarks

Many studies carried out *in vivo* and *in vitro* support the importance of Th2-like cells and Th2-type cytokines not only in IgE antibody synthesis, but also in the induction and maintenance of allergic inflammation. In patients with atopic disorders, Th2-like cells producing IL-4 and IL-5 but not, or limited amounts of, IFN-γ, are present in the blood and accumulate mainly in the target organs.

It should be noted that even in intrinsic and occupational asthma, particular subsets of T cells that are able to produce IL-5 in combination with other cytokines may play an important role. Nonallergic asthmatics had elevated levels of IL-2 and IL-5, but not IL-4, in bronchoalveolar lavage (BAL) fluid and in supernatants from PB and BAL lymphocytes (21). The majority of TCC derived from bronchial biopsies taken 48 h after positive specific provocation test in patients with isocyanate-induced asthma were CD8+ TCC able to produce IL-5 and IL-2, but not IL-4 (10). On the basis of these observations, it is possible to suggest that particular T cell subsets able to produce IL-5 and IL-2 or other cytokines, but not IL-4, may be involved in the induction and maintenance of different forms of nonatopic asthma.

The mechanisms responsible for the preferential expansion of Th2-like cells in atopic patients are currently under investigation. Particular class II molecules on APC have been shown to be involved in permissive binding with allergen peptides. In the genesis of atopy, a role for additional genes, not linked to MHC genes, which control the overall IgE responsiveness, has also been suggested. At present, there is a general consensus on the essential and dominant role played by IL-4 in the development of Th2-like cells. Evidence from both animal and human models suggests that IL-4 can strongly influence activated CD4+ T cells to differentiate into cells that produce the Th2 set of cytokines. In contrast, IFN-γ, IFN-α, and IL-12 (in part via induction of IFN-γ) exert the opposite regulatory effect by favoring the development of Th1 cells.

In atopics, some genetic alterations present at level of molecular mechanisms directly involved in the regulation of expression of IL-4 gene may be hypothesized (22, 23). In theory, these alterations may be present at the level of signal transduction pathways and/or at level of the molecular complexes formed by transcription factors and their corresponding promoter regulatory elements. These alterations may be responsible for the overexpression of the IL-4 gene in the cells which can provide this cytokine in the endogenous microenvironment. Furthermore, according to the findings previously reported, in atopics overexpression of not only the IL-4 gene, but also of other cytokine (IL-3, IL-5, GM-CSF) genes of the same family may be present. The overexpression of these genes may be the primary cause of the production by expanded Th2-like cells, and even by other cells, of the cytokines involved in airway allergic inflammation, and may explain its peculiar and persistent histological, pathophysiological, and clinical aspects. This overexpression may be due to alterations in the above-mentioned common regulatory mechanisms, may be genetically determined and related to the non-HLA linked "IgE regulating genes" responsible for the high levels of total serum IgE. In this connection, very recently, sib-pair analysis of 170 individuals from 11 Amish families revealed evidence for linkage of five markers in chromosome 5 q 31.1 with a gene controlling total serum IgE concentration (24).

Other hypothetical alterations may be due to deficient regulatory activity of the cytokines responsible for the inhibition of Th2-like cell development. According to some data, at least in patients with severe atopic disorders, defective NK and CD8$^+$ cell function might account for low IFN-γ production that favors Th2 differentiation (13). The above possibilities cannot be considered as mutually exclusive.

As previously reported, in different forms of nonatopic asthma the principal role in the induction and maintenance of airway inflammation may be played by particular subsets of T cells that can produce IL-2 and IL-5 but not IL-4 (21). If the pathogenetic role of different subsets of Th cells in non-atopic asthma is confirmed, the problem which will still need solving is what cytokines or other factors are responsible for the preferential expansion of these T cell subsets, and then for the overexpression of IL-5 and other cytokine genes, without any overexpression of IL-4 gene.

Address for correspondence:

Prof. Mario Ricci
Istituto di Clinica Medica III
Policlinico di Careggi
Viale Morgagni 85
I-50134 Florence
Italy

References

1. Ricci M, Rossi O. Dysregulation of IgE responses and airway allergic inflammation in atopic individuals. *Clin Exp Allergy* 1990; 20:601–609.

2. Ricci M, Rossi O, Bertoni M, Matucci A. The importance of Th2-like cells in the pathogenesis of airway allergic inflammation. *Clin Exp Allergy* 1993; 23:360–369.

3. Del Prete GF, De Carli M, Mastromauro C, Biagiotti R, Macchia D, Falagiani P, Ricci M, Romagnani S. Purified protein derivate (PPD) of *Mycobacterium tuberculosis* and excretory-secretory antigen(s) (TES) of *Toxocara canis* select human T cells clones with stable and opposite (Th1 or Th2) profile of cytokine production. *J Clin Invest* 1991; 88:346–350.

4. Piccinni MP, Macchia D, Parronchi P, Giudizi MG, Bani D, Alterini R, Grossi A, Ricci M, Maggi E, Romagnani S. Human bone marrow non-B, non-T cells produce interleukin 4 in response to cross-linkage of Fc-ε and Fc-γ receptors. *Proc Natl Acad Sci USA* 1991; 88:8656–8660.

5. Gauchat JF, Henchoz S, Mazzei G, Aubry JP, Brunner T, Blasey H, Life P, Talabot D, Flores-Romo L, Thompson J, Kishi K, Butterfield J, Dahinden C, Bonnefoy JY. Induction of human IgE synthesis in B cells by mast cells and basophils. *Nature* 1993; 365:340–343.

6. Parronchi P, Macchia D, Piccinni MP, Biswas P, Simonelli C, Maggi E, Ricci M, Ansari AA, Romagnani S. Allergen- and bacterial antigen-specific T-cell clones established from atopic donors show a different profile of cytokine production. *Proc Natl Acad Sci USA* 1991; 88:4538–4542.

7. Parronchi P, Manetti R, Simonelli C, Santoni Rugiu F, Piccinni MP, Maggi E, Romagnani S. Cytokine production by allergen (Der pI)-specific CD4$^+$ T cell clones derived from a patient with severe atopic disease. *Int J Clin Lab Res* 1991; 21:186–189.

8. Piccinni MP, Mecacci F, Sampognaro S, Manetti E, Parronchi P, Maggi E, Romagnani S. Aeroallergen sensitization can occur during fetal life. *Int Arch Allergy Immunol* 1993; 70:1–3.

9. Robinson D, Hamid Q, Ying S, Tsicopoulos A, Barkans J, Bentley A, Corrigan C, Durham S, Kay B. Predominant Th2 -like bronchoalveolar T-lymphocyte population in atopic asthma. *N Engl J Med* 1992; 326:298–304.

10. Del Prete GF, De Carli M, D'Elios M, Maestrelli P, Ricci M, Fabbri L, Romagnani S. Allergen exposure induces the activation of allergen-specific Th2 cells in the airway mucosa of patients with allergic respiratory disorders. *Eur J Immunol* 1993; 23:1445–1449.

11. Robinson DS, Ying S, Bentley AM, Meng Q, North J, Durham SR, Kay B, Hamid Q. Relationships among numbers of bronchoalveolar lavage cells expressing messenger ribonucleic acid for cytokines, asthma symptoms, and airway methacholine responsiveness in atopic asthma. *J Allergy Clin Immunol* 1993; 92:397–403.

12. Ricci M. T cells, cytokines, IgE and allergic inflammation. *Int Arch Allergy Appl Immunol* 1992; 99:165–171.

13. Romagnani S. Induction of Th1 and Th2 responses: A key role for the 'natural' immune response? *Immunol Today* 1992; 13:379–381.

14. Scott P. IL-12: Initiation cytokine for cell-mediated immunity. Science 1993; 260: 496–497.

15. Maggi E, Parronchi P, Manetti R, Simonelli C, Piccinni MP, Santoni Rugiu F, De Carli M, Ricci M, Romagnani S. Reciprocal regulatory effects of IFN-γ and IL-4 on the *in vitro* development of human Th1 and Th2 clones. *J Immunol* 1992; 148:2142–2147.

16. Szabo SJ, Gold JS, Murphy TL, Murphy KM. Identification of cis-acting regulatory elements controlling interleukin-4 gene expression in T cells: roles for NF-Y and NF-ATc. *Mol Cell Biol* 1993; 8:4793–4805.

17. Abe E, De Waal Malefyt R, Matsuda I, Arai KI, Arai N. An 11-base-pair DNA sequence motif apparently unique to the human interleukin 4 gene confers responsiveness to T-cell activation signals. *Proc Natl Acad Sci USA* 1992; 89:2864–2868.

18. Li-Weber M, Krafft H, Krammer PH. A novel enhancer element in the human IL-4 promoter is suppressed by a position-indipendent silencer. *J Immunol* 1993; 151:1371–1382.

19. Bruhn KW, Nelms K, Boulay JL, Paul WE, Lenardo MJ. Molecular dissection of the mouse interleukin-4 promoter. *Proc Natl Acad Sci USA* 1993; 90:9707–9711.

20. Masuda ES, Tokumitsu H, Tsuboi A, Shlomai J, Hung P, Arai KI, Arai N. The granulocyte-macrophage colony-stimulating factor promoter cis-acting element CLE0 mediates induction signals in T cells and is recognized by factors related to AP1 and NFAT. *Mol Cell Biol* 1993; 13:a-i.

21. Walker C, Bode E, Boer L, Hansel TT, Blaser K, Virchow J-C Jr. Allergic and nonallergic asthmatics have distinct patterns of T-cell activation and cytokine production in peripheral blood and bronchoalveolar lavage. *Am Rev Respir Dis* 1992; 148:109–15.

22. Ricci M., Matucci A., Rossi O. Recent advances in the pathogenetic mechanisms and genetic aspects of atopic diseases. *ACI News* 1994; 4: 103–108.

23. Ricci M. IL-4: a key cytokine in atopy. *Clin Exp Allergy* 1994; 24: 801–812.

24. Marsh DG, Neely JD, Breazeale DR, Ghosh B, Freidhoff LR, Ehrlich-Kautzky E, Schou C, Krishnaswamy G, Beaty TH. Linkage analysis of IL-4 and other chromosome 5q 31.1 markers and total serum immunoglobulin E concentrations. *Science* 1994; 264:1152–1255.

The Potential Role of IgA-Mediated Mucosal Immunity in the Prevention of Hypersensitivity Reactions in the Respiratory Tract

Jiri Mestecky*, Michael W Russell**, Mogens Kilian***

Keywords: Mucosal immunity, secretory IgA (S-IgA), eosinophils, oral immunotherapy, IgA functions

Mucosal membranes of the respiratory and intestinal tracts are protected against excessive stimulation with environmental antigens, including certain allergens, by humoral and cellular mechanisms. Mucosal antibodies, represented primarily by secretory IgA and IgA in serum, appear to play an essential role in the elimination of antigens by non-inflammatory means through their ability to inhibit both IgE-mediated processes and complement activation by other Ig isotypes. Results of several studies suggest that perturbations of IgA-mediated mucosal immunity (IgA deficiency or cleavage of S-IgA by proteases released by mucosal pathogens) enhance the incidence of allergic respiratory diseases.

The encouraging results of immunotherapy with allergens given by the oral route need to be further analyzed with respect to characterization of the mechanisms involved (enhanced mucosal humoral immunity and/or oral tolerance) using suitable antigen delivery systems intended to selectively downregulate allergic reactions.

Introduction

Complex interactions among cells (e. g., T and B lymphocytes, mast cells, eosinophils, and other cells) and their products (e. g., antibodies, cytokines, and inflammatory mediators) occur in the respiratory tact and are responsible for the pathogenesis and clinical manifestations of hypersensitivity reactions (1). In common with allergic disorders that affect the gastrointestinal and genitourinary tracts and the ocular system, allergies in the respiratory tract begin and progress in the special-ized microenvironment of the mucosal membranes. The large surface areas of the gastrointestinal and respiratory tracts are the major sites of stimulation of the entire immune system, including both the mucosal and systemic compartments, with environmental antigens and allergens (2). The characteristic feature of the mucosal immune system is the striking predominance of IgA-producing plasma cells and of polymeric IgA which is selectively transported through the epithelial cells (3, 4). It has been proposed by Heremans, and others (for reviews see 5, 6) that this secretory IgA (S-IgA) inhibits the absorption of antigens, including potential allergens, from mucosal membranes and may consequently prevent the development of as well as downregulate allergic reactions in mucosae.

What is the Function of IgA?

Extensive studies that were recently reviewed (7) clearly established the uniqueness of IgA among other Ig isotypes: in general, IgA antibodies bound to corresponding antigen do not initiate the chain of events resulting in inflammation with its potentially deleterious consequences (Table 1). On mucosal surfaces, S-IgA antibodies specific for haptens and protein antigens inhibit their absorption (8, 9), apparently by the formation of large complexes. Viruses and other biologically active antigens are effectively neutralized by IgA not only in external secretions but also within infected epithelial cells. In mucosal tissues, the anti-inflammatory activity

*   University of Alabama at Birmingham, Departments of Microbiology and Medicine, Birmingham, AL, USA.
**   University of Alabama at Birmingham, Department of Microbiology, Birmingham, AL, USA.
*** University of Aarhus, Institute of Medical Microbiology, Aarhus, Denmark.

Table 1. Potentially beneficial and detrimental functions of secretory and serum IgA in respiratory tract hypersensitivity reactions.

Beneficial effects
- Prevention of allergen absorption from the respiratory mucosa
- Elimination of antigens complexed to IgA
- Anti-inflammatory activity:
  - lack of complement activation
  - inhibition of complement activation by IgG
  - inhibition of IgE-mediated reactions
- Removal of immune complexes by Fcα receptor-bearing monocytes/macrophages and PMN

Detrimental effects
- Generation of immune complexes containing IgA and complement-activating Ig that induce tissue damage
- Degranulation of eosinophils with ensuing tissue damage due to the release of EDN, MBP, EOP, ECP

---

of IgA has been convincingly demonstrated (9): in contrast to IgG-containing immune complexes, IgA complexed to an antigen did not activate complement with its inflammatory consequences, and did not result in mucosal tissue damage and enhanced uptake of bystander antigen. This observation is of basic physiological importance and may be highly relevant to the tissue damage seen in mucosal allergic reactions. In the systemic compartment, the elimination of IgA-containing immune complexes by the hepatobiliary route (10, 11) occurs without the involvement of inflammatory mechanisms generated by complement activation.

The ability of IgA to activate complement, especially by the alternate pathway, has been controversial, but most evidence favors the view that IgA does not effectively activate either pathway (7, 12). In contrast, IgA antibodies strongly block classical pathway complement activation by IgG or IgM antibodies (12, 13), and a similar though less dramatic effect has been observed for the alternate pathway (12).

Furthermore, it has been shown that IgA can inhibit the development of cutaneous anaphylaxis, the Arthus reaction, and the IgE-mediated Prausnitz-Küstner reaction (14, 15). This observation is again relevant to the pathogenesis of asthma and other IgE-dependent hypersensitivity disorders. Although complement-dependent inflammatory reactions and tissue damage are inhibitable by IgA antibodies, recent studies have indicated that IgA, and particularly S-IgA, are highly effective as inducers of eosinophil degranulation (16, 17). In addition to macrophages/ monocytes and neutrophils, these cells also express Fcα receptors (FcαR) (18). Interestingly, the density of FcαR on eosinophils isolated from the peripheral blood of allergic patients is significantly increased compared to normal individuals (18). One may speculate that S-IgA, which may gain access to tissue eosinophils through an impaired mucosal epithelial barrier in atopic patients, further accentuates local damage due to the release of eosinophil-derived toxins (19). The ability of S-IgA-allergen immune complexes (20) and polymeric Fc fragments of S-IgA (generated by bacterial proteases; see below) to degranulate eosinophils and the involvement of carbohydrate-rich SC in this await further study.

The Role of S-IgA in Respiratory Tract Hypersensitivity Reactions

The ability of S-IgA to inhibit the absorption of macromolecules, including potential allergens, from mucosal surfaces has been well documented in several experimental systems (7–9, 21). Thus, one might predict that the absence of S-IgA from external secretions, due to IgA deficiency or functional impairment of S-IgA effector functions, would be accompanied by enhanced immune responses in other Ig isotypes. An increased incidence of atopic diseases in IgA-deficient individuals has indeed been observed (22–26). Furthermore, the absence of S-IgA from gastrointestinal secretions results in increased levels of antibodies to ingested milk proteins and immune complexes in sera of IgA-deficient individuals (27). By analogy, it is likely that the penetration of potential allergens through the mucosa of the respiratory tract may be enhanced in the absence of corresponding S-IgA antibodies (21).

Another important mechanism involved in the

development of respiratory tract allergies is likely to be associated with a functional defect of S-IgA due to its cleavage by specific proteases (7). The ability of S-IgA to cross-link macromolecular antigens and form large and poorly absorbed complexes due to the tetra- and octa-valency of S-IgA dimers and tetramers may be significantly impaired by its proteolytic cleavage with specific enzymes produced by resident bacteria. Secretions of the upper respiratory tract contain predominantly locally produced S-IgA1 molecules (28) that are uniquely sensitive to bacterial IgA1 proteases (7). Extensive studies of the nasopharyngeal microbiota of atopic children revealed that nasal secretions collected from such individuals contain Faba and $(Fc\alpha)_2\alpha SC$ fragments, and that IgA1-protease-producing bacteria, including *Streptococcus mitis* biovar 1 and *Haemophilus influenzae*, were present with increased frequency in the nasopharynx (29, 30). These results imply that a functional defect in S-IgA caused by the formation of monovalent (non-cross-linking) Fabα fragments by IgA1 protease-producing bacteria is reflected in an enhanced absorption of allergens and induction of IgE antibodies (29, 30).

The increased incidence of atopic diseases in IgA-deficient patients or in individuals with a functional defect in S-IgA molecules due to their proteolytic cleavage provides indirect evidence for the importance of S-IgA in mucosal defense mechanisms. Furthermore, these findings suggest that the induction of allergen-specific S-IgA antibodies in the respiratory tract may be of benefit for the prevention and treatment of atopic diseases.

Immunotherapy of Atopic Diseases and Its Relationship to Mucosal S-IgA Mediated Protection

Strategies used for the induction of S-IgA antibodies in respiratory secretions exploit the existence of the common mucosal immune system: ingestion of antigens results in the appearance of specific S-IgA antibodies in tears, saliva, milk, and nasal secretions (for review see 2). Thus, oral immunotherapy with allergens such as pollens has been used in several studies, with some success (see below). However, it is unclear whether the beneficial effect is due strictly to the induction of specific S-IgA antibodies in nasal secretions or other mechanisms such as oral tolerance. The latter phenomenon has recently received significant attention because of its therapeutic potential in the treatment of auto-immune disorders (31). Studies performed in humans and in animals indicate that the induction of S-IgA antibodies and of systemic unresponsiveness are not mutually exclusive: serum and secretory antibodies *and* the suppression of T cell responsiveness may be induced in parallel (32). Initial studies suggest that Th1 cells involved in delayed-type hypersensitivity reactions become tolerized, whereas Th2 cells, which are essential for the differentiation of B cells into Ig-secreting plasma cells, are not tolerized. These findings may explain why oral immunotherapy with allergens that induce delayed-type hypersensitivity (e. g., poison ivy) were often successful (33). The mechanisms responsible for the effectiveness of oral immunotherapy in antibody-mediated hypersensitivity reactions have not been elucidated, as there appears to be neither a decrease in IgE, nor an increase in S-IgA antibodies consistent with the clinical improvement (34–37).

Because of the low uptake of undigested antigens from the mucosa of the gastrointestinal tract, several approaches have been explored to maximize the mucosal immune response (for review, see 38). In this regard, cholera toxin (CT) and its B-subunit have been used as an adjuvant for highly effective delivery of antigens to mucosal surfaces (39). However, two recent studies performed in animal models suggest that in addition to heightened S-IgA responses, significant elevation of serum IgE levels occurs (40, 41). Although the levels of antigen-specific IgE antibodies in sera and in external secretions have not been determined, these results warrant cautious approaches and further evaluations in humans. The potential of alternative antigen-delivery systems, such as microspheres, expression of antigens in live vectors or plants, and mucosal DNA immunization (42), to induce IgE antibodies in addition to S-IgA, awaits further evaluation.

Acknowledgments

This work was supported by US PHS grants DE 08228, DE 08182, DE 09691, AI 15128, and AI 35991.

47

Address for correspondence:

Jiri Mestecky, MD
University of Alabama at Birmingham
Dept. of Microbiology – BBRB 757
845 – 19th St. South
Birmingham, AL 35294–2170
USA

References

1. Redington AE, Jones DB, Holgate ST. Mucosal immune function in asthma. In PL Ogra, J Mestecky, ME Lamm, W Strober, JR McGhee, J Bienenstock (Eds) *Handbook of Mucosal Immunology*. San Diego: Academic Press, 1994, p. 539.

2. Mestecky J. The common mucosal immune system and current strategies for induction of immune response in external secretions. *J Clin Immunol* 1987; 7:265.

3. Alley CD, Mestecky J. The mucosal immune system In G Bird, JE Calvert (Eds) *B Lymphocytes in Human Disease*. Oxford: Oxford University Press, 1988, p. 222.

4. Brandtzaeg P. Overview of the mucosal immune system. *Current Topics Microbiol Immunol* 1989; 146:13.

5. Heremans JF. Immunoglobulin A. In M Sela (Ed) *The Antigens* Vol II. New York: Academic Press 1974, p. 365.

6. Hobbs JR. IgA as a safer form of antibody response. *Protides Biol Fluids* 1978; 25:865.

7. Kilian M, Russell MW. Function of mucosal immunoglobulins. In PL Ogra, J Mestecky, ME Lamm, W Strober, JR McGhee, J Bienenstock (Eds) *Handbook of Mucosal Immunology*. San Diego: Academic Press, 1994, p. 127.

8. Walker WA, Bloch KJ. Intestinal uptake of macromolecules: *in vitro* and *in vivo* studies. *Ann NY Acad Sci* 1983; 409:593.

9. Tolo K, Brandtzaeg P, Jonsen J. Mucosal penetration of antigen in the presence or absence of serum-derived antibody. An *in vitro* study of rabbit oral and intestinal mucosa. *Immunology* 1977; 33:733.

10. Mazanec MB, Nedrud JG, Kaetzel CS, Lamm ME. A three-tiered view of the role of IgA in mucosal defense. *Immunol Today* 1993; 14:430.

11. Russell MW, Brown TA, Claflin JL, Shroer K, Mestecky J. Immunoglobulin A-mediated hepatobiliary transport constitutes a natural pathway for disposing of bacterial antigens. *Infect Immun* 1983; 42:1041.

12. Nikolova EB, Tomana M, Russell MW. All forms of human IgA antibodies bound to antigen interfere with complement (C3) fixation induced by IgG or by antigen alone. *Scand J Immunol* 1994; 39:275.

13. Russell-Jones GJ, Ey PL, Reynolds BL. The ability of IgA to inhibit the complement-mediated lysis of target red blood cells sensitized with IgG antibody. *Molec Immunol* 1980; 17:1173.

14. Ishizaka K, Ishizaka T, Hornbrook M. Blocking of Prausnitz-Küstner sensitization with reagin by normal human β_{2A} globulin. *J Allergy* 1963; 34:395.

15. Russell-Jones GJ, Ey PL, Reynolds BL. Inhibition of cutaneous anaphylaxis and Arthus reactions in the mouse by antigen-specific IgA. *Int Archs Allergy Appl Immunol* 1981; 66:316.

16. Abu-Ghazaleh RI, Fujisawa T, Mestecky J, Kyle RA, Gleich GJ. IgA-induced eosinophil degranulation. *J Immunol* 1989; 142:2393.

17. Tomassini M, Tsicopoulos A, Tai PC, Gruart V, Tonnel A-B, Prin L, Capron A, Capron M. Release of granule proteins by eosinophils from allergic and nonallergic patients with eosinophilia on immunoglobulin-dependent activation. *J Allergy Clin Immunol* 1991; 88:365.

18. Monteiro RG, Hostoffer RW, Cooper MD, Bonner JR, Gartland GL, Kubagawa H. Definition of immunoglobulin A receptors on eosinophils and their enhanced expression in allergic individuals. *J Clin Invest* 1993; 92:1681.

19. Gleich GJ, Adolphson CR. The eosinophilic leukocyte: Structure and function. *Adv Immunol* 1986; 39:177.

20. Johnson KJ, Wilson BS, Till GO, Ward PA. Acute lung injury in rat caused by immunoglobulin A immune complexes. *J Clin Invest* 1984; 74:358.

21. Stokes CR, Soothill JF, Turner MW. Immune exclusion is a function of IgA. *Nature* 1975; 255:745.

22. Kaufmann HS, Hobbs JR. Immunoglobulin deficiencies in an atopic population. *Lancet* 1970; ii:1061.

23. Taylor B, Norman AP, Orgel HA, Stokes CR, Turner MW, Soothill JF. Transient IgA deficiency and pathogenesis of infantile atopy. *Lancet* 1973; ii:111.

24. Stokes CR, Taylor B, Turner MW. Association of house-dust and grass-pollen allergies with specific IgA antibody deficiency. *Lancet* 1974; ii: 485.

25. van Asperen PP, Gleeson M, Kemp AS, Cripps AW, Geraghty SB, Mellis CM, Clancy RL. The relationship between atopy and salivary IgA deficiency in infancy. *Clin Exp Immunol* 1985; 62:753.

26. Cortesina G, Carlevato MT, Bussi M, Baldi C, Majore L, Ruffino C. Mucosal immunity in allergic rhinitis. *Acta Otolaryngol* 1993; 113:397.

27. Cunningham-Rundles C, Brandeis WE, Good RA, Day NK. Milk precipitin circulating immune complexes and IgA deficiency. *Proc Natl Acad Sci USA* 1978; 75:3387.

28. Kett K, Brandtzaeg P, Radl J., Haaijman JJ. Different subclass distribution of IgA-producing cells in human lymphoid organs and various secretory tissues. *J Immunol* 1987; 136:3611.

29. Sørensen CH, Kilian M. Bacterium-induced cleavage of IgA in nasopharyngeal secretions from atopic children. *Acta Path Microbiol Immunol Scand* Section C 1984; 92:85.

30. Kilian M, Husby S, Høst A, Halken S. Increased proportion of bacteria capable of cleaving IgA1 in the pharynx of infants with atopic disease. (submitted).

31. Weiner HL. Treatment of autoimmune diseases by oral tolerance. *Mucosal Immunol Update* 1993; 1:1.

32. Husby S, Mestecky J, Moldoveanu Z, Holland S, Elson CO. Oral tolerance in humans. T cell but not B cell tolerance after antigen feeding. *J Immunol* 1994; 152:4663.

33. Stevens FA. Status of poison ivy extracts. *J Am Med Assoc* 1945; 127:912.

34. Taudorf E, Laursen LC, Djurup R, Kappelgaard E, Pedersen CT, Søborg M, Wilkinson P, Weeke B. Oral administration of grass pollen to hay fever patients. *Allergy* 1985; 40:321.

35. Möller C, Dreborg S, Lanner Å, Björkstén B. Oral immunotherapy of children with rhinoconjunctivitis due to birch pollen allergy. *Allergy* 1986; 41:271.

36. Björkstén B, Möller C, Broberger V, Ahlstedt S, Dreborg S, Johansson SGO, Juto P, Lanner Å. Clinical and immunological effects of oral immunotherapy with a standardized birch pollen extract. *Allergy* 1986; 41:290.

37. Taudorf E, Møller C, Russell MW. Secretory IgA response in oral immunotherapy. Investigation in birch pollinosis. *Allergy* 1994 (in press).

38. Michalek SM, Eldridge JH, Curtiss III R, Rosenthal KL. Antigen delivery systems: new approaches to mucosal immunization. In PL Ogra, J Mestecky, ME Lamm, W Strober, JR McGhee, J Bienenstock (Eds) *Handbook of Mucosal Immunology*. San Diego: Academic Press, 1994, p. 373.

39. Holmgren J, Lycke N, Czerkinsky C. Cholera toxin and cholera B subunit as oral-mucosal adjuvant and antigen vector system. *Vaccine* 1993; 11:1179.

40. Marinaro M, Staats HF, Kiyono H, McGhee JR. Antibody isotype profiles associated with the use of cholera toxin (CT) as an oral adjuvant. *FASEB J* 1994; 8:A514 (abstr 2979).

41. Snider DP, Marshall JS, Perdue MH, Liang H. Production of IgE Ab and allergic sensitization of intestinal and peripheral tissues after oral immunization with protein Ag and cholera toxin. *J Immunol* 1994; 153:647.

42. McGhee JR, Mestecky J. Mucosal vaccines: Areas arising. *Mucosal Immunol Update* 1993; 1:1.

The Process of Airway Inflammation and its Relationship to Clinical Symptoms

Stephen T Holgate*

Keywords: Asthma, inflammation, cytokines

While most asthma is associated with atopy, there exist forms of the disease where no environmental allergens can be identified. Research has until recently focused on early and late phase allergen-induced inflammatory responses in asthma involving mast cells and eosinophils. However, recognising that asthma is a chronic inflammatory disorder, cytokine and mediator pathways are now being resolved that underlie the persistence of this inflammatory response.

Bronchial biopsy and lavage data have now provided convincing evidence from different types of asthma that airway inflammation underlies much of the disordered airway function (1). This inflammatory response is specifically characterised by infiltration with activated mast cells and eosinophils and appears to be largely T-cell driven, at least in the chronic persistent disease. A large number of epidemiological studies have established causality, with aeroallergen exposure (particularly to domestic mites) involving the upregulation of IgE, the sensitisation of mast cells and eosinophils and the subsequent allergen-induced release of both preformed and newly generated inflammatory mediators. In considering the underlying mechanisms involved in initiating airway inflammation that recruits these pathways, several steps require consideration.

Process of Sensitisation

In genetically susceptible individuals, primary sensitisation of the airways occurs through the participation of professional antigen presenting cells called dendritic cells. These cells, which line the bronchi both in the epithelium and in the submucosa, are identified by their cell surface presence

of a specific cell surface marker $CD1a^+$ and have the capacity to identify and subsequently process antigen (Figure 1). Augmentation of antigen recognition is facilitated by the presence of both a low affinity (CD23) and the high affinity (FcεR1) receptors on the surface of the dendritic cells. An increase in the number of dendritic cells co-staining for CD1a and the α chain of FcεR1 in the epithelium of patients with bronchial asthma suggests that these cells play a key role not only in terms of initiating primary sensitisation but also in maintaining this response once the disease has developed (2). Antigen presentation most likely takes place in the local lymphoid collections and involves a cognate interaction between dendritic cells and T lymphocyte and the participation of MHC class II at the T-cell receptor. Differentiation of T cells along the Th2-type pathway involving the upregulation of the IL4 gene cluster encoded on chromosome 5 (IL-13, IL-4, IL-5, IL-3, GM-CSF, and IL-9) is the prime stimulus for initiating the allergic inflammatory response so characteristic of asthma (3, 4).

Allergen Challenge: The Early and the Late Reaction

Once sensitised to specific allergens, subsequent exposure to this results in both early and late phases of airway obstruction and an acquired increase in bronchial hyperresponsiveness. The former is mediated through the cross linkage of FcεR1 by specific allergen and results in the release of three major bronchoconstrictor mediators: histamine, prostaglandin D_2 and the sulphodipeptide leukotrienes LTC_4 and LTD_4. Indeed, these mediators account for the majority of the so-called early

* University of Southampton, Southampton, UK.

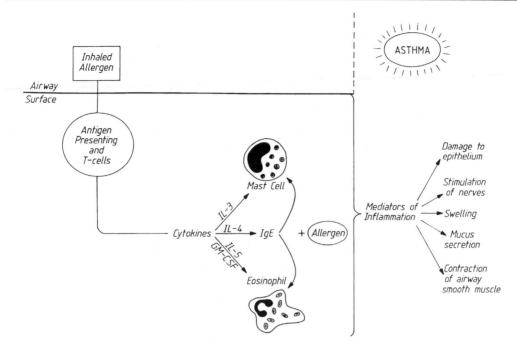

Figure 1. Schematic representation of the cellular events of allergic asthma.

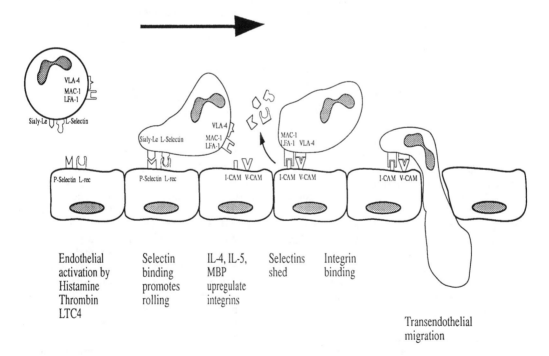

Figure 2. Sequence of events involved in the recruitment of inflammatory cells from the microvasculature in allergic inflammation.

asthmatic reaction which is largely airways smooth muscle dependent (5). Further amplification of this response may occur through the activation of local and central neural reflexes.

The late reaction ensues 4–6 h after antigen challenge and persists for anything up to 24 h. The airway obstruction has an important oedematous component to it, in addition to there being increased secretions in the airway and smooth muscle contraction. Bronchial biopsy taken at the onset of the late reaction demonstrates infiltration of the airway wall with neutrophils, eosinophils and T cells with migration of mast cells towards the airway surface (6, 7). Recruitment of leukocytes from the microvasculature involves upregulation of specific adhesion molecules, namely P-selectin, E-selectin, ICAM-1 and VCAM-1 (Figure 2). The latter three adhesion molecules are under the control of specific cytokines, namely interferon-γ, TNF-α and IL-1β with interleukin-4 augmenting VCAM-1 expression (7). We have recently found incontrovertible evidence that these adhesion molecules are upregulated between 6 and 24 h post challenge in parallel with recruitment of leukocytes bearing the reciprocal integrin molecules (6).

Since leukocyte recruitment is observed within 2–4 h following challenge, this does not give sufficient time for cytokines to be newly generated by T cells and other cells to upregulate the adhesion molecule pathways (8). An alternative source of cytokine is the mast cell. Immunohistochemical staining of bronchial biopsies of asthmatic airways shows the presence of TNF-α, IL-4, IL-5 and IL-6 within the secretory granules of human mast cells that can be released with cross-linkage of cell surface IgE (9–11). Immunologic activation also within 2 h initiates transcription of IL-4, IL-5 and TNF-α, but only in the presence of stem cell factor (12). IL-4 transcription remains elevated for 6–8 h, while that for IL-5 remains up to 48 h following a single allergen stimulus.

It seems highly probable that cross-linkage of IgE releases sufficient cytokine from these cellular stores to initiate the recruitment of leukocytes from the microvasculature, allergen specific T-cell responses occurring somewhat later (13). When it is recognised that every mast cell will respond to allergen by release of mediator, whereas only 1 in 300–2000 T cells are allergen specific, the role of the mast cell as an orchestrator of the allergic inflammatory response assumes greater importance.

The ability of drugs, such as sodium cromoglycate and nedocromil sodium, to inhibit both early and late phase responses and the acquired increase in bronchial hyperresponsiveness is in entire accord with the mast cell being responsible for releasing cytokines underpinning these reactions (14). The influence of corticosteroids in attenuating the late reaction when administered prior to antigen challenge can be accounted for by the effect of the expression of adhesion molecules on the microvasculature, whereas the inhibitory effect of β₂ agonists largely relates to their specific influence on mast cells and through their capacity to functionally antagonise the constrictor property of mast cell and eosinophil dependent mediators.

Allergic Asthma: A Model of Chronic Inflammation

Increasingly, we are recognising that patients with asthma have persistent airway inflammation even in the absence of allergen. This implies that other pathways are engaged in maintaining the inflammatory reaction other than mast cells and T cells. Nasal polyp and bronchial explants cultured *ex vivo* and stimulated in the presence of antigen result in survival of a population of cells for 4–7 days in culture, particularly epithelial cells, T cells, fibroblasts and eosinophils. Assessments of the potential growth factor capacity of the supernatant from these antigen stimulated explants indicate the presence of large quantities of GM-CSF, IL-5, IL-8 and IL-3, although the cellular prominence of these cytokines in such a model has not yet been elucidated. Nevertheless, the capacity of myofibroblasts to generate GM-CSF in the presence of TNF-α (15), the ability of the epithelium to generate GM-CSF, IL-6 and IL-8 when appropriately stimulated (16) and the synthetic capacity of Th2-like lymphocytes to generate and secrete IL-3, IL-5 and GM-CSF (3, 4) suggest that these are all important sources. Indeed, assays of the supernatant of these explants against the survival of highly purified human eosinophils indicate that there is sufficient reserve within the bronchial mucosa itself to maintain ongoing airway inflammation for a considerable period of time without additional cells being required from the microvasculature.

Thus, when considering airway inflammation in asthma as a chronic inflammatory disease, it is important to recognise that, in addition to the mast cell, eosinophil and T cell, there are matrix cells in the airway wall that are capable of contributing to the cytokine milieu which may or may not be antigen dependent. Such mechanisms may become particularly important in the chronic persistent form of the disease and even in that form not associated with an initial allergic stimulus (i. e., intrinsic asthma).

Concluding Comment

With respect to allergic asthma, experimental models now extend beyond early and late phase bronchoconstriction to evoke the concept of chronic airway inflammation involving not only cells of the immune system but also those of the airway wall. When coupled with the recent recognition of airway wall remodelling and utilisation of matrix proteins in leukocyte recruitment, these factors assume greater importance than previously recognised, and may well account for why asthma as a chronic disease occurs in humans and does not occur in other mammals.

By understanding in more detail the pathways whereby leukocytes are recruited and maintained within the inflammatory zone, it is likely that novel drug therapies will emerge which are more selective and more active against the special type of inflammation that underpins asthma.

Address for correspondence:

Prof Stephen T Holgate
Southampton General Hospital
Level D, Centre Block
Tremona Road
Southampton SO16 6YD
UK

References

1. Holgate ST. The Cournand Lecture. Asthma: Past, present and future. *Eur Resp J* 1993; 6:1507–1520.

2. Tunon-de-Lara JM, Bradding P, Redington AE, Goulding D, Church MK, Semper A, Holgate ST. Expression and cellular distribution of the a subunit of high affinity receptor for immunoglobulin E (FCeRI)

in normal and asthmatic airways. *Clin Exp Allergy* (submitted).

3. Van Leeuwen BH, Martinson ME, Webb GC, Young IG. Molecular organisation of the cytokine gene cluster, involving the human IL-3, IL-4, IL-6 and GM-CSF genes on human chromosome 5. *Blood* 1989; 73:1142–1148.

4. Walker C, Bode E, Boer R, Hansel TT, Blaser K, Virchow JC. Allergic and non-allergic asthmatics have distinct patterns of T-cell activation and cytokine production in peripheral blood and bronchoalveolar lavage. *Am Rev Respir Dis* 1992; 146:109–115.

5. Holgate ST, Robinson C, Church MK. Mediators of immediate hypersensitivity. In Middleton E Jr, Reed CE. Ellis EF, Adtkinson NF, Junginger JW, Busse WW (Eds) *Allergy: Principles and practice*, 4th edn. St. Louis: Mosby, 1993, pp. 267–301.

6. Montefort S, Gratziou C, Goulding D, Polosa R, Haskard DO, Howarth PH, Holgate ST, Carroll MP. Bronchial biopsy evidence for leucocyte infiltration and upregulation of leucocyte endothelial cell adhesion molecules 6 hours after local allergen challenge of sensitised asthmatic airway. *J Clin Invest* 1994; 93:1411–1421

7. Gratziou C, Carroll M, Montefort S, Teran L, Howarth PH, Holgate ST. Inflammatory and T-cell profile of sensitised asthmatic airways assessed by bronchoalveolar lavage 6 hours after local allergen provocation. (Submitted)

8. Springer TA. Adhesion receptors of the immune system. *Nature* 1990; 346:425–434.

9. Bradding P, Feather IH, Howarth PH, Mueller R, Roberts JA, Britten KM, Bews JPA, Hunt TC, Okayama Y, Heusser CH, Bullock GR, Church MK, Holgate ST. Interleukin-4 is localised to and released by human mast cells. *J Exp Med* 1992; 176:1381–1386.

10. Bradding P, Feather IH, Wilson S, Bardin PG, Heusser CH, Holgate ST, Howarth PH. Immuno-localisation of cytokines in the nasal mucosa of normal and perennial rhinitic subjects: The mast cell as a source of IL-4, IL-5 and IL-6 in human allergic mucosal inflammation. *J Immunol* 1993; 151:3853–3865.

11. Bradding P, Roberts JA, Britten KM, Montefort S, Djukanovic R, Heusser C, Howarth PH, Holgate ST. Interleukin-4, -5, -6 and TNFa in normal and asthmatic airways: Evidence for the human mast cell as an important source of these cytokines. *Am J Respir Cell Mol Biol* 1994; 10:471–480.

12. Okayama Y, Petit-Frére, Kassel O, Semper A, Quint D, Tunon de Lara JM, Bradding P, Holgate ST, Church MK. Expression of messenger RNA for IL-4 and IL-5 in human lung and skin mast cells in response to FCe receptor cross-linkage and the presence of stem cell factor. *J Immunol* (in press).

13. Bentley AM, Meng Q, Robinson DS, Hamid Q, Kay AB, Durham SR. Increases in activated T-lymphocytes, eosinophils and cytokine mRNA expression for interleukin 5 and granulocyte/macrophage colony stimulating factor in bronchial biopsies after allergen inhalation challenge in atopic asthmatics. *Am J Respir Cell Mol Biol* 1993; 8:35–42.

14. Edwards AM. Sodium cromoglycate (Intal) as an anti-inflammatory agent for the treatment of chronic asthma. *Clin Exp Allergy* 1994; 24:612–623.

15. Holgate ST. Djukanovic R, Howarth PH, Montefort S, Roche W. The T-cell and the airways fibrotic response in asthma. *Chest* 1993; 103:125S–128S.

16. Devalia JL, Campbell AM, Sapsford R et al. Effect of nitrogen dioxide on synthesis of inflammatory cytokines expressed by human bronchial epithelial cells. *Am J Respir Cell Mol Biol* 1993; 9:271–279.

Properties and Characteristics of Inflammatory and Resident Cells in Asthmatic Airways

AR Sousa, RN Poston, SJ Lane, TH Lee*

Keywords: Asthma, cytokines, epithelium, macrophages, eosinophils, T lymphocytes, mast cells, neutrophils

Bronchial asthma is a disease that is characterized by a history of episodic wheezing, by physiologic evidence of reversible airflow obstruction, either spontaneously or following bronchodilator therapy, and by pathologic evidence of inflammatory changes in the bronchial mucosa (1, 2). Early studies of deaths from status asthmaticus revealed marked inflammation in the bronchial tree (3). There was plugging of the lumen with mucus, epithelial cells, and eosinophils, shedding of the epithelium, basement membrane thickening, smooth muscle hypertrophy and an intense inflammatory cell infiltrate in the mucosa and submucosa, characterized by a predominantly eosinophilic infiltrate but also containing mononuclear cells and neutrophils. More recently, with the development of fibreoptic bronchoscopy, biopsy and lavage in asthmatic subjects has become possible. Bronchoalveolar lavage (BAL) fluid from asthmatic subjects, in the absence of bronchial provocation, contains increased numbers of mast cells, epithelial cells, eosinophils and neutrophils compared to that obtained from normal controls (4, 5). Elevated levels of eosinophil-derived major basic protein (MBP), histamine, prostaglandin D_2 (PGD_2) and of the peptidoleukotrienes have also been reported (5–7). Immunohistochemical analyses of bronchial biopsies confirm the presence of airway inflammation in subjects with mild to moderately severe asthma (8, 9) (Figure 1). Immunohistochemistry and *in situ* hybridization have shown that these cells are activated and are producing proinflammatory and chemotactic cytokines. The evidence is therefore compelling that airway inflammation is central to the pathogenesis of bronchial asthma, emphasizing the importance of understanding the properties and characteristics of inflammatory and resident cells in asthmatic airways.

Epithelial Cells and Basement Membrane

The bronchial epithelium is the primary interface between the lung and inspired air. It has long been recognized to be the primary barrier protecting the underlying tissues from inhaled irritants and noxious stimuli. It also controls airway humidity and the composition of airway fluid.

Loss of epithelial integrity is a recognized feature of asthma, and it has been suggested that this may be one of the causes of the increased bronchial hyper-reactivity characteristic of the disease. Laitinen and coworkers (11) found extensive damage of the epithelium and areas in which only basal cells were present. The ciliated epithelial cells were swollen and the intercellular spaces were widened. Several studies have reported the presence of increased numbers of bronchial epithelial cells recovered by bronchoalveolar lavage from asthmatic subjects when compared with those from normal subjects, and have established a positive relationship between epithelial cell counts and the extent of airway hyper-responsiveness (4). In recent years, it has become increasingly apparent that the role of the epithelial cell is not merely as a physical barrier, since it is considerably more metabolically active than was previously recognized. When stimulated, bronchial epithelium releases a number of arachidonic acid-derived metabolites (11). Also, it is possible that bronchodilator factors normally produced by healthy epithelium and that these are lost when the epithelium is shed.

Asthmatic bronchial epithelium has also been shown to produce mRNA, and protein, for several different inflammatory cytokines. mRNA tran-

* Department of Allergy and Respiratory Medicine; Department of Experimental Pathology, UMDS, Guy's Hospital, London, UK.

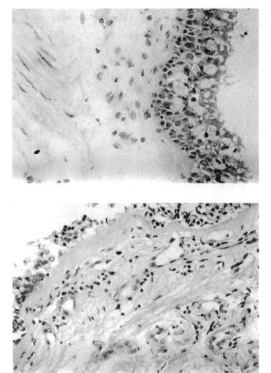

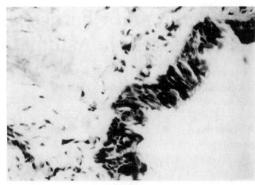

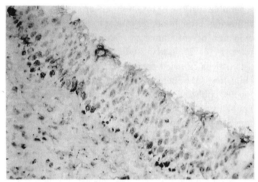

Figure 1. (a, above) Bronchial biopsy of a normal subject stained with hematoxylin and eosin. (b, below) Bronchial biopsy of an asthmatic subject stained with hematoxylin and eosin. There is an increased number of infiltrating inflammatory cells, basement membrane thickening and epithelial shedding.

Figure 2. (a, above) Bronchial biopsy of an asthmatic subject stained for GM-CSF by a polyclonal goat antibody using the avidin-biotin complex (ABC) immunoperoxidase method. The epithelium shows intense staining by the brown reaction product. (b, below) Bronchial biopsy from a control subject stained by the same method. The epithelium shows only weak staining (from reference 13).

scripts for GM-CSF, IL-6, IL-8, IL-1α and IL-1β (12) have been described in epithelial cells. Cultured epithelial cells from patients with asthma have enhanced generation of IL-1, IL-6, IL-8 and GM-CSF. Studies using fibreoptic bronschoscopy have shown increased protein expression of GM-CSF, MCP-1, TNF-α, IL-6 and IL-8 (13–15) (Figure 2). Recently, bronchial epithelium has also been shown to express the low-affinity receptor for IgE, FcεRII, suggesting a possible role for bronchial epithelium in antigen presentation. Bronchial epithelium is a potential target site for drug delivery. Corticosteroids are the most effective drugs used in the therapy of bronchial asthma, and several groups have demonstrated downregulation of several different cytokines, such as GM-CSF, on bronchial epithelium, which may explain their therapeutic efficacy (13).

Previous studies using light microscopy have described thickening and hyalinization of the epithelial basement membrane. Recent morphologic studies have shown that the bronchial epithelial basement membrane is of normal thickness in asthma, but there is dense deposition of collagen fibrils in the subepithelial region (16). Immunohistochemistry indicates the presence of collagen type IV, fibronectin and laminin in the true basement membrane, and the subepithelial collagen consists predominantly of collagen types II and V, together with fibronectin but not laminin (16). It has been proposed that the cellular source of the subepithelial collagen is the myofibroblast. Mast cells present in the airway lumen and mucosa are a potential source of growth factors, as are macrophages, eosinophils and the bronchial epithelial cell.

Macrophages and Monocytes

The classification of lung macrophages has traditionally divided them into two categories based upon their anatomic distribution: alveolar or interstitial. Alveolar macrophages (AM) are the ones collected in BAL. Interstitial macrophages are those present in the lung submucosa.

Most studies of BAL fluid have found that the numbers of mononuclear phagocytes present were not increased as compared to the control subjects. In contrast, immunohistochemistry of the bronchial biopsy specimens showed that the submucosa had a significantly increased activated heterogeneous macrophage population in asthmatic subjects (9) (Figure 3). In addition, the macrophage population had phenotypic characteristics of peripheral blood monocytes, suggesting that they had migrated recently into the lung. There was also heterogeneity of the macrophage/monocyte population. HLA class II antigen was expressed on the macrophages of the airway mucosa to a greater extent in the asthmatic subjects than in normal individuals. Hence, not only are there greater numbers of macrophages in asthmatic airways but they are also more activated. This macrophage activation is further confirmed by the upregulation of inflammatory cytokines such as GM-CSF, MCP-1, IL-1β and TNF-α.

Alveolar macrophages constitute the majority of cells recovered by BAL both in normal and in asthmatic subjects. Cultured AM have an increased respiratory burst as detected by chemiluminescence, when compared to normal controls. Analysis of BAL fluid from asthmatic patients following antigen challenge reveals increased amounts of β-glucuronidase, whereas corresponding macrophage intracellular levels were decreased, suggesting that the macrophage secretory process may be activated by allergen, acting through the FcεRII receptor (17). In atopic asthmatic subjects, the numbers of IgE FcεRII⁺ alveolar and tissue macrophages and peripheral blood monocytes are in-

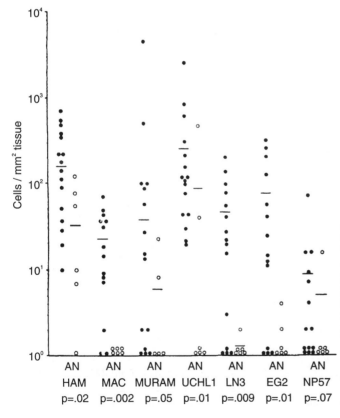

Figure 3. Graph showing individual cell counts in the submucosa of bronchial biopsies obtained from asthmatic (A) and normal (N) subjects defined by a panel of antibodies. HAM = HAM-56, a pan-macrophage marker; MAC387 = a recently blood-derived macrophage/monocyte marker; MURAM = an anti-muramidase (lysozyme) marker; UCHL1 = an anti-activated T memory cell (CD45Ro) marker; LN3 = an anti-HLA-DR class II marker; EG2 = an anti-eosinophil cationic protein marker; NP 57 = an anti-neutrophil elastase marker (from reference 8).

creased. Rankin and colleagues demonstrated that normal AM could be activated by monoclonal IgE and specific antigen to generate both LTC$_4$ and LTB$_4$ (18). Furthermore, IgE-antigen complexes can activate rat peritoneal macrophages to release lysosomal enzymes and superoxide anion. The existence of low-affinity FcεRII suggests that macrophages and their monocyte precursors may be directly involved in allergic responses in addition to their role in presenting antigens to T lymphocytes.

Monocytes and macrophages are necessary for the generation of cell-mediated immune responses by processing and presenting antigen to antigen specific lymphocytes, committing them to antigen specific division and cytokine generation. Human AM from normal subjects function poorly as accessory cells for the presentation of recall antigens to autologous peripheral blood T lymphocytes (19), and this may be important for the appropriate control of immune and inflammatory processes within the lung. Furthermore, there is evidence suggesting an association between AM accessory function and the presence of BAL lymphocytes in bronchial asthma (20). The reason for this association remains to be determined but it may be due to infiltration into the asthmatic lung of a functionally distinct subset of site and allergen-specific CD4$^+$ cells with a specific pattern of cytokine release. Alveolar macrophages can influence eosinophil function, as suggested by the fact that AM from asthmatic, but not from normal subjects enhance the capacity of eosinophils to produce LTC$_4$ (21). The enhancing activity appears to be due to GM-CSF.

Both alveolar and tissue macrophages are therefore capable of influencing the functions of other inflammatory cells, such as eosinophils and are, therefore, an important constituent of the inflammatory pathology of bronchial asthma.

Eosinophils

Bronchial asthma is known to be associated with eosinophilia of the blood and lung (22). Activated eosinophils release a number of mediators that are directly involved in the pathogenesis of asthma, a correlation being seen between the extent of eosinophilic inflammation in the airways and the clinical severity of the disease Eosinophils are able to metabolize histamine, inactive leukotrienes, and

platelet-activating factor (PAF), and are able to suppress histamine release. Hence, they were initially attributed a protective role in the allergic response. Subsequent research has suggested that they may serve a proinflammatory function since they are capable of secreting preformed and newly generated mediators capable of eliciting tissue damage. Their presence in the airway and ability to express FcεRII provides a means by which these cells can be activated via IgE-dependent mechanisms. The observation that human eosinophils produce IL-3 and GM-CSF when stimulated by ionophore or IFN-γ suggests that there are additional mechanisms by eosinophils may augment the local inflammatory response, including autocrine effects of IL-3 and GM-CSF upon eosinophil survival and function (23). An increased number of eosinophils in asthmatic airways has been seen by different groups (8, 24). Major basic protein (MBP) deposition has been observed in the bronchial wall and in the mucus in the asthmatic lung. The sites of MBP deposition coincide with areas of epithelial damage suggesting involvement of the eosinophil in epithelial damage. The levels of MBP in sputum correlate with disease severity and the levels decrease after treatment. Levels of eosinophils and eosinophilic cationic protein (ECP) in BAL fluid, and numbers of intraepithelial eosinophils also correlate with the severity of asthma. Davies and coworkers have noted that the number of activated intraepithelial eosinophils correlate with the levels of GM-CSF on bronchial epithelium, emphasizing the importance of the interrelationship between all the cells, resident and inflammatory, to the pathogenesis of asthma.

Lymphocytes

There is compelling evidence for the role of the T lymphocyte in the pathogenesis of bronchial asthma. There are increased numbers of T lymphocytes in asthmatic airways (8). In acute severe asthma, peripheral T helper (CD4$^+$) lymphocytes are activated on the basis of enhanced IL-2 receptor expression, increased elaboration of IFN-γ and soluble IL-2 receptor, and increased class II HLA DR and the very late activation antigen (VLA-1) (25). Analysis of BAL fluid 48 h following bronchial allergen challenge suggested recruitment of these cells to the lung. Bronchial biopsies from mild asthmatic subjects showed increased activated CD4[+] T cells (26). Robinson and coworkers (27) have shown increased levels of mRNA for IL-2, IL-3, IL-4, IL-5 and GM-CSF in BAL fluid from atopic asthmatic subjects when compared with those from healthy volunteers, but no differences were detected between the two groups in cells expressing mRNA for IFN-γ or IL-4, and IL-5 mRNA was predominantly localized to T cells. This profile of cytokine mRNA expression is compatible with predominant activation of the Th2 subset of T helper cells and is in accordance with studies in both murine and human T cell clones implicating the Th2-like cytokines in the immunopathology of allergic bronchial asthma. These data are further supported by the presence of Th2-like patterns of cytokine in both BAL fluid and bronchial biopsies 24 h after allergen challenge to the lung (28). Increased levels of IL-5 mRNA have also been reported in bronchial biopsies from asthmatic subjects, suggesting an important role for Th2 cytokines in T lymphocyte-eosinophil interactions *in vivo*.

Ackerman and coworkers have shown the protein expression of IL-3, IL-4, IL-5 and GM-CSF on CD4[+] T lymphocytes of bronchial biopsies from atopic asthmatic subjects, whereas CD4[+] T lymphocytes from nonatopic asthmatic subjects predominantly expressed IL-2, IL-3, IL-5 and GM-CSF (15).

Mast Cells

Mast cells can be seen in the bronchi of normal and asthmatic subjects. They are activated by IgE-dependent mechanisms, adenosine, cold air and exercise to release mediators such as histamine and prostaglandin D_2. Pulmonary mast cells are increased in number in chronic bronchial asthma and show enhanced spontaneous and IgE-stimulated release of mediators. Mast cells are, in addition, activated in the asthmatic lung (4, 24). Lung mast cells are characterized by storage of the neutral protease tryptase in their granules, as opposed to chymase which characterizes connective tissue mast cells. Several studies have demonstrated an increased concentration of histamine in the BAL fluid during the early reaction that follows endobronchial allergen challenge. The increase in histamine correlates with that of the unique mast cell protease tryptase, supporting the mast cell origin of

these mediators (29). *In vitro* IgE-dependent activation of mast cells leads to the production of arachidonic acid-derived metabolites (30). The most abundant cyclooxygenase product synthesized and released from the human lung mast cell is PGD_2 (30). After local airway challenge of asthmatic airways with allergen through a bronchoscope, there is a 150-fold increase in the concentration of PGD_2 in BAL fluid. Following allergen provocation, concentrations of leukotriene C_4 and its metabolite, LTE_4 have been found in increased concentrations in BAL fluid. LTE_4 has also been found in increased concentrations in the urine in and during natural exacerbations of the disease.

Recently, human mast cells have been shown to generate cytokines, such as TNF-α and IL-4 in response to cross-linkage of the high-affinity receptor FcϵR2 or to the calcium ionophore A23187 (31). In addition, human skin mast cells also seem to be expressing IL-5. It seems likely that human mast cells are capable, upon activation, of expressing the same range of cytokines as murine mast cells such as IL-1, IL-3, IL-6 and GM-CSF.

The emphasis on the mast cell as an essential cell in the pathogenesis of asthma has recently been tempered by the observation that albuterol, which is a very potent inhibitor of mast cell degranulation, had little effect on the allergic inflammation induced by allergen challenge. This has cast doubt over the hypothesis of the importance of the mast cell in the more prolonged and protracted phases of inflammation induced by allergic reactions. Mast cells play a pivotal role in the recruitment and priming of inflammatory cells following allergen challenge in sensitized subjects. The mast cell may play an important role in the recruitment and activation of T lymphocytes and eosinophils, and in the regulation of local IgE production within the airways in chronic asthma.

Neutrophils

Neutrophils have been reported to be associated with the transient bronchial hyper-responsiveness induced by ozone, but the evidence for the involvement of neutrophils in the mechanism of bronchial asthma is much less certain. Following allergen and exercise challenge, a peptide with neutrophil chemotactic activity (NCA) has been detected in the peripheral circulation (32). The release of this molecule is associated with increased expression of cell surface markers of neutrophil activation such as complement receptors and IgG Fc receptors (33). Therefore, asthmatic neutrophils seem to be activated. Enhanced neutrophil complement receptor expression has also been shown to accompany allergen induced EAR and LAR.

The reported numbers of neutrophils in BAL is controversial, depending on the lavage volume. Allergen provocation also results in varying numbers of neutrophils recovered in the BAL fluid that to some extent can be explained on the basis of differences in the timing of lavage. Thus BAL performed at 4 h post allergen challenge has shown an increase in both neutrophil and eosinophil numbers, with neutrophils subsiding and the eosinophil counts remaining elevated at 24 h (34). Further evidence of the involvement of the neutrophils in inflammation in asthma has been given by studies of occupational forms of asthma. After allergen challenge with diisocyanates, a marked rise in the number of neutrophils in BAL occurs in relation to the late asthmatic response with only modest increases in eosinophils (35).

Bronchial biopsies in mild asthmatics after bronchial provocation with common inhalant allergens has shown little evidence of neutrophil infiltration of the airway mucosa (4), although bronchial biopsies only provide limited information to a single moment in time and give no information about the very important cell dynamics.

Summary

There is considerable interest and research into the mechanisms underlying the pathogenesis and maintenance of the inflammatory response in asthma. The development and maintenance of the inflammatory response in asthma is likely to be a consequence of a complicated interaction between the various inflammatory and resident cells and the mediators they generate. There is a complex cytokine network operating in the asthmatic airways, both recruited and resident cells representing important sources of these substances. Through the release of these cytokines, resident cells may influence the recruitment and function of additional effector cells, particular macrophages, eosinophils and T lymphocytes. Recruited cells may then amplify the inflammatory loop by producing cytokines themselves. As the reactions progress further, cytokines from resident cells and from recruited and activated inflammatory cells may exert complex paracrine and autocrine effects on resident and infiltrating cell populations that ultimately result in the increased release of factors directly involved in the pathology of bronchial asthma.

Acknowledgments

The authors wish to acknowledge the financial support of the Wellcome Trust, National Asthma Campaign and the Special Trustees of Guy's Hospital.

Address for correspondence:

Prof TH Lee MD FRCP
Department of Allergy and
Respiratory Medicine
4th Floor, Hunt's House
Guy's Hospital
London SE1 9RT
UK

References

1. Arm JP, Lee TH. The pathobiology of bronchial asthma. *Adv Immunol* 1992; 51:323.

2. Djukanovic R, Roche WR, Wilson JW, Beasley CRW, Twentyman OP, Howarth PH, Holgate ST. Mucosal inflammation in asthma. *Am Rev Respir Dis* 1990; 142:434.

3. Dunnill MS. The pathology of asthma, with special reference to changes in the bronchial mucosa. *J Clin Pathol* 1960; 13:27.

4. Beasley R, Roche WR, Roberts JA, Holgate ST. Cellular events in the bronchi in mild asthma and after bronchial provocation. *Am Rev Respir Dis* 1989; 139:806.

5. Agius R, Godfrey RC, Holgate ST. Mast cell and histamine content of human bronchoalveolar lavage fluid. *Thorax* 1985; 40:760.

6. Liu MC, Bleecker ER, Lichtenstein LM, Kagey-Sobotka A, Niv Y, McLemore TL, Permutt S, Proud D, Hubbard WC. Evidence for elevated levels of histamine, prostaglandin D_2, and other bronchoconstricting prostaglandins in the airways of subjects with mild asthma. *Am Rev Respir Dis* 1990; 142:126.

7. Lam S, Chan H, LeRiche JC, Chan-Yeung M, Salari H. Release of leukotrienes in patients with bronchial asthma. *J Allergy Clin Immunol* 1988; 81:711.

8. Poston RN, Chanez P, Lacoste JY, Litchfield T, Lee TH, Bousquet J. Immunohistochemical characterization of the cellular infiltration in asthmatic bronchi. *Am Rev Respir Dis* 1992; 145:918.

9. Laitinen LA, Laitinen A, Haahtela T. Airway mucosa inflammation even in patients with newly diagnosed asthma. *Am Rev Respir Dis* 1993; 147:697.

10. Laitinen LA, Heino M, Laitinen A, Kava T, Haahtela T. Damage of the airway epithelium and bronchial reactivity in patients with asthma. *Am Rev Respir Dis* 1985; 131:599.

11. Hunter JA, Finkbeiner WE, Nadel JA, Goetzl EJ, Holtzman MJ. Predominant generation of 15-lipoxygenase metabolites of arachidonic acid by epithelial cells from human trachea. *Proc Natl Acad Sci USA* 1985; 82:4633.

12. Proud D. The epithelial cell as a target and effector cell in airway inflammation. In: Holgate ST, Austen KF, Lichtenstein LM Kay AB (Eds) *Asthma: Physiology immunopharmacology and treatment*. London: Academic Press (in press).

13. Sousa AR, Poston RN, Lane SJ, Nakhosteen JA, Lee TH. GM-CSF expression in bronchial epithelium of asthmatic airways: decrease by inhaled corticosteroids. *Am Rev Respir Dis* 1993; 147:1557.

14. Sousa AR, Lane SJ, Nakhosteen J, Yoshimura T, Lee TH, Poston RN. Increased expression of the monocyte chemoattractant protein-1 in asthmatic bronchi. *Am J Respir Cell Biol* 1994; 10:142.

15. Ackerman V, Marini M, Vittori E, Bellini A, Vassali G, Mattoli S. Detection of cytokines and their cell sources in bronchial biopsy specimens from asthmatic patients. Relationship to atopic status, symptoms, and level of airway hyperresponsiveness. *Chest* 1994; 105:687.

16. Roche WR, Beasley R, Williams JH, Holgate ST. Subepithelial fibrosis in the bronchi of asthmatics. *Lancet* 1989; 1:520.

17. Unanue ER, Allen PM. The basis for the immunoregulatory role of macrophages and other accessory cells. *Science* 1987; 236:551.

18. Rankin JA, Hitchcock M, Merrill W, Bach MK, Brashler JR, Askenase PW. IgE-dependent release of leukotriene C4 from alveolar macrophages. *Nature* 1982; 297(5864):329–331.

19. Gant VA, Shakoor ZS, Barbosa IL, Hamblin AS. Normal and sarcoid alveolar macrophages differ in their ability to present antigen and to cluster with autologous lymphocytes. *Clin Exp Immunol* 1991; 86:494.

20. Gant VA, Cluzel M, Shakoor Z, Rees J, Lee TH, Hamblin AS. Alveolar macrophage accessory cell function in bronchial asthma. *Am Rev Respir Dis* 1992; 146:900.

21. Howell CJ, Pujol JL, Crea AEG Davidson R, Gearing AJH, Godard P, Lee TH. Identification of an alveolar macrophage-derived activity in bronchial asthma which enhanced leukotriene C4 generation by human eosinophils stimulated by ionophore (A23187) as granulocyte macrophage colony-stimulating factor (GM-CSF). *Am Rev Respir Dis* 1989; 140:1340.

22. Bousquet J, Chanez P, Lacoste JY, Barneon G, Ghavanian N, Enander I, Venge P, Ahlstedt S, Simony-Lafontaine J, Godard P, Michel FB. Eosinophilic inflammation in asthma. *N Engl J Med* 1990; 323:1033.

23. Moqbel R, Hamid Q, Ying S, Barkans J, Hartnell A, Tsicopoulos A, Wardlaw AJ, Kay AB. Expression of mRNA and immunoreactivity for the granulocyte/macrophage colony-stimulating factor in activated human eosinophils. *J Exp Med* 1991; 174:749.

24. Djukanovic R, Wilson JW, Britten KM, Willson SJ, Walls AF, Roche WR, Howarth PH, Holgate ST. Quantification of mast cells and eosinophils in the bronchial mucosa of symptomatic atopic asthmatics and healthy control subjects using immunohistochemistry. *Am Rev Respir Dis* 1990; 142:863.

25. Corrigan CJ, Hartnell A, Kay AB. T lymphocyte activation in acute severe asthma. *Lancet* 1988; 1:1129.

26. Jeffery PK, Wardlaw AJ, Nelson FC, Collins JV, Kay AB. Bronchial biopsies in asthma. An ultrastructural, quantitative study and correlation with hyperreactivity. *Am Rev Respir Dis* 1989; 140:1745.

27. Robinson DS, Hamid Q, Ying S, Tsicopoulos A, Barkans J, Bentley AM, Corrigan C, Durham SR, Kay AB. Predominant TH2-like bronchoalveolar T-lymphocyte population in atopic asthma. *N Engl J Med* 1992; 326:298.

28. Bentley AM, Meng Q, Robinson DS, Hamid Q, Kay AB, Durham SR. Increases in activated T lymphocytes, eosinophils, and cytokine mRNA expression for interleukin-5 and granulocyte/macrophage colony-stimulating factor in bronchial biopsies after allergen inhalation challenge in atopic asthmatics. *Am J Respir Cell Mol Biol* 1993; 8:35.

29. Wenzel SE, Fowler AA 3rd, Schwartz LB. Activation of pulmonary mast cells by bronchoalveolar allergen challenge. *In vivo* release of histamine and tryptase in atopic subjects with and without asthma. *Am Rev Respir Dis* 1988; 137:1002.

30. Holgate ST, Robinson C, Church MK. Mediators of immediate hypersensitivity. In: Middleton E, Reed CE, Ellis EF, Adkinson NF, Yuninger JW (Eds) *Allergy: Principles and practice*. St. Louis: Mosby, 1988, p. 135.

31. Bradding P, Feather IH, Wilson S, Bardin PG, Heusser CH, Holgate ST, Howarth PH. Immunolocalization of cytokines in the nasal mucosa of normal and perennial rhinitic subjects. The mast cell as a source of IL-4, IL-5, and IL-6 in human allergic mucosal inflammation. *J Immunol* 1993; 151:3853.

32. Lee TH, Brown MJ, Nagy L, Causon R, Walport MJ, Kay AB. Exercise-induced release of histamine and neutrophil chemotactic factor in atopic asthmatics. *J Allergy Clin Immunol* 1982; 70:73.

33. Papageorgiou N, Carroll M, Durham SR, Lee TH, Walsh GM, Kay AB. Complement receptor enhancement as evidence of neutrophil activation after exercise-induced asthma. *Lancet* 1983; 2:1220.

34. Metzger WJ, Richerson HB, Worden K, Monick M, Hunninghake GW. Bronchoalveolar lavage of allergic asthmatic patients following allergen bronchoprovocation. *Chest* 1986; 89:477.

35. Fabbri LM, Boschetto P, Zocca E, Milani G, Pivirotto F, Plebani M, Burlina A, Licata B, Mapp CE. Bronchoalveolar neutrophilia during late asthmatic reactions induced by toluene diisocyanate. *Am Rev Respir Dis* 1987; 136:36.

Airway Hyper-Responsiveness as a Diagnostic Feature of Asthma

Frederick E Hargreave, Marcia M Pizzichini, Emilio Pizzichini*

Keywords: Airway responsiveness, asthma, peak expiratory flow, sputum

Measurement of airway responsiveness to histamine or methacholine is useful in patients in whom the diagnosis is clinically uncertain, who present with symptoms consistent with asthma but have normal spirometry. In such patients, the demonstration of normal responsiveness suggests that asthma is not present. The presence of hyper-responsiveness suggests that the symptoms are associated with asthma. Measurements of airway responsiveness is a valid alternative to measurement of diurnal variation of PEF and has a number of advantages.

However, like all of the other characteristics of asthma, the histamine or methacholine inhalation test is not a gold standard for the diagnosis. There are reasons for discrepancies between the test result and symptoms which need to be appreciated to interpret the result. For example, the demonstration of normal responsiveness does not exclude the condition of eosinophilic bronchitis, which will respond to treatment with corticosteroids. In addition, histamine or methacholine hyper-responsiveness is not diagnostic for asthma when there is chronic airflow limitation.

Introduction

When considering the diagnostic value of a test for asthma, the definition and gold standard for the diagnosis needs to be taken into account. Unfortunately, asthma can still not be defined precisely, and there is no gold standard for the diagnosis. Asthma is currently regarded as a syndrome with symptoms associated with variable airflow obstruction, airway hyper-responsiveness and airway inflammation (1). Airway inflammation is considered to be the cause of the other features but the characteristics of the inflammation and their relationship to the clinical characteristics has not been examined in enough detail. Other problems with defining asthma and identifying a gold standard for the diagnosis are that all of the features are variable from one time to another, and none of the clinical features, including airway hyper-responsiveness, are entirely specific for asthma. These points need to be kept in mind when considering airway hyper-responsiveness as a diagnostic feature.

A Controversial Issue

The value of the measurement of airway responsiveness for the diagnosis of asthma is controversial. In the past year, three articles from the UK have been critical of its use. Laszlo (2) concludes that "measurement cannot be used to diagnose asthma unless a definition is used which is so stringent that it becomes very insensitive." In fact, we will illustrate that the current definition of histamine or methacholine airway hyper-responsiveness is appropriate and sensitive. Pattemore and Holgate (3) conclude that "measurement is uninterpretable and unhelpful in those in whom the diagnosis is difficult clinically." However, there is evidence to the contrary that this is just the group of patients in whom measurement is most useful to exclude or support the diagnosis. Finally, Rogers and O'Connor (4) state that "in the diagnosis and management of asthma, measurement of airway responsiveness is no substitute for monitoring clinical parameters: symptoms, spirometric measures, serial peak flow readings and rate of consumption of β-agonists." In fact, there is evidence that serial measurements of peak expiratory flow (PEF) are only as good or as bad as measurements of responsiveness in making the diagnosis.

*   Asthma Research Group, Departments of Medicine and Paediatrics, St. Joseph's Hospital and McMaster University, Hamilton, Ontario, Canada.

Some Methodological Issues

One of the problems with measuring airway responsiveness is the number of stimuli that can be used (5). These stimuli either act directly on certain receptors on airway smooth muscle (e.g., histamine, methacholine, prostaglandins, and leukotrienes), or indirectly via the release of chemical mediators or the stimulation of nerves which then act on airway smooth muscle (e.g., exercise, eucapnic hyperventilation of cold dry air, or inhalation of hypo- or hypertonic saline, adenosine monophosphate (AMP), propranolol, bradykinin, neurokinin A, substance P, SO_{+2}, or metabisulfite). It has been hoped that the stimuli acting indirectly might be as sensitive but more specific for asthma than the direct stimuli; however, so far there have been only limited studies which have not confirmed this hope. The best standardized and investigated method is still the inhalation test with histamine or methacholine; responsiveness to these two agents correlate very closely.

The inhalation tests are performed in a dose-response manner (6, 7). The dose must be carefully regulated and the response, usually measured by FEV_1, must be measured correctly to accurately interpret results. When responsiveness is normal, the dose-response curve is placed to the right, i.e., a high dose is required to cause airway constriction, and there is a maximal response plateau, indicating that airway constriction is limited to a relatively mild degree. When responsiveness is heightened, the curve shifts to the left and the maximal response plateau is increased and eventually lost. The results are usually expressed as the position of the curve indicated by the provocation concentration (or dose) to cause a fall in FEV_1 of 20% (PC_{20} or PD_{20}). The lower the PC_{20}, the greater the responsiveness.

The cut point between normal and increased responsiveness has been derived from clinical studies using other measurements of variable airflow obstruction (8–12). The most appropriate cut point for the method we use is 8 mg/ml. However, it is probably better to include a gray area of a twofold difference in concentration around this point, i.e., between 4 and 16 mg/ml, where variable airflow obstruction may or may not be associated with symptoms. It is very unlikely to have variable airflow obstruction when the PC_{20} is greater than 16 mg/ml.

Histamine or Methacholine Airway Hyper-responsiveness and Other Physiological Measurements

When the degree of airway responsiveness to histamine is correlated with baseline FEV_1, the baseline FEV_1 is usually normal until responsiveness is moderately to severely increased (8). This indicates that the measurement of responsiveness is a more sensitive indicator of abnormal airway function than FEV_1 and will be useful to confirm or refute the diagnosis of asthma when symptoms are present but the FEV_1 is normal.

The relationship between FEV_1 and airway responsiveness to methacholine is different in cigarette smokers with chronic bronchitis (13). Here, there is a more direct linear relationship between FEV_1 and PC_{20}. When the FEV_1 is less than 70% predicted, the PC_{20} is usually reduced into the hyper-responsive range. Therefore, if the FEV_1 is reduced to this degree, a low PC_{20} is not necessarily specific for asthma.

Airway responsiveness to histamine or methacholine correlates very closely with the diurnal variation of PEF when this is expressed as the difference between the lowest pre-bronchodilator and the highest post-bronchodilator values over the highest value (8). If the post-bronchodilator value is not taken into account, the correlation can be poor, presumably because the extent of diurnal spontaneous reversal of airflow obstruction is incomplete in some subjects with asthma. The appropriateness of the PC_{20} cut point and gray area separating normal and hyper-responsiveness in relation to variable airflow obstruction has been demonstrated in comparisons of PC_{20} with diurnal variation of PEF (8–10). When airway responsiveness is increased, diurnal variation of PEF is usually increased even when there are no symptoms. When airway responsiveness is normal, diurnal variation of PEF is also normal. These results suggest that measurements of histamine or methacholine airway responsiveness are as good or as bad as measurements of diurnal variation of PEF.

However, they have a number of advantages over PEF. In particular, their performance is supervised so that the accuracy can be confirmed, compliance is not an issue, the expression and interpretation of results is better standardized, measurement of airway responsiveness is more sensitive and reproducible, and, finally, results can be obtained more quickly if the laboratory is organized to do the tests.

The degree of airway responsiveness to histamine or methacholine and indirect stimuli such as exercise (11, 14), isocapnic and hyperventilation of cold dry air (12, 15), and hypertonic saline (16, 17) correlate to a variable degree between studies. The degree of responsiveness to two indirect stimuli, such as distilled water and exercise, does not necessarily correlate (17). This is not surprising, since the different stimuli are causing airway narrowing through different mechanisms and the influence of these will vary in the subjects included in the different studies. In general, hyper-responsiveness to indirect stimuli seems to be less sensitive for the presence of asthma (11, 18, 19). There is a possibility that exercise (20) and eucapnic hyperventilation of cold dry air (21) are more specific for identifying the presence of asthma in patients with other airway disease; however, hyper-responsiveness to AMP (22,23) and hypertonic saline (24) are not. The specificity of hyper-responsiveness to indirect stimuli to asthma requires further investigation.

Poor Relationships Between the Degree of Airway Responsiveness, Symptoms, and Asthma

Epidemiological studies have shown that many people are hyper-responsive to histamine or methacholine but have no symptoms, while others with symptoms or a previous diagnosis of asthma have normal airway responsiveness (25–27). These observations have been the main reason why measurements of responsiveness to histamine and methacholine have been criticized as a diagnostic test. However, it is inappropriate to extrapolate such epidemiological results to clinical practice. In epidemiological studies, the details of symptoms and their relation with abnormalities of airway function and with past treatment are less carefully obtained, and comparisons are made between period prevalence of symptoms, usually within the past year, and point prevalence of airway responsiveness, rather than between the more recent oc-

currence of symptoms and the measurement of responsiveness (28). There are also other explanations for the discrepancies between symptoms and responsiveness.

Airway hyper-responsiveness without symptoms may be due to failure to recognize symptoms (29), to failure to recognize variable airflow obstruction (10, 30), and to an apparent absence of active airway inflammatory cell infiltration (29), as well as to chronic airflow limitation due to other airway disease (21). In a study comparing a group of normal older children with asymptomatic hyper-responsive children and symptomatic hyper-responsive children matched with the asymptomatic group for the degree of hyper-responsiveness, the degree of diurnal variation of PEF was the same between the two hyper-responsive groups, and different (increased) compared with the normal group (10). This illustrates the failure to recognize variable airflow obstruction in the asymptomatic hyper-responsive children. In another study comparing asymptomatic hyper-responsive older children with asthmatic hyper-responsive children matched for the degree of hyper-responsiveness with the asymptomatic group, the children were asked if they had symptoms during the methacholine test and whether they recalled similar symptoms in the past (29). Over half of the asymptomatic group recalled similar symptoms, illustrating a failure to recognize symptoms when initially questioned. In the same study, examination of sputum by methods demonstrated to give repeatable, responsive, and valid results, showed that the asymptomatic group had normal eosinophil differential counts while the asthmatic group had raised counts. When the two groups were treated with inhaled steroid, airway responsiveness only increased significantly in the asthmatic group. These observations identify the presence of inflammatory cell infiltration as a cause of symptoms. In keeping with these observations, Jones (31) has shown that 58% of asymptomatic children with a positive exercise test, when reassessed 6 years later, had developed symptomatic asthma. Further longitudinal studies are needed to investigate the outcome of children and adults with asymptomatic hyper-responsiveness.

There are also a number of reasons why symptoms might occur in the absence of histamine or methacholine airway hyper-responsiveness. Symptoms associated with variable airflow obstruction might occur if responsiveness is in the borderline normal gray area or, further into the normal range, if there is a stimulus to bronchoconstriction which causes an usually severe airway reaction, e. g., exposure to a chemical sensitizer at work (32). Symptoms, particularly cough and sputum, can also be caused by eosinophilic bronchitis without the physiological abnormalities of asthma but with reversal of the symptoms by treatment with corticosteroid (33, 34). However, most people with symptoms and normal airway responsiveness probably have some other cause for the symptoms. Symptoms are recognized to be nonspecific for the disease causing them. They may be due to some other cause of airway inflammation or to some other condition such as chronic hyperventilation, laryngeal dysfunction, unfitness, etc.

Address for correspondence:

Dr FE Hargreave
Firestone Regional Chest and Allergy Unit
St. Joseph's Hospital
50 Charlton Avenue East
Hamilton, Ontario L8N 4A6
Canada

References

1. Sheffer AL, Bousquet J, Busse WW, Clark TJH, Dahl R, Evans D, Fabbri LM, Hargreave FE, Holgate ST, Magnussen H, Partridge MR, Pauwels R, Rodriguez-Roisin R, Rubinfeld A, Sotes MR, Sears MR, Szczeklik A, Warner J. International consensus report on the diagnosis and management of asthma. *Eur Respir J* 1992; 5:601–641.

2. Laszlo G. European standards for lung function testing: 1993 update. *Thorax* 1993; 48:873–876.

3. Pattemore PK, Holgate ST. Bronchial hyperresponsiveness and its relationship to asthma in childhood. *Clin Exp Allergy* 1993; 23:886–900.

4. Rogers DF, O'Connor BJ. Airway responsiveness: Relation to asthma and inflammation. *Thorax* 1993; 48:1095–1096.

5. Joos GF, Kips JC, Pauwels RA. Direct and indirect bronchial responsiveness. *Respir Med* 1993; 87 (Suppl B):31–36.

6. Woolcock AJ, Salome CM, Yan K. The shape of dose-response curve to histamine in asthmatic and normal subjects. *Am Rev Respir Dis* 1984; 130:71–75.

7. Sterk PJ, Daniel EE, Zamel N, Hargreave FE. Limited bronchoconstriction to methacholine using partial flow-volume curves in nonasthamatic subjects. *Am Rev Respir Dis* 1985; 132:272–277.

8. Ryan G, Latimer KM, Dolovich J, Hargreave FE. Bronchial responsiveness to histamine: Relationship to diurnal variation of peak flow rate, improvement after bronchodilator, and airway calibre. *Thorax* 1982; 37:423–429.

9. Ramsdale EH, Morris MM, Roberts RS, Hargreave FE. Asymptomatic bronchial hyperresponsiveness in rhinitis. *J Allergy Clin Immunol* 1985; 75:573–577.

10. Gibson PG, Mattoli S, Sears MR, Dolovich J, Hargreave FE. Variable airway obstruction in asymptomatic children with methacholine airway responsiveness. *Clin Invest Med* 1988; 11:C105.

11. Anderton RC, Cuff MT, Frith PA, Cockcroft DW, Morse JLC, Jones NL, Hargreave FE. Bronchial responsiveness to inhaled histamine and exercise. *J Allergy Clin Immunol* 1979; 63:315–320.

12. O'Byrne PM, Ryan G, Morris MM, McCormack D, Jones NL, Morse JLC, Hargreave FE. Asthma induced by cold air and its relation to nonspecific bronchial responsiveness. *Am Rev Respir Dis* 1982; 125:281–285.

13. Ramsdale EH, Morris MM, Roberts RS, Hargreave FE. Bronchial responsiveness to methacholine in chronic bronchitis: Relationship to airflow obstruction and cold air responsiveness. *Thorax* 1984; 39:912–918.

14. Haby MM, Anderson SD, Peat JK, Mellis CM, Toelle BG, Woolcock AJ. An exercise challenge protocol for epidemiological studies of asthma in children: Comparison with histamine challenge. *Eur Respir J* 1994; 7:43–49.

15. Chandler Deal E, McFadden ER Jr, Ingram RH Jr, Breslin FJ, Jaeger JJ. Airway responsiveness to cold air and hyperpnea in normal subjects and in those with hayfever and asthma. *Am Rev Respir Dis* 1980; 121:621.

16. Smith CM, Anderson SD. Inhalational challenge using hypertonic saline in asthmatic subjects: a comparison with responses to hyperpnoea, methacholine and water. *Eur Respir J* 1990; 3:144–151.

17. Sont JK, Booms P, Bel EH, Vandenbroucke JP, Sterk PJ. The determinants of airway hyperresponsiveness to hypertonic saline in atopic asthma *in vivo*. Relationship with sub-populations of peripheral blood leucocytes. *Clin Exp Allergy* 1993; 23:678–688.

18. Ninan TK, Russel G. Is exercise testing useful in a community based asthma survey? *Thorax* 1993; 48:1218–1221.

19. Galdès-Sebalt M, McLaughlin FJ, Levison H. Comparison of cold air, ultrasonic mist, and methacholine inhalation as tests of bronchial reactivity in normal and asthmatic children. *J Pediatr* 1985; 107:526–530.

20. Godfrey S, Springer C, Novski N, Maayan CH, Avital

A. Exercise but not methacholine differentiates asthma from chronic lung disease in children. *Thorax* 1991; 46:488–492.

21. Ramsdale EH, Roberts RS, Morris MM, Hargreave FE. Differences in responsiveness to hyperventilation and methacholine in asthma and chronic bronchitis. *Thorax* 1985; 40: 422–426.

22. Pin I, Hepperle MJ, Wong BJO, Ramsdale EH, Hargreave FE. Methacholine (M) and adenosine monophosphate (AMP) airway hyperresponsiveness (AHR) in asthmatics and smokers with chronic airflow limitation (CAL). *Am Rev Respir Dis* 1991; 143:A413.

23. Oosterhoff Y, De Jong JW, Jansen MAM, Koëter GH, Postma DS. Airway responsiveness to adenosine 5'-monophosphate in chronic obstructive pulmonary disease is determined by smoking. *Am Rev Respir Dis* 1993; 147:553–558.

24. Anderson SD, Rodwell L, Du Toit JI. Airway response to non-isotonic aerosol (NIA) in subjects with chronic airflow limitation (CAL). *Eur Respir J* 1990; 3 (Suppl 10):74–75.

25. Sears MR, Jones DT, Holdaway MD, Hewitt CJ, Flannery EM, Herbison GP, Silva PA. Prevalence of bronchial reactivity to inhaled methacholine in New Zealand children. *Thorax* 1986; 41:283–289.

26. Salome CM, Peat JK, Britton WJ, Woolcock AJ. Bronchial hyperresponsiveness in two populations of Australian schoolchildren . I. Relation to respiratory symptoms and diagnosed asthma. *Clin Allergy* 1987; 17:271–281.

27. Pattemore PK, Asher MI, Harrison AC, Mitchell EA, Rea HH, Stewart AW. The interrelationship among bronchial hyperresponsiveness, the diagnosis of asthma, and asthma symptoms. *Am Rev Respir Dis* 1990; 142:549–554.

28. Cockcroft DW, Hargreave FE. Airway hyperresponsiveness. Relevance of random population data to clinical usefulness. *Am Rev Respir Dis* 1990; 142:497–500.

29. Pin I, Radford S, Kolendowicz R, Jennings B, Denburg JA, Hargreave FE, Dolovich J. Airway inflammation in symptomatic and asymptomatic children with methacholine hyperresponsiveness. *Eur Respir J* 1993; 6:1249–1256.

30. Brand PLP, Rijekan B, Shouten JP, Koëter GH, Weiss ST, Postma DS. Perception of airway obstruction in a random population sample. Relationship to airway hyperresponsiveness in the absence of respiratory symptoms. *Am Rev Respir Dis* 1992; 146:396–401.

31. Jones A. Asymptomatic bronchial hyperreactivity and the development of asthma and other respiratory tract illnesses in children. *Thorax* 1994; 49:757–761.

32. Hargreave FE, Ramsdale EH, Pugsley SO. Occupational asthma without bronchial hyperresponsiveness. *Am Rev Respir Dis* 1984; 130:513–515.

33. Gibson PG, Dolovich J, Denburg J, Ramsdale EH, Hargreave FE. Chronic cough: eosinophilic bronchitis without asthma. *Lancet* 1989; i:1346–1348.

34. Gibson PG, Hargreave FE, Girgis-Gabardo A, Morris MM, Denburg J, Dolovich J. Chronic cough with eosinophilic bronchitis: examination for variable airflow obstruction and response to corticosteroid. *Clin Exp Allergy* 1994; in press.

The T-Cell Receptor in Development and Activation

Charles A Janeway Jr, Fridrika Hardardottir, Soon-cheol Hong, Sang-wook Tim Yoon, Ruslan Medzhitov, Alexander Chervonsky, Stephanie Constant, Kim Bottomly*

Keywords: T-cell receptor, coreceptor, costimulation, T-cell subset

Adaptive immune responses, including those responsible for the production of IgE antibody and delayed-type hypersensitivity reactions, involve the antigen-specific activation of CD4 T lymphocytes. The specificity of this component of the adaptive immune response is determined by the antigen receptor on the CD4 T cell. This receptor is made up of two chains that are highly variable, called α and β, stably associated in the cell membrane with the CD3 γ, δ, and ε chains, and the ζ chains. This receptor recognizes antigen in the form of peptide fragments bound to class II molecules of the major histocompatibility complex (MHC) (1). During the recognition of peptide:MHC class II complexes by the αβ T-cell receptor, the CD4 molecule serves as a coreceptor, binding to the outer invariant face of the MHC class II molecule. This binding is important mainly to allow the CD4 molecule to participate in positively signaling to the T cell, from which the name coreceptor derives. In addition, the transmembrane tyrosine phosphatase CD45 is also known to participate both in signal transduction through the T-cell receptor and as a physical component of the complex of the T-cell receptor and CD4 (2–4). In this paper, we will briefly describe our findings relating to the role of the T-cell receptor in the ontogenetic development of T cells bearing CD4 molecules, in the activation of T cells by antigen, a process which involves the simultaneous delivery of a costimulatory signal, and interpretive behaviors of the T-cell receptor that allow distinct outcomes to arise from ligation of the same receptor by different amounts of ligand or by subtle changes in ligand structure.

The Role of the T-Cell Receptor in T-Cell Development

All T cells recognize antigen in the form of peptide fragments bound stably in the cleft at the outer end of an MHC molecule (1). CD8 T cells recognize peptides generated in cell cytosol and display them at the cell surface bound to MHC class I molecules, to which the CD8 co-receptor protein binds, while CD4 T cells recognize peptides generated in intracellular vesicles such as endosomes that are displayed at the cell surface by MHC class II molecules. The genes encoding MHC molecules are extensively polymorphic, there being at least 100 distinct alleles at some loci. Because a given T-cell receptor generally recognizes antigen only when it is bound to a particular allelic variant of a particular MHC class II molecule, a property known as MHC restriction, most of the T-cell receptors generated within an individual will presumably not be able to recognize antigen presented by that individual's MHC molecules. This suggested some time ago that those T cells whose receptors can recognize foreign peptides bound to self MHC molecules would in some way be positively selected to remain in the T-cell repertoire found in peripheral lymphoid organs (5). Additional evidence supporting this supposition was obtained from bone marrow chimeric and thymus grafted mice. However, the most dramatic demonstration of the importance and specificity of positive selection came from placing the rearranged genes encoding the α and β chains of a T-cell receptor of known specificity in the mouse genome (6). T cells bearing this receptor could be identified by monoclonal antibodies unique to that receptor, allowing the impact of the receptor on the development of αβ T cells to be determined.

We have performed studies of this type using the rearranged genes encoding an αβ T-cell receptor specific for a peptide of myelin basic protein, an autoantigen, bound to syngeneic MHC class II molecules. We have tested the ability of this receptor to lead to T-cell maturation in mice of varying

---

*   Section of Immunobiology, Yale University School of Medicine and Howard Hughes Medical Institute, New Haven, CT, USA.

MHC genotype. Our studies reveal that only the initial selecting MHC genotype, and none of eight others, can drive positive selection of this T-cell receptor (7). This indicates that positive selection is highly specific, and that most T cells which generate receptors restricted to other MHC genotypes will not mature within the thymus, so that these receptors are not expressed in the peripheral T-cell repertoire.

These studies confirm and extend earlier studies of a number of investigators on positive selection. These investigators have also noted that MHC class II-restricted receptors direct the maturation of T cells to become CD4+CD8- T cells, whereas MHC class I-restricted receptors direct their maturation to become CD8+ T cells. This process takes place in two steps (7–9). In the initial step, the interaction of the T-cell receptor with any self MHC molecule induces a downregulation in either CD4 or CD8. In the second step, if the receptor recognizes self MHC class II molecules and the T cell downregulated CD8, then CD4 and the T-cell receptor can cooperate in driving the final maturation of the T cell. However, half the time the wrong coreceptor is selected and when the T-cell receptor and the coreceptor cannot synergize, the cells eventually die without maturing and leaving the thymus (7). We have shown this by crossing our T-cell receptor transgenic mice to mice carrying a transgene encoding the apoptosis-inhibiting protein bcl-2. In such mice, cells that repress the expression of CD4 become CD4-CD8+ T cells. However, these cells are not fully mature, as they fail to emigrate from the thymus. Thus, the first step in positive selection apparently induces a choice of co-receptor molecule, but does not inhibit programmed cell death, whereas the second step inhibits cell death and in addition provides a signal to emigrate from the thymus. The signal inhibiting cell death is unlikely to be bcl-2 itself, since T cells can mature relatively normally in mice that do not express this protein (10). Studies show that interaction of the coreceptor with the T-cell receptor, mediated by joint recognition of a given MHC molecule, is required for maturation and emigration from the thymus. In the next three sections, we shall explore how the T-cell receptor recognizes its peptide:MHC ligand, and how the coreceptor participates in this process.

The Role of the T-Cell Receptor in T-Cell Activation

When the T-cell receptor binds to its MHC class II:peptide ligand, this transduces a signal into the cell (2). We have studied the interaction of the $\alpha\beta$ T-cell receptor with MHC class II molecules in some detail. Using the receptor from a cloned T-cell line, we have shown that the portion of the receptor encoded in the Vα gene segment, comprising the equivalent of complementarity-determining regions (CDR) 1 and 2 in antibody molecules, makes contact with the α helical region of the α chain of the MHC class II molecule (11). Residue 51 in the middle of the CDR2 loop is also influenced by the second residue of the bound peptide, which lies in this vicinity (12). This has allowed us to position the CDR2 loop of the T-cell receptor α chain roughly over the amino-terminal end of the antigenic peptide, while it and CDR1 make contact with the amino-terminal half of the α helical region of the MHC class II α chain.

Although this result applies to the T-cell receptor on the cloned T-cell line studied, it does not tell us anything about the orientation of other T-cell receptors to their MHC:peptide ligands. Recently, following early studies by Gascoigne, Malissen, and others (13–15), we have been exploring the selective expression of different Vα genes in CD4 and CD8 T cells (16). By comparing the sequences of Vα chains derived from CD4 and CD8 T cells, we have observed certain residues that are dimorphic between Vα domains of T-cell receptors expressed by CD4 T cells and Vα chains of T-cell receptors expressed by CD8 T cells. Although these residues are found at three separate locations along the linear sequence of Vα, they appear to be clustered in the complete folded Vα domain, forming a patch on the external surface of Vα close to the Cα domain. Because this patch of sequence difference cannot conceivably make contact with MHC molecules, we have proposed that this is the site at which coreceptors physically react with the T-cell receptors. It is important to note that Vβ domains appear not to segregate selectively with CD4 and CD8 except in rare circumstances.

Although these data suggest that the use of a particular Vα is dictated by its ability to interact with the coreceptor molecule, we also find that the CDR1 and CDR2 loops of Vα domains found on CD4 T cells are respectively about 1 and 2 amino acids shorter than those found on Vα domains of CD8 T cells. These data suggest that Vα genes are coevolving to have specificity for MHC class I or MHC class II molecules and simultaneously for their ability to interact with CD8 and CD4 molecules respectively, with each interaction using a different surface of this protein domain.

Other data also suggests that the Vα domain has a Vα site for coreceptors. Early studies on the physical association of CD4 with the T-cell receptor carried out by a variety of techniques in our laboratory suggested that the CD4 molecule would interact with Vα on the D10 cloned T-cell line (17). Second, activation of CD4 T cells by anti-Vβ antibody is not inhibited by anti-CD4 Fab fragments, whereas activation by anti-Vα antibody is readily inhibited by these Fab fragments (16). We believe this reflects a new example of the phenomenon we termed epitope interference, when antibodies to two molecules which must interact in order to produce an effect instead lead to steric inhibition that prevents their interaction. Finally, when T cells are raised in an MHC class II-negative animal, and then stimulated with MHC class II molecules, a strong association between Vα and coreceptor is observed. In this experimental scheme, the CD4 coreceptor can only function during positive selection by associating with the TCR, while during activation by MHC class II molecules, CD8 can only function by directly and physically interacting with the T-cell receptor. These data suggest that Vα2 and Vα11 make stable physical associations only with CD4, while Vα3 and Vα8 make stable associations only with CD8.

These data all suggest that a T-cell receptor must interact with its MHC ligands in a stereotypic fashion. This is based on the fact that MHC class I and MHC class II molecules differ in their α carbon backbones only in the vicinity in which CDR1 and CDR2 of the Vα domain bind (18). In addition, if CD4 physically interacts with both the T-cell receptor and the MHC class II molecule (19), then the receptor can only bind MHC class II molecules in a single orientation.

In Addition to T-Cell Receptor Ligation, Simultaneous Delivery of a Costimulatory Signal is also Required for Naive T-Cell Activation

When CD4 T cells are purified and separated into naive and memory cells on the basis of differential expression of CD45 isoforms, the memory cells will respond to anti-CD3 antibody bound to an insoluble matrix or displayed on the surface of fibroblasts expressing Fc receptors. By contrast, naive CD4 T cells will only respond to anti-CD3 antibody bound to Fc receptors on cells that express costimulatory signals (20). Expression of these costimulatory signals may be regulated by extrinsic agents such as microbial substances (21, 22) and by intrinsic signals delivered by T cells such as the gp39 or CD40 ligand expressed by activated CD4 T cells (23, 24). It is thought that this requirement for costimulation is important in preventing T-cell responses to antigens expressed exclusively on certain tissue cells. If this is correct, then it is equally important that the same cell must deliver both the peptide:MHC ligand and the costimulatory molecule. Were this not true, then T cells recognizing antigens expressed on peripheral tissue cells could subsequently be costimulated by a different cell bearing a costimulator but not the antigen. Moreover, by requiring one cell to express both ligand and costimulator, the presence of ligand can be coupled to recognition of microbial substances in a single cell, allowing the adaptive immune response to discriminate infectious nonself from noninfectious self (21).

To examine this, we studied the activation of naive T cells by fibroblasts transfected with genes encoding the Fcγ receptor, the costimulatory molecule B7, or both. Only fibroblasts cotransfected with the Fcγ receptor and B7 could costimulate the growth of CD4 T cells. Similar studies were carried out with naturally occurring antigen presenting cells (25). Thus, the requirement for costimulation helps to preserve self tolerance by linking antigen recognition to costimulation in a single antigen presenting cell, and similarly allows the immune system to discriminate antigens associated with potentially harmful pathogens from antigens encountered coincidentally in the environment.

Effects of Varying Ligand Structure or Ligand Density on CD4 T-Cell Responses

In the previous section, we learned that the outcome of T-cell receptor ligation is strongly influenced by whether or not a costimuatory signal is simultaneously delivered to the T cell. When this costimulatory signal is present, the T cell will grow in response to receptor ligation; when it is absent, the T cell will either become unresponsive to antigen, a state known as anergy, or will undergo programmed cell death. Thus, the presence or absence of a costimulatory molecule on the cell presenting antigen has an important impact on naive T cells (26).

Recently, it has come to be appreciated that not all ligands that bind the T-cell receptor produce an identical outcome, even when used under identical conditions of costimulation. The first studies to suggest this involved the use of monoclonal anti-T-cell receptor antibodies as ligands. In these studies, it was shown that antibodies had very different potencies for stimulation of a cloned T-cell line, depending upon which epitope on the T-cell receptor they bound. This function was independent of the antibody's affinity, since the results were calculated in terms of activity per molecule bound. Both high and low affinity antibodies could be either high or low potency. Interestingly, high potency antibodies always induced a physical association of CD4 with the T-cell receptor, whereas low potency antibodies did not. More importantly, monavalent Fab fragments of high potency antibodies could produce a similar effect, even though they could not activate the T cell by themselves, because they could not crosslink the receptor (27). More recently, several laboratories have observed that subtle modification in peptide structure can convert an activating peptide into a peptide that can competitively antagonize activation through the T-cell receptor. Indeed, some such antagonist peptides can actually induce anergy even when presented by cells with appropriate costimulatory activity. These data strongly suggest T-cell activation does not result simply from the T-cell receptor ligation, but rather from ligation in a special way (27, 28). That is, ligands may signal not only by receptor aggregation but also by producing conformational changes in the receptor upon binding.

In earlier studies of T-cell priming *in vivo*, we have demonstrated that the nature of the ligand can also control whether CD4 T cells differentiate into IL-4-secreting Th2 cells, crucial for the production of IgE antibody, or interferon-γ (IFN-γ) producing, Th1-like T cells that protect against atopic allergy by antagonizing IL-4 and mediate delayed-type hypersensitivity. Indeed, in one experimental system, a peptide presented by one MHC class II molecule led to pure Th1 responses, while the same peptide bound to a different MHC class II molecule generated a pure Th2 response (29). However, this did not show that the same peptide on the same T-cell receptor could lead to different fates in T-cell maturation.

New studies, carried out using *in vitro* priming of naive CD4 T cells from T-cell receptor transgenic mice have addressed this latter issue. Here, we have shown that very low doses of peptide antigen, presented by dendritic cells, lead to selective priming of Th2-like cells that produce IL-4 and not IFN-γ on restimulation in tissue culture. Alternatively, priming with much higher doses of antigen causes selective priming of IFN-γ-producing rather the IL-4-producing CD4 T cells. These results are particularly interesting in light of current models of allergy induction. They suggest that the very low doses of protein antigens likely to gain access to regional lymph nodes in the lung by transit across the respiratory epithelium are highly likely to induce Th2 responses that lead to IgE production. Higher doses, used for desensitization, may be able to convert this response to Th1-like cells or to generate a new round of Th1 cells that can now inhibit the action of Th2 cells in IgE production (30).

Conclusions

We have presented a model of T-cell receptor function in which the T-cell receptor binds to MHC molecules in a fixed orientation in association with a coreceptor molecule, CD4 for MHC class II-associated recognition and CD8 for MHC class I-associated recognition. We have also argued that peptide binding produces conformational changes in the T-cell receptor that are crucial to signaling through this receptor, and which are interpreted by the T cell. One way in which this might occur is through the induction of CD4 binding in the Vα domain of the T-cell receptor upon ligand binding. This would change the signaling properties of the

T-cell receptor by bringing CD4 into the complex. Although not discussed in this paper, we have also shown that CD45 is part of the signaling complex, and that its associations with the T-cell receptor may also be governed by the nature of the T-cell receptor ligand (4, 31). Thus, the T-cell receptor is a complex of signaling proteins that is assembled during antigen recognition, and whose assembly is influenced not only by binding to antigen, but also by the precise nature of the antigenic molecule. In addition, activation requires the appropriate delivery of costimulatory molecules, expressed most effectively on activated dendritic cells migrating out of peripheral tissues after ingesting antigen (32). Thus, the production of atopic reactions in response to inhaled allergens may reflect exposure of CD4 T cells to very low doses of peptide antigen bound to potent antigen presenting cells. Atopic individuals could reflect those that bind peptide best, if peptide supply is extremely limiting, or those that bind it worst if peptide levels are high. In this latter scenario, resistance to allergy mediated by Th1 cells, as recently demonstrated by Holt and his colleagues in rodent models (33), would be the norm, and failure to do so would be associated with atopy.

Acknowledgements

This work is supported by the Howard Hughes Medical Institute and grants from the NIH to CJ (AI-14579 and AI-26810) and KB (AI-26791 and CA-38350).

Address for correspondence:

Charles A Janeway
Section of Immunobiology
Yale University School of Medicine
and Howard Hughes Medical Institute
New Haven, CT 06510
USA

References

1. Germain RN. MHC-dependent antigen processing and peptide presentation: Providing ligands for T lymphocyte activation. *Cell* 1994; 76:287.

2. Weiss A, Littman DR. Signal transduction by lymphocyte antigen receptors. *Cell* 1994; 76:263.

3. Dianzani U, Luqman M, Rojo J, Yagi J, Baron JL, Woods A, Janeway CA Jr, Bottomly K. Molecular associations on the T cell surface correlate with immunological memory. *Eur J Immunol* 1990; 20:2249.

4. Novak TJ, Farber D, Leitenberg D, Hong S-C, Johnson P. Isoforms of the transmembrane tyrosine phosphotase CD45 differentially affect T cell recognition. *Immunity* 1994; 1:109.

5. Janeway CA, Wigzell H, Binz H. Hypothesis. Two different V gene products make up the T cell receptors. *Scand J Immunol* 1976; 5:993.

6. von Boehmer H. Positive selection of lymphocytes. *Cell* 1994; 76:219.

7. Hardardottir F, Baron J, Petrie H, Janeway CA Jr. Most developing T cells are lost because they fail positive selection. Submitted 1994.

8. Chan SH, Cosgrove D, Waltzinger C, Benoist C, Mathis, D. Another view of the selective model of thymocyte selection. *Cell* 1993; 73:225.

9. Davis CB, Killeen N, Crooks MEC, Raulet D, Littman DR. Evidence on a stochastic mechanism in the differentiation of mature subsets of T lymphocytes. *Cell* 1993; 73:237.

10. Hockenberry DM, Oltvai ZN, Yin XM, Milliman CL, Korsmeyer SJ. Bcl-2 functions in an antioxidant pathway to prevent apoptosis. *Cell* 1993; 75:241.

11. Hong SC, Chelouche A, Lin RH, Shaywitz D, Braunstein N, Gllimcher L, Janeway CA Jr. An MHC interaction site maps to the amino-terminal half of the T cell receptor alpha chain variable domain. *Cell* 1992; 69:999.

12. Yoon ST, Hong S-C, Janeway CA Jr. Identification of a contact site in the MHC:peptide ligand of a single amino acid in the second complimentarity determining region of the T cell receptor alpha chain. Submitted 1994.

13. Utsunomiya Y, Bill J, Palmer E, Golob K, Takagaki Y, Kanagawa O. Analysis of a monoclonal rat antibody directed to the alpha chain variable region (Vα3) of the mouse T cell antigen receptor. *J Immunol* 1989; 43:2602.

14. Jameson SC, Nakajima PB, Brooks JL, Heath W, Kanagawa O, Gascoigne NRJ. The T cell receptor Vα11 gene family. *J Immunol* 1991; 147:3185.

15. Jameson SC, Kaye J, Gascoigne NRJ. A T cell receptor Vα region selectively expressed in CD4+ cells. *J Immunol* 1990; 145:1324.

16. Chervonsky A, Medzhitov R, Hong S-C, Waterbury G, Yoon ST, Barlow A, Hayday AC, Janeway CA Jr. Structural and functional evidence for the co-evolution of MHC class recognition and co-receptor binding in T cell receptor Vα gene segments. Submitted 1994.

17. Dianzani U, Shaw A, Al-Ramadi BK, Kubo RT,

Janeway CA Jr. The physical association of CD4 with the T cell receptor. *J Immunol* 1992; 1548:678.

18. Brown JH, Jardetsky TS, Gorga JC, Stern LJ, Urban RG, Strominger JL, Wiley DC. Three dimensional structure of the human class 2 histocompatibility antigen HLA-DR. *Nature* 1993; 364:33.

19. Konig R, Huang LY, Germain RN. MHC class II interaction with CD4 mediated by a region analogous to the MHC class I binding site for CD8. *Nature* 1992; 356:796.

20. Luqman M, Bottomly K. Activation requirements for CD4+ T cells differing in CD45R expression. *J Immunol* 1992; 149:2300.

21. Janeway CA Jr. Approaching the asymptote?: evolution and revolution in immunology. *Cold Spring Harbor Symp Quant Biol* 1989; 54:1.

22. Liu Y, Janeway CA Jr. Microbial induction of costimulatory activity for CD4 T cell growth. *Intl Immunol* 1991; 3:323.

23. Ranheim EA, Kipps TJ. Activated T cells induce expression of B7/BB1 on normal or leukemic B cells through a CD40-dependent signal. *J Exp Med* 1993; 177:1047.

24. Kennedy MK, Mohler KM, Shanebeck KD, Baum PR, Picha KS, Ottens-Evans CA, Janeway CA Jr, Grabstein KH. Induction of B cell costimulatory function by recombinant murine CD40 ligand. *Eur J Immunol* 1994; 24:116.

25. Liu Y, Janeway CA Jr. Cells that present both specific ligand and costimulatory activity are the most effi-

cient inducers of clonal expansion of normal CD4 T cells. *Proc Natl Acad Sci USA* 1992; 89:3845.

26. Janeway CA Jr, Bottomly K. Signal and signs for lymphocyte responses. *Cell* 1994, 76:275.

27. Janeway CA Jr, Dianzani U, Portoles P, Rath S, Reich EP, Rojo JM, Yagi J, Murphy DB. Cross-linking and conformational change in T cell receptors: Role in activation and repertoire selection. *Cold Spring Harbor Symp Quant Biol* 1989; 54:657.

28. Evavold BD, Sloan-Lancaster J, Allen PM. Tickling the TCR: selective T cell functions stimulated by altered peptide ligands. *Immunol Today* 1993; 14:602.

29. Murray JS, Madri J, Tite J, Carding SR, Bottomly K. MHC control of CD4+ T cell subset activation. *J Exp Med* 1989; 170:2135.

30. Pfeiffer C, Murray J, Madri J, Bottomly K. Selective activation of Th1- and Th2-like cells in *in vivo* response to human collagen IV. *Immunol Rev* 1991; 123:65.

31. Janeway CA Jr. The T cell receptor as a multicomponent signaling machine: CD4/CD8 coreceptors and CD45 in T cell activation. *Annu Rev Immunol* 1992; 10:645.

32. Knight SC, Stagg AJ. Antigen-presenting cell types. *Curr Opin Immunol* 1993, 5:374.

33. McMenamin C, Holt PG. The natural immune response to inhaled soluble protein antigens involves major histocompatibility complex (MHC) class I-restricted CD8+ T cell-mediated but MHC class II-restricted CD4+ selective suppression of immunoglobulin E production. *J Exp Med* 1993; 178:889.

B-Cell Ontogeny, Repertoire Selection, and Tolerance

Fritz Melchers*

Keywords: Positive and negative selection of T and B cells, surrogate light chain, preB cell receptor complex, immature B cells, TcR and Ig gene rearrangements, RAG-1 and RAG-2 genes, SCID, life expectancy of lymphocytes, secondary rearrangements, lymphocyte differentiation without rearrangements

Differentiation of precursor B lymphocytes from early to late stages found in bone marrow can occur without Ig gene rearrangements. The role of the μH/surrogate L chain preB receptor and of μH chain/L chain containing igM receptors on immature and mature B cells is not to induce the next Ig gene rearrangements in line. Rather they select precursor and immature B cells for proliferative expansion, further cellular differentiation and altered life expectancy in the primary lymphoid organs, and, in the end, in the peripheral mature sites.

Lymphocytes of mouse and man are generated throughout life in primary lymphoid organs – T lymphocytes in the thymus, B lymphocytes in bone marrow. Progenitors which derive from pluripotent hematopoietic stem cells are induced to be committed towards the T or B lymphocytic pathway of differentiation. In the thymus, rearrangements of gene segments of the T cell receptor (TcRt) β and α, and of δ and γ loci are induced. In the bone marrow, immunoglobulin (Ig) heavy (H) and light (L) chain loci are rearranged. Rearrangements can occur in- and out-of-frame. Those cells which succeed in rearranging β and α, δ and γ, or H and L chain genes in-frame can express TcR and Ig on their surface.

Rearrangements are ordered in space and time during lymphocyte development. Dβ to Jβ rearrangements in TcR β chain gene loci, and D_H to J_H rearrangements in Ig H chain gene loci, precede Vβ to DβJβ and V_H to $D_H J_H$ rearrangements, respectively. These are then followed by Vα to Jα rearrangements in thymocytes, as well as Vκ to Jκ and, finally, Vλ to Jλ rearrangements in B cell precursors (1). Order in the rearrangements is imposed by molecular and cellular selection mechanisms. Molecular selections are thought to involve the opening of a

given TcR or Ig gene locus, its sterile transcription, and the recognition of specific heptamer/nonamer palindromic sequences next to the V, D, and J segments by the rearrangement enzyme complex. Cellular selections either suppress or enhance the proliferation of a given stage of precursor cell, or suppress or induce the transit of a cell from one compartment to the next by differentiation without proliferation. These cellular selections always appear to involve the expression of productively rearranged TcR or Ig gene loci on the surface of cells. Remarkable similarity exists between T lymphocyte development in the thymus and B lymphocyte development in bone marrow (2).

Differentiation of Precursor B Lymphocytes Without Ig Gene Rearrangements

The roles of TcR β and α chains and of Ig H and L chains in these cellular selections becomes most evident in mutant mice, such as SCID or RAG-1T or RAG-2T (3–5). "T" stands for targeted integration of a defective gene by homologous recombination into the germline, leading to mouse strains which are defective for the targeted (T) gene (6, 7). In SCID mice, TcR and Ig gene rearrangements are attempted but never productive; in RAG-1T or RAG-2T mice, they are not even attempted. In recent experiments from our laboratory it has been demonstrated that a cellular program of differentiation of B lineage cells from the earliest progenitor to the stage of an immature B cell can occur without productive, or even without any Ig gene rearrangements (8). Differentiation can be monitored by

---

* Basel Institute for Immunology, Basel, Switzerland.

changes in expression of preB cell-specific markers, by changes of *in vitro* growth properties, by the induction of apoptosis, and by the expression of sterile transcripts of the IgH and κL chain gene loci. Stromal cell/IL-7-reactive B220$^+$ B cell precursors are found in fetal liver and bone marrow of SCID, SCID/*bcl-2* transgenic, and RAG-2T mice in frequencies comparable to normal mice. Like cells from normal mice, they proliferate normally on stromal cells in the presence of IL-7, and differentiate *in vitro* upon IL-7 deprivation from c-kit$^+$, CD43$^+$, surrogate L chain$^+$, RAG-1$^+$, RAG-2$^+$, CD25$^-$ clonable preB cells into c-kit$^-$, CD43$^-$, surrogate L chain$^-$, RAG-1$^+$, RAG-2$^+$, CD25$^+$ immature B cells, which are no longer clonable on stromal cells and IL-7. Concomitantly, they enter a program of apoptosis, unless a *bcl-2* transgene is expressed. While long-term proliferating precursor B cells of RAG-2T express sterile transcripts of the μH, but little of the κL chain gene locus, *in vitro* differentiation to later stages of development induces sterile transcription of the κL chain gene locus. These findings suggest that B cell differentiation to the stage of immature B cells *in vivo* might be controlled by cell-to-cell contacts and by cytokines provided by the microenvironment in the bone marrow, but not by Ig gene rearrangements or Ig proteins expressed from them.

While differentiation of cells without Ig or TcR gene expression appears to be possible, the development of normal numbers of precursors in bone marrow and thymus is severely impaired in rearrangement-defective mice (and in similar human SCID patients) (9). They have at best 1% of the normal numbers of cells which express markers characteristic of the μH chain-expressing preB-II cells, or of the μH chain/L chain-expressing immature B cells in bone marrow, and have similarly at best 1% of the CD4$^-$ CD8$^-$ β chain-expressing, and of the CD4$^+$ CD8$^+$ double positive, α/β TcR-expressing thymocytes in the thymus. Hence, the expansion of precursor cells to fill the compartments in bone marrow and thymus with normal numbers of cells is impaired, and mature, peripheral T and B cells are missing.

The PreB Cell Receptor of Surrogate L Chain and μH Chain Positively Selects Productively V$_H$-D$_H$-J$_H$-Rearranged B Cell Precursors by Induction of Proliferation

One of the ways by which productive rearrangements of the H chain gene locus could be monitored by a precursor B cell would be to deposit D$_H$J$_H$Cμ proteins and μH chains in association with the surrogate L chain, encoded by the preB cell specific genes λ$_5$ and V$_{preB}$ into the surface membrane (10).

This view of B cell differentiation is supported by the analysis of mice carrying a targeted deletion of the exon coding for the transmembrane portion of the μH chain (μMT mice) (11) or a targeted deletion of the entire J$_H$ gene cluster of the IgH gene locus (J$_H$T mice) (12, 13). Both mutant mouse strains are devoid of peripheral, mature B cells, and are blocked in the development of B cell precursors at the transition for D$_H$J$_H$-rearranged preB-I to V$_H$D$_H$J$_H$-rearranged preB-II cells (for nomenclature used in this study, see 2). Mice with a targeted disruption of the λ$_5$ gene (λ$_5$ T mice) (14) are blocked at the same stage of B cell differentiation; however, they can generate B cells from the smaller pool of early preB-1 cells, so that peripheral B cells are produced, though at a slower rate (15). The analysis of B cell generation in λ$_5$ T mice shows that the surrogate L chain is not mandatory, but helpful for B cell development. It allows the expansion of precursor B cells with productive V$_H$D$_H$J$_H$ rearrangements and thereby the generation of a 20–100-fold larger preB-II cell compartment, which is large enough to secure the generation of sufficient numbers of sIg$^+$ B cells.

In support of this scenario, it has been shown by Decker et al. (16) that once a V$_H$ gene segment has been rearranged to D$_H$J$_H$ gene segments yielding a productive V$_H$D$_H$J$_H$ rearrangement, an estimated 5–6 divisions may occur. This would allow the estimated $2–5 \times 10^6$ pro/preB-I cells to expand to $30–50 \times 10^6$ cytoplasmic mH chain-positive preB-II cells *in vivo*. This preB-II compartment has been found to express CD25 (17).

T cell development could be guided by very similar proliferative expansion of productively V$_\beta$D$_\beta$J$_\beta$-rearranged CD4$^-$ CD8$^-$ precursor thymocytes, which have recently been shown to express a glycoprotein of 33 kDa molecular weight together with the TcR β chain on their surface (18). This 33 kDa protein might well serve the role of a "surrogate a chain" in T cell development.

Allelic Exclusion

One B cell makes only one H chain, and one T cell makes only one β chain. This phenomenon, called allelic exclusion, can be explained by a number of events contributing to the final representation of cells expressing only one of the two possible H and β chains, respectively. First, when the first productive $V_HD_HJ_H$ or $V_\beta D_\beta J_\beta$ rearrangement has been made in a preB-II cell or in a double negative thymocyte, while the second allele may either still be only D_HJ_H- or D_bJ_b-rearranged, or may already have made a $V_HD_HJ_H$ or $V_\beta D_\beta J_\beta$ rearrangement, though nonproductive, the expression of the μH chain/surrogate L chain preB cell receptor would lead to a 100-fold expansion by proliferation of this cell with only one productive rearrangement. Furthermore, however, it is well possible that the preB cell receptor or the preT cell receptor signals not only proliferative expansion but also inhibition of the rearrangement machinery and the transcriptional activity at the second allele.

Negative and Positive Selections of Immature Lymphocytes Expressing α/β TcR or μH/L Chain Ig Molecules on Their Surface

During the transit into the mature, peripheral compartments of the immune system, immature TcR$^+$ and sIg$^+$ cells are negatively and positively selected (2, 19). Negative selection deletes in primary lymphoid organs, and anergizes in the periphery, those cells which are autoreactive with high avidity for self-antigens.

Immature lymphocytes differ from mature, peripheral cells in their continued expression of the recombination-active genes RAG-1 and -2 (20, 21). Immature sIgM$^+$ sIgD$^-$ B cells generated from precursors "*in vitro*" therefore continue to rearrange κ and λ L chain gene loci. Mature B cells no

longer express RAG-1 and -2, no longer rearrange κ and λ L chain gene loci, express sIgM and sIgD, and have changed their life expectancy. In the primary lymphoid organs, practically all lymphoid precursors, i.e., all immature "in-frame"-rearranged, TcR or Ig-expressing, or out-of-frame-rearranged, TcR or Ig-negative cells have a short life to live, all around 3 days. Each day a small proportion (between 0.1% and 3%) of these immature cells transits from the primary to the secondary lymphoid organs. In the secondary organs only TcR$^+$ and Ig$^+$ cells, but not the TcR$^-$ and Ig$^-$ cells, are found, and they now are much longer lived. Their half-lives have been measured to be at least 6 weeks, and sometimes longer (22).

In the transition from immature to mature B cells, surface-bound Ig molecules could signal the downregulation of RAG-1 and -2 expression, the upregulation of surface IgD expression, and a change in the migratory patterns and life expectancy of these cells. It is not clear whether this transition from immature to mature cells is, again, accompanied by proliferative expansion.

Positive selection is well understood for T cells (19). Immature thymocytes expressing a TcR with intermediate avidity for self-MHC class I or II molecules and self-peptides bound into them are positively selected to fill the pool of peripheral, mature T cells in which all those with non-fitting, useless TcR are discarded. Positive selection of fitting T cells probably prolongs their life expectancy, while non-fitting T cells die within 3 days, as rapidly as those which never made a TcR due to out-of-frame rearrangements. As a result of this positive selection, a repertoire of self-MHC-restricted T cells is generated for the periphery. A foreign peptide, presented on the self-MHC molecules upon uptake and processing of the corresponding foreign antigen by antigen-presenting cells, will elicit the response of a T cell to proliferate and mature to effector functions whenever it manages to increase the avidity of a TcR on a peripheral mature T cell to the presenting complex of foreign peptide and self-MHC molecule.

Positive selection also occurs during transit from immature sIg$^+$ B cells in primary lymphoid organs to mature sIg$^+$ B cells in the periphery (2). It is not yet clear whether self-antigens can positively select, and if so, who can. The repertoires of peripheral, mature B cells at least do not give any evidence for dominant selecting self-antigens as MHC molecules are for T cells.

Positive selection of B cells certainly occurs

when they are stimulated by foreign antigens (23). This can occur with and without the help of T cells. Helper T cell-independent antigens stimulate B cells, mainly to proliferation and maturation into clones of IgM-secreting cells. No memory develops. Helper T cell-dependent antigens, on the other hand, stimulate not only proliferation and maturation to IgM secretion, but also induce the switching of IgH class expression and somatic hypermutations of variable (V) regions of Ig H and L chain genes. This occurs in germinal centers of secondary lymphoid organs. Memory to the antigenic experience develops. Some memory cells can be accounted for by an increase in antigen-specific T and B cells, by changes in the expression patterns of lymphokine genes in T_H cells, by changes in the class and the avidity of the Ig molecules specific for the antigen made by the B cells, and by different migratory patterns and increased life expectancies of the experienced antigen-specific T and B cells.

Acknowledgment

The Basel Institute for Immunology was founded and is supported by F. Hoffmann-La Roche Ltd., Basel, Switzerland.

Address for correspondence:

Dr Fritz Melchers
Basel Institute for Immunology
Grenzacherstrasse 487
CH-4005 Basel
Switzerland

References

1. Alt FW, Blackwell TK, DePinho RA, Reth MG, Yancopoulos GD. Regulation of genome rearrangement events during lymphocyte differentiation. *Immunol Rev* 1986; 89:5.

2. Rolink A, Melchers F. Generation and regeneration of cells of the B-lymphocyte lineage. *Curr Opin Immunol* 1993; 5:207.

3. Bosma GC, Custer RP, Bosma MJ. A severe combined immunodeficiency mutation in the mouse. *Nature* 1983; 301:527.

4. Mombaerts P, Iacomini J, Johnson RS, Herrup K, Tonegawa S, Papaioannou VE. RAG-1-deficient mice have no mature B and T lymphocytes. *Cell* 1992; 68:869.

5. Shinkai Y, Rathbun G, Lam, KP, Oltz EM, Stewart V, Mendelson M, Charron J, Datta M, Young F, Stall AM, Alt FM. RAG-2-deficient mice lack mature lymphocytes owing to inability to intiate V(D)J rearrangement. *Cell* 1992; 68:855.

6. Gu H, Zou Y-R, Rajewsky K. Independent control of immunoglobulin switch recombination at individual switch regions evidenced through Cre-*loxP*-medicated gene targeting. *Cell* 1993; 73:1155.

7. Chen J, Gorman JR, Stewart V, Williams B, Jacks T, Alt FW. Generation of normal lymphocyte populations by *Rb*-deficient embryonic stem cells. *Curr Biol* 1993; 3:405.

8. Melchers, F, Haasner D, Grawunder U, Kalberer C, Karasuyama H, Winkler T, Rolink AG. Roles of IgH and L chains and of surrogate H and L chains in the development of cells of the B lymphocyte lineage. *Annu Rev Immunol* 1994; 12:209.

9. Rolink A, Karasuyama H, Haasner D, Grawunder U, Mårtensson I-L, Kudo A, Melchers F. Two pathways of B-lymphocyte development in mouse bone marrow and the roles of surrogate L chain in this development. *Immunol Rev* 1994; 137:185.

10. Melchers F, Karasuyama H, Haasner D, Bauer S, Kudo A, Sakaguchi N, Jameson B, Rolink A. The surrogate light chain in B-cell development. *Immunol Today* 1993; 14:60.

11. Kitamura, D, Roes J, Kühn R, Rajewsky K. A B cell-deficient mouse by targeted disruption of the membrane exon of the immunoglobulin μ chain gene. *Nature* 1991; 350:423.

12. Chen J, Trounstine M, Alt FW, Young F, Kurahara C, Loring JF, Huszar D. Immunoglobulin gene rearrangement in B cell deficient mice generated by targeted deletion of the J_H locus. *Int Immunol* 1993; 5:647.

13. Ehlich A, Schaal S, Gu H, Kitamura D, Müller W, Rajewsky K. Immunoglobulin heavy and light chain genes rearrange independently at early stages of B cell development. *Cell* 1993; 72:695.

14. Kitamura D, Kudo A, Schaal S, Müller W, Melchers F, Rajewsky K. A critical role of λ_5 protein in B cell development. *Cell* 1992; 69:823.

15. Rolink A, Karasuyama H, Grawunder U, Haasner D, Kudo A, Melchers F. B cell development in mice with a defective λ_5 gene. *Eur J Immunol* 1993; 23:1284.

16. Decker DJ, Boyle NE, Koziol JA, Klinman NR. The expression of the Ig H chain repertoire in developing bone marrow B lineage cells. *J Immunol* 1991; 146:350.

17. Rolink A, Grawunder U, Winkler TH, Karasuyama H, Melchers F. IL-2 receptor α chain (CD25, TAC) expression defines a crucial stage in preB cell development. *Int Immunol* 1994; 6 (in press).

18. Groettrup M, von Boehmer H. A role for a preT-cell

receptor in T-cell development. *Immunol Today* 1993; 14:610.

19. von Boehmer H. Thymic selection: a matter of life and death. *Immunol Today* 1992; 13:454.

20. Rolink AG, Grawunder U, Haasner D, Strasser A, Melchers F. Immature sIg$^+$ B cells can continue to rearrange κ and λL chain gene loci. *J Exp Med* 1993; 178:1263.

21. Borgulya P, Kishi H, Uematsu Y, von Boehmer H. Exclusion and inclusion of α and β T cell receptor alleles. *Cell* 1992; 69:529.

22. Rajewsky K. B-cell lifespans in the mouse – Why to debate what? *Immunol Today* 1993; 14:40.

23. Clark EA, Ledbetter JA. How B and T cells talk to each other. *Nature* 1994; 367:425.

Environmental Impact on Hypersensitivity and Allergy

Terumasa Miyamoto*

Keywords: Indoor allergens, occupational allergens

House dust is the most important allergen which includes various house dust mites. Molds, pets, and various chemicals have become important in allergy. Allergic diseases related to occupation should be emphasized.

Introduction

The world is full of naturally occurring and man-made substances capable of causing reactions in susceptible individuals. Some act as irritants and others as allergens. There are various indoor allergens which produce allergic reactions. Among these, house dust is the most important allergen which includes various house dust mites. So far, 36 species of house dust mites have been identified. *Dermatophagoides pteronyssinus* and *D. farinae* are the most important causes of asthma. *Dermatophagoides* species reproduce between temperatures of 20 and 30°C and a relative humidity of 50–80% (see Figure 1). Various insects and spiders are found in house dust, as shown in Table 1, and some of these are also important allergens.

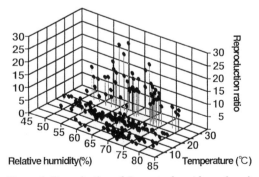

Figure 1. Reproduction of *Dermatophagoides* and environmental factors.

Table 1. Number of insects and spiders found in 12 house dust samples (per gram).

	No.		
	1–6	7–12	Total
Book lice	300	52	352
Two-winged flies	341	147	488
Midges	139	10	149
Others	202	127	329
Wasps, bees, ants	321	10	331
Ants	220	5	225
Others	101	5	106
Beetles	80	25	105
True bugs	57	5	62
Moths	15	0	15
Springtails	20	0	20
Thrips	0	7	7
Spiders	90	5	95
Unidentified	351	90	441
Total	1575	331	1906

Most of the insects found were a fragment(s), such as a part of the body, leg, wing, head, etc.

Various molds are found in houses, and some of these are also important allergens. Pets have become popular, and these too are important sources of allergens. Chemical pollutants are also discharged indoors from heaters. These sources of allergens should also be taken in to consideration, along with smoking, when treating respiratory ailments.

SO_2, NO, O_3, oxidants, acid rain, sulfuric acid mist, and SPM should be taken into consideration. From our studies, it has become clear that the SPM has an adjuvant effect in producing IgE antibody.

Allergic diseases related to occupation should be emphasized now more than ever. At the present time, about 120 types of occupational allergen have been reported, including industrial chemicals, material of vegetable and animal origin, inorganic

* National Sagamihara Hospital, Japan.

material, and synthetic substances. In the modern era, environmental allergens and irritants will increase and new substances will be synthesized to which human beings have never before been exposed. In order to stop the present increasing trend of allergic diseases, we must increase our attempts to control allergens or irritants.

This symposium is therefore very significant, and will provide much useful information. The contributors to this book are all experts in these subjects, and I am sure that readers will benefit greatly from reading their contributions.

Address for correspondence:

T Miyamoto
3-43-4, Ogikubo
Suginami-ku. Tokyo
Japan

The Role of Indoor and Outdoor Air Pollution in Allergic Diseases

Heidrun Behrendt*,**, Karl-Heinz Friedrichs**, Ursula Krämer**, Bettina Hitzfeld*,**, Wolf-M. Becker***, Johannes Ring****

Keywords: Air pollution, particulate matter, allergy, mediators, allergen carrier, epidemiology, allergotoxicology

The role of indoor and outdoor air pollution on the induction, elicitation, and maintenance of allergic inflammatory reactions ("allergotoxicology") is demonstrated by means of environmental epidemiology and experimental studies including human *in vitro* cell systems as well as pollen samples. We distinguish two types of air pollution: Type I air pollution is present predominantly in Eastern Europe and is associated with infectious and chronic inflammatory airway reactions; type II air pollution is present in the industrialized Western countries in both the indoor and outdoor environment and is composed of mainly NO/NO_2, O_3, VOCs, and fine particles. The latter is associated with allergic diseases and allergic sensitization: The risk of becoming sensitized is 2–3 times higher when living in a household near roads with heavy traffic or when unvented gas is used for cooking/heating. Substances adsorbed to airborne particles collected in West German regions are able to induce the release of mediators from human basophils and neutrophils, and exhibit priming effects on them. Airborne pollutants also interact with pollen grains as is shown by morphology as well as by immunochemistry. It is concluded that air pollutants interfere with parameters of allergy at the level of sensitization, elicitation of symptoms, and chronification of disease.

Environmental pollution has been recognized to be harmful to human health, especially with respect to cytotoxicity, mutagenicity, and cancerogenicity. In allergic reactions, air pollutants are proposed to be at least one important factor among others contributing to the overall increase of allergies worldwide. This suggestion is confirmed by experimental work showing that a variety of substances involved in air pollution, i.e., SO_2, NO_2, O_3, and particles (1, 2), are able either to exhibit adjuvant activity for allergen-specific IgE production in experimental animals (3–8) or to modulate mediator release (9–12) and to have irritant effects on effector organs in the allergic response (13 for ref.).

The Nature, Source, and Classification of Air Pollutants

Air pollution is not restricted to single substances or to single contaminated spots. It is a worldwide problem related to densely populated urban areas and to heavily industrialized regions. A great number of substances of either gaseous or particulate origin are emitted into either the outdoor or indoor environment or both (Tables 1, 2). Some contaminants are even found to occur at far higher concentrations indoors than outdoors (Table 2). Outdoor air pollutants have no respect for national boundaries and can affect regions far distant from the emission sources. Their concentration mostly depends on various factors such as emission pattern, removal processes, climate, and weather conditions (1).

According to Spengler (1), air pollutants may be classified as *primary*, such as those being emitted as such into the atmosphere (SO_2, NO, NO_2, volatile organic compounds, large particles, CO);

---

*   Department of Experimental Dermatology & Allergology, Universitätskrankenhaus Eppendorf, University of Hamburg, Hamburg, Germany.
**   Medical Institute of Environmental Hygiene at the University, Düsseldorf, Germany.
***   Division of Allergology, Research Institute Borstel, Borstel, Germany.
**** Department of Dermatology, Universitätskrankenhaus Eppendorf, University of Hamburg, Hamburg, Germany.

Table 1. Main outdoor air pollutants.

Gaseous agents:	SO_2
	CO
	NO/NO_2
	O_3
Volatile organic chemicals (VOC):	
	benzene
	toluene
	xylene
	methylene chloride
Particulates:	TSP
	PM_{10}
	$PM_{2.5}$
Metals:	AS, Cd, Cr,
	Cu, Pb, Hg, Ni

Table 2. Main indoor pollutants.

Source and type	Indoor concentration	Indoor/ outdoor ratio
Pollutants from outdoors		
Sulfur oxides	0–15 µg/m³	<1
Ozone	0–10 ppb	<<1
Pollutants from indoors and outdoors		
Nitrogen oxides	10–700 µg/m³	>>1
Carbon monoxide	5–50 ppm	>>1
Carbon dioxide	2000–3000 ppm	>>1
Particulate matter	10–1000 µg/m³	1
Pollutants from indoors		
Radon	0.01–4 pCi/L	>>1
Formaldehyde	0.01–0.5 ppm	>1
Synthetic fibers	0–1 fiber mL	1
Organic substances		>1
Polycyclic hydrocarbons		>1
Mercury		>1
Aerosols		>1
Microorganisms		>1
Allergens		>1

From Spengler (1992)

and as *secondary*, such as those being formed within the atmosphere by chemical or physical processes (ozone, fine particles <1µm). Both groups of pollutants have been shown to exhibit effects on the respiratory tract of asthmatics and nonasthmatics alike (14, 15), and they may even enhance and aggravate symptoms during the emission of peak concentrations of these pollutants (13, 16 for ref.). Outdoor air pollution – as is summarized in Table 1 – is represented by gaseous substances, by volatile organic compounds (VOCs), by particles, and by

metals usually adsorbed to the particles. All of these compounds are emitted by man-made sources: industrial processes including petrol refineries, metallurgy, and chemical plants. SO_2 and NO_x as well as particles are emitted by stationary combustion processes. Another source are waste-incinerating plants, which emit a great variety of substances including CO, NO_x, hydrocarbons, solvents, VOCs, aldehydes, toxic metals, and smoke. The major man-made source of outdoor air pollution today, however, is transportation, especially the automobile. Emissions from this source include gaseous compounds (CO, NO/NO_2, hydrocarbons) and particulates deriving from unburned fuel, fuel additives, or carbonaceous soot. Exposure to these pollutants may be measured by either detecting immission concentrations in the polluted region or by determination of internal body load using blood, urine, or teeth as vehicle (17). Table 2 gives an impression of the great variety of indoor air pollutants. It indicates that indoor contaminants may come in from the outdoors only, or may have both indoor and outdoor sources. In addition, more than 300 contaminants are known to occur only in the indoor environment, some of them being highly carcinogenic in nature. The concentration of indoor air pollutants varies and generally depends on the rate of ventilation, on additional sources of indoor contaminants, e.g., heating/cooking with unvented gas, and smoking, and on human activity.

As fas as air pollution in general is concerned, two types are to be distinguished at the moment (Figure 1):

– *Type I air pollution* is characterized by the existence of the primary pollutants SO_2, particles (total suspended matter TSP) and dust fall, and is emitted predominantely from outdoor sources. Today, this type is still present in the eastern part of Germany and in other countries of Eastern Europe. It is associated with adverse health effects on the airways, i.e., viral and bacterial airway inflammation and infectious diseases (18).

– *Type II air pollution* is characterized by the presence of primary and secondary pollutants, each of them being emitted from outdoor as well as from indoor sources. This type is found in the highly populated, industrialized urban areas in the Western world. And it is this type II air pollution that is predominantly associated with allergic sensitization in terms of prevalence rates. One has to keep in mind that the biological effects of environmental pollutants are generally

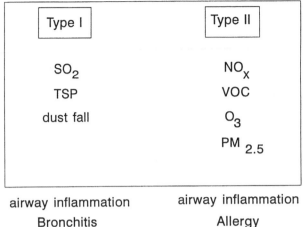

AIR POLLUTION

Figure 1. Classification of air pollution.

induced by the *repeated uptake of low doses of multiple agents* which coexist in the atmosphere and to which the individual is exposed either simultaneously or consecutively. Therefore, it still remains a problem to directly correlate ambient levels of toxic substances with chronic adverse health effects. As fas as allergic reactions are concerned, the situation is further complicated by the fact that the interaction between allergens and pollutants does not only occur within the exposed individuals but also at the level of the allergen carrier itself. The pollen being released into a polluted atmosphere will itself be exposed to the contaminants.

Epidemiological Evidence for an Association Between Type-II Air Pollution and Allergy

The aims of our epidemiological cross-sectional studies were to monitor the effects of air pollution on the health of children as a basis of control, and to establish dose-response relationships by studies in areas with highly different types and intensities of air pollution. For this purpose, more than 3600 preschool children, 5–6 years old, were investigated in reunited Germany during the Spring of 1991 in two areas with different types of pollution (Type I/East versus Type II/West) and with different intensities of pollution within these areas, including one control region for each type. Both study areas were comparable in geographic latitude, weather and climate conditions as well as in the genetic background of the population, but differed with respect to type and intensity of air pollution as well as living conditions (18, 19). The results obtained show that an association between emittants of type II air pollution and parameters of allergic sensitization can be observed in West Germany. This is true for the indoor source variable "Cooking/heating with unvented gas" as well as for the outdoor source variables "Living more than 2 years within 50 m of a road with heavy traffic" and "Staying/moving more than 1 hour per day on a road with heavy traffic" (20). When unvented gas is used in the household, the prevalence rates for children with total serum IgE elevation above $180 \, kU/L$ is 17% (control 8%), for children with specific IgE antibodies against grass or mite allergens it is 21% vs 6.5% and 24% vs 8,2%. The adjusted odds ratios indicating a positive and significant association between these two variables are given in Table 3.

A similar positive association between exposure and sensitization to at least one inhalable allergen or lifetime prevalence of allergic diseases has been found for outdoor sources of type II air pollution, automobile exhaust (Table 4). Therefore, in our studies, *the exposure to emission sources of type II air pollutants seem to be a risk factor for atopic sensitization* after controlling for other covariates.

Table 3. Indoor source of air pollution: Cooking/heating with unvented gas. Results from two studies in West Germany among preschool children in 1988 (n = 488) and 1991 (n = 1052).

	OR (95% CI)	n (year)
Serum IgE > 180 kU/l	2.90 (1.60, 4.20)	488 (1988)
	2.94 (1.47, 5.87)	593 (1991)
RAST grass	3.36 (1.52, 7.44)	590 (1991)
RAST mite	2.97 (1.45, 6.10)	590 (1991)
SPT mite	2.22 (1.29, 5.37)	1052 (1991)

adjusted for age, sex, passive smoking, family history of allergy, social status

Table 4. Outdoor source of air pollution: Automobile exhaust. 1052 preschool children, West Germany 1991. Adjusted for covariates.

lifetime prevalence	OR (95% CI)	p
bronchial asthma	1.7 (1.0, 2.9)	<0.05
hay fever	0.9 (0.5, 1.4)	
atopic eczema	1.4 (1.1, 1.8)	<0.05
allergy	1.2 (1.0, 1.5)	<0.1
sensitization (RAST max)	3.7 (1.4, 9.2)	<0.01

If this is true, what do we then learn from comparative studies in East- and West-German regions exhibiting different types and different intensities of air pollution? There is evidence from our own studies (18, 19, 20, 21) and from others (22) that the prevalence of viral and bacterial infections, tonsillitis, pneumonia, and bronchitis is higher in the East compared to the West, and within the East is higher the more the area is polluted with SO_2 and dust. In contrast, there were lower rates of doctor's diagnosed hay fever in the East. In skin-prick tests, the lowest rates of sensitization were found against birch pollen (18), being even lower than in the control area in West Germany, although the pollen counts did not differ between these areas (Behrendt, unpublished observation). The most striking difference between East and West, however, is the level of total serum IgE, the mean being about three times higher in East-German children, a fact not reflected by specific IgE values against seven common allergens in the RAST (19). The risk of having high serum IgE levels is significantly higher when living in East Germany, independent of the intensity of air pollution – even after controlling for all other relevant covariates including parasitic infestation. Therefore, elevated levels of total serum IgE do not necessarily reflect allergic sensitization; the reason for this has still to be elucidated and is not known at the moment.

Experimental Evidence for Airborne Particles as Priming Factors

Airborne particles seem to play a crucial role in provoking adverse health effects from air pollution. They contain a large number of chemical substances that can induce cytotoxic, mutagenic, and carcinogenic effects on mammalian cells. Substances adsorbed to airborne particles collected in a highly polluted region in West Germany were also able to release histamine from enriched human basophils in a nontoxic-dose-dependent fashion (23). They also show a priming effect on anti-IgE-induced release of histamine and LTC_4. The increase in mediator release is significantly higher in basophils from allergic donors than from nonallergic persons (10). This indicates that cells from atopic individuals are more sensitive to the particles associated with type-II air pollution, thus maybe describing a "risk population." Similar findings have been detected in purified human neutrophils after incubation with extracts of airborne particles: The cells are morphologically activated (10, 23). They show enhanced production of oxygen radicals in chemiluminescence, as is true for the generation and release of LTB_4, LTC_4, PGE_2, and interleukin-8 (10, 12). There was an interesting difference, however, in mediator release between allergic and nonallergic donors, namely, increased LTB_4 and decreased PGE_2 secretion in allergic donors as compared to normals.

From these *in vitro* experiments we conclude that substances adsorbed to airborne particles are able to interfere with cells involved in inflammatory processes and exhibit priming effects on them. Therefore, the exposure of individuals to adequate concentrations of particles may provoke enhancement of symptoms of allergic diseases and continuation of allergic inflammation.

Evidence for the Interaction Between Pollen and Air Pollutants

Pollen grains, which are the major source of outdoor aeroallergens, also incorporate pollutants when released into a polluted atmosphere. They are able to accumulate heavy metals e.g., lead, cadmium, and mercury as well as sulfur, and the amount of sulfur per pollen dry weight seems to be a bioindicator for the burden of the atmosphere with sulfuric aerosols (24 for ref.). We investigated the behavior of pollen grains that had been collected from four differently polluted regions in Northrhine-Westphalia (West Germany) by means of Burkhard traps and/or high volume samplers (24, 25). The results obtained show that there is an overall higher concentration of pollen grains in polluted urban areas than in rural regions, independent of weather conditions. In addition, emission peaks of SO_2, NO/NO_2, or atmospheric fine dust – but not of O_3 – usually precede peaks of high pollen concentrations. Pollen grains collected from industrial regions polluted with high amounts of organic substances are agglomerated with airborne particles (Figure 2). The same holds true for hazel pollen collected from trees near a road with heavy traffic, but not for pollen from park trees (25). The particles agglomerated to the pollen surface are heteromorphic, smaller than 5 µm in diameter, and may be aggregated. A substantial amount of them belongs to the submicronic range. Agglomeration of particles to pollen surfaces in areas with emission of organic compounds deriving from the fuel industry is supported by semiquantitative data confirming both a high degree of agglomeration as well as a high number of defective and destroyed pollen grains (24, 26). Based on these observations, we investigated whether pollen-particle interactions affect allergen formation and release at the level of the carrier itself. Results obtained from *in vitro* experiments with native *Dactylis glomerata* pollen and extracts of airborne particulate matter show that substances present in the aqueous phase of the particles induce the release of proteins from pollen grains and give rise to the formation of submicronic particles (24). Using SDS-polyacrylamide gel electrophoresis and immunoblotting, an alteration of allergenic protein bands, i.e., shifting of binding pattern intensity of IgE reactive bands to the acidic side, has been demonstrated (25). The altered allergens, however, do not prove the altered allergenicity *per se*.

The conclusion from these experiments is that organic substances adsorbed to airborne particles mediate the agglomeration of particles onto pollen surfaces followed by local preactivation of the coated pollen. Under appropriate conditions, aqueous compounds may then induce local allergen release resulting in either allergenic extrusions followed by the generation of allergenic aerosols or in adsorption of pollen-derived proteins to airborne particles. In regions with high air pollution, particles may therefore carry not only pollutants, but also allergens, and pollen host not only allergens, but also pollutants. Therefore, pollen counts may not necessarily reflect the actual load of the atmosphere with outdoor allergens within polluted regions. Methods have to be developed to directly measure allergens in the outdoor environment.

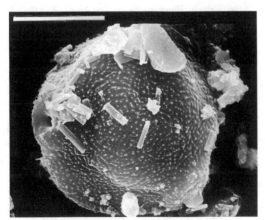

Figure 2. Agglomeration of airborne particles onto the surface of a birch pollen collected in a highly polluted region. Scanning electron micrograph, bar 10 µm.

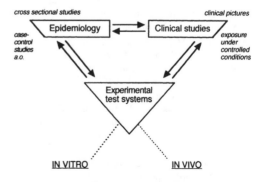

Figure 3. Course of investigation in allergotoxicology.

In order to further elucidate the role of indoor and outdoor air pollution in the induction, elicitation, and maintenance of allergic inflammatory reactions ("allergotoxicology," 27) a huge interdisciplinary effort has to be undertaken including environmental epidemiology, *in vitro* experiments, and clinical investigations (Figure 3).

Acknowledgements

Supported by a grant of the BMFT (07ALL04) and by a grant of MURL/NRW.

Address for correspondence:

Prof. Dr. Heidrun Behrendt
Abt. für Experimentelle
Dermatologie und Allergologie
Universitätskrankenhaus Eppendorf
Martinistr. 52
D-20246 Hamburg
Germany

References

1. Spengler JD. Outdoor and indoor air pollution. In AB Tarcher (Ed) *Principles and Practice of Environmental Medicine.* New York: Medical Book Co., 1992, 21

2. Quackenboss JJ, Lebowitz MD, Crutchfield CD. Indoor-outdoor relationships for particulate matter: Exposure classifications and health effects. *Environment International* 1989; 15:353.

3. Riedel F, Krämer M, Scheibenbogen C, Rieger CHL. Effects of SO₂ exposure on allergic sensitization in the guinea pig. *JACI* 1988; 82:527.

4. Osebold JW, Zee YC, Gershwin LJ. Enhancement of allergic lung sensitization in mice by ozone inhalation. *Proc Soc Exp Biol Med* 1988; 188:259.

5. Muranaka M, Suzuki S, Koizumi K, Takafuji S, Miyamoto T, Ikemori R, Tokiwa H. Adjuvant activity of diesel-exhaust particulates for the production of IgE antibody in mice. *JACI* 1986; 77:616.

6. Takafuji S, Suzuki S, Koizumi K, Tadokoro K, Miyamoto T, Ikemori R, Muranaka M. Diesel-exhaust particulates inoculated by the nasal route have an adjuvant activity for IgE production in mice. *JACI* 1987; 79:639.

7. Takafuji S, Suzuki S, Koizumi K, Tadokoro K, Ohashi H, Muranaka M, Miyamoto T. Enhancing effect of suspended particulate matter on the IgE antibody production in mice. *Int Arch Allergy Appl Immunol* 1989; 90:1.

8. Yanai M, Ohuri T, Aikawa T, Okayama H, Sekizawa K, Maeyama K, Sasaki H, Takashima T. Ozone increases susceptibility to antigen inhalation in allergic dogs. *J Appl Physiol* 1990; 68:2267.

9. Behrendt H, Wieczorek M, Wellner S, Winzer A. Effect of some metal ions (Cd, Pb, Mn) on mediator release from mast cells *in vivo* and *in vitro*. In NH Seemayer, W Hadnagy (Eds) *Environmental hygiene.* Berlin-Heidelberg: Springer 1988, p. 105.

10. Hitzfeld B, Friedrichs KH, Behrendt H. In vitro interaction between human basophils and polymorphonuclear granulocytes: Effect of airborne particulate matter. *Int Arch Allergy Immunol* 1992; 99:390.

11. Raulf M, König W. In vitro effects of polychlorinated biphenyls on human platelets. *Immunol* 1991; 72:287.

12. Hitzfeld B, Friedrichs KH, Tomingas R, Behrendt H. Organic atmospheric dust extracts and their effects on functional parameters of human polymorphonuclear leukocytes (PMN). *J Aerosol Sci* 1992; 23 (Suppl 1):S531.

13. Pierson WE, Koenig JQ. Respiratory effects of air pollution on allergic disease. *JACI* 1992; 90:557.

14. Molfino NA, Wright SC, Katz I, Tarlo S, Silverman F, McClean PA, Szalai JP, Raizenne M, Slutsky AS, Zamel N. Effect of low concentrations of ozone on inhaled allergen responses in asthmatic subjects. *Lancet* 1991; 338:199.

15. Magnussen H, Jörres R, Wagner HM, von Nieding G. Relationship between the airway response and inhaled sulphur dioxide, isocapnic hyperventilation and histamine in asthmatic subjects. *Int Arch Occup Environ Health* 1990; 62:485.

16. Ruszak C, Devalia JL, Davies RJ. The impact of pollution on allergic disease. *Allergy* 1994; 49:21.

17. Jermann E, Hajimiragha H, Brockhaus A, Freier I, Ewers U, Roscovanu A. Exposure to benzene, toluene, lead, and carbon monoxide of children living in a central urban area with high traffic density. *Zbl Hyg* 1989; 189:50.

18. Schlipköter HW, Krämer U, Behrendt H, Dolgner R, Stiller-Winkler R, Ring J, Willer HJ. Impact of air pollution on children's health – Results from Saxony-Anhalt and Saxony as compared to Northrhine Westphalia. In *Health and ecological effects. Critical issues in the global environment*, Vol 5. Pittsburgh, PA: Air & Waste Management Association 1992, IUA 2103.

19. Behrendt H, Krämer U, Dolgner R, Hinrichs J, Willer H, Hagenbeck H, Schlipköter HW. Elevated levels of total serum IgE in East German children: atopy, parasites, or pollutants? *Allergo J* 1993; 2:31.

20. Krämer U, Behrendt H, Dolgner R, Kainka-Stänicke E, Oberbarnscheidt J, Sidaoui H, Schlipköter HW.

Auswirkung der Umweltbelastung auf allergologis-che Parameter bei 6jährigen Kindern. In J Ring (Ed) *Epidemiologie allergischer Erkrankungen.* München: MMV, 1991, 165.

21. Ring J, Behrendt H, Schäfer T, Vieluf D, Krämer U. Impact of pollution on allergic diseases: Clinical and epidemiological studies. *This volume.*

22. von Mutius E, Fritzsch C, Weiland SK, Röll G, Magnussen H. Prevalence of asthma and allergic disorders among children in united Germany: a descriptive comparison. *Br Med J* 1992; 305:1395.

23. Behrendt H, Friedrichs KH, Fischer I, Tomingas R. Airborne particulate matter induces histamine release from and degranulation of enriched human basophils. *ACI News* 1991 (Suppl) 1:218.

24. Behrendt H, Friedrichs KH, Kainka-Stänicke E, Darsow U, Becker WM, Tomingas R. Allergens and pol-lutants in the air – a complex interaction. In J Ring, B Przybilla (Eds) *New trends in allergy III.* Berlin-Heidelberg: Springer, 1991, 467.

25. Behrendt H., Becker WM, Friedrichs KH, Darsow U, Tomingas R. Interaction between aeroallergens and airborne particulate matter. *Int Arch Allergy Immunol* 1992; 99:425.

26. Kainka-Stänicke E, Behrendt H, Friedrichs KH, Tomingas R. Morphological alterations of pollen and spores induced by airborne pollutants: observations from two differently polluted areas in West Germany. *Allergy* 1988; 43 (suppl 7):57.

27. Behrendt H. Allergotoxikologie: Ein Forschungskon-zept zur Untersuchung des Einflusses von Um-weltschadstoffen auf die Allergieentstehung. In J Ring (Ed) *Allergieforschung: Probleme, Strategien und klinische Relevanz.* München, MMV, 1992, 123.

Dose-Response Relationships Between Asthma and Exposure to Indoor Allergens

Thomas AE Platts-Mills, Richard B Sporik, George W Ward, Peter W Heymann, Martin D Chapman*

Keywords: Asthma, mites, cat, cockroach, indoor allergen exposure

Over the last 30 years there has been a complete change in understanding of asthma, and today exposure to allergens is seen as an important cause of the characteristic eosinophil-rich inflammation of the bronchi (1–3) (see Table 1). While many experiments have contributed to this understanding, they can be attributed to three different discoveries:

1. The discovery of IgE by Ishizaka, Bennich and Johansson lead to understanding both of the control of IgE production and of the pathophysiology of immediate and delayed events following exposure to allergens.
2. The identification of dust mites by Voorhorst and Spieksma lead to analysis of the immunochemistry of house dust and an understanding of the role of indoor allergens in asthma (4).
3. In 1970 Altounyan first reported that nonspecific bronchial hyperreactivity (BHR) could be increased by seasonal exposure to pollen (5). Progressive reductions in BHR were subsequently reported by several groups when mite allergic asthmatics moved from their houses either to high altitude sanatoria or allergen-free rooms in a hospital (6–9).

Table 1. Criteria for causality# and the evidence supporting a causal link between mite allergen exposure and the development of asthma.*

---

1. The strength of association is large (2)
    - (i)   Population studies (12, 17, 34)
    - (ii) Control studies (13, 21, 23, 24))
    - (iii) prospective studies (15, 34)
2. Repeated observations in different populations have consistent findings: (see 2, 3, 10)
    - (i)   UK (15)
    - (ii)   Europe (4, 11, 13)
    - (iii) USA (19, 21, 23)
    - (iv) Other
3. A cause leads to a specific event (i. e., asthma)
4. There is a dose response gradient
5. There is experimental evidence
    - (i) Avoidance studies (6, 7, 8, 9, 24)
    - (ii) Challenge studies
6. There are analogous explanations and the mechanism is biologically plausible

---

#Hill AB. *Proc Roy Soc Med* 1965;58:295; *Sporik et al. *Clin Exp Allergy* 1992; 22:897; for full list of references see (1).

While the case for a causal relationship is dependent on many different experiments, an important issue is whether there is evidence for a dose-response relationship between exposure and disease. In evaluating the relationship between a potentially toxic gas (or an airborne dust) and human disease, it has become normal to examine evidence for a dose-response and also to identify a threshold below which exposure does not carry any risk of disease. The situation with allergens is more complex for several reasons:

- Exposure to allergens is to particles which because of their size (i. e., > 10 µm) can fall rapidly; consequently, airborne levels vary with the level of disturbance. Because of this, most exposure measurements have to be based on the concentration of allergen in reservoir samples of dust (see International Workshop Reports, 2, 10).
- The relationship between exposure to allergens and disease includes two interdependent steps. Prolonged exposure leads to sensitization of genetically at-risk individuals. Continued exposure can lead to inflammation of the lungs and the associated BHR (Figure 1). However, this second phase is restricted to individuals who have first developed immediate hypersensitivity.
- The relationship between exposure to allergens and disease is complicated by several other factors, including intercurrent viral infection, use of

---

*   Asthma and Allergic Disease Center, University of Virginia, Charlottesville, VA, USA.

ETIOLOGY OF BRONCHIAL REACTIVITY IN ADULTS

Figure 1. Etiology of bronchial reactivity in adults.

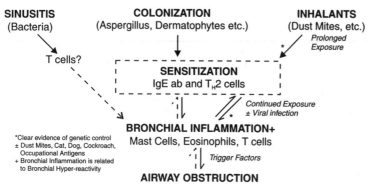

β_2-agonists, tobacco smoke and outdoor air pollution.

Finally, there are many other etiological factors that can contribute to asthma and will thus tend to confuse any simple relationship between exposure to allergens and diseases. Simple examples are: chronic sinusitis, *Aspergillus* infection of the lungs; *Trichophyton* and other fungal colonization of the skin or mucosal surfaces away from the lungs; food or coloring substances. Thus, it is not surprising that although there is a clear dose-response relationship between exposure to indoor allergens and sensitization, the evidence for a simple dose-response relationship between exposure and symptoms of asthma is less clear.

Sensitization to Mite Allergens

In the original publications on dust mites, it was proposed that 100 mites/g of dust was a significant levels of exposure and that 500 mites/g of dust was

commonly associated with disease (4). These values are important first because 100 mites/g has been supported by several subsequent studies (11, 12) and because the concentration of mites in reservoir dust was used as the index of exposure. In more recent studies, measurement of group I mite allergen/g of dust has been used as the index of exposure. However, there is good agreement between 100 mites/gram and the now recognized threshold of $2\,\mu g$ group I/g dust (2, 10, 13, 14):

– Studies on patients presenting with asthma suggest that mite sensitization is common among asthmatics who are living in houses where mite allergen levels are $> 2\,\mu g/g$ (13, 15, 16).
– Population studies on school age children clearly show progressively higher prevalence of sensitization in direct relationship to mite allergen exposure levels (15–17) (see Table 3).
– In Australia, France, Sweden and the United States the prevalence of sensitization to mite antigens is very low in low humidity areas where the mean levels of mite allergen are less than $2\,\mu g/g$.

Table 2. Sensitization and exposure to mite allergens.

Country	Comparison	Threshold*	Authors
UK	Within Poole	> 2 μg/g#	Sporik et al., *NEJM* 1990; 323:502
Australia	Coastal vs. inland	> 2 μg (> 100 mites/g)#	Peat et al., *Clin Exp Allergy* 1993;23:812
Sweden	South vs. North	> 2 μg/g	Wickman et al., *ARRD* 1993;148:58
		[1 μg/g]	[Dreborg, Bjorksten, Munir, Aberg]
Denmark	Within Aarhus	> 100 mites/g#	Korsgaard, *ARRD* 1983; 128:231
France	Marseilles vs. Briancon	> 2 μg/g	Charpin et al, *ARRD* 1991; 143:983
Germany	Different towns	> 2 μg/g#	Lau et al., *J All Clin Imm* 1989; 84:718
USA	Virginia vs New Mexico	> 2 μg/g	Sporik, Pollart et al., in press

* Threshold concentration of group I mite allergen/g dust; # evidence for a progressive effect of increasing dose.

Table 3. Influence of mite concentration in house dust on sensitization and the relationship of sensitization to asthma in school children.

	Lismore†	Moree†	Los Alamos*
Children with current asthma %**	11.3	8.3	6.3
Mite sensitization of population %	28	25	18 (6%)#
Mite sensitization as a risk factor for asthma (odds ratio)	(18)	(5)	(<1.5)
Cat sensitization of population %	6	5	31
Mean mite allergen in house dust: Group I µg/g	83.0	11.2	<0.5

† Modification from Peat et al., *Clin Exp Allergy* 1993; 23:812; * from Sporik, Ingram, Honsinger et al. 1994, submitted; # children born in Los Alamos; ** asthma defined as symptomatic BHR.

– A prospective study in the UK not only confirmed the dominant role of mite sensitization, but also showed a quantitative relationship between exposure in the first two years of life and sensitization (15).

Sensitization to Other Indoor Allergens

The data for allergens other than mite is much less complete, but simple conclusions are possible for cat, dog, and cockroach allergens. In communities where cats are not kept indoors (e. g., Sao Paulo Brazil or inner city Atlanta), the levels of cat allergen are low (i. e., < 1 µg Fel d I/g dust) and cat sensitization is present in less than 10% of asthmatics (18, 19). By contrast, in towns where up to 50% of houses have indoor animals, both cat and dog allergens are present in almost all houses. For example, in a community such as Los Alamos, NM, cat and dog sensitization are present in ~60% of asthmatics. In this town the houses with cats have between 8 µg and 1,000 µg Fel d I/g dust, while almost all the houses have > 1 µg Fel d I/g dust (17). Whether children who currently live in a house without an animal become sensitized to animal allergens because of occasional exposure to high levels in the past or from prolonged exposure to levels between 1 and 8 µg/g is not clear.

Although there are great advantages to expressing allergen levels in absolute units, the levels of cat and mite allergen are almost certainly not equivalent in that the form in which cat allergen becomes airborne is very different from mite. Furthermore, for airborne cat allergen the relative roles of reservoirs such as carpets or the cat itself is still not well defined (20). In some communities mites are not relevant because of low humidity, and cat or dog sensitization is strongly associated with asthma, e. g., the mountain states of the USA and Northern Sweden. Since asthma is still common in these areas, the implication is that important changes have occurred in houses in addition to those that have increased mite growth.

There is abundant evidence for an association between cockroach sensitization and asthma (21, 22). This risk is restricted to communities where cockroach (generally *Blattella germanica*) infestation is common (19, 23). Thus, at a simple level it is clear that there is a dose-response relationship, but measurements of exposure are still rather limited. The assays for Bla g I and Bla g II are standardized in arbitrary units, and there is only very limited evidence for a threshold level (19, 21, 23).

Relationship of Exposure to Asthma

It is now assumed that the major role of indoor allergens in asthma is in causing inflammation of the bronchi. Furthermore, it is clear that bronchial challenge of allergic individuals can produce both the characteristic eosinophil infiltration of the bronchi and increased BHR. However, at present there is no method of measuring inflammation simple enough for epidemiological investigation. Thus, symptoms of asthma or BHR are used as surrogate measurements of inflammation. On the other hand, it is by no means clear that there is a simple quantitative relationship between measurements of inflammation and symptoms or BHR. In all studies, a significant proportion of children and young adults who become allergic to mites do not have symptoms of asthma (1, 2, 10, 16). Thus, sensitization is a risk factor for asthma but does not have a simple relationship, even among children who remain in the same houses with similar levels of exposure (15). The implication is that the level of exposure necessary to induce inflammation and BHR varies over a wide range (Figure 1). Thus, some allergic individuals will only develop symptoms if they are exposed to high levels of allergen (e. g., > 10 µg group I/g dust), while others who have similar levels of IgE antibody only require modest exposure (e. g., ~1 µg group I/g dust) to maintain symptoms.

In 1984, Korsgaard reported a strong correlation between asthma and the number of mites/g of dust in houses in Aarhus (11). Subsequent studies have confirmed that most of the allergic asthmatics presenting to hospital are exposed at home to relevant allergens (3, 10, 19, 23). However, when the houses of asthmatics were compared to those of random controls in the same community, the levels of allergen were very similar. This was true for mite allergen, animal dander, and cockroach allergens in separate studies (17, 19, 23). The implication is that once patients have become sensitized, the existing levels of allergen in their community are sufficient to maintain BHR and asthma symptoms in at least a proportion of cases.

It is unethical to test experimentally whether patients exposed chronically to higher levels of allergen become symptomatic. Many studies have addressed the question of whether reduction of exposure can reduce symptoms. If patients are moved from their house to an "allergen-free" environment, studies consistently show decreased symptoms and decreased BHR (6–10). In some of these studies it is possible to define the quantitative reduction in exposure that is associated with improvement. This was possible in our study in London (7), in comparison between Marseilles and Briancon (8), and also in the avoidance study carried out by Ehnert et al. in apartments in Berlin (24). In each case the concentration of mite allergen in the low allergen environment was < 2 µg group I mite allergen/g dust and the estimated reduction in exposure was ~95%. These results strongly support the idea that continued exposure is essential for the maintenance of BHR and symptoms, but they cannot be said to establish a dose-response or a specific threshold.

Recently, we have evaluated children who moved from a high mite environment (i. e., coastal states of the USA) to one with no mites (i. e., 7,200 feet high in New Mexico). Among these children, mite sensitization was not a significant risk factor for current BHR (17). Thus, the levels of mite allergen (< 1 µg/g) appear to be too low to maintain BHR in sensitized individuals. The implication of these results for treatment is obvious. Indeed, simple physical measures to reduce exposure to mite allergens have become a normal part of asthma treatment (25). Questions about house design are in the long run far more important and are not resolved. If increased temperature, decreased ventilation, increased humidity and increased furnishings (e. g., fitted carpets) have caused the increased prevalence of allergy to indoor allergens and associated increase in asthma, then changing the design of houses and particularly children's bedrooms may be the best approach to controlling asthma.

Interaction Between Allergen Exposure and Other Factors that can Exacerbate/cause Asthma

That the prevalence of asthma has increased is difficult to deny. Evidence has been obtained from many parts of the developed world, and over this same period it has become increasingly recognized that the large majority of asthmatics are allergic to indoor allergens. This leaves two questions: (1) Is the dominant association between asthma and mites a new phenomenon, or has mite sensitization always been common? and (2) Are changes in houses a convincing explanation of the increased prevalence of asthma? Other explanations that have been advanced include: the increased use of inhaled adrenergic agonists; environmental tobacco smoke (ETS); intercurrent viral infection; and air pollution. Our own studies and those of others suggest that ETS is an important factor for acute respiratory diseases among children under 2 (or 3) years old, but appears to be less relevant among older children or adults (19, 23, 26, 27, 28). Indeed, it is difficult to assign a major role for ETS given that the dramatic fall in smoking among middle class Americans has not been matched by a parallel decrease in asthma. Viral infection has been shown to be an important factor for acute episodes of airway obstruction. Among children under 2 years old this is predominantly RSV and unrelated to allergy, while among older children or young adults, rhinovirus and coronavirus are more important (26, 29,

30). The experimental data with rhinovirus generally does not show a direct effect on the lung, but rhinovirus infection can upregulate the eosinophil response to allergen challenge (31). In keeping with that, Duff et al. reported that the strongest risk factor for asthma among children over 2 years old presenting to an emergency room was the combination of rhinovirus infection and sensitization to indoor allergens (26).

The possibility that adrenergic agonists could play a harmful role in asthma was first proposed in the 1960s during the epidemic of asthma deaths associated with isoprenaline forte inhaler use in the UK and New Zealand. However, 25 years later it is still not clear whether the problem is restricted to a subgroup of less selective agonists, i. e., fenoterol and Isoprenaline, or is a general property of high dose β-agonists. In some areas of the world inhalers are prescribed to as many as 18% of school age children. Despite this, asthma remains strongly associated with sensitization to indoor allergens. This implies that β-agonists are not creating BHR in nonallergic individuals. Use of inhalers could be increasing BHR either because bronchodilation allows allergic individuals to inhale more allergen or by having an upregulating effect on some aspect of bronchial inflammation. Recently, Cockcroft et al. reported an increased response of the lung to allergen challenge in patients given 2 weeks β_2-agonist (32). Similarly, ozone has been reported to increase the response of the lung to allergens (33). Taken together the results suggest that many of the associated factors actually interact with allergen exposure. If so, it is possible that the increase in asthma is really due to the multiplicative interaction between increased allergen exposure, viral infections and widespread use of β_2-agonists.

Conclusions

Among children and young adults, sensitization to common indoor allergens is the strongest predictor of either chronic symptoms or acute attacks of asthma (1, 2, 16, 34, 35). Comparing different communities within a country, it is clear that the mean allergen levels in houses can predict the prevalence of sensitization. In addition, there are at least 3 studies where a dose-response relationship is clear within a community. The evidence for either threshold levels or a dose-response relationship be-

tween exposure and symptoms among sensitized individuals is less clear. There appear to be several reasons for this:
1. There is a very wide range of allergen exposure which is necessary to induce symptoms.
2. Intercurrent virus infection plays an important role in exacerbating symptoms, but this is predominantly among allergic individuals.
3. Treatment, especially with inhaled steroids or cromolyn (which can reduce BHR) or β_2-agonists (which can increase BHR) can alter symptoms so as to obscure a simple relationship.

On the other hand, the results of avoidance experiments strongly support the view that continuing exposure to allergen is necessary for continuation of symptoms and BHR. Despite some difficulties with avoidance measures, reducing exposure to mite and/or other allergens should be seen as a primary anti-inflammatory treatment for asthma. In addition, it is likely that changes in houses have played an important role in the increased prevalence of asthma over the last 30 years. This implies that true control of our current epidemic of asthma would best be achieved by increasing ventilation, decreasing temperature and reducing furnishing in houses, and particularly in children's bedrooms.

Address for correspondence:

Thomas AE Platts-Mills
Asthma and Allergic Disease Center
University of Virginia
Box 225
Charlottesville, VA 22908
USA

References

1. Sporik RB, Chapman MD, Platts-Mills TAE. House dust mite exposure as a cause of asthma (Editorial). *Clin Exp Allergy* 1992; 22:897–906.
2. Platts-Mills TAE, De Weck A. Dust mite allergens and asthma – A world wide problem. *Bull WHO* 1989; 66:769–780.
3. Platts-Mills TAE, Chapman MD. Dust mites: immunology, allergic disease, and environmental control [Review]. *J Allergy Clin Immunol* 1987; 80:755–775.
4. Voorhorst R, Spieksma FTM, Varekamp N. House dust mite atopy and the house dust mite *Dermato-*

phagoides pteronyssinus (Troussart, 1897). Leiden: Stafleu's Scientific Publishing, 1969.

5. Altounyan RE. Changes in histamine and atropine responsiveness as a guide to diagnosis and evaluation of therapy in obstructive airways disease. In: Pepys J, Frankland AW (Eds) *Disodium chromoglycate in allergic airways disease*. London: Butterworth, 1970, pp. 47–53.

6. Kerrebijn KF. Endogenous factors in childhood CNSLD: Methodological aspects in population studies. In Orie NGM, van der Lende R (Eds) *Bronchitis III*. The Netherlands: Royal Vangorcum Assen, 1970, pp. 38–48.

7. Platts-Mills TAE, Tovey ER, Mitchell EB, Moszoro H, Nock P, Wilkins SR. Reduction of bronchial hyperreactivity during prolonged allergen avoidance. *Lancet* 1982; 2:675–678.

8. Vervloet D, Penaud A, Razzouk H, Senft M, Arnaud A, Boutin C, Charpin J. Altitude and house dust mites. *J Allergy Clin Immunol* 1982; 69:290–296.

9. Piacentini G, Martinati L, Fornari A, Comis A, Carcereri L, Boccagni P, Boner AL. Antigen avoidance in a mountain environment: Influence on basophil releasability in children with allergic asthma. *J Allergy Clin Immunol* 1993; 92:644–650.

10. Platts-Mills TAE, Thomas WR, Aalberse RC, Vervloet D, Chapman MD, Co-Chairmen. Dust mite allergens and asthma: Report of a 2nd international workshop. *J Allergy Clin Immunol* 1992; 89:1046–1060.

11. Korsgaard J. Mite asthma and residency. A case-control study on the impact of exposure to house-dust mites in dwellings. *Am Rev Resp Dis* 1983; 128:231–235.

12. Peat JK, Britton WJ, Salome CM, Woolcock AJ. Bronchial hyperresponsiveness in two populations of Australian schoolchildren. III. Effect of exposure to environmental allergens. *Clin Allergy* 1987; 17:297–300.

13. Lau S, Falkenhorst G, Weber A, Werthman I, Lind P, Bucttner-Goetz P, Wahn U. High mite-allergen exposure increases the risk of sensitization in atopic children and young adults. *J Allergy Clin Immunol* 1989; 84:718–725.

14. Charpin D, Birnbaum J, Haddi E, Genard G, Lanteaume A, Toumi M, Faraj F, van der rempt X, Vervloet D. Altitude and allergy to house dust mites: A paradigm of the influence of environmental exposure on allergic sensitization. *Am Rev Resp Dis* 1991; 143:983–986.

15. Sporik R, Holgate ST, Platts-Mills TAE, Cogswell J. Exposure to house dust mite allergen (Der p I) and the development of asthma in childhood: A prospective study. *N Engl J Med* 1990; 323:502–507.

16. Peat JK, Tovey E, Millis CM, Leeder SR, Woolcock AJ. Importance of house dust mite and Alternaria al-

lergens in childhood asthma: an epidemiological study in two climatic regions of Australia. *Clin Exp Allergy* 1993; 23:812–820.

17. Sporik RB, Price W. Sussman JH, Honsinger R, Platts-Mills TAE. Association of asthma with serum IgE and skin-test reactivity to allergens among children living at high altitude: Tickling the dragon's breath. Submitted.

18. Arruda K, Rizzo MC, Chapman MD, Fernandez-Caldas E, Baggio D, Platts-Mills TAE, Naspitz CK. Exposure and sensitization to dust mite allergens among asthmatic children in Sao Paulo, Brazil. *Clin Exp Allergy* 1991; 21:433–439.

19. Call RS, Smith TF, Morris E, Chapman MD, Platts-Mills TAE. Risk factors for asthma in inner city children. *J Pediatr* 1992; 121:862–866.

20. Luczynska CM, Li Y, Chapman MD, Platts-Mills TAE. Airborne concentrations and particle size distribution of allergen derived from domestic cats (*Felis domesticus*): Measurements using cascade impactor, liquid impinger and a two site monoclonal antibody assay for Fel d I. *Am Rev Resp Dis* 1990; 141:361–367.

21. Pollart S, Smith TF, Morris EC, Gelber LE, Platts-Mills TAE, Chapman MD. Environmental exposure to cockroach allergens: Analysis with monoclonal antibody-based enzyme immunoassays. *J Allergy Clin Immunol* 1991; 87:505–510.

22. Kang B. Study on cockroach antigen as a probable causative agent in bronchial asthma. *J Allergy Clin Immunol* 1976; 58:357–365.

23. Gelber LE, Seltzer LH, Bouzoukis JK, Pollart SM, Chapman MD, Platts-Mills TAE. Sensitization and exposure to indoor allergens as risk factors for asthma among patients presenting to hospital. *Am Rev Resp Dis* 1993; 147:573–578.

24. Ehnert B, Lau-Schadendorf S, Weber A, Buettner P, Schou C, Wahn U. Reducing domestic exposure to dust mite allergen reduces bronchial hypersensitivity in sensitive children with asthma. *J Allergy Clin Immunol* 1992; 90:135–138.

25. Platts-Mills TAE. Allergen-specific treatment for asthma: III. *Am Rev Respir Dis* 1993; 148:553–555.

26. Duff AL, Pomeranz ES, Gelber LE, Price GW, Farris H, Hayden FG, Platts-Mills TAE, Heyman PW. Risk factors for acute wheezing in infants and children: viruses, passive smoke, and IgE antibodies to inhalant allergens. *Pediatrics* 1993; 92:535–540.

27. Roorda RJ, Gerritsen J, Van Aalderen WM, Schouten JP, Veltman JC, Weiss ST, Knol K. Risk factors for the persistence of respiratory symptoms in childhood asthma. *ARRD* 1993; 146:1490–1495.

28. Martinez FD, Cline M, Burrows B. Increased incidence of asthma in children of smoking mothers. *Pediatrics* 1992; 89:21–26.

29. Johnston SL, Bardin PG, Pattemore PK. Viruses as precipitants of asthma symptoms III. Rhinoviruses: Molecular biology and prospects for future intervention. *Clin Exp Allergy* 1993; 23:237–246.

30. Nicholson KG, Kent J, Ireland DC. Respiratory viruses and exacerbations of asthma in adults. *Brit Med J* 1993; 307:982–986.

31. Lemansky RF, Dick EG, Swenson CA, Busse WW. Rhinovirus upper respiratory infection increases airway reactivity in late asthmatic reactions. *J Clin Invest* 1989; 83:1.

32. Cockcroft DW, McParland CP, Britto SA, Swystun VA, Rutherford BC. Regular inhaled salbutamol and airway responsiveness to allergen. *Lancet* 1993; 342:833–837.

33. Molfino NA, Wright SC, Katz I, Tarlo S, Silverman F, McClean PA, Szalai JP, Raizenne M, Slutsky AS, Zamel N. Effect of low concentrations of ozone on inhaled allergen responses in asthmatic subjects. *Lancet* 1991; 338:199–203.

34. Sears MR, Hervison GP, Holdaway MD, Hewitt CJ, Flannery EM, Silva PA. The relative risks of sensitivity to grass pollen, house dust mite, and cat dander in the development of childhood asthma. *Clin Exp Allergy* 1989; 19:419–424.

35. Wickman M, Nordvall SL, Pershagen G, Korsgaard J, Johansen N. Sensitization to domestic mites in a cold temperate region. *Am Rev Respir Dis* 1993; 148:58–62.

Genetic and Environmental Interaction in Children

Bengt Björkstén*

Keywords: Asthma, hyperreactivity, genetics, environment, infants, children, prevention, prediction, pollution

Sensitization and manifest allergic disease is the final result of environmental influences in genetically susceptible individuals. Several environmental risk factors have been identified which enhance sensitization and the appearance of allergic manifestations. In young children, exposure to tobacco smoke is by far the most important factor. Other factors include air pollution from industry and traffic, poorly ventilated homes, and certain viral infections.

Experimental, epidemiological, and clinical observations strongly support the concept that the conditions under which the primary encounter with an allergen takes place influences the immune response, i.e., whether tolerance or sensitization is triggered. There seems to be a period during which primary sensitization takes place, resulting in allergic manifestations later in life. Although environmental factors undoubtedly play a major role in the development of allergic disease, the mechanisms as well as the individual factors are unknown.

Recent studies in formerly socialist countries of Europe, where the lifestyles are similar in many respects to those of Western Europe some 30–40 years ago, lend strong support to the notion that allergies are on the increased. It is not known whether Western lifestyle is associated with an introduction of new unknown adjuvants enhancing sensitization, or whether factors that are necessary for the induction of tolerance are lacking.

Introduction

Several epidemiological studies in recent years indicate that the prevalence of allergic diseases is increasing, at least in children and young adults (1, 2). There is increasing experimental and clinical evidence that the conditions under which an allergen is encountered in infancy may have consequences for many years, perhaps even for life (3, 4). If this is indeed true, then the prevalence in adults would continue to increase for many years, even after institution of effective allergy-preventive measures in childhood.

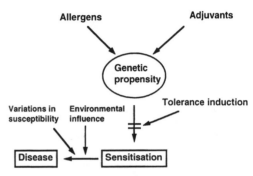

Figure 1. Schematic representation of the interaction between allergen exposure, nonspecific "adjuvant" factors and genetic propensity for sensitization and manifest allergic disease. The chain of events is usually interrupted in nonatopic individuals by the induction of tolerance.

The etiology of allergy is multifactorial and depends on the interaction in genetically susceptible individuals between the time and amount of allergen exposure and the presence of nonspecific "adjuvant" factors, including air pollution (Figure 1). The propensity for the sensitization and even more so for the manifestation of allergic disease does not only vary between individuals, but also over time in an individual. In most individuals, repeated exposure to an allergen results in the induction of tolerance. This is less likely to occur in atopic persons.

Environmental factors that influence the development of allergic disease are either specific or nonspecific. In order to develop an allergy, the individual has obviously to be exposed to the allergen. Allergens are present in almost every part of the world, though the relative importance of the in-

*   Department of Paediatrics, Faculty of Health Sciences, University Hospital, Linköping, Sweden.

97

dividual allergens varies, depending on climatic conditions. In subarctic regions, like the Nordic countries, house dust mites used to be absent, but there is now evidence for an increasing prevalence (5). This may, at least partly, be due to modern technology used for building houses and energy conservation measures (6).

It has traditionally been assumed that air pollution primarily occurs outdoors. A number of studies have shown, however, that indoor concentrations of some pollutants may be far in excess of outdoor concentrations (7). There is probably no air outdoors that is so polluted as that in a room where people are smoking. In many countries, outdoor air pollution has decreased over the past decades. Furthermore, there is no clear relation between air pollution and the prevalence of allergy. On the contrary, Swedish studies have reported a higher prevalence of allergy in the northern, less polluted part of the country than in the southern, more industrialized parts, which are also more affected by pollution from central Europe (2). The indoor environment, therefore, probably plays an equally large, or even larger, role in the development of allergic sensitization and the appearance of allergic disease in the sensitised individual.

This review discusses some aspects of the genetic and environmental interaction, e.g., that the effects of allergen exposure and nonspecific adjuvants in the environment are particularly important in the genetically susceptible individual, rather than in the general population.

Variations in Susceptibility

The relative risk for allergic disease and the tendency to develop allergic disease early in life are both strongly influenced by genetic factors and a family history of allergic disease. The genetics of atopy, however, is not fully understood. A recent report (8) suggesting that atopy and excessive IgE antibody formation are associated with a gene on the short arm on chromosome 11 has not been confirmed (9, 10). Very recently, an association to chromosome 5 was reported (11). Since atopy is associated with several biochemical and immunological aberrations that could explain parts of the phenotypic expression of allergy, it is perhaps not even reasonable to expect a simple inheritance involving only one or a few genes.

There are a number of immunochemical, biochemical, and clinical tests available for the identification of subjects at high risk of developing allergy (reviewed in 12). Unfortunately, none of the procedures for allergy prediction have both a satisfactory sensitivity *and* specificity. Furthermore, some of the tests are complicated and poorly standardized, and therefore they are not very useful in clinical routine. Presently, the most reliable predictive test for future allergy is the demonstration of IgE antibodies in a clinically healthy infant, either by skin-prick tests or in serum (13). A temporary low-level IgE antibody formation is a normal part of the primary immune response and is commonly seen in healthy infants and children during the first years of life (14) against common allergens. In atopic individuals, however, the duration of the IgE antibody formation is often long and the levels are high.

An individual's likelihood of developing allergic disease is not constant over time, even if the general propensity is genetically determined. Thus, the risk of sensitization is affected by the time for, and the conditions under which, exposure to allergens takes place. There seems to be a period in early life during which an infant is particularly susceptible to sensitization (summarized in 4 and 15). A higher incidence of allergy to birch and grass pollen has thus been reported in children born in the spring (16). This relationship between season of birth and development of allergy seems to be limited to children with a congenital propensity to develop allergic disease (17). Similarly, early feeding with foreign proteins is associated with an increased risk for allergic disease, but mostly so in genetically susceptible individuals (18).

Variations in individual susceptibility to sensitization over time may also partly be explained by respiratory tract infection, as sensitization occurs more easily during an infection (19).

Nonspecific, Environmental Factors ("Adjuvants")

Various environmental factors may enhance sensitization and also trigger an allergic reaction in a sensitized individual (Table 1). While allergy is rare to most of the compounds listed in the table, they do play a role both in the sensitization process and in the appearance of clinical symptoms. It is not

Table 1. Adjuvant factors thought to be involved either in sensitization or manifestations of allergic disease.

Air pollution and sources:
  Tobacco smoke
  Industry and traffic; solid particles, SO_2, NOx
  Combustion by-products; CO_2, CO, SO_2, NO_2, NO, formaldehyde, volatile vapours
  Photochemical reactions; ozone, NO_2
Building materials; formaldehyde, decoration and paints; solvents, furnishings
Tight, poorly ventilated homes
Pesticides and consumer products; organic substances, aerosols
Respiratory tract infections; viral, pertussis
Ongoing allergic reaction (facilitates sensitisation to new allergens)

entirely clear exactly how these adjuvants act. Possibly, an inflammatory reaction is induced in the airways which facilitates the penetration of allergens or enhances antigen presentation.

Three studies of individuals belonging to the same ethnic group but living under different conditions clearly demonstrate that the incidence of allergic disease is higher in industrialized countries than in rural areas of developing countries (20, 21). Such environmental differences are also present in industrialized countries, i.e., between urban and rural areas. As an example, the relative risk for a positive skin-prick test is 70% higher among 11-year-old children living in a moderately polluted town in northern Sweden than among children living in the neighbouring countryside (22).

Passive smoking is by far the best identified risk factor for the development of allergic disease. This is particularly true in early childhood – independent of how "allergy" is defined. Numerous epidemiological studies demonstrate an association between exposure to tobacco smoke and recurrent wheezing (summarized in 4), bronchial hyperreactivity, as well as a diagnosis of asthma. An association between passive smoking and an increased risk for sensitization to environmental allergens has also been demonstrated, both in clinical studies and in animal experiments. There is little doubt that exposure to tobacco smoke is the most important environmental risk factor for childhood allergy and respiratory disease identified so far. The long-term effects of childhood exposure to tobacco smoke are unknown.

Modern, well-insulated houses have been associated with an increased risk for the development of allergic manifestations, as well as with sensitization. In temperate climates, where house dust mites used to be scarce, the increased humidity in modern energy-saving homes has resulted in an increase prevalence of mite allergy. In a large epidemiological study, comprising 5300 children living in a defined geographical area, it was found that living near an air-polluting paper pulp plant, living in homes with a dampness problem, and having smoking parents were all strong risk factors for allergic disease (23). This relationship was particularly pronounced in children with a family history of allergy. Children living in a house with dampness problems and having smoking parents had an increased prevalence of asthma compared to children not exposed to these risk factors. This was particularly obvious in children with a family history of allergy, in whom 22% had manifest asthma if exposed to the two risk factors (Figure 2).

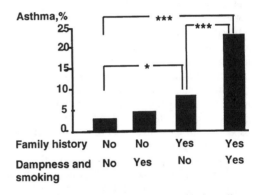

Figure 2. Exposure to tobacco smoke and indoor climate (living in tight buildings with a dampness problem) as risk factors for childhood asthma in children with and without a family history of allergy. The proportion of children in each group who developed asthma is shown.

An understanding of the role of environmental factors has been complicated by some recent observations. Air pollution is a major problem in many formerly socialist countries in central and Eastern Europe, yet the prevalence of atopy among children is much lower than in Western Europe. As an example, the prevalence of positive skin-prick tests in Leipzig in former East Germany is less than half of that among children of the same age living in Munich in West Germany (24). Similarly, atopic sensitization is much lower in Konin in central Poland (25) and in Estonia than in northern Sweden. Mirroring the observed differences in

Table 2. Prevalence of positive skin prick tests among 11–12 year old school children in five locations in the Baltic Sea region.

| | Sundsvall, Sweden | | Poland | Estonia | |
	Rural	Urban	Konin	Tallinn	Tartu
n	289	351	358	597	637
≥1 pos SPT, %	24.2	35.3	13.7	12.9	8.3
crude OR	1	1.71	0.49	0.46*	0.28*
95% CI		1.2–2.4	0.3–0.7	0.3–0.7	0.2–0.4

Odds ratio for a positive skin prick test in Tallinn (coastal, industrialized town), as compared to Tartu (university town) was 1.81.

skin-prick test positivity in an urban and rural area of Sweden, the prevalence of at least one positive skin-prick test was significantly higher in Tallinn, an industrialized coastal city than in Tartu, which is an inland university town (Table 2). Thus, although air pollution does seem to play a role in the development of atopy, other factors connected with Western lifestyle prove to be much more important. The nature of these factors is unknown.

In addition to the introduction of many new chemicals into the environment, there have been many changes in lifestyle in industrialized countries over the past decades. The type of foods eaten has changed dramatically with the introduction of new industrial products with numerous additives. Even fresh food items differ in many respects from those available only a few decades ago. As an example, through genetic manipulation and use of various chemical compounds, the storage time of food has been much prolonged, often allowing a shelf life of months (e. g., apples). Virtually nothing is known regarding the possible influence on childhood allergy of such changes in the diet.

Psychological factors may also influence the immune system. As an example, family interaction is often disturbed in the families of asthmatic children, with family therapy improving the asthma. A recent prospective study addressed the question whether the disturbed family interaction is a primary finding or a consequence of disease (26). The study included the families of 100 infants with a strong family history of allergy. The entire family participated in a standardized family test when the children were 3 and 18 months old, assessing ability to adapt to changing circumstances ("adaptability") and the balance between emotional closeness and distance ("cohesion"). An unbalanced family interplay was common at 3 months (37%), though it was not predictive for respiratory illness.

At 18 months, a dysfunctional interaction was significantly more common in families of children with eczema and obstructive symptoms, as compared to families of healthy children. The study indicates that a dysfunctional family interaction is the result, rather than a cause of recurrent wheezing in infancy.

The role of infections, notably in the respiratory tract, as risk factors for the development of childhood allergic disease is complex. An infection induces an inflammatory reaction in the respiratory mucosa, which in turn modifies the local immune response. To what extent this enhances sensitization to inhaled allergens is not fully understood, although there are studies indicating that this is the case for at least some viruses, notably respiratory syncytial virus. Animal experiments support the clinical observations, showing an enhanced IgE production after allergen exposure and concomitant viral infection. Also, it is common knowledge that infections may trigger clinical symptoms in already sensitized individuals, and that infections increase bronchial hyperreactivity.

The relationship between bronchiolitis caused by respiratory syncytial virus (RSV) during the first 6 months of life and the development of asthma was recently studied prospectively in 47 infants (27). Two matched controls were selected for each child, making a study population of 140 participants in the follow-up at 3 years. Asthma, defined as three episodes of bronchial obstruction verified by a physician, was found in 11 of the 47 children with RSV bronchiolitis (23%) and in only one of 93 controls. A positive test for IgE antibodies against a mixture of allergens were recorded in 32% of the RSV children and 9% of the controls (p = 0.02). Of particular interest was the observation that among the former, 6 of the 11 children with a family history of allergy developed asthma, compared to only 5 of 36 without such a history. Thus, the risk for asthma after RSV bronchiolitis was much higher in infants with a genetic propensity to allergy.

As summarized in (4), *Bordetella pertussis* is of particular interest among the infectious agents, as it is a well-established adjuvant for the induction of IgE antibody formation in experimental animals. Furthermore, whooping cough is associated with bronchial hyperreactivity for several months. It has also been shown that IgE antibodies to pertussis toxin appear after an infection and after immunization against pertussis. The latter observation raises the question about a possible role of vaccinations as a risk factor for allergic disease. This notion is further strengthened by the fact that aluminum, which is used as an adjuvant in many vaccines, is also one of the most potent adjuvants for IgE antibody synthesis in animals. Properly designed epidemiological studies are needed to clarify a possible relationship between routine immunizations of infants and the development of atopic disease.

Pre- and Postnatal Risk Factors

During fetal life and infancy there is a close immunological interaction between the mother and her offspring, through the placenta and the breast milk. Relatively little is known about the exchange of immunological information (28). Very recently we found that elevated levels of IgG anti-IgE antibodies in the cord blood were associated with less allergy during the first 18 months of life (29). This was particularly obvious in babies with a strong family history of allergy (Figure 3). This finding and reported individual variations in the composition of human milk would indicate that maternal immunity may be an important environmental factor influencing the risk for allergic manifestations in her child, even many years later.

Since some newborn babies who will later develop allergic disease can be identified already at birth by an elevated level of IgE in cord blood, the question has been raised whether sensitization may take place already during fetal life. This is, however, only rarely the case. The IgE antibodies in cord serum seem more to be the consequence of nonspecific spontaneous IgE synthesis, perhaps lack of suppression, than of antigen stimulation. This notion would be supported by the negative outcome of randomized studies of the manipulation of maternal diet during pregnancy (30). On the

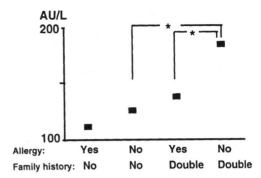

Figure 3. Levels of IgG anti-IgE antibodies in cord blood in relation to development of allergic disease in infants with and without a strong (at least two affected members of the immediate family) family history of allergy.

other hand, there have been some recent studies in which antigen-specific T-cell responses were recorded in cord blood. These studies, however, did not control for several alternative possibilities, so that they are not conclusive. The possible role of intrauterine sensitization therefore remains an open question.

It has also been suggested that perinatal stress factors could represent environmental influences that would increase the risk for later appearing allergic disease. These studies (summarized in 3) were retrospective, however, and did not control for various other possibilities. In unpublished studies, we have not seen any indication for prematurity as a risk factor for atopic sensitization.

There has been much interest over the past 10 years regarding the possibility of preventing allergic disease, notably asthma, by avoiding primary sensitization in early life. The efforts have focused on various allergen-avoidance procedures, including administration of infant formulae with reduced allergen content.

The original hypothesis for allergy prevention was that allergic disease could be avoided by preventing the onset of the "allergic march" in early infancy. Thus, by preventing the development of food allergy and eczema in early life, the later onset of asthma and then allergic rhinoconjunctivitis would be avoided. Recent prospective studies of infants with a genetic propensity toward allergic disease have not confirmed this hypothesis. In these studies, exposure of infants to allergenic foods during the first months of life, notably cow milk and egg, was avoided (30); the mothers of breast-fed babies adhered to a diet free of cow milk, egg, and certain other allergenic foods, and any supplementary feeding of the babies was in the form of extensively hydrolyzed products with low allergenicity. The dietary manipulation of breast feeding mothers and infants was associated with a lower incidence of allergic manifestations and demonstrable IgE antibodies to foods. The effect, however, was limited to the first, or possibly second, year of life and to eczema, while the incidence of respiratory symptoms and allergic manifestations appearing later were not affected. The results are not surprising in light of the more recent knowledge concerning the primary sensitization, showing that the effects of avoidance of exposure to allergens during the period of particular susceptibility in early life is antigen specific (15). Thus, dietary restrictions would not be expected to have an effect on sensitization to inhaled allergens, nor to reduce the incidence of sensitization to food antigens not avoided.

Address for correspondence:

Bengt Björkstén
Department of Paediatrics
Faculty of Health Sciences
University Hospital
S-581 85 Linköping
Sweden

References

1. Burney PG, Chinn S, Rona RJ. Has the prevalence of asthma increased in children? Evidence from the national study of health and growth 1973–86. *Brit Med J* 1990; 300:1306–10.

2. Åberg N. Asthma and allergic rhinitis in Swedish conscripts. *Clin Exp Allergy* 1989; 19:59–63.

3. Björkstén B, Kjellman, N-I. Perinatal environmental factors influencing the development of allergy. *Clin Exp Allergy* 1990; 20:3–8.

4. Björkstén B. Risk factors in early childhood for the development of atopic diseases. *Allergy* 1994; 49:400–407.

5. Wickman M, Nordvall SL, Pershagen G, Sundell J, Schwartz, B. House dust mite sensitization in children and residential characteristics in a temperate region. *J Allergy Clin Immunol* 1991; 88:89–95.

6. Munir AKM, Björkstén B, Einarsson R, Ekstrand-Tobin A, Warner A, Kjellman, N-IM. Environmental influence on mite allergens in homes of asthmatic children. *J Allergy Clin Immunol* 1994;

7. Munir AKM, Björkstén B. Indoor air pollution and allergic sensitization. In H Knöppel and P Wolkoff (Eds) *Chemical microbiological health and comfort. Aspects of indoor air quality.* Brussels: ECSC, EEC, 1992, 181–199.

8. Young RP, Sharp PA, Lynch JR, Faux JA, Lathrop GM, Cookson WO, Hopkin, JM. Confirmation of genetic linkage between atopic IgE responses and chromosome 11q13. *J Med Genet* 1992; 29:236–8.

9. Amelung P, Panhuysen C, Postma, D. Atopy and bronchial hyperresponsiveness. Exclusion of linkage of markers on chromosome 11q and 6p. *Clin Exp Allergy* 1992; 22:1077–1084.

10. Rich S, Roitman-Johnson B, Breenberg B, Roberts S, Blumenthal M. Genetic analysis of atopy in three large kindreds: no evidence of genetic linkage to D11S97. *Clin Exp Allergy* 1992; 22:1070–1076.

11. Marsh DG, Neely JD, Breazeale DR, Ghosh B, Freidhoff LR, Ehrlich-Kautzky E, Schon L, Krishnaswamy G, Blaty TH. Linkage analysis of IL-4 and other chromosome 5g 31.1 markers and total serum immunglobulin E concentrations. *Science* 1994; 264: 1152–1156.

12. Kjellman N-IM, Croner S, Fälth Magnusson K, Odelram H, Björkstén, B. Prediction of allergy in infancy. *Allergy Proc* 1991; 12:245–9.

13. Kjellman N-IM. IgE determinations in neonates is not suitable for general screening. *Pediatr Allergy Immunol* 1994; 5:1–4.

14. Hattevig G, Kjellman B, Björkstén B. Appearance of IgE antibodies to ingested and inhaled allergens during the first 12 years of life in atopic and nonatopic children. *Pediatr Allergy Immunol* 1993; 4:110–117.

15. Holt P, McMenamin C, Nelson D. Primary sensitization to inhalant allergens during infancy. *Pediatr Allergy Immunol* 1990; 1:3–13.

16. Björkstén F, Suoniemi I. Time and intensity of first pollen contacts and risk of subsequent pollen allergies. *Acta Med Scand* 1981; 209:299–303.

17. Croner S, Kjellman, N-IM. Predictors of atopic disease: cord blood IgE and month of birth. *Allergy* 1986; 41:68–70.

18. Björkstén B. Does breast feeding prevent the development of allergy? *Immunol Today* 1983; 4:215–217.

19. Frick OL, German DF, Mills J. Development of allergy in children. 1. Association with virus infections. *J Allergy Clin Immunol* 1979; 63:228–241.

20. Asseyr A, Botan A, Ziruolo M, Businco L. Atopic dermatitis and breast feeding of Somali children living in Somalia and in Italy. *Pediatr Allergy Immunol* 1991; 2:141–143.

21. Waite D, Eyles E, Tonkin S, O'Donnell T. Asthma

prevalence in Tokelauan children in two environments. *Clin Allergy* 1980; 10:71–75.

22. Bråbäck L, Kälvesten L. Urban living as a risk factor for atopic sensitization in Swedish school children. *Pediatr Allergy Immunol* 1991; 2:14–19.

23. Andrae S, Axelson O, Björkstén B, Fredriksson M, Kjellman N-IM. Symptoms of bronchial hyperreactivity and asthma in relation to environmental factors. *Arch Dis Child* 1988; 63:473–8.

24. von Mutius E, Martinez F, Fritzsch C, Nicolai T, Thiemann H. Difference in the prevalence of asthma between east and west Germany: The role of atopic sensitization. *Eur Resp J* 1993; 6 (Suppl)17:224s.

25. Bråbäck L, Breborowicz A, Dreborg S, Knutsson A, Pieklik H, Björkstén B. Atopic sensitization and respiratory symptoms among Polish and Swedish schoolchildren. *Clin Exp Allergy.*

26. Gustafsson PA, Björkstén B, Kjellman N-IM. Family dysfunction in asthma – A prospective study of illness development. *J Pediatrics* 1994, in press.

27. Sigurs N, Bjarnason R, Sigurbergsson F, Kjellman B, Björkstén B. Asthma and IgE antibodies after respiratory syncytial virus bronchiolitis: a prospective cohort study with matched controls. *Pediatrics* 1994, in press.

28. Duchén K, Björkstén B. Sensitization via the breast milk. In J Mestecky (Ed) *Immunology of milk and the neonate.* New York: Plenum Press, 1991, 427–436.

29. Vassella C, Odelram H, Kjellman N-IM, Borres M, Vanto T, Björkstén B. High anti-IgE levels at birth are associated with a reduced allergy incidence in early childhood. *Clin Exp Allergy* 1994.

30. Businco L, Dreborg S, Einarsson R, Giampietro G, Høst A, Keller K, Strobel S, Wahn U, Björkstén B, Kjellman N-IM, Sampson H, Zeiger RN. Hydrolysed cow's milk formulae. Allergenicity and use in treatment and prevention. An ESPACI position paper. *Pediatr Allergy Immunol* 1993; 4:101–11.

Occupational Asthma

Anthony J Newman Taylor*

Keywords: Asthma, occupation, environment

Occupational asthma is now the single most commonly reported cause of new cases of occupational lung disease in United Kingdom, with an estimated annual incidence of hypersensitivity induced induced occupational asthma of some 1500 cases per annum. Isocyanates are the single most frequent reported cause accounting for some 22% of cases.

Investigation of working populations exposed to causes of occupational asthma, including enzymes, laboratory animals, acid anhydrides and platinum salts, have shown that sensitisation and asthma occur primarily during the first 1–2 years of exposure, and their induction during this period is dependant on intensity of exposure, modified by atopy and tobacco smoking. A study in Barcelona corroborated these findings, identifying the same factors as determinants of epidemic asthma caused by community exposure to soya bean.

The HLA haplotype DR3 is closely associated with induction of specific IgE in those exposed to trimellitic and possibly tetrachlorophthalic but not phthalic anhydrides.

Nature of Occupational Asthma

Occupational asthma is asthma induced by an agent inhaled at work. The defining clinical characteristics of asthma – variable airflow limitation and airway hyper-responsiveness – which distinguish it from other less reversible causes of airflow limitation are believed to be manifestations of a characteristic pattern of airway inflammation – desquamative eosinophilic bronchitis. Agents inhaled at work can induce airway inflammation and initiate asthma by causing toxic damage to the airway epithelium (irritant inducers) or as the outcome of a specific hypersensitivity response (hypersensitivity inducers).

Irritant inducers are respiratory irritants such as chlorine, sulphur dioxide and ammonia which, when inhaled in sufficient concentration, cause airway injury and inflammation by a direct toxic action. *Hypersensitivity inducers* include inhaled proteins (such as animal excreta, flour and enzymes) other complex biological molecules (such as wood resin acids and microbe derived antibiotics) and low molecular weight chemicals (such as isocyanates and acid anhydrides) which bind covalently to proteins to form hapten-protein conjugates. Airway inflammation occurs as the outcome of a specific hypersensitivity (probably immune dependent) response. Irritant induced asthma (or reactive airways dysfunction syndrome, ARDS) has no latent interval between irritant inhalation and the development of asthma, which occurs within hours of exposure; a latent interval of months or years is characteristic of hypersensitivity induced asthma.

Although the subject of increasing interest, irritant induced asthma is a considerably less reported cause of occupational asthma and to date the subject of less investigative interest. This paper will focus on hypersensitivity induced occupational asthma which is the cause of the great majority of reported cases and has been the subject of considerable research interest. Indeed, the term occupational asthma has been defined in United Kingdom for the purposes of statutory compensation as "asthma induced by sensitisation to an agent inhaled at work."

Causes of Hypersensitivity-Induced Occupational Asthma

Some of the more important causes of occupational asthma are shown in Table 1. The proteins and complex biological molecules may be encountered in a wide variety of circumstances which include agriculture; storage and transport of vegetable

* National Heart & Lung Institute, London, UK.

crops; food production; forestry; carpentry; the use of laboratory animals; and the commercial exploitation of microbes as sources of food, antibiotics and enzymes. Isocyanates are used in the manufacture of rigid and flexible foams, inks, adhesives, varnishes and paints. Acid anhydrides are used as curing agents for epoxy and alkyd resins. Complex platinum salts are essential intermediates in platinum refining and reactive dyes are used to bind a colour (chromophore) covalently to textiles.

Table 1. Some agents responsible for "hypersensitivity-induced" occupational asthma.

	Proteins	Low molecular weight chemicals
Animal	Excreta of rats, mice etc.; locusts, grain mites	
Vegetable	grain/flour castor bean green coffee bean ispaghula latex	plicatic acid (Western red cedar) colophony (pinewood resin)
Microbial	harvest moulds	antibiotics, e. g., penicillins, cephalosporins
"Mineral"		acid anhydrides isocyanates complex platinum salts polyamines reactive dyes

The SWORD (Surveillance of Work and Occupational Respiratory Diseases) scheme, to which the great majority of respiratory and occupational physicians in the United Kingdom report *new* cases of occupational lung disease, has provided information about the relative important of occupational asthma and its causes and has allowed estimation of the incidence of the disease in different occupational groups. The estimated incidence of new cases of occupational lung disease in 1992 was around 3500 (1). Asthma, which accounted for 28% of cases, was the single most frequent diagnostic category. Isocyanates have been consistently the most frequently reported agent, accounting for 22% of cases; flour/grain dust, wood dust, solder flux and laboratory animals together accounted for a similar proportion (22%). The overall annual incidence was $22/10^6$ working population. The occupational groups with the highest incidence were coach and other spray painters ($658/10^6$/year), chemical processors ($364/10^6$/ year), plastic workers ($337/10^6$/year) and bakers ($334/10^6$/year).

By comparison, the incidence of occupational asthma in Finland as reported to a register of occupational disease was some six times higher than the rate reported to SWORD in the United Kingdom (2). This was probably due at least in part to more complete case ascertainment through all physicians and not only specialists as in the UK. The most common cause of occupational asthma in Finland was allergy to cow epithelium, a reflection of the greater proportion employed in agriculture and with animal contact; similarly, the incidence of allergic alveolitis was several times higher in Finland than the UK.

Determinants of Hypersensitivity Induced Occupational Asthma

Three major factors have been identified as contributing to the development of occupational asthma in working populations exposed to its causes: exposure, atopy and tobacco smoking. The contribution of HLA haplotype has also recently been investigated.

Exposure

Although the factor most directly amenable to control, exposure has to date received less attention than atopy and smoking as a determinant of occupational sensitisation and asthma. Nonetheless, several studies, both of incidence and prevalence of sensitisation and of asthma measured as work related respiratory symptoms or measurable airway hyper-responsiveness or both), have found evidence for an exposure-response gradient. The development of skin test reactions in enzyme detergent works to *B. subtilis* enzyme primarily occurred during the first two years of exposure, with the highest incidence amongst those most heavily exposed (3). In a study of manufacturers of the pharmaceutical cimetidine Coutts et al. found the prevalence of work related nasal and lower respiratory symptoms increased with increasing frequency of exposure to cimetidine at work (4). In a study of bakery workers, the prevalence of work related respiratory symptoms and airway hyper-responsiveness was greatest among those who had ever worked in the dustiest conditions (5), and a gradient of work related respiratory symptoms was found in relation to measured airborne colophony in a workforce involved in soft solder manufacture (6). A recent study of laboratory animal workers has found a gradient of both new work related nose, chest and skin symptoms, and of skin test reactions to rat urine protein in relation to measured airborne rat urine protein concentrations (7).

Atopy

Atopy, usually defined in immunological terms as one or more skin test reactions to common inhalant allergens (which in the UK would include grass pollen, *D. pteronyssinus* and cat fur) has been found to be associated with an increased frequency of sensitisation and asthma caused by several agents, notably laboratory animals, enzymes and platinum salts. Several studies have found asthma to be some five times more common in atopic than non-atopic laboratory animal workers (8, 9). The incidence of skin test reactions was greater in atopic individuals to *Alcalase* in enzyme detergent workers in each category of exposure (3) and to the complex platinum salt ammonium hexachloroplatinate in platinum refinery workers (10). On the other hand, for several of its causes, such as isocyanates, colophony and plicatic acid, occupational asthma occurs no more frequently among atopics than non-atopics.

HLA Haplotype

One case-referent study has examined the relationship between HLA haplotype and the development of specific IgE to acid anhydrides. A significant excess of HLADR3 was found among cases with IgE to trimellitic anhydride and possibly also to tetrachlorophthalic anhydride (TCPA), but not phthalic anhydride (11). Studies of possible HLA associations need to be extended both to other occupational allergens to determine their inter-relationship between HLA haplotype, exposure and other risk factors such as atopy and smoking.

Tobacco Smoking

Tobacco smoking is associated with an increased risk of specific IgE and asthma in those exposed to several, but not all, of the causes of occupational asthma. Specific IgE either measured in serum or inferred from an immediate skin test response has been found some four to five times more frequently in smokers than non-smokers exposed to TCPA (12), green coffee bean and ispaghula (13), and ammonium hexachloroplatinate (14). The risk of developing asthma is also increased, although less among smokers: all seven cases of asthma caused by TCPA in one factory outbreak were smokers (15) and the risk of asthma in a platinum refinery (14) and snow crab processing workers (16) was some twofold greater in smokers than non-smokers.

Comparison of Occupational with Community Acquired Asthma

The important risk factors for the development of occupational asthma identified to date are intensity of exposure and for agents, such as rat urine proteins, complex platinum salts and acid anhydrides, which are associated with the development of specific IgE antibody, atopy and smoking. The asthma epidemic in the city of Barcelona which was caused by allergy to soya beans disseminated from the harbour provided an opportunity to determine whether similar risk factors were important in community acquired asthma caused, as with occupational asthma, by exposure to a single sensitising agent. The risk factors identified were proximity to the harbour (a surrogate for intensity of exposure), atopy and smoking (17) (Table 2), consistent with those observed in occupational asthma caused by laboratory animals (7) and acid anhydrides (12).

Table 2. Odds ratio for Barcelona epidemic asthma cases.

Soybean exposure*	SPT	Odds ratio Non-smokers	Smokers
> 4 km	−	1.0	1.5
≤ 4 km	−	1.4	2.9
> 4 km	+	2.4	3.2
≥ 4 km	+	2.8	7.9

* Distance of home or workplace from harbour. After Sunyer et al. 1992 (17)

Address for correspondence:

Prof Anthony J Newman Taylor
OBE FRCP FFOM
National Heart & Lung Institute
1 b Manresa Road
London SW3 6LR
UK

References

1. Sallie BA, Ross DJ, Meredith SK, McDonald JC. SWORD'93. Surveillance of work-related and occupational respiratory disease in the UK. *Occup Med* 1994; (in press).

2. Keskinen H. Registers for occupational disease. *Br Med J* 1991; 303:597–598.

3. Juniper CP, How MJ, Goodwin BFJ, Kinshott AK. Bacillus subtulis enzymes: A seven year clinical epidemiological and immunological study of an industrial allergen. *J Soc Occ Med* 1977; 27:3–12.

4. Coutts II, Lozewicz S, Dally MD, Newman Taylor AJ, Burge PS, Flynd AC, Rodgers DJH. Respiratory symptoms related to work in a factory manufacturing cimetidine tablets. *Br Med J* 1984; 288:14–18.

5. Musk AW, Venables KM, Crook B, Nunn AJ, Hawkins R, Crook GDW, Graneek BJ, Tee RD, Farrer N, Johnston DA, Gordon DJ, Darbyshire JH, Newman Taylor AJ. Respiratory symptoms, lung function and sensitisation to flour in a british bakery.*Br J Ind Med* 1989; 46:636–642.

6. Burge PS, Edge G, Hawkins ER, White V, Newman Taylor AJ. Occupational asthma is a factory making flux cord solder containing colophony. *Thorax* 1981; 86:828–834.

7. Cullinan P, Lowson D. Nieuwenhuijsen M et al. Work-relation symptoms, sensitisation and estimated exposure in workers not previously exposed to laboratory animals. *Occup Env Med* 1994; (in press).

8. Slovak AJM, Hill RN. Laboratory animal allergy: A clinical survey of an exposed population. *Br J Ind Med* 1981; 38:38–41.

9. Venables KM, Tee RD, Hawkins ER, Gordon DJ, Wale CJ, Farrer NM, Lam TH, Baxter PJ, Newman Taylor AJ. Laboratory animal allergy in a pharmaceutical company. *Br J Ind Med* 1988; 455:660–666.

10. Dally MD, Hunter JV, Hughes EG, Stewart M, Newman Taylor AJ. Hypersensitivity to platinum salts: A population study. *Am Rev Respir Dis* 1980; 121:230 a.

11. Young RP, Barker RD, Pile KD, Cookson WOCM, Newman Taylor. The association of HLA-DR3 with specific IgE to inhaled acid anhydrides. *Am J Respir Crit Care Med* 1994; (in press).

12. Venables KM, Topping MD, Howe W, Luczynska CM, Hawkins R, Newman Taylor AJ. Interaction of smoking and atopy in producing specific IgE antibody against a hapten protein conjugate. *Br Med J* 1985; 290:201–204.

13. Zetterstrom O, Osterman K, Machado L, Johannson SGO. Another smoking hazard reused serum IgE concentrations and increased risk of occupational allergy. *Br Med J* 1991; 283:1215–1217.

14. Venables KM, Dally MB, Nunn AJ, Stevens JF, Stephens R, Farrer N, Hunter JV, Stewart M, Hughes EG, Newman Taylor AJ. Smoking and occupational allergy in a platinum refinery. *Br Med J* 1989; 299:939–942.

15. Howe W, Venables KM, Topping MD, Dally MD, Hawkins ER, Law SJ, Newman Taylor AJ. 1983 Tetrachlorophthalic anhydride asthma: evidence for specific IgE antibody. *J Allergy Clin Immunol* 71:5–11.

16. Cartier A, Malo JL, Forrest F et al. Occupational asthma in snow-crab processing workers. *J Allergy Clin Immunol* 1984; 74:261–269.

17. Sunyer J, Anto JM, Sabria J, Rodrigo MJ, Roca J, Morell F, Rodriguez-Roisin, Codina R. Risk factors of soybean epidemic asthma. *Am Rev Respir Dis* 1992; 145:1098–1102.

Overview of Therapeutic Strategies in Allergy and Bronchial Asthma

A Oehling*

Keywords: Bronchial asthma, therapy overview, allergy

For those of us who for almost 40 years have been treating allergic and asthmatic patients, it has been with satisfaction that we have been able to watch the progress of therapy. As far as treatment of the allergic response is concerned, it is during the two last decades that substances able to inhibit allergic response at the cell membrane level have appeared. Sodium chromoglycate, Ketotifen, and more recently Nedochromil stand out. We have already showed how Ketotifen was able in *in vitro* tests to increase methyltransferase activity, at the same time avoiding the antigen-antibody reaction taking place on the cellular membrane, and so inhibiting the delivery of mediators (1).

It is very important to remember when using these drugs that they are innocuous substances, with no toxic effects on the different organs or systems. On the other hand, we must highlight the new third generation antihistamines, which have been bringing much greater efficacy than the antihistamines of the first and second generations, with hardly any secondary effects, in the treatment of allergic diseases as well as atopic asthma. We consider that substances such as Cetirizine, Terfenadine, and Loratidine have a very important part to play in the treatment of pollinosis, urticaria, etc.

Other contributions here are dealing with new topics in the therapy of allergic diseases and asthma. Here, I would like to summarize an aspect which seems really worrying to me, related to the therapeutic strategy in bronchial asthma.

Faced with any disease, a physician feels it is his ethical duty to analyze the usefulness and the risk of any treatment he starts with the patient, who puts all his trust and faith in the physician's professionalism. That is why the therapeutic approach must not only consider the symptoms and the appropriate treatment to get rid of them, but must also look at the causal or etiopathogenic factors. Thus, on one hand, the use of drugs to inhibit the asthmatic response are needed and, on the other, from the causal point of view, we should start a therapy and prophylaxis that will at the same time inhibit the causal factor or factors.

In general, the primary care for the asthmatic patient consists of eliminating the cardinal symptom of asphyxia or dyspnea. Preferable here is the use of broncholytics and anti-inflammatory drugs. Nevertheless, if we consider the basic elements of the asthmatic reaction (Table 1), we find that there

Table 1. Targets in bronchial asthma treatment.

Bronchoconstriction	Bronchodilators
Inflammation	Corticosteroids
Obstruction	Mucolytics
Infection	Antibiotics

are four basic points to examine in the asthmatic patient: bronchoconstriction, inflammation, obstruction, and infection. Of course, in genuine atopic asthma, infection should theoretically not be relevant, and so it is often not considered further. However, in a high percentage of patients (in our experience and that of many other authors, from 60 to 80%) the infection should in fact take all our attention (2, 3) (Figures 1 and 2).

It is precisely in these regards that the progress of therapy has not, in my opinion, gone down the best road, since not all factors are considered in the treatment of bronchial asthma.

*   Departamento de Alergologia e Inmunologia Clinica, Clinica Universitaria, Facultad de Medicina, Universidad de Navarra.

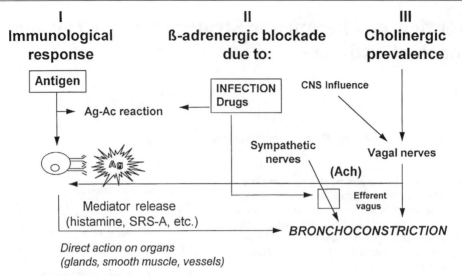

Figure 1. Mechanisms of bronchial hyperreactivity.

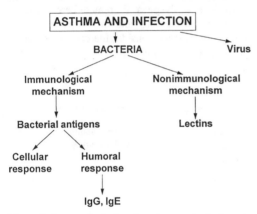

Figure 2. Immunological and nonimmunological mechanisms in infectious asthma.

In the following, I comment briefly on each one of these aspects.

Bronchoconstriction

Logically, since the main aim is to eliminate the most important symptom that is oppressing the patient as soon as possible, i. e., the dyspnea or asthma, the use or broncholytics is the first step. Theophyline, Salbutamol, Salmeterol, etc., are the most common, and they provide useful help. Their administration will always be needed as long as the causal factor is not eliminated. Therefore, treatment lasting months or years will indicate the impossibility of eliminating the cause. Of course, I am not referring here to very exceptional cases of extreme bronchial hyperactivity.

Inflammation

Anti-inflammatory therapy can act in parallel to broncholytics. Here, the best drugs are the corticosteroids, from prednisolone with 5 anti-inflammatory units, to betametasone, with 35 anti-inflammatory units. Once the acute inflammation phase is over, the use of other corticosteroids such as Budesonide, Beclometasone, administered in aerosol form, can be considered. However, nowadays we are seeing how, once the cardinal clinical problem is solved, many doctors pay no attention to the causal factors. "Asthma maintenance" and a long, excessive, and unnecessary corticoid treatment result. It has been during recent years since different corticoid preparations in aerosol form appeared that this tendency to "asthma maintenance" has increased. The pharmaceutical industry and thankful speakers tell us of the excellent results of using corticosteroids in aerosol form, orally, over long periods, but do not take into account the secondary effects of these, and there is no control of the suprarenal activity. That is, the high percentage of suprarenal insufficiency and many other secondary effects are overlooked, generating a "drug iatrogenia." On the other hand, we must consider that the inhaled corticosteroids are usually deposited mainly in the central airways, normalizing the lung function (4). Nevertheless, it seems that in the peripheral airways they do not inhibit the inflammation and the epithelial damage enough, and this could produce irreversible chronic lung disease (5). With all this I am only reflecting what we see day after day in the clinic.

Obstruction

The problem raised by the discrinia with the consequent worsening and accumulation of mucous secretion is often forgotten, not taking into account the actions of mucolytics such as Bromexine, Ambroxol, and others in making fluid, thus facilitating the expulsion of mucous and decreasing the obstruction. This aspect is sufficiently well known for me not to continue further.

Infection

It is here, in fact, where the biggest mistakes are being made. As mentioned above, infection is not important in atopic asthma, but in the remaining cases it plays an important role, existing at the same time as sinupathy and the rhinosinubronchial syndrome. Many authors, including Norn (6) and others, have emphasized in recent years the importance of this factor (Figure 3), as it forms part of the vicious circle of the breathing limitation. According to Wilson, the best way of breaking this circle is antibiotic treatment. That is the reason why for many years we have repeatedly asked the question: Where does long-term treatment with broncholytics and corticosteroids lead us, if we do not eliminate the infectious agent, which is well kept in the upper or lower airways, in a more or less larval way, and will lead to an asthmatic crisis if it becomes acute again? (Figure 4)

The persistent infection of the airways leads to a lesion of the bronchiolar tissue, which in turn leads to a decrease in mucociliary clearance and to the maintenance of the inflammatory response. This vicious circle leads to the insidious progression of the respiratory problems. Chronic bronchitis resolves with the corresponding asthmatization. To break this vicious circle, it is absolutely necessary to use

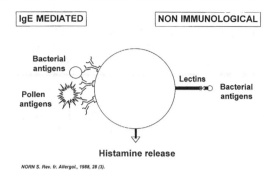

NORN S. Rev. fr. Allergol., 1988, 28 (3).

Figure 3. Role of bacterial antigens and lectins in the asthmatic reaction.

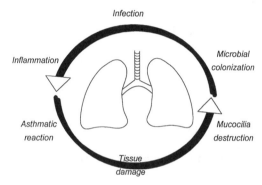

Figure 4. The vicious circle in the asthmatic reaction.

antibiotics, if possible wide spectrum ones, such as the modern macrolids, which are more efficient than the betalactamides. Ciprofloxacine, quinolone, and the macrolids Roxitromicine and Claritromicine, and more recently Ceftibuten, should be considered. Logically, the ideal would be to give antibiotic therapy after seeing the antibiogram of the sputum culture, which would give some indication of the most suitable antibiotic.

In this overview of therapeutic strategy, I would like to again emphasize an aspect that in our experience, and in that of many other authors, continues being completely ignored, thus contributing not to healing asthmatic people, but rather to keeping them asthmatic: infection. More attention must be paid to infection. We consider irresponsible to create an international consensus on the treatment of asthma following one-sided criteria, and not taking into account an etiopathogenic factor that can clearly be influenced.

I am absolutely convinced that the new drugs in the fight against bronchospasm and inflammation

111

will contribute greatly to the treatment of allergic diseases and asthma. According to the studies we have been doing over recent years on the control of immunotherapy by means of immunologic parameters, we are absolutely convinced of the benefits of such treatment, as long as it is done for more than three years (7). However, I insist that we must not forget that the most important phase in the treatment of these diseases is the etiologic factor.

Address for correspondence:

A Oehling
Departamento de Alergologia e
Inmunologia Clinica
Clinica Universitaria, Facultad de Medicina
Universidad de Navarra
Apartado 4209
E-31080 Pamplona
Spain

References

1. Castillo JG, Gamboa PM, Santos F, Oehling A. Effect of ketotifen on the methyltransferase activity of asthmatic patients. *Allergol Immunopathol* 1990; 18/5:255–259.

2. Madamba A, Baena Cagnani CE, Oehling A. Etiological factors in child bronchial asthma. *Allergol Immunopathol* 1980; 8:673–678.

3. Beck E, Slapke J, Müller S, Meiske W, Glende M. Upper respiratory track infection (URI) is a potent trigger factor for asthma manifestation in predisposed individuals: Preliminary results of a retrospective case control study. *Atemw Lungenkrkh* 1990; 16/1 (Suppl 22):24.

4. Laube BL, Norman PS, Adams GK. The effect of aerosol distribution on airway responsiveness to inhaled methacholine in patients with asthma. *J Allergy Clin Immunol* 1992; 89:510–518.

5. Lundgren R, Soderberg M, Horsteat P, Stenlin R. Morphological studies on bronchial mucosal biopsies from asthmatics before and after ten years of treatment with inhaled steroids. *Eur Respir J* 1988; 1:883–889.

6. Clementsen P, Kristensen KS, Norn S. Microorganisms and exacerbation of chronic obstructive pulmonary diseases: pathophysiological mechanisms. *Allergy* 1992; 47: 195–202.

7. Oehling A, Sanz ML, Garcia BE. Immunological parameters in the immunotherapy follow-up. *Int Arch Allergy Immunol* 1992; 99:474–477.

Ion Channels as Therapeutic Targets in Asthma Therapy

Peter J Barnes*

Keywords: K⁺ channel, Ca²⁺ channel, calcium antagonists, potassium channel openers, chloride channels

Ion channels regulate many cellular activities in the airways. Voltage- and receptor-operated calcium channels are important in regulating the concentration of intracellular calcium ions (Ca^{2+}) in many cell types, although in airway smooth muscle and inflammatory cells the release of Ca^{2+} from intracellular stores appears to be more important. Calcium antagonists that block voltage-operated calcium channels have not proved to be useful as bronchodilators or anti-asthma drugs. Potassium channels are important in regulation of cell activity and several types of K⁺ channel are now recognized pharmacologically. In airway smooth muscle calcium-dependent and ATP-sensitive K⁺ channels are important in bronchodilatation. ATP-sensitive K⁺ channel openers are effective in relaxing human airway smooth muscle *in vitro*, but are not useful clinically because of cardiovascular side effects. Whether openers of calcium-dependent K⁺ channels may be more useful remains to be determined. Chloride channels are poorly characterized, but blockade of Cl⁻ channels may inhibit the release of mediators from inflammatory cells and may inhibit sensory neurotransmission. Cl⁻ channel blockade may account for the anti-asthma effects of inhaled cromones and frusemide.

Introduction

The concentration of intracellular ions, such as calcium (Ca^{2+}) and potassium (K⁺) ions, has a profound influence on cell activity. The intracellular concentrations of these ions are partly determined by their passage through specific ion channels at the cell surface. Ions channels are protein-lined pores in the cell membrane, several of which have now been cloned. Most channels are made up of distinct subunits which are grouped together in the cell membrane. Whether the channel is open or closed depends on different factors for each channel, but may be determined by receptor activation, the polarization of the cell membrane or the presence of particular ligands which interact directly with the channel. Drugs which open or block these channels have now been discovered (such as highly specific naturally occurring toxins) or developed through pharmaceutical research, leading to an enormous increase in our understanding of the role of these channels in different cell types. It has also raised the possibility that these drugs may be useful therapeutically.

Airway calibre is largely determined by the tone of airway smooth muscle and airway smooth muscle contraction is determined by the intracellular Ca^{2+} concentration ($[Ca^{2+}]_i$). Drugs with block calcium channels should therefore be bronchodilator if airway smooth muscle cells behave in the same manner as vascular smooth muscle cells, in which calcium antagonists are potent vasodilators. A reduction in intracellular K⁺ leads to hyperpolarization of smooth muscle cells and thus to relaxation, suggesting that drugs which open K+ channels (KCOs) may also act as bronchodilators.

In addition to airway smooth muscle, many other cells contribute to airway obstruction in asthma and chronic obstructive airway diseases. Release of neurotransmitters from airway nerves and inflammatory mediators from inflammatory cells, such as mast cells, eosinophils, neutrophils, macrophages and T-lymphocytes may also be determined by Ca^{2+} and K⁺ channels, so that calcium antagonists or KCOs may have additional effects to bronchodilatation.

This chapter reviews the possible roles of Ca^{2+} channels and K⁺ channels in airway disease, with particular emphasis on therapeutic potential in the treatment of airway obstruction.

* Department of Thoracic Medicine, National Heart and Lung Institute, London, UK.

Calcium Channels

Several types of calcium channels have now been identified on the basis of drug selectivity. electrophysiological properties and from molecular cloning.

Voltage-Operated Channels

Voltage-operated channels (VOCs) or *L-type* channels (for long-lasting) open in response to depolarization of the cell, resulting in influx of Ca^{2+} to increase intracellular Ca^{2+} concentration; these channels are blocked by dihydropyridines (such as nifedipine and nimodipine), by verapamil and by diltiazem. Several subtypes of L-type channel have now been recognized in different tissues (1). Each consists of five subunits. Voltage-sensitive calcium channels are important is contractile responses of pulmonary vascular smooth muscle, but are less important in the contractile response of airway smooth muscle or in the activation of inflammatory cells. T-type calcium channels are also opened by depolarization but are insensitive to dihydropyridines. Electrophysiological studies have revealed the presence of both L- and T-channels in airway smooth muscle, although the L-channels are less sensitive to dihydropyridines than the L-channels in the myocardium (2). N-type channels, which are largely restricted to neurons, are also sensitive to depolarization and insensitive to dihydropyridines, but are blocked by the toxin omega-conotoxin.

Receptor-Operated Channels

Receptor-operated channels (ROCs) are envisaged as channels which open in response to activation of certain receptors; these receptors are not well defined but drugs that block ROCs, such as SK&F 96365, have been developed. ROCs may be regulated by signals from intracellular stores and by inositol phosphates, so that Ca^{2+} enters via ROCs to fill intracellular stores.

Airway Smooth Muscle

Activation of an airway smooth muscle cell by a spasmogen results in a rapid rise in $[Ca^{2+}]_i$ from a resting level of about 0.1 nM to 10–100 nM. Studies with fluorescent markers of $[Ca^{2+}]$, such as aequorin and fura-2 in airway smooth muscle cells show a rapid elevation and return to baseline within a minute. The rise in $[Ca^{2+}]_i$ leads to contraction by activating a series of enzymes. The source of calcium for contraction may derive from extracellular Ca^{2+}, which enter the cell through calcium channels down electrochemical and concentration gradients, or from intracellular stores.

Both VOCs and ROCs have been differentiated in airway smooth muscle cells (2, 3). Depolarization of airway smooth muscle with potassium chloride (KCl) solutions results in a contraction which is due to influx of Ca^{2+} through VOCs. This contractile response is blocked by calcium antagonists, such as verapamil, nifedipine and diltiazem. The dihydropyridine calcium *agonist* BAY K8644 augments KCl-induced contractions of airway smooth muscle, by increasing calcium entry. Patch clamp studies of airway smooth muscle cells indicate that both T- and L-channels are present, although the L-channels are less sensitive to dihydropyridine agonists and antagonists than the classical L-channels in myocardium.

Functional studies indicate that VOCs mediate contraction due to depolarization of airway smooth muscle, but the role of VDCs in response to endogenous mediators and neurotransmitters is questionable. Contraction of airway smooth muscle in response to agonists, such as acetylcholine and histamine, is independent of external Ca^{2+} and is not associated with ^{45}Ca uptake, suggesting that calcium entry is not important for *initiation* of contractile responses. Entry of Ca^{2+} via ROCs may be important in refilling intracellular stores and in the maintenance of increased tone, however. Calcium antagonists have only weak effects against contraction of human airway smooth muscle induced by histamine or methacholine, although they are apparently more effective in *reversing* the contraction induced by these agents (4). This may indicate that calcium antagonists are not important in the initiation of contraction, but may play a more important in the maintenance of tone.

Most spasmogens contract airway smooth muscle in the absence of extracellular calcium, suggesting that the source of Ca^{2+} for contraction must be intracellular. It is now evident that release of calcium from intracellular stores is controlled receptor-coupled phosphoinositide hydrolysis (5).

Other Cells

A rise in $[Ca^{2+}]_i$ is important in the secretion of inflammatory mediators from inflammatory cells, such as mast cells, neutrophils and eosinophils. Calcium antagonists, such as nifedipine, have no significant inhibitory effect on mediator release from these cells, however, suggesting that calcium release from intracellular stores may be more important. The nature of the calcium channels in inflammatory cells such as eosinophils has not been explored in detail. Agonists, such as platelet activating factor (PAF) cause a transient rise in $[Ca^{2+}]_i$ which is not blocked by dihydropyridines, but is blocked by EDTA, suggesting that a ROC is involved (6). Whether ROCs are involved in the activation and secretion of mediators from inflammatory cells implicated in asthma is currently under investigation.

Similarly calcium antagonists have no significant effect on the release of neurotransmitters, since calcium entry into nerve terminals is dependent on N-channels that are not susceptible to calcium antagonists such as dihydropyridines.

Calcium antagonists have little effect on airway microvascular leakage induced by inflammatory mediators, and therefore are unlikely to have an inhibitory effect on airway oedema formation (7). The potent vasodilator action of calcium antagonists could theoretically increase plasma exudation, by increasing the delivery of blood to leaky post-capillary venules.

Calcium Antagonists in Asthma

Although calcium antagonists, which block VDCs, have been found to be very effective in cardiovascular disease, their use in asthma has proved to be disappointing (4, 8).

Calcium antagonists are only weakly effective in human airways *in vivo*. They do not cause bronchodilatation in either normal or asthmatic subjects, and give only weak protection against histamine-, methacholine-, allergen- or exercise-induced bronchoconstriction. For this reason calcium antagonists are of no value in the clinical management of obstructive airway disease. However they may be safely used to treat hypertension and ischaemic heart disease in patients with asthma in whom even selective b-blockers are contraindicated.

Potassium Channels

Recovery of cells after depolarization depends on the movement of K^+ out of the cell via K^+ channels

in the cell membrane. This results in hyperpolarization of the cell with relaxation of smooth muscle and inhibition of cell activity. Conversely blockade of K^+ channels with drugs as tetraethylammonium (TEA) and 4-aminopyridine (4-AP) results in increased excitability or hyperresponsiveness of cells. Many different types of K^+ channel have now been defined, using selective toxins, patch-clamping techniques and cloning (9).

Differentiation of K^+ Channels

Although more than 10 different types of K^+ channel have been described, they may be subdivided into four main classes.

Voltage-Gated Channels

These are the delayed rectifier channels (K_{dr}) which open on depolarization of the membrane which and return the cell membrane to its previous polarized state. This is a diverse group of channels, some of which are blocked by a-dendrotoxin. TEA and 4-AP effectively block all K_{dr}.

Ca^{2+}-Activated Channels

Ca^{2+}-activated channels (K_{Ca}) open in response to elevation of intracellular Ca^{2+} concentration. Large conductance (maxi-K) K^+ channels are found in smooth muscle and neurons and are blocked by the scorpion venoms charybdotoxin and iberiotoxin. Small conductance channels, some of which are blocked by apamin, are found predominantly in neurons, although they are also found on some types of smooth muscle.

Receptor-Coupled Channels

Receptor-coupled channels are opened by certain receptors via a G-protein, but no specific blockers have been found.

ATP-Sensitive Channels

ATP-sensitive channels (K_{ATP}) are opened by a fall in intracellular ATP concentration. These channels are found in smooth muscle and in the islet cells of the pancreas. They are blocked by sulphonylureas such as glibenclamide and are opened by drugs such as cromakalim (BRL 34915), its active enantiomer levcromakalim (BRL 38227), aprikalim (RP 53891) and HOE 245.

115

Airway Smooth Muscle

K$^+$ channels play an important role in relaxation of airway smooth muscle (10, 11). β-Agonist induced bronchodilatation is markedly inhibited by charybdotoxin and iberiotoxin (12, 13), indicating that opening of a maxi-K channel is involved in the relaxant response. Neither apamin nor glibenclamide have any inhibitory effect on the relaxation response to β-antagonists, however. A rise in intracellular cyclic AMP causes opening of maxi-K channels in airway smooth muscle, but there is also evidence from patch-clamping studies that β-adrenoceptors are directly coupled, via G$_s$, to maxi-K channels (14). This suggests that it may be possible for airway smooth muscle to relax in response to β-antagonists without an increase in intracellular cyclic AMP. Since charybdotoxin appears to have a greater inhibitory effect at low concentrations of β-agonists, and no effect at high concentrations, this suggests that maxi-K channels may be directly opened via β-receptor coupling at low concentrations of agonist, but as concentrations rise there is an increase in cyclic AMP which leads to relaxation via other mechanisms.

KCOs, which open ATP-sensitive K$^+$ channels, relax animal and human airways *in vitro* (15, 16). Thus levcromakalim and HOE 234 almost completely relay human airway smooth muscle *in vitro*. The relaxant effect of KCOs in airway smooth muscle is competitively inhibited by the K$_{ATP}$ blocker glibenclamide. This indicates that the channel involved belongs to the ATP-sensitive K$^+$ channel class, although the low sensitivity to glibenclamide distinguishes it from the high affinity ATP-sensitive K$^+$ channel typical of pancreatic islets. Glibenclamide itself has no effect on airway smooth muscle tone, and may only bind to the channel when it is in the open state. KCOs appear to act as functional antagonists, as they reverse with equal potency contraction induced by cholinergic agonists, histamine and neurokinin A (15). This is somewhat surprising, since contraction due to these spasmogens is mediated by Pl hydrolysis and intracellular Ca^{2+} release, rather than via depolarization of the cell, and this is why Ca antagonists are not effective. The efficacy of K$^+$ channel activation in airway smooth muscle may indicate that these drugs have additional effects other than repolarizing or hyperpolarizing cells. It is possible that they may also act on endoplasmic reticulum to pump Ca^{2+} back into intracellular stores, thus lowering [Ca^{2+}]$_i$. KCOs are also effective bronchodilators *in vivo*, both after intravenous administration and via inhalation and reach the efficacy of β-agonists. KCOs may therefore form a new class of bronchodilator for use in asthma.

Effects on Neurotransmission

K$^+$ channels are also involved in the release of neurotransmitters from peripheral nerves, including airway nerves. In anaesthetized guinea pigs cromakalim has an inhibitory effect on cholinergic neurotransmission and the release of neuropeptides from sensory nerves in airways (17). The inhibitory effect on neuropeptide release has also been demonstrated in guinea-pig airways *in vitro* (18), and is presumably due to hyperpolarization of the nerve ending which prevents the release of neurotransmitters. This suggests that KCOs may reduce neurogenic inflammation in the airways, and there is evidence that these drugs have an inhibitory effect on neurogenic airway microvascular leakage and vagus nerve-induced mucus secretion form goblet cells (19, 20).

Modulation of neurotransmission is also mediated by opening of maxi-K channels, since charybdotoxin reverses the modulatory effect of many agonists, including opioids, neuropeptide Y and a-agonists on neuropeptide release from airway sensory nerves (18). Similarly charybdotoxin also blocks the modulatory effect of pre-junctional inhibitors of cholinergic nerves in guinea-pig and human airways (21). Charybdotoxin increases cholinergic nerve-induced contraction of airway smooth muscle, via inhibition of the inhibitory effects of acetylcholine on muscarinic M$_2$-autoreceptors (21).

Effects on Other Cells

It is likely that K$^+$ channels are important in the regulation of inflammatory cell activation and secretion, although the nature of the K$^+$ channels in inflammatory cells, such as mast cells, eosinophils, T-lymphocytes and macrophages remains to be defined. KCOs appear to have little or no inhibitory effects on the release of mediators from inflammatory cells. Thus cromakalim has no effect on IgE-dependent release of mediators from sensitized human lungs. KCOs similarly have no inhibitory effect on airway microvascular leakage. In rat basophil leukaemia cells K$_{Ca}$ appear to be involved in degranulation and histamine release. A recent study suggests that small conductance K_{Ca} channels may be involved in the activation of mast cells in the airway, since apamin has an inhibitory effect on allergen-induced constriction of guinea pig airways *in vitro*, but has no effect on the direct contractile response to histamine (22).

Clinical Studies in Asthma

The potent relaxant effect of KCOs in airway smooth muscle *in vitro* suggests that these drugs may be useful as novel bronchodilators in asthma (10, 23). Orally administered cromakalim has a small inhibitory effect on histamine-induced bronchoconstriction in normal individuals, but there is evidence for a small protective effect against the nocturnal fall in lung function in asthmatic patients (24). By contrast orally administered levcromakalim had no significant bronchodilator effect, nor any protective effect against histamine or methacholine-induced bronchoconstriction in asthmatic patients (25). The highest dose of levcromakalim administered has significant adverse effects, with postural hypotension and headaches, as a consequence of its vasodilator action. This suggests that this class of drug is not likely to be useful via the oral route, since vasodilator side effects will limit the dose that can be given. One way to overcome this problem may be the use of inhaled preparations and animal studies indicate that this rout of administration is effective (26). However, if the drug is absorbed from the lung into the systemic circulation there may still be a problem of side effects.

KCOs such as cromakalim and levcromakalim have cardiovascular side effects that limit their development as anti-asthma therapies. In the future it is possible that KCOs that have a greater selectivity for airway K_{ATP} channels may be developed. The KCO BRL 55834 appears to have less cardiovascular effects than levcromakalim, indicating that such selectivity may be possible (26). The K^+ channel which appears to play a major role in relaxation of airway smooth muscle is the maxi-K channel, suggesting that drugs that selectively open this channel may be more useful than K^{ATP} openers. Extracts from a medicinal help used in asthma therapy in Ghana appear to have a selective effect on maxi-K channels (27). The most active ingredient is dehydrosoyasaponin I (DHS-I) which reversibly activates maxi-K channels in tracheal smooth muscle preparations and may form the basis of a new class of bronchodilator therapy.

Chloride Channels

Little is known about chloride channels in the airways. Although several types of Cl^- channels can be distinguished electrophysiologically, these are not well defined and selective inhibitors and activators are lacking. An inwardly directed calcium-activated Cl^- channel has been described in airway smooth muscle cells, but the functional role of this channel are not yet clear.

The loop diuretic frusemide was observed to inhibit exercise-induced asthma, and subsequently several other indirect challenges, suggesting that such drugs may have potential as anti-asthma compounds (28, 29). The protective effect in indirect challenges and the lack of effect against bronchoconstriction induced directly by spasmogens, such as histamine and methacholine, are analogous to the effects of sodium cromoglycate and nedocromil sodium. The mechanism of action of frusemide is still uncertain. The fact that bumetanide, a more potent loop diuretic, does not share the same anti-asthma effects as frusemide suggests that inhibition of the $Na^+/K^+/Cl^-$ cotransporter is unlikely to account for its anti-asthma effects. Frusemide, unlike bumetanide, appears to block Cl^- channels in certain cells. Thus the inhibitory effects of frusemide may be mimicked by Cl^- channel blockers such as DIDS and NPPB (30). It is of interest that nedocromil sodium also appears to block Cl^- transport in nerves. This indicates that cromones may also work through inhibition of certain Cl^- channels. In the future development of more potent and selective inhibitors may help to define these channels more clearly and lead to the development of new anti-asthma drugs in the future.

Address for correspondence:

Prof. PJ Barnes
Department of Thoracic Medicine
National Heart and Lung Institute
Dovehouse St
London SW3 6LY
UK

References

1. Tsien, RW, Tsien RY. Calcium channels, stores and oscillations. *Annu Rev Biol* 1990; 6:715–760.

2. Kotlikoff, MI. Calcium currents in isolated canince airway smooth muscle cells. *Am J Physiol* 1988; 254: C793–901.

3. Murray RK, Kotlikoff MI. Receptor-activated calcium influy in human airway smooth muscle cells. *J Physiol* 1991; 435:123–144.

4. Löfdahl C-G, Barnes PJ. Calcium channel blockade and asthma – the current position. *Eur J Respir Dis* 1985; 67:233–237.

5. Hall I, Chilvers ER. Inositol phosphates and airway smooth muscle. *Pulm Pharmacol* 1989; 2:113–120.

6. Kroegel C, Pleass R, Yukawa T, Chung KF, Westwick J, Barnes PJ. Characterization of platelet-activating factor-induced elevation of cystolic free calcium concentration in eosinophils. *FEBS Lett* 1989; 243:41–46.

7. Boschetto P, Roberts NM, Rogers DF, Barnes PJ. The effect of antiasthma drugs on microvascular leak in guinea pig airways. *Am Rev Respir Dis* 1989; 139:416–421.

8. Barnes PJ. Clinical studies with calcium antagonists in asthma. *Br J Clin Pharmacol* 1985; 20:289S–298S.

9. Cook NS. The pharmacology of potassium channels and their therapeutic potential. *Trends Pharmacol Sci* 1988; 9:21–24.

10. Black JL, Barnes PJ. Potassium channels and airway function: new therapeutic approaches. *Thorax* 1990; 45:213–218.

11. Kotlikoff MI. Potassium currents in canine airway smooth muscle cells. *Am J Physiol* 1990; 259:L384–L395.

12. Miura M, Belvisi MG, Stretton CD, Yacoub MH, Barnes PJ. Role of potassium channels in bronchodilator responses in human airways. *Am Rev Respir Dis* 1992; 146:132–136.

13. Jones TR, Charette L, Garcia ML, Kaczorowski GJ. Interaction of iberiotoxin with β-adrenoceptor agonists and sodium nitroprusside on guinea pig trachea. *J Appl Physiol* 1993; 74:1879–1884.

14. Kume H, Kotlikoff MI. Muscarinic inhibition of single K_{Ca} channels in smooth muscle cells by a pertussin-sensitive G protein. *Am J Physiol* 1991; 261:C1204–12049.

15. Black JL, Armour CL, Johnson PRA, Alouan LA, Barnes PJ. The action of a potassium channel activator BRL 38227 (lemakalim) on human airway smooth muscle. *Am Rev Respir Dis* 1990; 142:1384–1389.

16. Miura M, Belvisi MG, Ward JK, Tadjkarini M, Yacoub MH, Barnes PJ. Bronchodilatory effects of the novel potassium channel opener HOE 234 in human airways *in vitro*. *Br J Clin Pharmacol* 1993; 35:318–320.

17. Ichinose M, Barnes PJ. A potassium channel activator modulates both noncholinergic and cholinergic neurotransmission in guinea pig airways. *J Pharmacol Exp Ther* 1990; 252:1207–1212.

18. Stretton CD, Miura M, Belvisi MG, Barnes PJ. Calcium-activated potassium channels mediate prejunctional inhibition of peripheral sensory nerves. *Proc Natl Acad Sci USA* 1992; 89:1325–1329.

19. Lei Y-H, Barnes PJ, Rogers DF. Inhibition of neurogenic plasma exudation and bronchoconstriction by K^+ channel activator BRL 38227 in guinea pig airways *in vivo*. *Eur J Pharmacol* 1993; 239:257–259.

20. Kuo H-P, Rohde JAL, Barnes PJ, Rogers DF. K^+ channel activator inhibition of neurogenic goblet cell secretion in guinea pig trachea. *Eur J Pharmacol* 1992; 221:385–388.

21. Miura M, Belvisi MG, Stretton CD, Yacoub M, Barnes PJ. The role of K^+ channels in the modulation of cholinergic neural responses in guinea pig and human airways. *J Physiol* 1992; 455:1–15.

22. Yamauchi H, Miura M, Ichinose M, et al. Involvement of aspirin sensitive K^+ channels in antigen-induced spasm of guinea-pig isolated trachea. *Br J Pharmacol* 1994; 112:958–962.

23. Buckle DR. Prospects for potassium channel activators in the treatment of airways obstruction. *Pulm Pharmacol* 1993; 6:161–169.

24. Williams AJ, Lee TH, Cochrane GM, et al. Attenuation of nocturnal asthma by cromakalim. *Lancet* 1990; 336:334–336.

25. Kidney JC, Fuller RW, Worsdell Y-M, Lavender EA, Chung KF, Barnes PJ. Effect of an oral potassium channel activator BRL 38227 on airway function and responsiveness in asthmatic patients: Comparison with oral salbutamol. *Thorax* 1993; 48:130–134.

26. Bowring NE, Arch JRS, Buckle DR, Taylor JF. Comparison of the airways relaxant and hypertensive potencies ofthe potassium channel activators BRL 55834 and levcromakalin (BRL 38227) *in vivo* in guinea pigs and rats. *Br J Pharmacol* 1993; 109:1133–1139.

27. McManus OB, Harris GH, Giangiacomo KM, et al. An activator of calcium-dependent potassium channels isolated from a medicinal herb. *Biochemistry* 1993; 32:6128–6133.

28. Bianco S, Pieroni MG, Refini RM, Robuschi M, Vaghi A, Sestini P. Inhaled loop diuretics as potential new anti-asthmatic drugs. *Eur Resp J* 1993; 6:130–134.

29. Barnes PJ. Diuretics and asthma. *Thorax* 1993; 48:195–197.

30. Perkins RS, Dent G, Chung KF, Barnes PJ. Effects on anion transport inhibitors and chloride ions on eosinophil respiratory burst activity. *Biochem Pharmacol* 1992; 43:2480–2482.

Lipid Mediator Antagonists

Paul M O'Byrne*

Keywords: Leukotrienes, 5-lipoxygenase, receptor antagonists, synthesis inhibitors, asthma, broncho-constriction, thromboxane, platelet activating factor

Asthma is an inflammatory airway disease with activated eosinophils, lymphocytes, and an increased number of mast cells in the airways, as well as characteristic structural changes of the airway wall. Mediators released from these cells are responsible for the structural changes in asthmatic airways and for the development of the physiological abnormalities that characterize asthma. Among these, are lipid mediators that are produced from arachidonic acid. The best studied of these in asthma are the cysteinyl leukotrienes (LT) C_4, and D_4, thromboxane A_2, and platelet activating factor (PAF). The development of mediator receptor antagonists or synthesis inhibitors has been essential for proving a role for the mediator in the pathogenesis of asthma and may also provide a novel therapy for asthma. Studies with a variety of leukotriene receptor antagonists and synthesis inhibitors indicate a pivotal role for the cysteinyl leukotrienes in induced bronchoconstriction in clinical models of asthma, such as exercise- and allergen-induced bronchoconstriction. Leukotriene receptor antagonists also acutely improve lung function in asthmatic subjects. The result of clinical trials in asthma suggest that leukotriene antagonists and synthesis inhibitors are very likely to have role in asthma therapy, even in patients with severe disease. However, their precise place in asthma therapy, and when and how they should be used, is not yet known. In contrast to the efficacy of the leukotriene antagonists and synthesis inhibitors in asthma, studies of thromboxane and PAF inhibitors do not support an important role for these mediators in the pathogenesis of asthma, and make it unlikely that these classes of compounds will be useful in treating asthma.

Introduction

Asthma is a common disease which affics at least 10% of the population of most countries in which its prevalence has been established. Asthmatic patients usually complain of variable symptoms such

as dyspnea, wheezing, chest tightness, and cough, which are caused by variable airflow obstruction. The variable airflow obstruction is, in part, a consequence of airway hyperresponsiveness to a variety of chemical bronchoconstrictor stimuli and physical stimuli such as exercise and hyperventilation of cold dry air (1), which is present in all patients with symptomatic asthma.

More recently, it has been recognized that asthma symptoms, variable airflow obstruction and airway hyperresponsiveness occur as a consequence of the characteristic form of cellular inflammation and structural changes in the airway wall (2) (Figure 1). The inflammation consists of a presence of activated eosinophils, lymphocytes, and an increased number of mast cells, which have been described both in bronchoalveolar lavage and airway biopsies from asthmatic subjects (3, 4), as well as characteristic structural changes of the airways (5, 6).

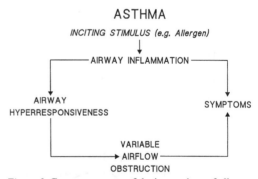

Figure 1. Current concepts of the interactions of allergen inhalation, airway inflammation, and the clinical manifestation of asthma.

Lipid Mediators in Asthma

The presence of activated inflammatory cells in the airways of asthmatics has led to the speculation that

---

* Department of Medicine, McMaster University, Hamilton, Ontario, Canada.

effector mediators released from these cells are responsible for the structural changes in asthmatic airways and for the development of the physiological abnormalities that characterize asthma. A large number of potential candidate mediators have been suggested to be important. Included in these are lipid mediators that are produced from arachidonic acid released by the action of a family of phospholipases (particularly phospholipase A_2) from the cell membrane. Arachidonic acid is subsequently metabolized by the enzyme cyclooxygenase, to produce prostaglandins (PGs) and thromboxane (Tx), or by 5-lipoxygenase to produce leukotrienes (LTs). The release of arachidonic acid can also result in the production of platelet activating factor (PAF) and a variety of other lipid mediators depending on the activity of a variety of intracellular enzyme systems (Figure 2).

Identifying a role for a these mediators in asthma has relied on the collection of various types of evidence. Generally, when the structure of the mediator is identified, and it is synthesized, the mediator is given (usually by inhalation) to asthmatics, to identify whether it can mimic some component of the asthmatic response. Then, when

assays for its measurment are available, efforts are made to measure it in biological fluids, to determine whether it is released during asthmatic responses. The availability of selective antagonists or synthesis inhibitors allow studies to be conducted to inhibit components of the asthmatic responses in clinical models of asthma. The final, *and most difficult,* step is to determine whether the mediator antagonists or synthetase inhibitors are useful in treating asthmatic patients, thereby proving that the mediator has an important role in this pathogenesis.

The development of mediator receptor antagonists or synthesis inhibitors is essential for proving a role for the mediator in the pathogenesis of asthma and may also provide a novel therapy for asthma. Once an antagonist or synthesis inhibitor has been demonstrated to be active in animal model of asthma, studies of its activity in humans usually begin. It is important to recognize, however, that activity in clinical models of asthma does not necessarily result in efficacy in clinical trials of asthma, nor does evidence of efficacy in clinical trials always mean the drug will be particularly useful in the management of asthma in clinical practice. The first approach to establish activity can be done

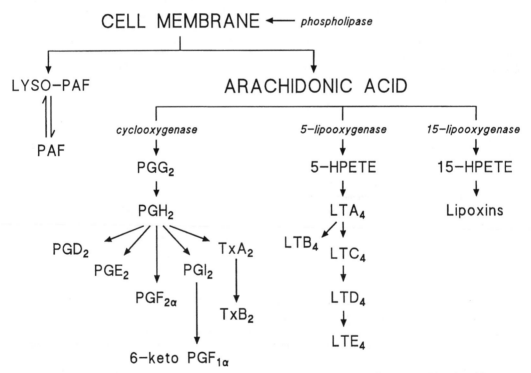

Figure 2. The production of products of cyclooxygenase, 5–lipoxygenase and of PAF from arachidonic acid.

by examining the ability of a synthesis inhibitor to prevent the production of the mediator *in vivo*. The activity is studied in clinical models of asthma. The most widely used are exercise-, hyperventilation-, and allergen-induced bronchoconstriction.

Allergen inhalation has been recognized as an important (perhaps the most important) stimulus which causes the characteristic airway inflammation, airway hyperresponsiveness, variable airflow obstruction, and symptoms in asthmatics. More than 50 years ago, the importance of slow reacting substance of anaphylaxis (SRS-A) in the events occurring after immunological challenge of the lungs was identified (7). Later, Brocklehurst demonstrated that SRS-A was released from lung segments from an asthmatic subject, when these segments were exposed to allergen (8). SRS-A was thought to be an important cause of symptoms after allergen exposure in atopic subjects, because it was a potent constrictor of airway smooth muscle with a longer duration of action than histamine. SRS-A is now known to consist of the cysteinyl leukotriene LTC_4, D_4, and E_4 (9).

Leukotrienes in the Pathogenesis of Asthma

The cysteinyl leukotrienes were initially demonstrated to be very potent constrictors of human airway smooth muscle *in vitro* (10), being at least 1000 times more potent than histamine. Inhaled LTC_4 and LTD_4 have also been demonstrated to be potent bronchoconstrictors in both normal and asthmatic subjects (11), being up to 10,000 times more potent than methacholine in some normal subjects, with a longer duration of action than inhaled histamine (12). The bronchoconstrictor effects of inhaled LTD_4 are resolved within 1–2 hours. LTE_4 increases airway hyperresponsiveness to histamine (13), and also, in a recent study, has been demonstrated to cause influx of eosinophils into asthmatic airways, an effect not seen with another bronchoconstrictor agonist, methacholine (14). These results with LTE_4 suggest that endogenously released cysteinyl leukotrienes may

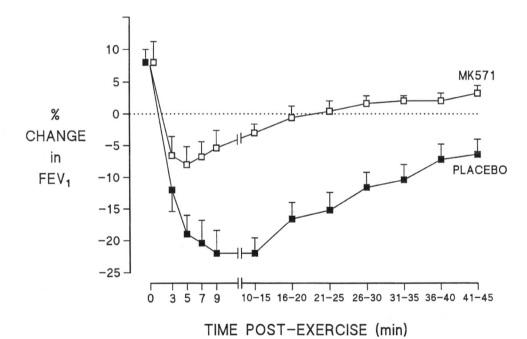

Figure 3: The percentagechange in FEV_1 (mean and SEM) over time post–exercise following treatment with placebo (solid squares) or MK–571 (open squares). Measurements were made in all subjects immediatly after exercise, then at 3 minutes and every 2 minutes until the FEV_1 began to improve. Treatment with MK–571 significantly reduced the maximal fall in FEV_1 after exercise (p<0.001) and shortened the recovery time (p<0.001). (Reprinted with permission from Manning et al., *New England Journal of Medicine* 1990; 323:1736–1739.)

have effects on airway function which persist long after their bronchoconstrictor effects have resolved.

Increases in urinary LTE_4 after exercise have been demonstrated in one (15), but not another study (16). By contrast, several investigators have demonstrated increases in urinary LTE_4 after allergen-induced bronchoconstriction (17, 18). The increases in urinary LTE_4 were significantly correlated, in one study, with the magnitude of the bronchoconstriction (17). Aspirin ingestion, which causes severe bronchoconstriction in aspirin sensitive asthmatics, also caused significant increases in urinary LTE_4 (19), and increases in urinary LTE_4 have been demonstrated to occur during acute spontaneous asthma (18), which decline as the asthma is treated and the bronchoconstriction resolves.

Activity of Leukotriene Inhibitors in Clinical Models of Asthma

A variety of different chemicals are available which interfere with the production or action of the cysteinyl leukotrienes. Three classes of compounds have been developed. These are receptor antagonists, the most advanced in development being ICI 204,291 (Accolate) (20), 5-lipoxygenase inhibitors, the most advanced in development being Zileuton (21), and antagonists of 5-lipoxygenase activating protein (FLAP), such as MK-0591 (22) and BAYx 1005 (23). These compounds attenuate the bronchoconstrictor responses after exercise (Figure 3), cold air and allergen (20–24). These studies have indicated that LTD_4 inhibitors can inhibit exercise-induced bronchoconstriction by a mean of between 50–70%, and indeed, in some asthmatic subjects, completely inhibit the response (24). Similarly, both LTD_4 antagonists and leukotriene synthesis inhibitors attenuate allergen-induced early responses by up to 80% (20, 23), and also attenuate the late response by up to 50% (20, 23). Aspirin-induced bronchoconstriction is also almost completely abolished by treatment with leukotriene synthesis inhibitors (25). These results, taken together, indicate a pivotal role for the cysteinyl leukotrienes in induced bronchoconstriction in these clinical models of asthma.

Leukotriene receptor antagonists also acutely improve lung function in asthmatic subjects who were selected to have bronchoconstriction prior to beginning treatment with the antagonists (26). The magnitude of the improvement in lung function that was achieved was much less than that achieved with optimal doses of an inhaled β_2-agonist. However, in both studies, the magnitude of the improvement with the antagonist and the β_2-agonist together was significantly greater than the β_2-agonist alone. These results suggest that the cysteinyl leukotriene are, in part, responsible for spontaneous bronchoconstriction in asthma.

Efficacy of Leukotriene Inhibitors in Asthma

The success of the leukotriene antagonists and synthetase inhibitors in attenuating bronchoconstriction in the clinical models of asthma suggested that these compounds were likely to be successful in the management of clinical asthma. The earliest clinical study, with a relatively less potent leukotriene receptor antagonist, LY171883, demonstrated that asthmatic subjects do receive clinical benefit from treatment with the compound (27). This was demonstrated by improvements in lung function, as well as a reduction in the use of inhaled β_2-agonists for symptom relief.

Subsequent studies, using more potent receptor antagonists and synthesis inhibitors, have confirmed that clinical benefit can be achieved with these compounds in patients with moderately severe asthma. A recently published study (28) has compared the 5-lipoxygenase inhibitor, Zileuton, with placebo for 4 weeks, in patients with mild to moderate asthma, who were not taking inhaled corticosteroids to control symptoms. Zileuton significantly improved the clinical outcome parameters, including symptoms, the forced expired volume in 1 sec (FEV_1), morning peak expired flow rates (PEFR), and B_2-agonist use, in a dose-dependent fashion. In another study, the FLAP-antagonist, MK-0591, was compared to placebo in patients with severe asthma not optimally controlled in moderate doses of inhaled corticosteroids (29). Once again, there was significant, and probably clinically useful, improvements in FEV_1, PEFR, and B_2-agonist use.

These results of clinical trials in asthma suggest that leukotriene antagonists and synthesis inhibitors are very likely to have role in asthma therapy, even in patients with severe disease. However, their precise place in asthma therapy and when and how they should be used, is not yet known. No direct head-to-head comparisons have yet been made with other drugs, particularly inhaled corticosteroids, known to be very effective in the management of asthma in most patients. Also, no information exists as to whether drugs of this class influence the inflammatory events that occur in asthmatic airways, and that are thought to be important in the pathogenesis of asthma.

Other Lipid Mediator Inhibitors in Asthma

Thromboxane and PAF are two other lipid mediators which have been extensively studied in asthma, and for which mediator inhibitors have been developed and tested in clinical models of asthma.

Studies have examined the effects of a thromboxane receptor antagonist and a synthetase inhibitor on airway responses after allergen challenge (30, 31). Both of these compounds slightly but significantly inhibited the magnitude of allergen-induced early asthmatic responses by 20–25%. However, the thromboxane synthetase inhibitor did not inhibit allergen-induced late asthmatic responses nor allergen-induced histamine airway hyperresponsiveness measured at 24 h post allergen (30). These studie taken together, suggest that thromboxane may be released following allergen challenge, and be partly responsible for the early asthmatic response, but is not important in causing airway hyperresponsiveness following allergen inhalation. The TxA_2 synthetase inhibitor, OKY 046, administered orally, reduces acetylcholine airway hyperresponsiveness in stable asthmatic subjects (32). However, these studies were uncontrolled, and need to be repeated in a placebo controlled double-blind study before the results can be properly interpreted. There are no published studies on the clinical efficacy of thromboxane receptor antagonists or synthetase inhibitors in the management of asthma. However, the weak activity in protecting against allergen-induced asthmatic responses would suggest that these compounds are unlikely to have a major clinical effect.

A variety of PAF receptor antagonists have become available for clinical study. Several of these are very potent and selective. Until recently, the "gold standard" compound has been the thienotriazolodizaepine, WEB 2086 (33). This compound

has been used to characterize the PAF receptor, and has been shown to prevent PAF-induced bronchoconstriction in human subjects (34). WEB 2086 is completely ineffective in its ability to inhibit allergen-induced early or late asthmatic responses or allergen-induced airway hyperresponsiveness (35). This results have been confirmed with another very potent PAF antagonist, UK 74,505 (36). Thus, PAF does not appear to be important in the pathogenesis of allergen responses in asthma. Thus, it is very unlikely that PAG antagonists will have any role in the treatment of asthma.

Conclusions

Inhaled LTC_4 and LTD_4 are the most potent bronchoconstrictors yet studied in human subjects. Potent and selective leukotriene antagonists are available for studies in asthmatic subjects. These studies have supported an important role for the cysteinyl leukotriene in clinical model of asthma, such as exercise, allergen and aspirin-induced asthma. Also, leukotriene release is, in part responsible for spontaneous bronchoconstriction in asthma. Lastly, studies of the leukotriene antagonists and synthesis inhibitors have demonstrated clinical efficacy in asthma. This proves that the cysteinyl leukotrienes are involved in the pathogenesis of asthma, and suggests that this class of drugs will be useful in the treatment of asthma. However, the eventual place of these drugs in treating asthma awaits studies comparing their efficacy to the drugs which are currently known to be effective in the treatment of asthma. In contrast to the efficacy of the leukotriene antagonists and synthesis inhibitors in asthma, studies of thromboxane and PAF inhibitors do not support an important role for these mediators in the pathogenesis of asthma, and make it unlikely that these classes of compounds will be useful in treating asthma.

Address for correspondence:

Paul M O'Byrne
McMaster University
Faculty of Health Sciences
Department of Medicine
1200 Main Street West
Hamilton, Ontario, L8N 3Z5
Canada

References

1. Hargreave FE, Ryan G, Thomson NC, O'Byrne PM, Latimer K, Juniper EF, Dolovich J. Bronchial responsiveness to histamine or methacholine in asthma: measurement and clinical significance. *J Allergy Clin Immunol* 1981; 68:347–355.

2. Djukanovic R, Roche WR, Wilson JW, Beasley CRW, Twentyman OP, Howarth PH, Holgate ST. State of the Art: Mucosal inflammation in asthma. *Am Rev Resp Dis* 1990; 142:434–457.

3. Kirby JG, Hargreave FE, Gleich GJ, O'Byrne PM. Bronchoalveolar cell profiles of asthmatic and non-asthmatic subjects. *Am Rev Resp Dis* 1987; 136:379–383.

4. Jeffery PK, Wardlaw AJ, Nelson FC, Collins JV, Kay AB. Bronchial biopsies in asthma. An ultrastructural, quantitative study and correlation with hyperreactivity. *Am Rev Resp Dis* 1989; 140:1745–1753.

5. Dunnill MS, Massarell GR, Anderson JA. A comparison of the quantitive anatomy of the bronchi in normal subjects, in status asthmaticus, in chronic bronchitis and in emphysema. *Thorax* 1969; 24:176–179.

6. Laitinen LA, Heino M, Laitinen A, Kava T., Haahtela T. Damage of the airway epithelium and bronchial reactivity in patients with asthma. *Am Rev Resp Dis* 1985; 131:599–606.

7. Kellaway CH, Trethewie ER. The liberation of a slow-reacting smooth muscle-stimulating substance in anaphylaxis. *Q J Exp Physiol* 1940; 30:121–145.

8. Brocklehurst WE. The release of histamine and formation of a slow-reactingsubstance (SRS-A) during anaphylatic shock. *J Physiol* 1960; 151:416–435.

9. Lewis RA, Austen KF. The biologically active leukotrienes. Biosynthesis, metabolism, receptors, functions and pharmacology. *J Clin Invest* 1984; 73:889–897.

10. Dahlen SE, Hedqvist P, Hammarstrom S, Samuelsson B. Leukotrienes are potent constrictors of human bronchi. *Nature* 1980; 288:484–486.

11. Adelroth E, Morris MM, Hargreave FE, O'Byrne PM. Airway responsiveness to leukotrienes C_4 und D_4 and to methacholine in patients with asthma and normal controls. *N Engl J Med* 1986; 315:480–484.

12. Barnes NC, Piper PJ, Costello JF. Comparative effects of inhaled leukotriene C_4, leukotriene D_4 and histamine in normal human subjects. *Thorax* 1984; 39:500–504.

13. Lee TH, Arm JP, Spur BW. Leukotriene E_4 (LTE_4) enhances airways histamine responsiveness in asthmatic subjects. *J Allergy Clin Immunol* 1987; 79:256A.

14. Laitinen LA, Laitinen A, Haahtela T, Vilkka V, Spur BW, Lee TH. Leukotriene E_4 and granulocytic infiltration into asthmatic airways. *Lancet* 1993; 341:989–990.

15. Kikawa Y, Miyanomae T, Inoue Y et al. Urinary leukotriene E_4 after exercise challenge in children with asthma. *J Allergy Clin Immunol* 1992; 89:1111–1119.

16. Taylor IK, Wellings R, Taylor GW, Fuller RW. Urinary leukotriene E_4 excretion in exercise-induced bronchoconstriction. *Am Rev Resp Dis* 1992; 145:A15.

17. Manning PJ, Rokach J, Malo JL, Ethier D, Cartier A, Girard Y, Charleson S, O'Byrne PM. Urinary leukotriene E_4 levels during early and late asthmatic responses. *J Allergy Clin Immunol* 1990; 86:211–220.

18. Taylor GW, Black P, Turner N, Taylor I, Maltby NH, Fuller RW, Dollery CT. Urinary leukotriene E_4 after antigen challenge and in acute asthma and allergic rhinitis. *Lancet* 1989; i:584–587.

19. Knapp HR, Sladek K, FitzGerald GA. Increased secretion of leukotriene E_4 during aspirin-induced asthma. *J Lab Clin Invest* 1992; 119:48–51.

20. Taylor IK, O'Shaughnessy KM, Fuller RW, Dollery CT. Effect of a cysteinyl leukotriene receptor antagonist, ICI 204–219 on allergen-induced bronchoconstriction and airway hyperreactivity in atopic subjects. *Lancet* 1991; 337:690–694.

21. Israel E, Dermarkarian R, Rosenberg M et al. The effects of a 5-lipoxygenase inhibitor on asthma induced by cold, dry air. *N Engl J Med* 1990; 323:1740–1744.

22. Ford-Hutchinson AW. Leukotriene antagonists and inhibitors as modulators of IgE-mediated reactions. *Springer Semin Immunopathol* 1993; 15:37–50.

23. O'Byrne PM, Watson RM, Strong HA, Wylie G. The effect of treatment with a 5-lipoxygenase inhibitor, BAYx 1005, on allergen-induced asthmatic responses. *Am J Resp Crit Care Med* 1994; 149:A532.

24. Manning PJ, Watson RM, Margolskee DJ, Williams V, Schartz JI, O'Byrne PM. Inhibition of exercise-induced bronchoconstriction by MK-571, a potent leukotriene D_4 receptor antagonist. *N Engl J Med* 1990; 323:1736–1739.

25. Israel E, Fischer AR, Rosenburg MA, Lilly CM, Shapiro J, Cohn J, Rubin R, Drazen JM. The pivitol role of 5-lipoxygenase products in the reaction of aspirin-sensitive asthmatics to aspirin. *Am Rev Resp Dis* 1993; 148:1447–1451.

26. Gaddy J, Bush RK, Margolskee D, Williams VC, Busse W. The effects of a leukotriene D_4 (LTD_4) antagonist (MK-571) in mild to moderate asthma. *Am Rev Resp Dis* 1992; 146:358–363.

27. Cloud ML, Enas GC, Kemp J, Platts-Mills T, Altman LC, Townley R, Tinkelmann D, King T, Middleton E, Sheffer AL, McFadden ER Jr, Farlow DS. A specific LTD_4/LTE_4-receptor antagonist improves pul-

monary function in patients with mild, chronic asthma. *Am Rev Resp Dis* 1989; 140:1336–1339.

28. Israel E, Rubin P, Kemp J et al. The effect of inhibition of 5-lipoxygenase by Zileuton in mild-to-moderate asthma. *Ann Int Med* 1993; 119:1059–1066.

29. Chapman KR, Friedman BS, Shingo S, Heyse J, Reiss T, Spector R. The efficacy of an oral inhibitor of leukotriene synthesis (MK-0591) in asthmatics treated with inhaled steroids. *Am J Resp Crit Care Med* 1994; 149:A215.

30. Manning PJ, Stevens WH, Cockcroft DW, O'Byrne PM. The role of thromboxane in allergen-induced asthmatic responses. *Eur Resp J* 1991; 4:667–672.

31. Beasley RCW, Fetherstone RL, Church MK, Rafferty P, Varley JG, Harris A, Robinson C, Holgate ST. Effect of a thromboxane receptor antagonist on PGD$_2$- and allergen-induced bronchoconstriction. *J Appl Physiol* 1989; 66:1685–1693.

32. Fujimura M, Sasaki F, Nakatsumi Y, Takahashi Y, Hifumi S, Taga K, Mifune J-I, Tanaka T, Matsuda T. Effects of a thromboxane synthetase inhibitor (OKY-046) and a lipoxygenase inhibitor (AA-861) on bronchial responsiveness to acetylcholine in asthmatic subjects. *Thorax* 1986; 41:955–959.

33. Casals-Stenzel J, Muacevic G, Weber K-H. Pharmacological actions of WEB 2086, a new specific antagonist of platelet activating factor. *J Pharmacol Exp Ther* 1987; 241:974–981.

34. Adamus WS, Heuer HO, Meade CJ, Schilling JC. Inhibitory effects of a new PAF acether antagonist WEB 2086 on pharmacologic changes induced by PAF inhalation in human beings. *Clin Pharmacol Ther* 1990; 47:456–462.

35. Freitag A, Watson RW, Matsos G, Eastwood C, O'-Byrne PM. The effect of a platelet activating factor antagonist, WEB 2086, on allergen-induced asthmatic responses. *Thorax* 1993; 48:594–599.

36. Kuitert LM, Hui KP, Uthayarkumar S, Burke W, Newland AC, Uden S, Barnes NC. Effect of a platelet activating factor (PAF) antagonist, UK 74,505 on allergen-induced early and late responses. *Am Rev Resp Dis* 1993; 147:82–86.

Hyposensitization and Allergen Avoidance: Better than Drugs?

Hans-Jørgen Malling*

Keywords: Allergen-specific treatment, allergen avoidance, asthma, clinical efficacy, immunotherapy, patient compliance, pharmacotherapy, quality of life, rhinitis

Allergic diseases may be treated using different approaches. The optimal situation is to avoid initiation of the allergic inflammation, by avoiding exposure to the offending allergen. Using allergen avoidance exclusively only has relevance in a few patients. Specific treatment by allergen injections has a documented anti-inflammatory effect, and the clinical efficacy has been shown in a number of controlled studies. Uncertainty as to the use of allergen specific immunotherapy relates to the risk of inducing systemic side effects, the long-term efficacy, and preventive aspects. Drug treatment seems in short-term studies to be effective, with a low frequency of adverse effects. The long-term capacity to prevent disease progression and permanent destructive change is unknown. The aims of treating allergic patients are to reduce symptoms, to interfere with disease progression, to avoid treatment-related side effects, and to improve patient compliance and quality of life. The optimal treatment strategy includes informing the patient about the nature of the disease, symptom deterioration, and the potential for intervention. Interference at different levels in the allergic cascade by combining allergen avoidance, immunotherapy, and drug treatment may potentially have the advantage of being more successful as well as eliciting less side effects. The treatment strategy has to be individually tailored, based on the offending allergens and how the patient copes with the disease.

Introduction

The optimal treatment of allergic diseases can not be defined simply by saying that a specific treatment modality is the best one in all situations. Also to be considered are the severity of the disease, the duration of symptoms, the offending allergens, the practicability of allergen avoidance, the response to drug treatment, the cost and adverse effects of different treatments, the psychological handling of the disease and of individual treatments, quality of life, etc. The optimal treatment has to be individualized, based on a precise knowledge of the advantages and disadvantages of each treatment modality, combined with a psychosocial evaluation of the patient, taking into consideration the expectations of, and prejudice against, various kinds of treatments. In this context, not only strict scientific evidence, but also psychological aspects play a major role. The availability of a highly effective drug is of little value if the patient does not want to undergo drug treatment. This paper will try to argue why access to various treatment modalities is likely to give the best results and to have the highest clinical success.

Treatment of Allergic Diseases

The allergic inflammatory cascade is induced by the exposure of mucosal IgE-bearing mast cells to allergens. The release of allergic mediators from mast cells, and the activation of inflammatory cells, results in symptoms which are due to the activation of target receptor cells (1). Because of the inflammatory nature of allergic diseases, treatment should not only be directed at reducing or diminishing symptoms but at reducing or even eliminating the inflammation, i.e., an anti-inflammatory treatment (2). In a highly simplified form, treating or reducing allergic symptoms can be approached from three different angles (Figure 1).

---

* Allergy Unit, National University Hospital, Copenhagen, Denmark.

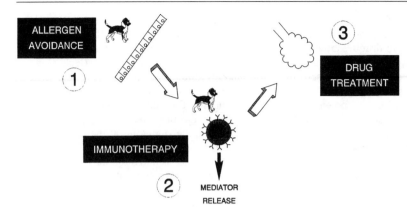

Figure 1. Possible interventions in the allergic inflammatory cascade. The most rational is to avoid contact with allergens (1). The next possibility is to reduce the release of allergic mediators, which seems to be the main action of immunotherapy (2). The ultimate approach is to inhibit the mediator-induced activation of target organ receptors by anti-allergic drugs (3).

Allergen Avoidance

The most logical approach to circumventing symptoms is to avoid the offending allergen coming into contact with mucosal IgE-bearing mast cells, as this will prevent activation of the allergic inflammation and thereby the symptoms. House dust-allergic asthmatic patients who have been moved to an allergen-free environment show a reduction in clinical symptoms and a significant reduction in inflammatory eosinophil markers (3). Basically, it seems easy to avoid allergens, or at least to reduce the exposure to the triggering allergens. In practice, full control of symptoms by allergen avoidance is very hard to obtain without extensive restrictions in the patient's life (4). Allergens like pollens or mold spores are ubiquitous in the air for long periods of the year. Animal dander allergens may be avoided by instructing the patients not to have pets and to avoid contact with furred animals. Unless the patient's life is to become severely restricted, it is not possible to totally eliminate the indirect allergen contact of the patient by exposure to animal allergens in connection with school, work, public transport, social contacts, etc. (4). The emotional unwillingness to get rid of a beloved pet is a particular problem. In theory, elimination of house dust mites is possible, but in practice it has proven difficult to reduce the number of mites by ordinary cleaning (5). Extensive mechanical ventilation might diminish the relative humidity to a level incompatible with the survival of mites, but does not remove the reservoir of mite pellets (6). Dry cleaning (7) and encasing mattresses (8) reduce mite allergens, but the clinical effect on symptoms is unknown. When discussing allergen avoidance, both a careful allergy diagnosis and

monitoring of allergen exposure before and during avoidance measures are crucial.

Hyposensitization = Allergen-Specific Immunotherapy

Allergen-specific immunotherapy was the cornerstone of specific treatment of allergic diseases until the introduction of highly efficacious anti-allergic drugs during the last decades. The decline in the use of specific treatment is probably a result of several factors. The use of immunotherapy is critically dependent on the establishment of a specific diagnosis, allergic symptoms being caused by a few dominant allergies, the availability of high-quality allergen extracts, physician's education and confidence in this kind of treatment, and the motivation of the patient (4). To many patients the advantages of immunotherapy are related to the mechanisms of action (9). Immunotherapy has shown an anti-inflammatory capacity in a number of studies. Mediator release as estimated by TAME-esterase, histamine, and PGD_2 decreases significantly in actively treated patients (10, 11), as does the recruitment of eosinophils in the late-phase nasal reaction (11, 12). Immunotherapy prevents the seasonal rise in spontaneous and ragweed-induced histamine-releasing factor production (13), and may induce an increase in BAL CD4+ (T-helper) cells (14). Using the late-phase skin reaction as a model in hay-fever patients successfully treated with grass pollen, a reduction in infiltrating CD4+ cells and activated eosinophils was observed, and immunotherapy induced significant cytokine mRNA expression for IL-2 and IFN-γ (15), i.e., expression

127

of a Th1-type cytokine profile (1). The clinical efficacy, i.e., a significant reduction in symptoms and the need for anti-allergic drug treatment, has been shown in a number of studies (4, 16). Furthermore, patients are pleased with the concept of trying to interfere with the pathophysiological mechanisms of the disease, i.e., the potential for treating the cause of the disease and not only the symptoms. Hypothetically, immunotherapy might work by accelerating the natural process, resulting in symptoms that either disappear or reduce in severity with age. Although still a matter of controversy, some follow-up studies seem to indicate that immunotherapy over a sufficiently long period of time (3–5 years) results in long-lasting clinical efficacy (4),in contrast to drug treatment that has to be continued "lifelong." In contrast to drug treatment, immunotherapy exclusively reduces symptoms induced by the allergen used for injection, i.e., it has no effect on symptoms caused by other allergens and symptoms induced by nonspecific triggers (4). This also implies that immunotherapy should only be considered in patients who are allergic to a few dominant allergens, and with minimal symptoms caused by nonspecific hyper-reactivity (4). To put this into perspective, immunotherapy should probably be considered in only 15–20% of allergic individuals, and when the proportion of allergy-induced symptoms is high, with children as the primary target group. The disadvantages of immunotherapy are primarily related to the risk of inducing systemic side effects (16). In fact this risk may represent the only real argument against immunotherapy, while all other arguments (such as the lack of clinical efficacy and poor patient compliance) are merely justifications for not running the rather limited risk of immunotherapy. This is not an attempt to ignore the fact that immunotherapy does indeed involve a risk of inducing severe life-threatening side effects or even death (17). The risks must, however, be put into perspective by comparing the frequency of severe life-threatening side effects (4) with the risk of not treating the allergic disease properly (18, 19) and the risk of pharmacotherapy (20). It is worth noting that more patients have died due to the toxicity of theophylines, which are still widely used in many parts of the world, than those who have received immunotherapy. Identifying the real risk of immunotherapy in a routine fashion is difficult, because of the lack of scientific evidence. In controlled studies, often investigating high-potency extracts and rapid dose increase regimens, the risks have

been reported to range from zero to a very low percentage; the majority of side effects have been rather mild, and very few have been life-threatening (4). The risk of inducing side effects may be substantially diminished by adhering to practical guidelines on monitoring patients, reducing doses or omitting injections depending on the reaction to the previous injection, the time interval between injections, and the symptoms at the time of injection (4). Careful monitoring of the patient for 30 min after injection, and initiation of treatment in the early phase of a reaction with appropriate drugs, primarily adrenaline supplied with corticosteroids and antihistamines, may reduce the risk to a minimum (4). Careful education of the treating physician and the availability of drugs and equipment for treating anaphylactic reactions are essential (21).

Pharmacological Treatment

Drug treatment has during the last few decades become the treatment of choice for allergic diseases. The availability of highly efficacious drugs is a major advantage for allergic patients. We must, however, realize that drug treatment alone does not seem to solve some of the major concerns of allergic diseases, such as the increase in asthma morbidity and mortality (22). Likewise, childhood asthma frequently persists in adolescence. Follow-ups of asthmatic children after 15 years (actual age at follow-up 21–29 years; mean age 25 years) confirmed the rather poor prognosis of childhood asthma, since 76% of subjects still had respiratory symptoms in adulthood (23). During the last decade, the importance of anti-inflammatory drug treatment has been emphasized (2). But many asthmatics are still treated primarily with β_2-agonists, and the majority of hay fever patients use antihistamines (treating the symptoms not the inflammation). Topically administered corticosteroids are recommended as the treatment of choice even for mild to moderate disease severity (2, 24). Their clinical efficacy in rhinitis has been documented by more than 70 placebo-controlled double-blind studies (24), and also in asthma their efficacy is evident (25). At least four essential questions regarding topical corticosteroids emerge:

1. Patient compliance: True patient compliance is only half of the expected level, indicating that patients do not take the drug at all, or take it in-

termittently or in a reduced dose. This limits the usefulness of an efficacious drug in daily clinical practice.

2. The administration of sufficiently high doses to target receptor cells: In allergic rhinitis this problem might not be important, but in asthma the delivery of drugs to epithelial cells in the most peripherally small airways is uncertain. Studies using labeled drugs or small particles do not demonstrate drug delivery to the peripheral airways convincingly enough (26). As inflammation also involves mucous membranes in the small airways, treating only the larger airways might mask the development of chronic irreversible structural changes in the smaller airways. Lung function tests such as peak flow or FEV1 only measure large airway function, and do not therefore elucidate the true scope of the problem.

3. Clinical efficacy: Although topical corticosteroids are effective, complete freedom from symptoms is not the rule, unless unacceptably high doses are used, implying an increased risk of side effects. A recent study investigating rather low doses of fluticasone and beclomethasone in adult asthmatics showed an increase in symptom-free days from about 20% to about 35%, an increase in symptom-free nights from 50% to 60%, and an increase in rescue-free days from 20% to 35%, but definitely not complete relief from symptoms (27). A study of intranasal corticosteroids (400 µg beclomethasone daily) in perennial allergic rhinitis resulted in a 45% reduction in total rhinitis score, in contrast to a 32% reduction with placebo (28). In other words, when the placebo effects are subtracted, the clinical benefit from a potent drug administered in a high dose was a 13% further reduction in symptoms, but the mean rhinitis score in actively treated patients was not reduced to half of the baseline values!

4. Long-term side effects of topical corticosteroids: In general, the use of topical steroids is considered to be safe. Short-term studies of intranasal corticosteroids only rarely resulted in side effects that made it necessary to discontinue the treatment (24). Long-term treatment with low to moderate doses is likewise safe, while the use of larger doses may result in systemic side effects. Inhaled corticosteroids are typically used in the treatment of asthma at higher doses that might give rise to concern about the long-term side effects (20). In severe asthma, the

risk:benefit ratio of inhaled corticosteroids has to be balanced against the alternative systemic corticosteroids, as the use of high-dose inhaled steroids implies a reduced intake of oral corticosteroids. An apparent individual susceptibility to side effects not necessarily related to the clinical efficacy confounds the evaluation of the safety of inhaled corticosteroids. One side effect indicating that inhaled corticosteroids have a systemic effect is the high frequency of easy bruising (29), which is not always reflected in hypothalamo-pituitary-adrenal (HPA) function (30). The long-term consequences of inhaled corticosteroids in the treatment of asthma, in relation to both preventing the accelerated decline in lung function (19) and the side effects in patients continuously treated with these drugs for 30–50 years, are unknown (20). Although no serious adverse effects have been observed in patients treated only with inhaled corticosteroids, the evidence pointing to disturbed HPA axis function is sufficiently impressive to raise concern about the use of these drugs. The current trend to use inhaled corticosteroids in larger doses in young patients calls for some caution in view of our lack of knowledge of how serious the side effects may turn out to be with long-term use (20). There is thus an obvious need for more longitudinal studies investigating the differences among various corticosteroids, delivery systems, and disease severities.

Conclusion

The treatment strategy for allergic diseases needs re-evaluation, using a holistic view and taking into consideration not only stringent scientific data, but also psychological aspects, such as how the patient copes with the disease and his or her expectations of the treatment. Patients often have insufficient knowledge as to the nature of the disease, the availability of different treatment concepts, the advantages and disadvantages of possible treatments, the inconvenience and cost of anti-allergic treatment, etc. Education of patients and information about possible treatment alternatives is crucial, as is involving the patient in the care of his or her disease and the treatment. The better the patient understands the disease and the potentials for intervention, the better the chances are of obtaining a

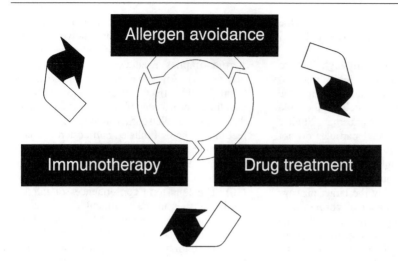

Figure 2. Integrated approach to the treatment of allergic diseases. Individual treatment modalities may be used in mild, uncomplicated disease. In more severe diseases, individual tailoring of the intervention strategy is important, combining allergen avoidance, immunotherapy, and drug treatment (for further explanation see text).

good result, increasing the patient's compliance and improving the quality of life.

The aims of treating allergic patients are to:
- Reduce symptoms to a degree allowing patients to live without limitations in normal daily activities
- Interfere with the natural progression of the disease, and, if possible, to prevent chronic irreversible structural changes
- Avoid or minimize treatment-related side effects
- Improve the patient's knowledge of the disease and treatment, resulting in improved patient compliance, awareness of the disease, and quality of life

The holistic approach to treating allergic diseases is highly demanding for the physician. It requires a comprehensive knowledge of the availability, advantages, and disadvantages of different treatment modalities, as well as a profound knowledge of the patient, taking into consideration the patient's education and psychosocial background, how well he or she copes with the disease, etc., as well as time for informing the patient, regular follow-ups, and adjustment of the treatment. Just supplying the patient with a prescription will not solve the tremendous socioecomomic and human impact of allergic diseases. The key point in this issue is the allergist, with his education and knowledge of "pros and cons" of the different treatments available.

The main issue in treating allergic disease is to use an approach interfering as broadly as possible in the pathophysiological mechanisms of the allergic cascade (Figure 2). Interference at different lev-

els in the allergic cascade may have the advantage of being more successful, and eliciting fewer side effects, than a single treatment modality. It would of course be preferable if allergen avoidance could eliminate symptoms completely, as the side effects induced by other treatments could then be avoided. The practicability and efficacy are, however, often extremely limited, and allergen avoidance has to be combined with other approaches. Drug treatment for mild and intermittent symptoms is often an acceptable option, based on patient compliance and side effects. In more bothersome cases, individual tailoring of the intervention strategy is essential, involving the patient in the process of decision-making. The advantages of combining allergen avoidance, immunotherapy, and drug treatment require further investigations focusing on patient compliance, long-term preventive aspects, and cost/effectiveness/side effect calculations. The question raised in the title of the paper can therefore only be answered by stating that all treatment modalities have advantages and disadvantages, and that the best practical treatment of allergic diseases is a combination of separate intervention methods acting at different levels of the allergic cascade.

Address for correspondence:

Hans-Jørgen Malling, MD
Allergy Unit 7551
National University Hospital
Tagensvej 20
DK-2200 Copenhagen N
Denmark

References

1. Ricci M, Rossi O, Bertoni M, Matucci A. The importance of Th2-like cells in the pathogenesis of airway allergic inflammation. *Clin Exp Allergy* 1993; 23: 360–369.

2. International Consensus Report on diagnosis and management of asthma. *Allergy* 1992; 47 (Suppl 14).

3. Boner AL, Peroni DG, Piacentini GL, Venge P. Influence of allergen avoidance at high altitude on serum markers of eosinophil activation in children with allergic asthma. *Clin Exp Allergy* 1993; 23:1021.

4. Malling H-J, Weeke B (Eds). EAACI Immunotherapy Position Paper. *Allergy* 1993; 48 (Suppl 14):9.

5. Platts-Mills TAE, Thomas WR, Alberse RC, Vervloet D, Chapman MD. Report of the second international workshop. *J Allergy Clin Immunol* 1992; 89:1046.

6. Wickman M, Emenius G, Egmar A-C, Axelsson G, Pershagen G. Reduced mite allergen levels in dwellings with mechanical exhaust and supply ventilation. *Clin Exp Allergy* 1994; 24:109.

7. Vandenhove T, Soler M, Birnbaum J, Chapin D, Vervloet D. Effect of dry cleaning on mite allergen levels in blankets. *Allergy* 1993; 48:264.

8. Wickman M, Nordvall SL, Pershagen G, Korsgaard J, Johansen N, Sundell J. Mite allergens during 18 months of intervention. *Allergy* 1994; 49:114.

9. Durham SR, Varney V, Gaga M et al. Immunotherapy and allergic inflammation. *Clin Exp Allergy* 1991; 21:206.

10. Hedlin G, Silber G, Naclerio R et al. Comparison of the in-vivo and in-vitro response to ragweed immunotherapy in children and adults with ragweed-induced rhinitis. *Clin Exp Allergy* 1990; 20:491.

11. Iliopoulos O, Proud D, Adkinson NF et al. Effects of immunotherapy on the early, late, and rechallenge nasal reaction to provocation with allergens: Changes in inflammatory mediators and cells. *J Allergy Clin Immunol* 1991; 87:855.

12. Furin MJ, Norman PS, Creticos PS et al. Immunotherapy decreases antigen-induced eosinophil cell migration into the nasal cavity. *J Allergy Clin Immunol* 1991; 88:27.

13. Brunet C, Bédard P-M, Lavoie A et al. Allergic rhinitis to ragweed pollen. II. Modulation of histamine-releasing factor production by specific immunotherapy. *J Allergy Clin Immunol* 1992; 89:87.

14. Rak S, Hallden G, Sörensen S et al. The effect of immunotherapy on T-cell subsets in peripheral blood and bronchoalveolar lavage fluid in pollen-allergic patients. *Allergy* 1993; 48:460.

15. Varney VA, Hamid QA, Gaga M et al. Influence of grass pollen immunotherapy on cellular infiltration and cytokine MRNA expression during allergen-induced late-phase cutaneous responses. *J Clin Invest* 1993; 92:644.

16. Bousquet J, Hejjaoui A, Michel F-B. Specific immunotherapy in asthma. *J Allergy Clin Immunol* 1990; 86:292.

17. Reid MJ, Lockey RE, Turkeltaub PC, Platts-Mills TAE. Survey of fatalities from skin testing and immunotherapy 1985–1989. *J Allergy Clin Immunol* 1993; 92:6.

18. Buist S. Asthma mortality: What we have learned? *J Allergy Clin Immunol* 1989; 84:273.

19. Bousquet J, Chanez P, Lacoste JY, et al. Asthma, a disease remodelling the airways. *Allergy* 1992; 47:3.

20. Dukes MNG, Holgate ST, Pauwels RA. Report of an international workshop on risk and safety of asthma therapy. *Clin Exp Allergy* 1994; 24:160.

21. AAAI Board of Directors. Guidelines to minimize the risk from systemic reactions caused by immunotherapy with allergenic extracts (Position statement). *J Allergy Clin Immunol* 1994; 93:811.

22. Sly RM. Mortality from asthma 1979–1984. *J Allergy Clin Immunol* 1988; 82:705.

23. Roorda RJ, Gerretsen J, van Aalderen WMC, et al. Follow-up of asthma from childhood to adulthood: Influence of potential childhood risk factors on the outcome of pulmonary function and bronchial responsiveness in adulthood. *J Allergy clin Immunol* 1994; 93: 575.

24. Mygind N. Glucocorticosteroids and rhinitis. *Allergy* 1993; 48:476.

25. Szefler SJ. Glucorticoid therapy for asthma. Clinical pharmacology. *J Allergy Clin Immunol* 1991; 88:147.

26. Summers QA. Inhaled drugs and the lung. *Clin Exp Allergy* 1991; 21:259.

27. Leblanc P, Mink S, Keistinen T, et al. A comparison of fluticasone propionate 200 µg/day with beclomethasone dipropionate 400 µg/day in adult asthma. *Allergy* 1994; 49:380.

28. Watson WTA, Becker AB, Simons FER. Treatment of allergic rhinitis with intranasal corticosteroids in patients with mild asthma: Effect on lower airway responsiveness. *J Allergy Clin Immunol* 1993; 91:97.

29. Mak VHF, Melchor R, Spiro SG. Easy bruising as a side-effect of inhaled corticosteroids. *Eur Respir J* 1992, 5:1068.

30. Padfield Pl, Teelucksingh S. Inhaled corticosteroids – the endocrinologist's view. *Eur Respir Rev* 1993; 3:494.

T Cells, Immunosuppression and Asthma

Sara H Lock, AB Kay*

Keywords: T lymphocytes, immunosuppression, corticosteroids, cyclosporin A, asthma

Asthma is a chronic inflammatory disorder characterized by infiltration of the bronchial mucosa with inflammatory cells, predominantly T lymphocytes and eosinophils. Increasing evidence suggests that increased numbers of CD4 T lymphocytes are activated in asthma. They release lymphokines which are relevant to the accumulation and activation of eosinophils in the bronchial mucosa, e. g., IL-3, IL-5, and GM-CSF. Parameters of disease severity have been related to the numbers of infiltrating lymphocytes and eosinophils and their activation status.

Glucocorticoids are the mainstay of modern therapy for asthma and have been shown to reduce T lymphocyte activation and cytokine production. Patients with severe disease may require long term oral glucocorticoid therapy and are at risk from developing long term side effects, particularly osteoporosis. There is also a group of patients who are clinically resistant to glucocorticoid therapy and whose T lymphocytes are not inhibited by these drugs *in vitro*. These two groups of patients may benefit from additional immunosuppressive therapy. The central role of the T lymphocyte in orchestrating inflammation in asthma suggests that drugs which target these cells may prove beneficial.

Cyclosporin A (CsA) inhibits T lymphocyte activation and proliferation by inhibiting the transcription of lymphokine mRNA. Clinical studies of CsA in chronic severe asthma have suggested a corticosteroid sparing effect with improvement in lung function. Other immunosuppressants which inhibit T lymphocytes may be of benefit in the treatment of chronic asthma in the future (e. g., FK506, rapamycin).

Introduction

Asthma affects between 5 and 10% of the population and the incidence appears to be increasing. Despite development of modern medications there are still 2000 deaths/year due to asthma in the UK.

Asthma is now accepted to be an inflammatory disorder characterized by an eosinophilic desquamative bronchitis. In this paper we will discuss the role of the T lymphocyte in the pathogenesis of asthma and the role of immunosuppressive agents in treatment for asthma.

T Cells

T cells have specific receptors which recognize antigen processed by and presented on the surface of antigen-presenting cells. Antigen binding in association with cell-cell interaction via MHC molecules leads to activation of CD4 "helper" T cells which can release a large number of proinflammatory lymphokines. The latter have many overlapping functions and can orchestrate different inflammatory responses (e. g., interleukin-5 [IL-5] promotes the differentiation of, primes and increases the survival of eosinophils).

Role of T Cells in Mucosal Inflammation

Early post-mortem studies of patients dying of acute asthma revealed mucous plugging of the airways and intense infiltration of the bronchial mucosa by inflammatory cells, particularly eosinophils and T lymphocytes (1). The technique of fibreoptic bronchoscopy, allowing bronchial biopsy and bronchoalveolar lavage, has enabled volunteers with mild asthma to be studied and compared with atopic non-asthmatics and normal controls. These studies have revealed chronic inflammatory changes in the bronchial mucosa, in these subjects with apparently well-controlled disease, that have similar characteristics to those found in patients dying due to asthma. In an electron micros-

* Department of Allergy and Clinical Immunology, Royal Brompton/National Heart & Lung Institute, London, UK.

copy study of such biopsies, elevated numbers of infiltrating lymphocytes were found to be irregular, suggesting activation in asthmatics compared to atopic non-asthmatics and normal controls (2). Evidence for airway T-lymphocyte activation has been provided by immunocytochemistry studies demonstrating increased expression of the interleukin-2 receptor (IL-2R) on bronchial mucosa T cells (3). In this study and others the total numbers of CD4 and CD8 T lymphocytes in the bronchial mucosa were comparable to normal controls, but activation of these cells, suggested by IL-2R expression, was only present in asthmatics (3–5). A study utilizing the technique of double-immunostaining demonstrated that the majority of IL-2R-positive cells in the bronchial mucosa were T lymphocytes (6). Infiltrating eosinophils have also been shown to be activated using the monoclonal antibody EG2- which binds to the secreted form of eosinophil cationic protein (ECP) (3). These studies have demonstrated a relationship between numbers of activated T lymphocytes and the total numbers of eosinophils and the numbers of activated eosinophils in the bronchial mucosa (3–5). There is evidence to suggest that activation of T lymphocytes and eosinophil recruitment into the bronchial mucosa with subsequent secretion of the latter's products may contribute to epithelial damage and possibly bronchial hyper-responsiveness in asthma (7). Thus circumstantial evidence is accumulating to support the hypothesis that activated CD4 T lymphocytes determine the numbers and activation status of eosinophils in the bronchial mucosa in asthma which may affect disease severity.

T Cell Cytokine Production

Studies in mice have revealed two subsets of CD4 T-lymphocytes, Th1 and Th2, differentiated by their cytokine profile (8). Th1 cells can elicit delayed-type hypersensitivity reactions and secrete IL-2, IL-3, IFN-γ, TNF-α, TNF-β, and GM-CSF, whilst Th2 cells secrete IL-3, IL-4, IL-5, IL-6, IL-10, and GM-CSF and are implicated in allergic inflammation. Studies of cutaneous late-phase and delayed-type hypersensitivity reactions have provided evidence that similar subsets may exist in man (9,10). Serum and culture supernatants of unstimulated peripheral-blood mononuclear cells from asthmatics, but not controls, have been found to prolong the survival of cultured eosinophils *in*

vitro (11). This effect was partially inhibited by specific antibodies against IL-3, IL-5 and GM-CSF, providing evidence for the presence of these lymphokines in asthmatic serum and suggesting their spontaneous secretion by T lymphocytes *in vivo*. Using the technique of *in situ* hybridization to detect cytokine, mRNA studies have demonstrated that IL-5 mRNA is present in cells in the bronchial mucosa of some mild asthmatics, but not normal controls (12). The numbers of activated CD4 T lymphocytes and eosinophils in these bronchial biopsies could be correlated with the amount of IL-5 mRNA. Cells retrieved from bronchoalveolar lavage (BAL) fluid in a group of mild asthmatics have been found to express significantly increased amounts of mRNA encoding IL-2, IL-3, IL-4, IL-5, and GM-CSF, but not interferon-γ, as compared with normal controls (13). Separation of T lymphocytes from the remainder of the BAL cells using immunomagnetic beads revealed that 98% of the IL-4 and IL-5 mRNA was associated with these cells (13). Thus, cytokine-mediated interactions between lymphocytes and eosinophils may be important in the regulation of airway inflammation in asthma.

Effects of Glucocorticoids on T Cells in Disease

An increased percentage of peripheral blood CD4 T lymphocytes were shown to express activation markers (IL-2R, VLA-1 and HLA-DR) in patients with acute severe asthma using the technique of flow cytometry (14). The expression of IL-2R and HLA-DR decreased following oral corticosteroid therapy, and the reduction in IL-2R correlated with clinical improvement (15). Oral corticosteroid therapy has also been shown to reduce numbers of peripheral blood memory (CD45RO) CD4 T lymphocytes (16). A proportion of patients in this study had elevated serum concentrations of IL-5, which was not present in control serum nor in the patients' serum following treatment with oral corticosteroids. A recent double-blind placebo-controlled study of corticosteroid therapy in moderate asthma found decreased bronchial hyperresponsiveness associated with decreased expression of mRNA for IL-4 and IL-5 by BAL cells in subjects receiving corticosteroids as compared with placebo (17). This suggests that the beneficial effects of corticosteroids in asthma may result from modulation of T-lymphocyte activation and cytokine production.

Effects of Glucocorticoids on T Cells In Vitro

Some patients have been demonstrated to be clinically unresponsive to corticosteroids and termed corticosteroid-resistant (18). The effect of corticosteroids on T-cell activation markers and serum cytokines has been investigated in patients with corticosteroid-resistant and corticosteroid-sensitive asthma (19). It was found that patients with corticosteroid-resistant asthma had increased expression of activation markers on CD4 T lymphocytes compared to corticosteroid-sensitive patients despite corticosteroid therapy. Furthermore, proliferation of T lymphocytes from corticosteroid-resistant patients was not inhibited by therapeutic concentrations of dexamethasone *in vitro*, but was moderately inhibited by cyclosporin A (CsA). Similarly, the production of IL-2 and IFN-γ by T lymphocytes was not inhibited by dexamethasone, but was inhibited by CsA. This suggests that other "anti-T lymphocyte" agents, such as CsA, may be of benefit in severe asthma.

Immunosuppression

Glucocorticoids

The beneficial effects of glucocorticoids in the management of asthma are well established (20). Inhaled glucocorticoids are recommended therapy for chronic asthma, and in severe asthma oral glucocorticoids are often required to control symptoms (21). Patients with severe asthma taking oral glucocorticoid therapy are at risk from developing the unwanted side effects of long-term administration of glucocorticoids, particularly osteoporosis, and may remain symptomatic with impaired lung function. Those patients who require oral glucocorticoids to control their disease, or who are clinically resistant to glucocorticoids, may benefit from additional or alternative immunosuppressive agents to improve disease control and reduce adverse effects.

Glucocorticoids bind to a cytosolic receptor which then translocates to the nucleus to interact with glucocorticoid receptive elements which can stimulate or inhibit gene transcription. They are known to inhibit T-lymphocyte proliferation and cytokine production *in vitro* (22). Present evidence suggests that in most subjects T lymphocytes and antigen-presenting cells are inhibited by corticosteroids, but that B lymphocytes, granulocytes (especially eosinophils) and mast cells are not (23). This, in conjunction with the evidence above, suggests that the activated CD4 T lymphocyte may be an important target for glucocorticoid therapy in asthma. Drugs such as cyclosporin A known to act on T lymphocytes and modulate cytokine production might therefore be of therapeutic value in severe asthma.

Previously Assessed Corticosteroid Sparing Agents

Azathiaprine, methotrexate and gold salts have been studied as potential corticosteroid sparing agents in asthma. Double-blind, placebo-controlled studies of azathiaprine, a purine antagonist, in chronic severe asthma did not demonstrate any significant benefit and azathiaprine therapy was associated with unwanted effects (24). Purine antagonists have relatively little effect on T-lymphocyte proliferative responses *in vitro*. Their primary mechanism of action appears to be at the level of killer cell activity and antibody production.

The precise mode of the anti-inflammatory action of gold salts is uncertain, although *in vitro* studies have demonstrated inhibition of mitogen-induced proliferation of T lymphocytes. Both parenteral and oral preparations have been evaluated in asthma. Parenteral gold is associated with significant adverse effects (e. g., proteinuria), and a blinded crossover study, whilst suggesting some benefit, concluded that side effects may preclude its continued use (25). A more recent study of oral gold salts has shown a significant corticosteroid sparing effect of 4 mg in the auranofin-treated group as compared with 0.3 mg in the placebo group (26). Lung function (FEV_1) improved by 6.4%, but two patients were withdrawn because of serious exacerbations of constitutional eczema.

The anti-metabolite methotrexate (MTX) is a folic acid antagonist inhibiting synthesis of purine and thymidine. There have been several studies evaluating MTX in chronic severe asthma. Low-dosage therapy (15 mg/wk) over 24 weeks in double-blind controlled study has been shown to produce an average reduction in corticosteroid dosage of 50%, as compared with 14% in controls (27). However, there were no significant effects on lung function and its use as a corticosteroid sparing agent is limited by side effects such as hepatic toxicity and nausea.

Cyclosporin A: Mechanisms of Action

Cyclosporin A (CsA) is a lipophilic, cyclic undecapeptide which was derived from fungal cultures of *Tolypocladium inflatum* in the 1970s. Like corticosteroids, CsA is thought to exert its immunosuppressive effects predominantly via inhibition of T lymphocytes, although it does have effects on other cells (e. g., mast cells and basophils). It inhibits T-lymphocyte proliferation, but is not myelotoxic and is now widely used in transplantation medicine. It has been evaluated in many autoimmune diseases, such as rheumatoid arthritis, psoriasis and more recently asthma. CsA inhibits T-lymphocyte activation at an early stage in the cell cycle ($G_0 \rightarrow G_1$), being most effective if added less than 2 h after activation. It inhibits the calcium-dependent cell signalling pathway and results in inhibition of cytokine mRNA transcription (28). CsA binds to a ubiquitous cytoplasmic protein, cyclophilin (29), which has peptidyl-prolyl *cis-trans* isomerase (PPIase) activity that is inhibited on binding CsA. However, this inhibition does not relate directly to CsA's immunosuppressive properties, as CsA derivatives which inhibit this PPIase activity are not effective immunosuppressive agents and vice versa. The CsA-cyclophilin complex binds to another cytoplasmic protein, calcineurin, which is a calcium- and calmodulin-dependent serine threonine phosphatase (30). Evidence has suggested that the cytoplasmic subunit of a transcription factor, NF-AT (nuclear factor of activated T lymphocytes), requires this phosphatase activity in order to translocate to the nucleus where it combines with its nuclear subunit to become an active transcription factor (31, 32). Thus, CsA-cyclophilin complexes prevent formation of active NF-AT in the nucleus, reducing the binding of NF-AT to cytokine gene promoter regions and hence reducing the transcription of mRNA for various cytokines (e. g., IL-2, IL-3, GM-CSF, IFN-γ). T cells have relatively low levels of calcineurin in their cytoplasm, which may explain their sensitivity to CsA.

Cyclosporin A in Chronic Severe Asthma

The increasing evidence for the central role of the T lymphocyte in the pathogenesis of asthma and the predominantly T lymphocyte effects of CsA led to the initiation of a double-blind, placebo-controlled crossover study of CsA in chronic severe asthma (33).

Thirty-three chronic severe asthmatics taking oral corticosteroids for at least 3 months in a dosage of at least 5 mg were given 12 weeks of CsA (5 mg/kg/day) and identical placebo in random order. Subjects were non-smokers with no contraindications to CsA therapy whose FEV_1 and/or PEFR was < 75% of predicted and who had shown ≥20% reversibility in lung function in response to bronchodilator (5 mg nebulised salbutamol) or spontaneously. Maintenance corticosteroid therapy was kept constant throughout the entire study period unless it was increased to treat disease exacerbations. One female patient withdrew from the study because of hypertrichosis and two patients failed to complete the protocol. CsA therapy resulted in a mean increase above placebo of 12% in morning PEFR (p < 0.004) and 17.6% in FEV_1 (p < 0.001). There was a mean reduction in diurnal variation in PEFR of 27.6% (p = 0.04). The frequency of disease exacerbations requiring an increased prednisolone dosage was reduced by 48% in patients taking CsA as compared with placebo (p < 0.02). In view of these encouraging results and the fact that CsA was well tolerated during the 12-week treatment phase, a study of CsA as a corticosteroid sparing agent was initiated. This double-blind, placebo-controlled, parallel group study has recently been completed. Thirty-nine corticosteroid-dependent asthmatics participated; 19 received CsA (5 mg/kg/day) and 20 received identical placebo. The patients kept daily diary cards recording daily prednisolone dosage, PEFR (pre and post bronchodilator), bronchodilator usage and symptom score. There was a 4 week run-in period during which prednisolone dosage was kept stable at minimum maintenance levels and then a 36 week treatment phase. An attempt was made to reduce prednisolone dosage at 14 day intervals if patients' asthma had been stable or improved as judged from the diary cards and spirometry. Three patients withdrew during the first 12 weeks of the study (1 exacerbation requiring high dose prednisolone, 1 hypertrichosis, and 1 non-asthma-related death); they were all taking CsA. In the remaining patients there was a median reduction in prednisolone dosage of 62% in the CsA-treated group as compared with 25% in the placebo-treated group (p = 0.043). Morning PEFR pre-bronchodilator increased in the CsA-treated group by a mean of 12% despite the reduction in their prednisolone dosage (p < 0.001) as compared with no significant change in the group taking placebo (p = 0.026 between groups). The major side effects of CsA are nephrotoxicity and hypertension, whilst less serious adverse effects include hyper-

135

trichosis and gum hypertrophy. There is evidence that renal toxicity remains largely reversible provided that trough blood concentrations are maintained in the range 100–200 µg/ml (average concentrations in the two studies described were 152 ng/ml and 144 ng/ml). During the corticosteroid reduction study, eight patients taking CsA and one taking placebo required treatment for hypertension, and there was a small rise in diastolic blood pressure (mean 5.48 mmHg, p <0.01). These studies suggest that cyclosporin A is an effective corticosteroid sparing agent and improves lung function in corticosteroid-dependent asthmatics. It was also well tolerated over a 36 week period, and although expected rises in blood pressure, urea and creatinine occurred they resolved on cessation of CsA therapy. Groups treating patients with transplanted lungs have been investigating the feasibility of using nebulised cyclosporin A (34). There are technical difficulties due to the lipophilic nature of the drug, but as with inhaled corticosteroids inhaled CsA therapy should have less systemic side effects and increase the range of asthmatics who could be treated with this medication.

Newer Immunosuppressant Agents

FK506 is a macrolide derived from a soil organism, *Streptomyces tsukudaiensis,* which, despite having a different structure to CsA, has similar immunosuppressant properties, although it is more potent (35). It also binds to a cytoplasmic protein named FK binding protein (FKBP) which has PPIase activity. The FK506-FKBP complex also binds to calcineurin, inhibiting its serine threonine phosphatase activity and thus reducing both the nuclear translocation of the cytoplasmic subunit of NF-AT and transcription of cytokine mRNA (30–32). FK506 is being evaluated in transplantation medicine, but its increased potency may be outweighed by similarly increased toxicity.

Rapamycin is also a macrolide which is derived from *Streptomyces hygroscopius* which binds to FKBP in competition with FK506 (36). Despite these similarities, rapamycin has a different site of action to FK506. It inhibits the cell cycle moving from the G_1 to the S phase and is effective even when added 12 h after activation. Hence, unlike CsA and FK506, it can inhibit T lymphoblasts which have already been activated, and this theoretically might result in a faster onset of therapeutic benefit in inflammatory disease. Cal-

cium-independent cell signalling pathways are affected, in contrast to CsA and FK506, which inhibit calcium-dependent pathways. It inhibits the cell signal transduction pathway following cytokine (e. g., IL-2) binding to cytokine receptor (IL-2R). The site of action for rapamycin may be a serine-threonine kinase which is required for progression into the S phase of the cell cycle. T lymphocytes are sensitive to rapamycin as they rely on IL-2/IL-2R interactions for proliferation. There is evidence to suggest that CsA and rapamycin may have synergistic effects, leading to increased therapeutic potential for this combined drug regimen.

Other new immunosuppressive agents such as brequinar sodium and mycophenolic acid which are inhibitors of *de novo* synthesis of pyrimidine and purine synthesis, respectively, are being studied as potential advances in transplantation therapy and may be evaluated for use in other autoimmune diseases in the future (37).

Alternative approaches to immunosuppression in asthma include inhibition of CD4 T lymphocytes with humanized anti-CD4 antibodies, anti-cytokine antibodies and soluble cytokine receptors.

Conclusion

Considerable support exists for the hypothesis that asthma represents a specialized form of cell-mediated immunity in which cytokines secreted by activated T lymphocytes lead to the specific accumulation and activation of eosinophils in the bronchial mucosa. Investigation of drugs inhibiting T-lymphocyte function has led to the discovery of a new therapeutic option in severe asthma, namely cyclosporin A. Development of related agents, the possibility of synergism between these agents and the emergence of technology allowing topical administration of these drugs may contribute to improved treatment for asthma in the future.

Address for correspondence:

AB Kay, Professor and Director
Department of Allergy and Clinical Immunology
National Heart & Lung Institute
Dovehouse Street
London, SW3 6LY
UK

References

1. Dunnill MS. The pathology of asthma with special reference to changes in the bronchial mucosa. *J Clin Pathol* 1960; 13:27–33.

2. Jeffery PK, Wardlaw AJ, Nelson FC, Collins JV, Kay AB. Bronchial biopsies in asthma: an ultrastructural, quantitative study and correlation with hyperreactivity. *Am Rev Respir Dis* 1989; 140:1745–1753.

3. Azzawi M, Bradley B, Jeffrey PK, Frew AJ, Wardlaw AJ, Knowles G, Assoufi B, Collins JV, Durham SR, Kay AB. Identification of activated T lymphocytes and eosinophils in bronchial biopsies in stable atopic asthma. *Am Rev Respir Dis* 1990; 142:1410–1413.

4. Bradley BL, Azzawi M, Assoufi B, Jacobson M, Collins JV, Irani A, Schwartz LB, Durham SR, Jeffery PK, Kay AB. Eosinophils, T lymphocytes, mast cells, neutrophils and macrophages in bronchial biopsies from atopic asthmatics: comparison with atopic non-asthma and normal controls and relationship to bronchial hyperresponsiveness. *J Allergy Clin Immunol* 1991; 88:661–674.

5. Bentley AM, Menz G, Storz C, Robinson DR, Bradley B, Jeffery PK, Durham SR, Kay AB. Identification of T lymphocytes, macrophages and activated eosinophils in the bronchial mucosa in intrinsic asthma:relationship to symptoms and bronchial responsiveness. *Am Rev Respir Dis* 1992; 146:500–506.

6. Hamid Q, Barkans J, Robinson DS, Durham SR, Kay AB. Coexpression of CD25 and CD3 in atopic allergy and asthma. *Immunology* 1992; 75:659–663.

7. Laitinen LA, Heino M, Laitinen A, Kava T, Haahtela T. Damage of airway epithelium and bronchial reactivity in patients with asthma. *Am Rev Respir Dis* 1985; 131:599–606.

8. Mosman TR, Coffman RL. Th1 and Th2 cells: different patterns of lymphokine secretion lead to different functional properties. *Annu Rev Immunol* 1989; 7:145–73.

9. Kay AB, Ying S, Varney V, Gaga M, Durham SR, Moqbel R, Wardlaw AJ, Hamid Q. Messenger RNA expression of the cytokine gene cluster IL-3, IL-5, GM-CSF in allergen-induced late-phase reactions in atopic subjects. *J Exp Med* 1991; 173:775–778.

10. Tsicopoulos A, Hamid Q, Varney V, Ying S, Moqbel R, Durham SR, Kay AB. Preferential messenger RNA expression of Th1-type cells (IFN-γ IL-2) in classical delayed-type (tuberculin) hypersensitivity reactions in human skin. *J Immunol* 1992; 48:2058–2061.

11. Walker C, Virchow J-C, Bruijnzeel PLB, Blaser K. T cell subsets and their soluble products regulate eosinophilia in allergic and non-allergic asthma. *J Immunol* 1991; 146:1829–1835.

12. Hamid Q, Azzawi M, Ying S, Moqbel R, Wardlaw AJ, Corrigan CJ, Bradley B, Durham SR, Collins JV, Jeffery PK, Quint DJ, Kay AB. Expression of mRNA for interleukin-5 in mucosal bronchial biopsies from asthma. *J Clin Invest* 1991; 87:1541–1546.

13. Robinson DR, Hamid Q, Ying S, Tsicopoulos A, Barkans J, Bentley AM, Corrigan CJ, Durham SR, Kay AB. Evidence for a predominant "Th-2-type" bronchoalveolar lavage T-lymphocyte population in atopic asthma. *N Engl J Med* 1992; 326:298–304.

14. Corrigan CJ, Hartnell A, Kay AB. Tlymphocyte activation in acute severe asthma. *Lancet* 1988; i:1129–1131.

15. Corrigan CJ, Kay AB. CD4 T lymphocyte activation in acute severe asthma: relationship to disease severity and atopic status. *Am Rev Respir Dis* 1990; 141:970–977.

16. Corrigan CJ, Haczku A, Gemou-Engesaeth V, Doi S, Kikuchi Y, Takatsu, Durham SR, Kay AB. CD4 T-lymphocyte activation in asthma is accompanied by increased serum concentrations of interleukin-5: effect of glucocorticoid therapy. *Am Rev Respir Dis* 1993; 147:540–547.

17. Robinson DS, Hamid Q, Ying S, Bentley AM, Assoufi B, Meng Q, Durham SR, Kay AB. Prednisolone treatment in asthma is associated with modulation of bronchoalveolar lavage cell interleukin-4, interleukin-5 and interferon-gamma cytokine gene expression. *Am Rev Respir Dis* 1993; 148:420–426.

18. Carmichael J, Paterson IC, Diaz P, Crompton GK, Kay AB, Grant IWB. Corticosteroid-resistance in chronic asthma. *Br Med J* 1981; 282:1419–1422.

19. Corrigan CJ, Brown PH, Barnes NC, Tsai JJ, Kay AB. Glucocorticoid resistance in chronic asthma: Peripheral blood T-lymphocyte activation and a comparison of the T-lymphocyte inhibitory effects of glucocorticoids and cyclosporin A. *Am Rev Respir Dis* 1991; 144:1026–1032.

20. Barnes PJ. A new approach to the treatment of asthma. *N Engl J Med* 1989; 321:1517–1527.

21. British Thoracic Society. Guidelines for management of asthma in adults. Statement by the research unit of the Royal College of Physicians of London, King's Fund Centre, National Asthma Campaign. *BMJ* 1990; 142:434–357.

22. Gillis S, Crabtree GR, Smith KA. Glucocorticoid-induced inhibition of T cell growth factor production. I. The effect on mitogen-induced lymphocyte proliferation. *J Immunol* 1979; 123:1624.

23. Schleimer RP. Effects of glucocorticosteroids on inflammatory cells relevant to their therapeutic applications in asthma. *Am Rev Respir Dis* 1990; 141:S59–69.

24. Hodges NG, Brewis RAL, Howell JBL. An evaluation of azathioprine in severe chronic asthma. *Thorax* 1971; 26:734–739.

25. Klaustermeyer WB, Noritake DT, Kwong FK. Chrysotherapy in the treatment of corticosteroid-dependent asthma. *J Allergy Clin Immunol* 1987; 79:720–725.

26. Nierop G, Gijzel WP, Bel EH, Zwinderman, Dijkman JH. Auranofin in the treatment of steroid dependent asthma: A double blind study. *Thorax* 1992; 47:349–354.

27. Shiner RJ, Nunn AJ, Chung FK, Geddes DM. Randomised, double-blind, placebo-controlled trial of methotrexate in steroid-dependent asthma. *Lancet* 1990; 336:137–140.

28. Granelli-Piperno A, Inaba K, Steinman RM. Stimulation of lymphokine release from T lymphoblasts: Requirement for mRNA synthesis and inhibition by cyclosporin A. *J Exp Med* 1984; 160:1792–1802.

29. Merker M, Handschumacher RE. Uptake and nature of the intracellular binding of cyclosporin A in a murine thymoma cell line, BW5147. *J Immunol* 1984; 132:3064.

30. Liu J, Farmer JD, Lane WS, Frieman J, Weissman I, Schreiber SL. Calcineurin is a common target of cyclophilin-cyclosporin A and FKBP-FK506 complexes. *Cell* 1991; 66:807–815.

31. Flanagan WM, Corthesy B, Bram RJ, Crabtree GR. Nuclear association of a T-cell transcription factor blocked by FK506 and cyclosporin A. *Nature* 1991; 352:803.

32. McCaffrey PG, Perrino BA, Soderling TR, Roa A. NF-ATp, a T lymphocyte DNA-binding protein that is a target for calcineurin and immunosuppressive drugs. *J Biol Chem* 1993; 268:3747.

33. Alexander AG, Barnes NC, Kay AB. Trial of cyclosporin in corticosteroid-dependent chronic severe asthma. *Lancet* 1992; 339:324–328.

34. Iacono AT, Keenan RJ, Duncan SR et al. Aerosolized cyclosporine as additional therapy for the treatment of refractory chronic rejection in lung transplant recipients. *Am Rev Resp Dis* 1994; 149(4):A730.

35. Schreiber SL, Crabtree GR. The mechanism of action of cyclosporin A and FK506. *Immunol Today* 1992; 13:136–141.

36. Nolan NH, Dumont FJ. Cyclosporin A, FK506, and rapamycin: Pharmacological probes of lymphocyte signal transduction. *Annu Rev Immunol* 1992; 10:519–560.

37. Thomson AW, Starzl TE. New immunosuppressive drugs: Mechanistic insights and potential therapeutic advances. *Immunol Rev* 1993; 136:71–98.

Patient Self-Management: Goals and Limits

Tony Foucard*

Keywords: Self-management, compliance

Asthma, eczema, and chronic rhinitis, with or without allergy, are suitable disorders for self-management as they are chronic and variable in course and severity. To obtain a good treatment result demands a well-informed patient with a good ability to comply with suggested treatment and prophylactic regimens, and to adjust them within given limits in relation to variations of symptoms or of exposure to allergens and irritants. The education and continuous support of the patient needs time, competence, enthusiasm, and accessibility of the medical team. This includes not only the doctor and nurse but sometimes also the physiotherapist, psychologist, social welfare officer, and dietitian.

Every year, medical societies, drug committees, and consensus groups meet to discuss therapeutic approaches to allergic diseases. This is important to achieve and maintain a good medical standard. These efforts stand in great contrast to the time we use to discuss means of achieving good patient compliance with suggested treatment regimens. We all know how difficult it is to get a patient to take penicillin for a full 7- or 10-day course. It is even more difficult to obtain good compliance in patients with a chronic disease treated using drugs with effects of such a type that no acute problems are noticed when single doses are omitted. Good compliance is even more difficult to achieve in chronic disorders characterized by better and worse periods, where the patients are expected to adjust the treatment in relation to the severity of the disease. This is the situation for most patients with eczema or asthma, and for some patients with rhinitis.

We all know why so little time is spent discussing these problems – there are no simple ways of achieving good compliance, and no single method is suitable for all patients. In spite of this it is important to define the problems and to discuss ways to obtain the best possible result.

Asthma and noninfectious rhinitis are more or less strongly influenced by exogenous factors. These include allergens such as animal danders, house dust mites, pollens, molds, and foods, but also respiratory tract infections, exercise, tobacco smoke, perfumes, or air polluted in other ways. These disorders have a varying severity and course. Some patients only notice symptoms on contact with defined substances, while others have mild chronic symptoms with exacerbations now and then. A smaller group has more severe chronic symptoms with better and worse periods. Since these disorders are chronic and variable, they are most suitable for self-treatment.

The best way to handle allergies and asthma is to prevent their onset. This is only possible if the person at risk can be identified, and unfortunately prevention is possible in only a minority of such identified individuals. The atopic trait is inherited. It is probably of polygenic inheritance with a varying degree of penetration. Furthermore, the proneness to asthma also seems to be inherited. Thus, it is possible to identify most children at risk of subsequent allergy or asthma. For risk infants, the best preventive measures are to breast-feed them for a longer period, preferably 6 months or more, and to withhold the introduction of strongly allergenic foods such as egg and fish up to at least 12 months. Furthermore, and this is important for children at risk, the indoor environment should be kept free of tobacco smoke and furry pet animals, and it should be made as uncomfortable as possible for house dust mites by maintaining adequate ventilation and good dust-cleaning routines. If sensitization cannot be prevented, the next best step is to prevent symptoms by eliminating or at least reducing contacts with relevant allergens and irritants. An early diagnosis is necessary for such secondary prevention, and especially when the patient is exposed to the allergen in his or her daily environment. It is also important with an early diagnosis to achieve an op-

---

* Department of Pediatrics, University Hospital, Uppsala, Sweden.

timal therapy, as it is easier to obtain a good result in mild cases than in severe ones and before chronic changes have developed.

The most severely handicapped patients are found among those who suffer from asthma, severe eczema, or severe food hypersensitivity to several daily foods. Although rather many infants and young children suffer from severe eczema and severe food hypersensitivity, the prognosis is fairly good and such patients usually improve within a few years. If these patients are not treated as well as possible, the quality of life for the family will be affected, and the child with severe hypersensitivity may experience life-threatening acute reactions or in the long run undernutrition. Otherwise, the long-term prognosis for these patients is probably not much worse than if they had been treated more vigorously. If a child with asthma is not treated optimally, chronic changes of the bronchial wall will develop in time, and such changes probably make the long-term prognosis worse. We are a little worried about the results from a recent study of deaths of asthma in Sweden. In the age group 15–24 years, deaths due to asthma occurred almost exclusively in patients with severe asthma during the 1970s and

Table 1. Estimated severity of asthma in 6 months preceding death from asthma.

| | 1–14 years | | 15–24 years | |
	mild	severe	mild	severe
1973–75	0	6	0	5
1980–81	0	6	3	12
1986–88	1	9	8	9

early 1980s (Table 1). During the period 1986–1988, 8 out of 17 deaths occurred in patients with seemingly mild asthma (1). In this study, asthma was defined as severe if the patient was treated with oral or inhaled corticosteroids or cromoglycate combined with oral β_2-agonists or theophyllins, or with oral β_2-agonists and theophyllins on a regular basis, used inhaled β_2-agonists five times per day or more, or was admitted to hospital for acute asthma during the 6 months preceding the final attack. All these patients with mild asthma who died had suffered from severe asthma for many years, but had improved during adolescence. It may indicate that chronic changes in the bronchial wall are a risk factor even when the asthma has improved so much that it is no longer regarded as severe. If this is true,

asthma remains the most important severe chronic disease in children as well as in adults.

Most efforts to teach patients how to cope with their disease are devoted to asthma. Although this is true we must not forget to show patients with eczema or severe food hypersensitivity proper time and interest. I have been told by more than one family who has a child with all three manifestations that they may well cope with the asthma, but it is much more difficult with the eczema or the food hypersensitivity.

From the patient's point of view, a complete cure as soon as possible is the best option. When a patient is told that this is not possible, a more realistic goal is to get an optimal quality of life with a minimal risk of complications and a minimal risk of developing new allergies or other sensitivities causing a clinical deterioration. For the average patient, an optimal quality of life probably means no or as few symptoms as possible. This goal should be achieved by moderate and acceptable improvements of the immediate environment, in combination with a simple and efficient pharmacotherapy without disturbing side effects. The risk of complications can be kept to a minimum by a satisfactory monitoring of the disease and good compliance with the suggested treatment regimen. Furthermore, contact with common symptom-precipitating factors should be avoided as much as possible. If these aims can be achieved, the risk of developing new allergies or other sensitivities of clinical importance will be kept at a minimum.

To obtain a good treatment result, the patient must be well informed about his or her disease, be cooperative, and comply with the treatment regimen. The patient must know how to prevent symptoms, why it is important to treat even mild asthma symptoms, how to recognize a deterioration early, and which measures (including improved pharmacotherapy) should be taken. Both oral and written information about the suggested treatment regimen, including measures for emergency situations, should be given.

To give all this information, and also convey an attitude that makes the patient motivated to take responsibility for his or her disease and its treatment and prophylaxis, is not an easy task. First of all, it takes time. To inform a patient and the family about asthma or eczema, their causes, prophylactic measures, treatment and prognosis takes at least three quarters of an hour at the first visit, and at least half an hour at the following visits. Since not only oral but also written information should be given to the patient or the family, it takes extra time. To give written information is especially important when the treatment includes more than two drugs. Otherwise there is a risk of misunderstanding.

Another corner-stone is knowledge. The doctor should be able to make clear to the patient all important aspects of the disease, why prophylactic treatment is important, how to recognize early symptoms, and how to vigorously treat them. During childhood it is highly desirable that both parents accompany their child to the doctor. The treatment of allergy, asthma, and eczema not only includes drugs but also prophylactic measures that can be very hard to accept, e. g., getting rid of a beloved dog or cat or stopping smoking. If recommendations about restrictions of the family life are given by the doctor and only one parent is present, it is often very difficult for this parent to convince the absent parent that the recommended measures must be executed.

Considering the great amount of information given, one parent often cannot remember all details, but if both are there, they may at least to some extent remember different things, and thus complement each other. To have at least two adults present is also desirable when the patient is an adolescent or an adult. More information is retained, and the companion may help the patient to interpret and remember the information given.

The prerequisites for being a good "informer" are not only good knowledge of the subject but also engagement, which is the third corner-stone. Without enthusiasm in conveying the message to the patient, one cannot expect that a prophylactic treatment will be maintained in the way the doctor expects. It is fairly easy to persuade the patient to treat ongoing symptoms, but it is much more difficult to motivate him or her for a long-term prophylactic treatment.

The fourth corner-stone is continuity. The patient should see the same doctor or team at all regular visits, which is necessary in order to optimize therapy and prophylaxis and maintain one and the same strategy. It also makes the patient feel more secure and facilitates questions and advice since the doctor does not need to have the patient's casebook available at an occasional consultation.

The fifth corner-stone is accessibility. When the patient realizes that the problems regarding therapy are beyond his/her own abilities, it should be possible to get in contact with the doctor or the nurse within a reasonable time. This gives the patient a feeling of security, a feeling that is a good basis for

the building-up of a competent patient who is self-confident regarding the disease.

In order to give the patient all the information necessary for successful treatment and prophylaxis, it may be wise to organize special lectures or courses about asthma, eczema, and food allergy, in many countries called asthma or eczema schools. The teachers in such asthma schools should not only include the doctor but also the nurse, the physiotherapist, the social welfare officer, the psychologist, and in selected cases a dietitian. Such schools also give a possibility for patients to meet others with similar problems. This may result not only in psychological support but also in the exchange of information that is of practical value in daily life.

Special problems are encountered at different ages. During infancy and childhood the parents take responsibility for the daily therapy and prophylactic measures regarding their child. This may involve special problems, as some young children are not very cooperative with inhalation devices and therefore suggested treatments may be difficult to accomplish. Poor cooperation can range from unwillingness to try to inhale, to an inadequate inhalation technique, which means that considerable less drug than expected is inhaled.

In eczema, an unwillingness to be treated with ointments may depend on whether they contain substances that cause itching or irritation of the eczematous skin. Carbamide at a concentration of 5% or more, and sometimes the preservative in common steroid ointments, may cause such problems. If the cause can be identified, a better tolerated alternative can be given and the child will probably accept the treatment much better.

As the child grows older, the parents will more and more frequently let the child carry out the treatments on his or her own. The child's motivation for treatment is often present only as long as the symptoms are troublesome, which means that there is a substantial risk that the maintenance and prophylactic treatment will not be carried out as carefully as expected. Many teenagers have to be constantly reminded about their daily treatments. This frequent reminding is considered as nagging by some teenagers, and if excessive may have the opposite effect. During adolescence, the problems may become even worse. The adolescent is trying to create an identity of his or her own and is attempting to free him- or herself from the family. He or she often listens more to friends than to parents, and tries to deviate as little as possible from the ideals regarding clothes, hair style, and behavior expressed by the peer group or other groups. There is a substantial risk that the adolescent in this situation will deny the symptoms, or at least describe them as milder and less frequent than they are. Consequently, he or she tends to undertreat the disease and accept symptoms that should not be accepted, and may adopt harmful habits, e. g., start tobacco smoking.

For the treating doctor it is one of the greatest challenges in pediatrics to be a good guide and help to the patient during these years. There is no simple way of achieving this that will suit all patients. A good start is to treat the adolescent as an adult, letting the accompanying mother or father sit in the waiting-room, to be a good listener, not to criticize too much but rather encourage and support, and to try to find compromise solutions acceptable to both parties. If this is done in a positive spirit and with a sense of humor, the patient may feel not only that the doctor is worth listening to, but that it is probably also wise to follow the recommendations, and that further check-ups are valuable. With time, the adolescent will mature, and hopefully, take more responsibility for his or her treatment.

Some of the problems met during adolescence may persist in adulthood. It may be difficult to make the patient as observant as desired of early and mild signs of deterioration. It is understandable that a patient who has been satisfied with a lung function level of about 70% of capacity will be very pleased to reach a function level of 90%. As the patient has never experienced 100%, at least not for many years, he or she does not know how it feels to have a quite normal lung function. Therefore, the motivation for even more intense treatment is often rather poor.

It is thus a very demanding task to teach the patient with asthma or eczema enough about the disease, its treatment, and risk factors, and to convince him or her to take responsibility for good compliance with the treatment regimen. This is not only desirable, but a prerequisite for good treatment results. As allergy specialists with many years of experience, we still find it difficult to achieve this goal. How will it then be possible for a less experienced general practitioner to convey knowledge and motivation to the patient?

Because of the large numbers involved, it is necessary that a large percentage of patients with asthma, eczema, and allergy be taken care of by general practitioners. Some of them will have good knowledge about these disorders and be interested and stand up for their patients, but others have less knowledge and interest and the risk of a poor result is much greater. Continuous education and training of general practitioners in the care of patients with asthma, eczema, and allergies is necessary to obtain good treatment results, and the allergy specialist has to take an active part in this work. The quality of care of patients with allergy and asthma in a given area depends more on the competence of the average general practitioner than on the competence of the few allergy specialists.

Address for correspondence:

Tony Foucard
Department of Pediatrics
University Hospital
S-751 85 Uppsala
Sweden

Reference

1. Foucard T, Graff-Lonnevig V. Asthma mortality rate in Swedish children and young adults 1973–88. *Allergy* 1994; 49: 616–619.

Asthma Runs in Families, but Does Not Ruin Them

AA Kaptein*

Keywords: Asthmatic child, families of asthmatic children, illness behaviour, parent-child interaction, psychology, self-management training

Asthma is a somatic condition whereby, as in any physical illness, the reaction of the patient toward the illness is a co-determinant of the medical and behavioural outcome of the illness. A patient's reaction to asthma constitutes the major area of study for behavioural scientists in the field of respiratory diseases.

In this chapter three topics will be discussed. First, an outline of current views with regard to the relationship between psychology and asthma is given. Second, psychological and social problems that face the family with an asthmatic child are reviewed. Finally, suggestions are presented on how the clinician – pulmonary physician, allergist, family physician – may be able to assist in helping the asthmatic child and his/her family in minimizing the psychological and social consequences of asthma.

Psychology and Asthma

Many clinicians will have experienced the mother of an asthmatic child. Cautiously and somewhat ashamedly, she finally has the courage to ask her physician whether she has done anything wrong in the upbringing of her child. It is her belief that she may somehow have caused her child's asthma. These notions of "psychosomatic" factors are still present in the minds of many mothers of asthmatic children, as well as physicians and psychologists – even in 1994.

Approximately fifty years ago, Alexander delineated various somatic illnesses which in his view were "psychosomatic". The "holy seven" of Alexander (neurodermatitis, duodenal ulcer, rheumatoid arthritis, ulcerative colitis, essential hypertension, hyperthyroidism, and asthma) were viewed as being caused by specific psychopathological processes in the mother-child interaction. With regard to asthma, a conflict involving the wish to be independent would, if frustrated, be translated into an asthmatic attack, this representing a suppressed cry for help. As stated by Alexander, "The nuclear psychodynamic factor is a conflict centering in an excessive unresolved dependence on the mother. The content of this dependence is the wish to be protected – to be encompassed by the mother or the maternal image ... The asthma attack represents a suppressed cry for the mother" (1). It follows that, in psychosomatic theory, therapy for asthma entailed bringing the unconscious conflict into consciousness, which would lead to a resolution of the conflict and disappearance of asthma altogether in the patient.

In the last twenty years, a wealth of empirical data has demonstrated that mothers with an asthmatic child are no more psychologically disturbed than mothers without an asthmatic child. Children with asthma are similar to children without asthma, as far as psychological morbidity is concerned (2). There is no empirical basis whatsoever for "blaming the victim," i.e., accusing the asthmatic child and his or her mother of being responsible for the suffering (3).

As a psychologist, one cannot help but feel ashamed about the damage that has been done to patients with asthma and their family members by "psychosomatic" notions about asthma. Fortunately, research by behavioural scientists has demonstrated the contribution psychology can make in the care for patients with asthma. Based on a rather straightforward theoretical model that is outlined below (Figure 1), modern psychology may help the child, his/her family and the clinician in the assessment and treatment of behavioural problems that result from inadequate illness behaviour (4).

Any organic illness elicits a psychological response in the afflicted person. This response, encompassing affective, (overtly) behavioural and cognitive domains, is defined as illness behaviour (adequate vs. inadequate). Shame, reluctance to use

*   Medical Psychology, Leiden University, The Netherlands

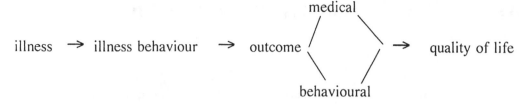

Figure 1. Relationships between illness and quality of life.

asthma medication in public and the idea that "asthma will go away if I do not think about it" are examples of the responses psychologists would label as inadequate illness behaviour. Applying relaxation techniques, avoiding contact with allergic stimuli and adopting ideas about how to control asthmatic symptoms are other examples, this time of responses which psychologists would label as adequate illness behaviour. Considerable research has demonstrated that inadequate illness behaviour is associated with an unfavourable medical outcome (e. g., more frequent hospitalizations, more severe medication) and behavioural outcome (e. g., higher levels of anxiety, school absenteeism or feelings of social isolation) (4). The combination of medical outcome with behavioural outcome may be conceptualised as "quality of life" (5). Illness behaviour, therefore, has a pivotal role between the illness itself and the impact of the illness on the patient's daily life. Objective characteristics of an illness with respect to pulmonary function or degree of hyperreactivity predict to some extent quality of life in the asthmatic child. However, the illness behaviour of the patient is a major contributor to quality of life as well (6, 7). Assuming optimal medical care, it is vital that physicians of asthmatic children pay appropriate attention to the illness behaviour of the patient. Illness behaviour may be

conceptualized as being determined by three key factors: the illness, the patient, and the environment (Figure 2):
- Characteristics of the illness: severity, prognosis, nature of symptoms (intermittent, as in asthma, or continuous, as in emphysema)
- Characteristics of the patient: knowledge, attitude, cognitions, coping skills concerning asthma
- Characteristics of the environment: degree of social support experienced by the patient, the way the family reacts towards the patient, nature of the physician-patient relationship, the image of an illness in a society

Using the concept of illness behaviour as a starting point, it should now be clear that some children with asthma display inadequate illness behaviour. The evidence for this can be seen in daily medical practice: poor control of symptoms, inappropriate attitudes toward asthma (anxiety, indifference or denial), panic, lack of medication compliance, inappropriate use of inhalation equipment, malingering, disruptions in schooling, family activities, sleep patterns or parental schedules (8, 9). In addition to these, the asthmatic child may evoke unexplained feelings in the physician (e. g., anger, rejection, protectiveness). These consequences of asth-

Illness behaviour

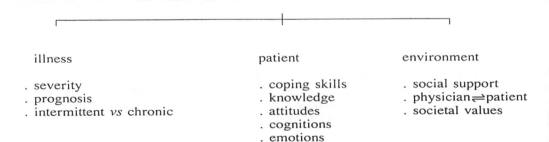

Figure 2. Illness behaviour and its determinants.

ma reflect inadequate illness behaviour, which increases the negative impact of asthma on the child (11).

Interactions of the Asthmatic Child and His/Her Family

Before discussing self-management, I will review how asthma in the child may affect the family, and vice versa. In six papers, from 1988 to 1993, data have been reported on the effects of the asthmatic child on family interactions. After careful review of this literature one still has to agree with Carson and Schauer: "Although the literature on childhood

asthma has mushroomed in the past decade, there remains a relative lack of data concerning relationships between asthmatic children and their parents" (12, p. 1139). Table 1 summarizes the six studies.

One conclusion stands out firmly: asthmatic children and their parents do not suffer major psychological damage or family problems. Results of these studies should be interpreted with caution. Methodological weaknesses are rather prominent, such as patient selection, confounding effects of severity of asthma, measures with unknown psychometric properties and improper control groups. As Renne and Creer noted in 1985: "There is an inverse relationship between reported differences (in personality patterns or traits) between asthmatic children and other populations, and the reliability and validity of assessment instruments" (2).

Table 1. Studies on consequences of asthma for child-parent interaction.

First author ref no, year	Subjects	Measures	Results
Carson (12) 1992	41 asthma 28 b, 13 g 8 to 13 years mean 11.2 years	Mother-Child Relationships Parenting Stress Index	Overindulgence ↑ asthma ↑ *vs* norm
Eiser (13) 1991	37 asthma 25 b, 12 g mean 4.5 years 37 healthy controls	Social Maturity Scale British Ability Scales Style of Discipline	NS
Kashani (14) 1988	56 asthma 36 b, 20 g 7 to 16 years 56 healthy controls	DICA NS DICA-P Child Behaviour Checklist	
MacLean (15) 1992	81 asthma 48 b, 33 g 6 to 14 y mean 9.8 years	Child Behaviour Checklist Life Event Checklist	NS
Perrin (16) 1989	46 asthma 27 b, 19 g 5 to 16 years	Health Resources Inventory	NS
Townsend (10) 1991	100 asthma 59 b, 41 g 7 to 18 years mean 11.3 years	Interviews with patients and parents listing the problems with management of asthma	Children: respiratory symptoms and asthma attacks (fear, anger) Parents: – helplessness – concern with long-term drug effects on child

Note. b = boys; g = girls; NS = no significant differences; ↑ = significantly higher; DICA = Diagnostic Interview for Children and Adolescents, (–P) = Parent Version.

145

Self-Management for Children with Asthma

There are children with asthma who find it hard to cope with their illness. Warning signs, such as disproportionate school absenteeism, disruptions of daily activities, excessive health care utilization and feelings of stigma and social isolation should be a reason for concern. In addition to individual care by the physician, the above-mentioned problems seem to be amenable to improvement by self-management training programmes (11, 17).

The following study on self-management training illustrates the potentially substantial impact it may have on the illness behaviour of children with asthma. Perrin, MacLean, Gortmaker and Asher described a randomized controlled trial of a combined education and stress management programme among children aged 6 to 14 years with asthma (18). The intervention consisted of four consecutive weekly meetings, each lasting 2 hours. The educational portion consisted of lessons during which knowledge concerning breathing, symptom recognition, attack management and coping were discussed. Parents and children participated together during the educational component. The stress-management activity, which included relaxation training and coping strategies, was carried out with the participating children alone. Children in the control group received a post-trial intervention programme which duplicated that received by the children in the treatment group. In this way they too could benefit from the intervention programme. Results indicated that the children in the experimental condition improved significantly on scales which measured behaviour problems, breathing knowledge and daily chores.

Fireman, Friday, Gira, Vierthaler and Michaels were the first authors to report a study in which the positive effects of self-management training in children with asthma were demonstrated (19). The Perrin et al. study builds on the now 10-year-old tradition of research about intervening in the illness behaviour of asthmatic children (18). Self-management training in children with asthma focuses on changing inadequate illness behaviour and therefore improves the medical and behavioural outcome. This, in turn, has a positive effect on the quality of life of the patients and their families. Further research is needed in order to identify more precisely those children and families in need of self-management training in order to develop more cost-effective interventions. As pointed out by Bailey et al., there is a need for the development of sound measures to operationalize asthma management practices of patients and their families (20). Clark and Starr-Schneidkraut's review of the management of asthma by patients and their families is a highly useful basis for future research in this area whereby the cooperation between patients, physicians and psychologists is a conditio sine qua non (21). As the title of this chapter suggests, "Asthma runs in families, but does not ruin them." Hopefully, this will be further supported by clinical and scientific evidence in the future.

Acknowledgment

The author wishes to express his gratitude to Barry d'Arnaud, Ann Ferrara, Jolie van den Heuvel, Jos Leenes, and Riet Wijen for their help.

Address for correspondence:

AA Kaptein, PhD
Medical Psychology
Department of Psychiatry
Leiden University
P.O. Box 1251
NL-2340 BG Oegstgeest
The Netherlands

References

1. Alexander F. *Psychosomatic medicine. Its principles and applications*. London: Allen & Unwin, 1949.

2. Renne CM, Creer TL. Asthmatic children and their families. In Wolraich ML, Routh DK (Eds) *Adv dev behav pediatr*, Vol 6. Greenwich, Conn.: Jai Press, 1985, p. 41.

3. Kronenfeld JJ. Self care as a panacea for the ills of the health care system: An assessment. *Soc Sci Med* 1979; 13A:263.

4. Kaptein AA, Ploeg HM van der, Garssen B, Schreurs PJG, Beunderman R (Eds). *Behavioural medicine: Psychological treatment of somatic disorders.* Chichester: Wiley & Sons, 1990.

5. Spilker B (Ed). *Quality of life assessments in clinical trials*. New York: Raven Press, 1990.

6. Kaptein AA, Brand PLP, Dekker FW, Kerstjens HAM, Postma DS, Sluiter HJ, the Dutch CNSLD group. Quality of life in a long-term multicentre trial

in chronic non-specific lung disease: Assessment at baseline. *Eur Respir J* 1993; 6:1479.

7. Schrier AC, Dekker FW, Kaptein AA, Dijkman JH. Quality of life in elderly patients with chronic non-specific lung disease seen in family practice. *Chest* 1990; 98:894.

8. Townsend M, Feeny DH, Guyatt GH, Furlong WJ, Seip A, Dolovich J. Evaluation of the burden of illness for pediatric asthmatic patients and their parents. *Ann Allergy* 1991; 67:403.

9. Creer TL, Marion RJ, Creer PP. Asthma Problem Behavior Checklist: Parental perceptions of the behavior of asthmatic children. *J Asthma* 1983; 20:97.

10. Fritz GK. Psychological issues in assessing and managing asthma in children. *Clin Rev Allergy* 1987; 5:259.

11. Rachelefsky GS. Review of asthma self-management programs. *J Allergy Clin Immunol* 1987; 80:506.

12. Carson DK, Schauer RW. Mothers of children with asthma: Perceptions of parenting stress and the mother-child relationship. *Psychol Rep* 1992; 71:1139.

13. Eiser C, Eiser JR, Town C, Tripp JH. Discipline strategies and parental perceptions of preschool children with asthma. *Br J Med Psychol* 1992; 64:45.

14. Kashani JH, König P, Shepperd JA, Wilfley D, Morris DA. Psychopathology and self-concept in asthmatic children. *J Pediatr Psychol* 1988; 13:509.

15. MacLean WE, Perrin JM, Gortmaker S, Pierre CB. Psychological adjustment of children with asthma: Effects of illness severity and recent stressful life events. *J Pediatr Psychol* 1992; 17:159.

16. Perrin JM, MacLean WE, Perrin EC. Parental perceptions of health status and psychological adjustment of children with asthma. *Pediatrics* 1989; 83:26.

17. Clark NM, Feldman CH, Evans D, Duzey O, Levison MJ, Wasilewski Y, Kaplan D, Rips J, Mellins RB. Managing better: Children, parents, and asthma. *Pat Educ Couns* 1986; 8:27.

18. Perrin JM, MacLean WE, Gortmaker SL, Asher KN. Improving the psychological status of children with asthma: A randomized controlled trial. *Dev Behav Pediatr* 1992; 13:241.

19. Fireman P, Friday GA, Gira C, Vierthaler WA, Michaels L. Teaching self-management skills to asthmatic children and their parents in an ambulatory care setting. *Pediatrics* 1981; 68:341.

20. Bailey WC, Wilson SR, Weiss KB, Windsor RA, Wolle JM. Measures for use in asthma clinical research. *Am J Respir Crit Care Med* 1994; 149:S1.

21. Clark NM, Starr-Schneidkraut J. Management of asthma by patients and families. *Am J Respir Crit Care Med* 1994; 149:S54.

The Role of the UK Asthma Training Centre and its Relevance to Allergy

Greta R Barnes*

Keywords: Teamwork, asthma clinics, nurse's role, ATC/RCGP Asthma Diploma, training activities, allergy training programme for primary care teams

Community asthma clinics became officially recognised in the UK in 1990, and many practice nurses now play a major role in the delivery of care as well as being major providers of asthma education for patients. Health professionals with an extended role require special training and rigorous assessment; this has been provided in the main by the Asthma Training Centre (ATC). The Asthma Training Centre/Royal College of General Practitioner's Diploma in Asthma Care was introduced in 1990 and has now been undertaken by over 5000 health professionals. The teaching of the diploma programme and subsidiary courses is carried out by a national training network of nurses and doctors.

The British Society of Allergy and Clinical Immunology (BSACI) approached the ATC to promote the importance and significance of allergic diseases in the community. ATC/BSACI pilot allergy courses, designed to have a particular relevance to community asthma clinics, were developed for ATC/RCGP Diplomees and GPs. The initial teaching was carried out by BSACI members. Four ATC Trainers undertook further training and gained practical expertise, and were then in a position to provide allergy training for other community health care professionals.

In the early 1980s it was becoming increasingly apparent in the UK that asthma was not being adequately diagnosed or treated (1). The management of asthma was chiefly reactive, and there was no consistent approach to care. Much of the criticism was directed at general practitioners, though it was generally agreed that asthma was a condition that should, in the main, be managed in primary care (2).

One of the major factors in providing good asthma care is having sufficient time. A full assessment is required in order to arrive at a correct diagnosis. Rational treatment needs to be prescribed tailored to the individual and the respective situation. Time has to be spent organising a comprehensive review system to include planned follow-up and monitoring. Productive and interactive time is required to demonstrate and check inhaler technique and to introduce written customised care plans and guided self-management (3, 4, 5). Relevant patient and family asthma education and counselling also needs to be introduced and established (6).

The health professional's chief objective of care should be to provide a logical systematic anticipatory approach to enable the patient to maintain optimum control of their asthma so it has a minimal effect on their lives.

Preliminary work carried out in a general practice in Stratford-upon-Avon in 1983 found that whilst improving the care of asthma certainly benefitted the patient, it also increased the workload of the practice. A shared-care approach was implemented by introducing a nurse-run asthma clinic; the results showed a ten-fold reduction in the number of patients nebulised for acute asthma during a 12-month period and a great increase in the number of patients prescribed prophylactic therapy. Patients were very satisfied with the clinic and with the service it provided (7). Charlton et al. also found a marked drop of acute attacks of asthma during the 6 months after setting up a nurse-run asthma clinic in one practice (8).

The mere existence of a special asthma clinic within the general practice setting, however, does not necessarily equate with improved care for patients. If a nurse is to play a major role in asthma care and to work with autonomy, she requires a high level of clinical expertise and motivation. In addition, it is important that she be an effective communicator and possess organisational and managerial skills. Of perhaps even greater importance is

---

*   Director, Asthma Training Centre, Stratford-upon-Avon, UK.

that she knows her limitations and is prepared to be accountable for her actions. To what extent the role of the individual nurse will expand depends on many factors, largely upon the nurse's ability and what is acceptable to her medical colleagues as well as available time and resources. Of all the qualities required, knowledge is the most important – something that can only be achieved by undertaking specialised training programmes.

Prior to the establishment of the Asthma Training Centre (ATC) in 1987, there was no specialised asthma training available in the UK. The Centre, which has charitable status, started because a need was identified. The original aim was, and still is, to provide training for health professionals in order to improve the care of asthma patients in the com-

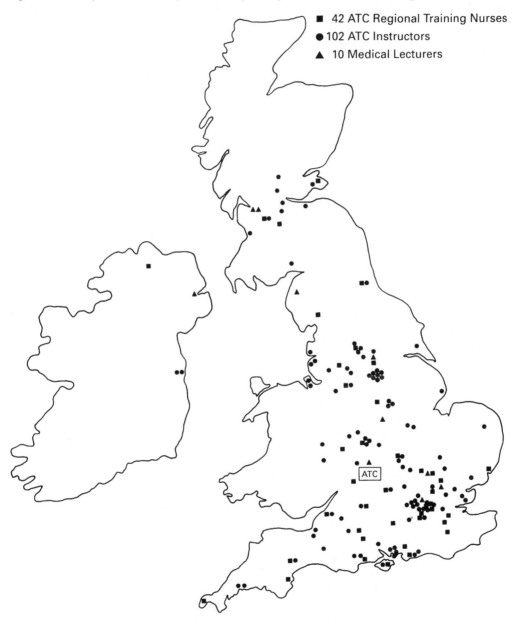

■ 42 ATC Regional Training Nurses
● 102 ATC Instructors
▲ 10 Medical Lecturers

Figure 1. Asthma Training Centre regional training network (September 1993).

149

munity. The Centre's activities extended rapidly, largely because of the introduction of the 1990 GP Contract and the 1993 New Health Reforms, which allowed general practitioners to claim re-imbursement for running asthma clinics in their practices. The reforms set out a requirement for the training of staff working in the clinics.

From September 1990 onwards, a diploma course developed in conjunction with the Royal College of General Practitioners (RCGP) was introduced (9). Attainment of the diploma is achieved by taking a practical and theoretical examination representing the culmination of a 6-month period of study. This involves distance learning, practical activities, and contact teaching as well as a 2-day intensive course (the second day attended by the GP) at the ATC or a local centre.

The ATC is linked with the University of Central England, which has validated and accredited the Asthma Diploma under the Credit Accumulation and Transfer Scheme (CATS). Since the diploma was introduced in 1990, over 5,000 health professionals have completed the programme.

To date there are 42 ATC Regional Nurse Trainers who are lecturer/practitioner nurses, 102 ATC Regional Nurse Instructors, and 10 medical lecturers (Figure 1). All three groups have undertaken additional intensive training programmes specific to their needs. The trainers teach students up to diploma level as well as general practitioners. The instructors act as mentors for students undertaking the diploma, and the medical lecturers fulfil an additional important role by teaching their GP colleagues.

Although the ATC/RCGP Diploma Course continues to be the major programme offered, over the years the number of other courses developed by the ATC has increased. Asthma courses are now in place for school nurses and hospital-based general and paediatric nurses as well as courses for general practitioners. Regular update programmes are held for post ATC/RCGP Asthma Diploma students throughout the UK, and allergy courses are about to be introduced.

Primary-care physicians in the UK are not, in general, greatly interested in allergy in relation to asthma. Some of this lack of interest could be due to the diminished role of skin-prick testing – brought about chiefly because desensitizing programmes in the UK have not been permitted in general practice since 1986. However, the main reason is probably because modern asthma drug treatments are very effective and have been strong-ly promoted in the UK by chest physicians and respiratory pharmaceutical companies. The practice of any form of avoidance measures in order to improve asthma care has played a minor role.

This may now change: The Government White Paper, entitled Health of the Nation, published in 1992 (11), highlighted the significance of allergic diseases, and the recently revised Guidelines on the Management of Asthma (12) have recommended for the first time that, where possible, provoking factors should be avoided. In addition, the British Society of Allergy and Clinical Immunology (BSACI) has acknowledged the relevance of health care moving from secondary to primary care, and has felt it important to spend time educating and delivering practical messages to those who work with patients in the community.

The ATC was approached by the BSACI in 1992 to discuss the role of asthma-trained nurses in relation to allergy and in the context of asthma clinics. Whilst the initiative was welcomed, it was evident that the lack of allergy expertise within the ATC needed addressing before advancement could be made. Allergy workshops were held for all the ATC Training Nurses, and four nominees received further in-depth training and practical allergy experience.

Pilot allergy courses were developed and held for ATC/RCGP Diploma Nurses and GPs. These courses, which were theoretically and practically based, included the role of allergy and allergens, basic mechanisms, allergy diagnosis, skin-prick testing,

Table 1. Allergy in the context of an asthma clinic.

Role of the Nurse

Minimum involvement:
• Take a structured formal allergy history
Patient always sees doctor for diagnosis, treatment and management

Medium involvement: – as Minimum PLUS
• Carry out skin prick testing – *refer back to doctor*
• Give basic advice and allergy education
• Provide explanatory allergy literature
• Establish regular follow-up
• Spot poor control – *refer back to doctor*

Maximum involvement: – as Medium PLUS
• Carry out allergy assessment relevant to general practice setting and make diagnosis
• Decide on management and treatment
• Give comprehensive allergy advice

allergy avoidance and the prevention of allergy as well as immunotherapy and anaphylaxis. The necessity of taking a careful clinical history was highlighted as well as the importance of identifying allergic patients and confirming offending allergens. The nurse participants agreed to participate in an allergy skin-prick test study to determine whether the result of the test altered their judgement about the role of allergy in a patient with asthma, and whether the skin tests altered the type of allergen avoidance advice given.

The courses showed that there was indeed a need for allergy training in relation to asthma, rhinitis, and atopic dermatitis, and that the nurse can have a developing role in allergy management (Table 1).

The first two pilot courses were led by BSACI members and the second two by the allergy-trained ATC trainers. The course is now ready to be offered to ATC post ATC/RCGP Asthma Diploma Students and their GPs. It will be interesting to note the response, though whatever the outcome, the Asthma Training Centre can, at last, truly say it now has a relevance to allergy.

Acknowledgements

Special thanks are due to BSACI members Stephen Durham, David Hide, Martin Church, and Samantha Walker for their expertise and enthusiasm.

Address for correspondence:

Greta R Barnes
The National Asthma Training Centre
Winton House, Church Street
Stratford-upon-Avon
Warwickshire CV37 6HB
UK

References

1. Clark T, Rees J, Dunitz M. Practical management of asthma. 1985.

2. Speight ANP, Lee DA Hay EN. Under diagnosis. Undertreatment of asthma in childhood. *BMJ* 1983; 286:1253–1258.

3. Maiman L et al. Education for self treatment by adult asthmatics. *J Amer Med Assoc* 1979; 241:1919–1922.

4. Beasley R et al. Self management plan in the treatment of adult asthma. *Thorax* 1989; 44:200–204.

5. Bone R C. The bottom line in asthma management is patient education. *Amer J Med* 1993; 94:561–563.

6. Fireiman P et al. Teaching self-management skills to asthmatic children and their parents in an ambulatory care setting. *Paediatrics* 1981; 68:341–348.

7. Pearson R and Barnes G. Asthma clinics in general practice: A practice approach. In Levy M (Ed) *Asthma in practice*. London: Royal College of General Practitioners, 15–20.

8. Charlton I et al. Audit of the effect of a nurse-run asthma clinic or workload and patient morbidity in a general practice. *Brit J Gen Prac* 41; 227–31.

9. Barnes G. Care of patients with asthma. *Nursing in General Practice – Clinical Care* 1990; 65–87.

10. Asthma Training Centre/Royal College of General Practitioners Diploma in Asthma Care. Asthma Training Centre, Winton House, Church Street, Stratford upon Avon.

The German Allergy Documentation and Information Center

Karl-Christian Bergmann*

Keywords: Museum of Allergology, information center, patient education, documentation, history of medicine

In 1991 an Allergy Documentation and Information Center was opened in Germany. The aims of the Center are twofold: (1) To be an Museum of Allergology collecting and preserving relevant historical artifacts from the field of allergy. (2) To work as an Information Center providing appropriate information and answers to allergy sufferers, the medical profession, the mass media, and others who are involved in controlling allergies.

The main elements of the institution are: (1) an exhibition including the history of allergology, presentation of allergic diseases, indoor and outdoor allergens, diagnostic procedures, prevention, prophylaxis, and therapy of allergies; (2) patient education courses and information material; (3) a library, specializing on patient information including a videothek; (4) an educational computer-software (Allergy Information System); (5) an electronic mailbox. The institution is sponsored by the Bad Lippspringe Treatment and Research Institute and supported by its own society. The advisory council includes the presidents of the German Society for Allergy and Immunity Research and the Physicians Society for German Allergologists, a medical historian and other outstanding allergologists.

Since its opening the Center has been very well accepted by about 5000–6000 visitors per year, and over 5000 home-users of the allergological software and electronic mailbox.

Allergy is a worldwide problem. In Germany alone, more than 15 million people have allergies. That means nearly one out of five people experience an allergic disorder in their lifetime.

As our understanding of allergy has grown, great diagnostic and therapeutic progress has been made and continues to be made every year. The time is ripe to collect and preserve materials demonstrating the history and progress of the field of allergy.

Patients who understand their allergies are more compliant and suffer less than uninformed patients. Therefore, the benefits of patient information and education are accepted worldwide. Several programs, e. g., for asthma schools, have been developed, but in Germany their use is still restricted to some places.

In the Summer of 1990, the Bad Lippspringe Treatment and Research Institute (Kuranstalten und Forschungsinstitute Bad Lippspringe GmbH) decided to contribute to the fight against allergic disorders by creating an Allergy Documentation and Information Center. On June 3, 1991, the Center was opened to the public. One of the key speakers in the opening ceremony was Professor Zoltan Ovary (New York), an important figure in the history of allergology, who dedicated the institution as the first international museum of allergy in the presence of more than 300 guests.

Aims of the Center

The aims of the Center are twofold:
- To collect, preserve, and display relevant materials from the field of allergy, including pictures, books, movies, congress materials, devices, instruments, allergens, and personal notes.
- To provide appropriate information and answers to allergy sufferers, their families and colleagues, teachers and school children, Employees' Liability Insurance Associations, the medical profession, pharmaceutical companies, the mass media, and others who are involved in controlling allergies.

* Allergy and Asthma Clinic Wilhelm Gronemeyer, Bad Lippspringe, Germany.

The Building and the Exposition

The home of the museum is a three-story, newly renovated villa built in 1916 (Figure 1). An elevator was added outside the building to maximize space within the building for exhibitions, while also providing easy access.

On the ground floor lie an information desk and exhibition showing milestones in allergy from ancient times, the Middle Ages, and modern times using pictures, figures, and short expositions (room 1). A presentation of the most common allergic diseases is given explaining etiology, symptoms, diagnostic, and therapeutic procedures (room 2). Indoor and outdoor allergens including occupationally derived allergic triggers (room 3) and relevant diagnostic procedures are presented (room 4). The last room (room 5) gives an introduction to the prevention, prophylaxis, and therapy of allergic disorders.

Since its opening the exposition has been visited by about 400 to 500 persons per month from all over the country with increasing rates.

The second floor houses a lecture room and a slide and video room, both of which are used constantly by patient education groups (asthmatics), who receive a structured program for 5 days, 2 hours per day. The "asthma school" includes information on allergies and is offered to and used by 700–900 out- and inpatients per year.

The library specializes in patient information material and has a mailbox. The secretariat sends books, pamphlets, and videos to persons unable to visit the Center personally. The bureau of the "German Pollen Information Service," which collects data from the 62 pollen traps in the country, and the "German League for the Fight against Airway Diseases" are also located in the Center.

The Allergy Information System (AIS)

The AIS is a PC educational software for physicians, medical students, and medical staff. It offers basic allergologic knowledge including pathophysiology, diagnosis, and treatment of allergic diseases. Also, in additional service modules it offers organizational aids for the medical practice. The program was sponsored by UCB Chemie GmbH, Germany.

Offering current allergologic fundamentals in an attractive way on the PC basically means that these contents are processed and presented differently from traditional print products. A PC screen is not suitable for reading longer texts without causing fatigue. Therefore, the AIS has a text/image ratio of 1:1, i.e., as a rule, not more than half of each display page contains textual information. Some 700 of the total of about 1000 display pages were supplied with test-adapted graphs.

The use of the AIS software requires an IBM-compatible personal computer with a hard disk and the MS-DOS operating system. In addition, a 3.5- or

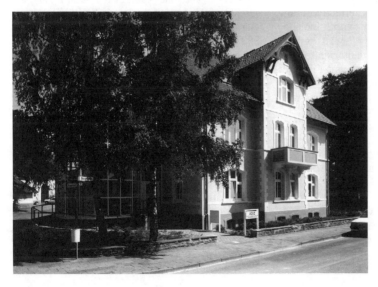

Figure 1. General view of the Allergy Documentation and Information Center in Bad Lippspringe, Germany.

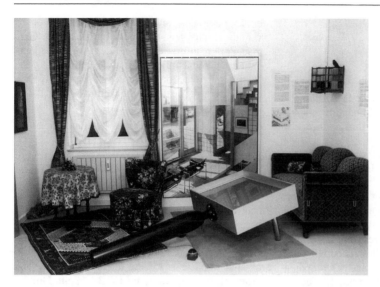

Figure 2. The indoor-allergen room with enlarged mites (magnifying-glass), cat, budgerigars, and other allergen sources.

5.25-inch floppy disk drive and a Microsoft-compatible mouse must be available. The AIS needs 8.3 MB storage capacity on the hard disk. Personalized letters for patients with allergy-specific recommendations can be printed out with any printer.

Since being offered to the public in the Autumn of 1992, the AIS software has been employed by more than 4000 users from the Center.

The Electronic Mailbox

The conventional approach to educating allergic patients how to minimize their exposure to allergens, to use metered dose inhalers correctly, or how allergen-specific immunotherapy works includes counseling and furnishing of relevant printed material. Huss and colleagues demonstrated the positive effects of supplementary computer instruction in house dust mite-avoidance measures on adherence to implementing measure in patients with mite-associated asthma (1).

This was just one of several reasons why a PC-based mailbox was opened in the Center in September 1993. This "allergy mailbox" is designed to provide information on allergic and airway diseases to everyone 24 hours a day.

The Main Menu offers data from the German Pollen Information System, the German League for the Fight against Airway Diseases, literature services for physicians, etc. The Message Menu allows the user to send and receive messages from other users.

To access the mailbox, the user needs a personal computer and a telephone modem. In the first 6 months of its existence, the mailbox phone number 05252/930295 has logged in more than 5000 calls from nearly 1000 regular users.

Support

The Bad Lippspringe Treatment and Research Institute, which runs seven clinics with 1300 beds, was the sponsor and initial financial supporter of the Center. The renovation of the building and assembly of the exposition cost 2.7 million German marks. The operational costs per year are about 250,000 German marks including salaries.

The institution is also supported by its own society, the "Society for the Promotion of Allergology and Information to the Public," which invites individuals and institutions to become members.

The scientific advisory council includes the presidents of the German Society for Allergy and Immunity Research and the Physicians Society of German Allergologists, a medical historian and other outstanding allergologists.

The Center is in close contact with and supports the activities of the UCB Institute of Allergy in Germany.

We ask all readers for contributions in form of allergologically relevant literature (books and reprints before 1960), instruments, devices, pictures, movies, and other historical material.

General information

Address

Allergy Documentation and Information Center
Burgstrasse 12
D-33175 Bad Lippspringe
Phone: 05252/954502
Fax: 05252/954501

Hours of Operation

Tuesday–Friday 10.00–12.00 and 14.00–17.00 o'clock, Saturday and Sunday 10.00–13.00 o'clock

Admission

Admission to the Center is free during normal hours.

Facilities for the disabled

A ramp provides easy access to the ground floor. Other floors may be reached by the lift.

Car parking

Limited car and bus parking space is available in front of and near the Center.

Photography

Photography with hand-held equipment is permitted for private purposes only. Flash may be used. Photography for commercial purposes and any requiring ancillary equipment is permitted only by prior arrangement with the Center.

Education service

Schools and other groups are invited to apply for guided tours by a physician.

Information desk

Information material in the form of books, pamphlets and videos for persons with allergies and/or respiratory tract diseases is avialable.

Address for correspondence:

Prof. Dr. K.-Ch. Bergmann
Allergy and Asthma Clinic Wilhelm Gronemeyer
Lindenstrasse 26
D-33175 Bad Lippspringe
Germany

Reference

1. Huss K, Squire EN, Carpenter GB, Smith LJ, Huss, RW, Salata K, Salerno M, Agostinelli D, Hershey J. Effective education of adults with asthma who are allergic to dust mites. *J Allergy Clin Immunol* 1992; 89:836–43.

Patient Education in the United States

Peter Socrates Creticos*

Keywords: Patient education, asthma education, United States

Asthma is a difficult and at times troublesome disease. The development of various health education resources has significantly improved our ability to manage this disease. One of the most important advancements in this field in the United States has been the implementation of the National Asthma Education Program's constructs. These and other educational approaches will be reviewed in this article.

reviewed the existing scientific literature, debated the merits of various therapeutic approaches, and through their consensus of opinions developed a set of general guidelines that would or should provide a logical framework for management of asthma by the various members of the health care team in conjunction with the patient (1).

Introduction

Successful management of the patient with asthma requires an integrated approach that incorporates environmental control, judicious use of medications, and involvement of the patient in his/her disease. This latter point cannot be overemphasized, as an uninformed or disinterested patient is apt to spell failure for any long term management strategy.

Therefore, the key to success in asthma management is the patient. An appropriate analogy is the diabetic – simply writing a set prescription of insulin without regard for the patient's total picture has been shown to be not only counterproductive but also likely to result in inadequate control of the underlying disease. In contrast, by having the patient take control of his/her management decisions and be responsible on a day-to-day basis for checking the blood glucose levels (e. g., finger stick) and adjusting the insulin dose accordingly through the day, that patient "suddenly" becomes a team player.

One of the more important steps taken to accomplish this goal in the US was the empowerment of a multidisciplined task force by the National Heart, Lung, and Blood Institute with the express purpose of developing guidelines to improve the diagnosis and treatment of asthma (1).

This expert panel convened under the guise of the National Asthma Education Program (NAEP),

Concept

One of the most important realizations by the task force was that successful management of asthma requires a partnership between the patient and the health care team (1). This is not simply a "contract" between the clinician and the patient. Rather, it is an active process that is built upon open communication between the health care provider and the patient. This active dialogue should encourage a more effectual learning process for the patient (Table 1) (1–5).

Table 1. Building a successful partnership.

– Open communication
– Active dialogue/Active process
– Active learning
– Integrated approach
– Joint development of a treatment plan

Inherent in this concept is the appreciation that patient education is not simply "rote memorization." Rather, it is an active learning process towards which end the patient becomes an active participant in the management of his/her disease.

* Johns Hopkins Asthma & Allergy Center, Baltimore, MD, USA.

Objectives of Patient Education

The objectives of this education process should be clearly stated for the patient (Table 2). They include: (1) helping the patient understand his or her asthma in terms that are simple to grasp; (2) providing the opportunity to learn and to practice the skills necessary to become adept at managing asthma; (3) providing the positive feedback and necessary behavior modification to further improve the implementation of the management strategy; (4) development of and adherence to a treatment plan (1, 6).

Table 2. Objectives of patient education.

– Helping patients understand their asthma
– Learning/practicing the skills necessary to manage asthma
– Positive feedback/imaging/behavior modification
– Adherence to treatment plan

Multidisciplined Approach

Much mention has been made of the health care team in this partnership. The management of asthma involves an integrated approach of a number of disciplines. Medical personnel, community support personnel, and the family members are all vital participants in ensuring patient acceptance and implementation of the management plan (Table 3).

Table 3. Integrated/multidisciplined approach.

– Patient
  Family
– Medical Personnel
  Physician
  Nurse
  Health educators
– Community Support
  Teachers
  Social workers

The medical team encompasses the physician – with whom the patient must develop a solid rapport and trust, the nurse – who oftentimes is the lead liaison in implementing treatment plan changes or encouraging the patient, and the nurse educator – who may be working closely with the patient during the learning curve.

Ancillary to this medical team is the role of the community support personnel usually involved with a patient. This would include school personnel, in particular those teachers closely involved with an asthmatic child/student. Depending upon the home situation, this could also involve various community organizations ranging from psychosocial personnel to church workers.

Perhaps most important is the role of the close family members in ensuring the success of any educational program. The family's support, encouragement, and positive attitude are crucial to any program's success. This may involve participation of various family members in the educational process to both reinforce the learning process at home and to provide the necessary positive feedback to the patient.

Components

The NAEP developed a specific clinician's guide entitled "Teach Your Patient about Asthma" which is designed to help physicians, physician assistants, nurses, health educators, and other related health professionals teach the asthmatic adult or child with asthma, and family members or parents of asthmatics about the management of asthma. The guide provides a stepwise teaching approach with sequential teaching units built upon each other, asthma "learning records" to allow the patient and medical team to monitor progress in the program, and worksheets with which the patient can begin to implement the learned skills and foster self-confidence in the self-management of his/her asthmatic condition (7). This guide can be obtained from the NAEP, Office of Prevention Education and Control, NHLBI, Bethesda, Maryland 20892 (USA) (Publication No. 92–2737, October, 1992).

The American Academy of Allergy and Immunology, in conjunction with the NAEP, provided a supplement "Advances in Asthma Care" which delineates the various components of a successful management program (6). These include but are not limited to:
1. Basic concepts: (a) defining asthma; (b) teaching the patient to recognize the signs/symptoms of asthma; (c) teaching the patient to recognize the triggers of asthma and to learn how to either avoid or implement procedures designed to reduce the allergen burden.

2. Therapeutics: (a) developing a treatment strategy for acute therapy, longitudinal care, preventive therapy; (b) learning correct techniques of administration of medications; (c) learning how to prevent and when to premedicate; (d) developing an individualized, written out treatment or "action plan."

3. Expanded therapeutics: (a) initiating treatment; (b) adjusting medications; (c) recognizing and treating adverse events associated with medication therapy, d) knowing indications for ER visits; (e) understanding the use/role of peak-flow monitoring.

4. Circumferential aspects: (a) allaying fears and dispelling myths sometimes associated with asthma; (b) improving the patient's self image; (c) fostering family support and understanding; (d) implementing community interaction – school nurse, associated school personnel (e. g., gym instructor, classroom teacher), work colleagues; (d) fostering relationships with support groups (AAFA, ALA, NONA) (6).

Tangential to these defined components of patient education, it is also important to provide the patient with or access to resources related to further developments in the field of asthma (Table 4) (8–12).

Table 4. Resources for asthma patients.

– Reading Resources
  NHLBI Asthma Reading & Resource List
  Asthma Resources Directory
  Asthma Education in the Schools Pamphlet
– Support Groups
  AAFA
  ALA
  NAAN

Teaching Module

Our approach at the Johns Hopkins Asthma and Allergy Center is based upon the recognition that not all patients learn alike. Some patients are visual learners while others are auditory learners. Some learn better in an individualized self-contained program, while others need active group support for learning.

Therefore, we have developed a multitiered program for patient education that incorporates each of these modalities (Table 5). Indeed, our oppor-

Table 5. Teaching module: The multitiered approach to patient education.

– Patient Workbook
  Guide developed by the National Asthma
  Education Program of the NHLBI
– Monthly Interactive Teaching Sessions
  Asthma Education Series
– Audio Visual Resources
  Unit coordinated videotapes
– Clinical appointments
  Reinforcement sessions

tunity to be selected as one of the several clinical care sites to test the Clinician's Guide developed by the National Asthma Education Program and provide feedback related to its contents and usability to the National Heart, Blood, and Lung Institute was invaluable in determining our approach to education of the asthmatic patient.

Each asthma patient evaluated at the JHAAC is provided the opportunity to matriculate through our asthma teaching module. At the initial patient visit, the constructs of the teaching program are laid out and the worksheets related to the management of that patient's asthma are given in a package to the patient.

At regularly scheduled follow-up visits or as deemed necessary by our nurses at prearranged educational visits, the teaching material that we have selected for the patients is reviewed and expanded upon.

Our teaching units are built around those suggested by the NAEP's Clinician's Guide. We have attempted to meet both our patient's needs and our health care provider's schedule through a series of interactive teaching sessions that are given sequentially over a 6-month period (Table 6). These evening sessions (6–7:30 pm) are provided on a continuous rotating basis; therefore, no matter when the patient enrolls in the cycle, he/she can complete the program.

These sessions are designed to highlight the major components of successful asthma management as outlined in the teaching guide, reinforce the patient's asthma management skills, and explore patient concerns or questions through an interactive dialogue session.

Tangential to this is an audiovisual resource program in which tapes have been developed to coordinate with the components (units) of our asthma education series. This further expands our education base by allowing patients to review asthma

Table 6. Johns Hopkins Asthma & Allergy Center Asthma Education Series.

Lecture 1: *Symptoms and Triggers of Asthma*
– Recognize the symptoms of asthma
– Recognize the triggers of asthma
Lecture 2: *Basic Treatment of Asthma*
– Understand the proper use of bronchodilator medications to treat asthma symptoms
– How to use "spacers" in conjunction with asthma metered dose inhalers
– Management of exercise-induced asthma
Lecture 3: *Preventive Treatment of Asthma*
– Understanding the concept of preventive therapy in the management of asthma
– Teaching the use of peak flow meters for the home self-monitoring of asthma
– Development of a specific medication plan tailored to the individual patient
Lecture 4: *Issues Related to Asthma Management*
– Recognizing the side effects that may be associated with the use of asthma medications
– Drug interactions that may complicate asthma
– Solving asthma problems in school/work setting
– The role of immunotherapy in treating allergic asthma
Lecture 5: *Treatment of Rhinitis*
– Understanding the relationship of symptoms of allergic rhinitis to asthma
– Understanding the proper use of "preventive" and "rescue" medicine in controlling allergic rhinitis
– Side effects associated with nasal medications
Lecture 6: *Review Session*
– A session to review the major points brought out in each of the topics related to the self-management of asthma
– Review of the patient's written asthma management plan
– A glimpse into the future of asthma management

management material while waiting at a scheduled follow-up office visit or by providing the opportunity to review a tape's contents on a loaner basis in the home library.

Conclusions

It is the goal of the National Asthma Education Program to provide to the clinician and the asthmatic patient the educational resources and skills necessary to successfully manage asthma. The methodologies developed under the auspices of the NHLBI and put at our disposal have given the health care provider in the United States a wonderful opportunity to work with the patient to master this difficult and at times troublesome disease.

Address for correspondence:

Peter S Creticos
John Hopkins Asthma & Allergy Center
5501 Hopkins Bayview Circle
Baltimore, MD 21224
USA

References

1. National Heart, Lung and Blood Institute, National Asthma Education Program. *Expert Panel Report: guidelines for the diagnosis and management of asthma.* NIH publication no. 91–3042, Bethesda, MD, 1991.

2. Feldman CH, Clark NM, Evans D. The role of health education in medical management in asthma. *Clin Rev Allergy* 1987; 5:195–205.

3. Mellins RB. Patient education is key to successful management of asthma. *J Respir Dis* 1989; S47–S52 (Suppl).

4. Schulman BA. Active patient orientation and outcomes in hypertensive treatment. *Med Care* 1979; 17:267–280.

5. Clark NC. Asthma self-management education: Research and implications for clinical practice. *Chest* 1989; 95:1110–1113.

6. *Advances in asthma care; participant workbook.* New York: NYSCP Communications, 1991 (developed in cooperation with the NAEP and the AAAI).

7. NHLBI, NAEP. *Teach your Patients about asthma: A Clinician's Guide.* Bethesda, MD: NIH publication no. 92–2737.

8. Parcel GS, Nader PR, Tieman K. A health education program for children with asthma. *J Dev Behav Pediatr* 1980; 1:128–132.

9. Lewis CE, Rachelefsky GS, Lewis MA, et al. A randomized trial of A.C.T. (asthma care training) for kids. *Pediatrics* 1984; 74:478–486.

10. National Heart, Lung and Blood Institute. *Air power: Self-management of asthma through group education.* Bethesda, MD: NIH publication no. 85–2362, 1984.

11. National heart, Lung and Blood Institute. *Living with asthma: Part 1: Manual for teaching parents the self-management of childhood asthma: Part 2: Manual for teaching children the self-management of Asthma.* Bethesda, MD: NIH publication no. 85–2364, 1984.

12. Weiss J, American Lung Association. Superstuff. In *National Institute of Allergy and Infectious Diseases: Self-management educational programs for childhood asthma, Vol II.* Bethesda, MD: NIH, 1981, pp. 273–294.

Education of Patients in Japan

Terumasa Miyamoto*

Keywords: Patient education, asthma diary, allergic rhinitis diary, peak flow

An asthma diary or an allergic rhinitis diary is a quick, convenient way of monitoring the patient's condition. Peak flow is valuable for patient self-assessment.

Education of Patients in Japan

Education of patients and their families is a very important part of the management of asthma and allergic disease in order to prevent symptoms and improve quality of life.

When we see patients in our clinic, we explain the possible causes of their asthma and allergic disease, the importance of allergen avoidance, such as house dust, moulds, and pets, and the importance of compliance with their medication. Aerosol inhalation techniques and the use of the holding chamber are also explained to the patient.

We give an asthma diary or allergic rhinitis diary to each patient, instruct them on how to complete the diary, and ask them to bring it with them on each visit to the clinic. Looking at the diary is a quick, convenient way of monitoring the patient's condition. We ask asthmatic patients to measure their PEF, before taking any medication or using an inhaler, shortly after they wake up, and just before they go to bed. They then record the value on the diary card for self-assessment. The red zone, yellow zone, and green zones are explained, and individualized instructions to increase or decrease their drugs according to these values are given to the patient.

There are two associations concerned with allergy in Japan. One is the Japanese Society of Allergy, which is an organization of physicians dedicated to promoting medical advancement and scientific achievement. The other is the Japanese Allergy Foundation, whose members include both physicians and lay people. The Allergy Foundation has eight branch offices which cover the whole of Japan. Both the main office and the branch offices hold lecture meetings for allergic patients. In addition, TV and video programs and radio broadcasts help patients and their families to understand their ailments. There are many books and pamphlets explaining allergic diseases and available treatments. While the patients are waiting at the outpatient clinic, a video is shown to them to explain various aspects of their diseases, such as the causes of allergic conditions, the mechanism of diseases, avoidance of allergens, and how to use their inhalers.

Address for correspondence:

T Miyamoto
3-43-4, Ogikubo
Suginami-ku. Tokyo
Japan

---

* National Sagamihara Hospital, Japan.

Patient Education in Mediterranean Countries: Italian Experience of an Education Program in Atopic Families

Luisa Businco, Barbara Bellioni, Arnaldo Cantani*

Keywords: Allergic disease, infants at risk of atopy, preventive measures

The main goal of modern medicine is the prevention of chronic and severe diseases. Atopic diseases in infants and children are common, disabling, chronic, and even life-threatening. Food allergy and atopic dermatitis may negatively interfere with the child's life and his/her physical and physiological development. Sensitization to foods occurs more commonly early in life; however, occasionally, it may even occur prenatally. Asthma is a very common pathology. Morbidity and mortality continue to be a major concern for physicians, particularly with children.

A recent epidemiological survey conducted in Italy shows that 22% of Italian children suffer from one or more atopic disease, the prevalence of atopic diseases being as follows: asthma 9%, atopic dermatitis 5%, urticaria 3%, oculorhinitis 3%, food allergy 1%, rhinitis 1%, anaphylaxis 0.1%. An environmental factor significantly associated with asthma was passive smoking.

The possibility of preventing such disorders in predisposed children has stimulated investigators' imaginations since the beginning of this century when atopic diseases were not as common as they are now. However, the possible influence of early diet on later food allergy and of allergen exposure in the first months of life on the development of asthma has received much attention only in the last decade. A number of triggering factors such as maternal smoking in pregnancy, occasional meals with milk-based formulas during the neonatal period, no breast-feeding, early weaning, passive smoking, pets at home, mite exposure early in life, living in a polluted area, and early social contacts have proved to play an important role in modulating the phenotypic expression of atopic disease in genetically predisposed infants. Infants at risk are identified through a history of atopic disease in one or both parents and/or one of the siblings.

Education of the family on the triggering environmental factors is the prerequisite to the primary and secondary prevention of atopic disease. In the 1980s we initiated an education program devoted to atopic-prone families in order to reduce the risk of sensitization in the neonate (1–2). Twenty maternity hospitals from all over Italy now participate in this educational program.

Table 1. Education program for atopic families.

Medical Staff:
– Pediatric Allergists
– Gynecologists
– Neonatologists
– Pediatricians
– Nurses
– Midwifes

Gynecologists, neonatologists, nurses and midwifes are trained to identify high-risk families and to give the educational support to parents (Table 1). Each center is supervised by a pediatric allergist skilled in allergy prevention. During pregnancy, parents are invited to participate in the education program for the prevention of atopic diseases in offsprings (Table 2). Parents are discouraged to smoke and to have pets at home. A number of preventive measures are also given to reduce proliferation of house dust mites in the home: removal of carpets and curtains as well as the use of encased mattresses and pillows are suggested; in addition we give advice about the temperature and humidity in the home. The mite presence in the home is investigated (Acarex), and if positive the use of an

* Allergy and Clinical Immunology Division, Department of Pediatrics, University "La Sapienza" of Rome, Italy.

Table 2. Education program for atopic families.

– Stop smoking
– No pets at home
– Measures for decreasing the proliferation of mites
  in the home
– Use of acaricide when needed
– Breast-feeding promotion and support
– Exclusively breast-feeding in the first 6 months
– No weaning before the 6th month of age

Table 3. Education program for atopic families: Promotion of breast-feeding.

Information on:
– physiology of mammary glands and lactation
– unique qualities of colostrum and human mik
– only small quantities of milk are produced and
  needed for the first few days after delivery
– more sucking makes more milk
– early supplements of cow's milk formulas depress
  milk production

Table 4. Education program for atopic families: Promotion of breast-feeding.

– Mothers are encouraged to hold and suckle their
  babies within 2 hours of delivery
– Babies stay in their mothers' rooms and are fed on
  demand
– No complementary or supplementary feeds for
  infants are allowed before the age of 6 months
– Use of pacifiers is discouraged as well as of bottle
  feeding

Table 5. Education program for atopic families: Results.

| | Education program | |
	Yes	No
Smokers at home	33%	48%
Pets at home	6%	22%
Breast-feeding in the first 6 months	68%	18%

acaricide (Acarosan) is encouraged, before the delivery and every six months, when necessary.

The education is given to small groups of parents with the help of slides, films, cassettes and pamphlets. In addition, an education program to support and encourage breast-feeding according to the UNICEF guidelines is given as follows (Table 3): Mothers receive appropriate information about the physiology of mammary glands and lactation, especially that colostrum is beneficial; that only small quantities of milk are produced and needed for the first few days after delivery; that more sucking produces more milk; that early supplements of cow's milk formulas depress milk production. In addition, mothers are informed about the unique qualities of human milk, and supported and assisted to establish lactation; mothers are encouraged to hold and suckle their babies within 2 hours of delivery; babies stay in their mothers' rooms and are fed on demand; no complementary or supplementary feeds for infants are allowed before the age of six months (Table 4). The use of pacifiers is discouraged as well as of bottle feeding.

At present 2,271 high risk babies have been enrolled in this education program. The results show that a great effort was made by most families to comply with the program we suggested in comparison with controls. As shown by Table 5, the number of pets at home was drastically reduced as well as the number of active smokers. The number

of babies breast-fed in the first 6 months of age also strikingly increased in the group of infants of families attending the education program.

In conclusion, our study indicates that education programs for atopic families show excellent compliance. Information regarding the triggering factors of atopic disease has a fundamental importance to the prevention of early sensitization in at-risk infants, as demonstrated by our education program.

Address for correspondence:

Prof. Luisa Businco
Allergy and Clinical Immunology Division
Department of Pediatrics
University "La Sapienza" of Rome
Viale Regina Elena 324
I-00161 Rome
Italy

References

1. Businco L, Marchetti F, Pellegrini G, Cantani A, Perlini R. Prevention of atopic disease in at risk nwborns by prolonged breast-feeding. *Ann Allergy* 1983; 51:296–299.

2. Businco L, Cantani A, Meglio P, Bruno G. Prevention of atopy: results of a long-term (7 months to 8 years) follow-up. *Ann Allergy* 1987; 59:183–186.

Contributions of Asthma Foundations in Latin American Patient Education

Natalio Salmun*

Keywords: Patient, education, foundation, knowledge, fears

One of the main objectives of Asthma Foundations in Latin America is education of the asthmatic patient and his family. We have organized lectures, and the media is often contacted, frequently utilizing posters, handouts, videos and booklets to facilitate it. The goals of education are: to make patients aware of early asthma symptoms and of appropriate therapy to be used; the detection of risk factors; increasing self management; decreasing morbidity and mortality; and to facilitate the asthmatic patient's return to a normal social life. This education is geared to patients and their families, general practitioners, and other health related professionals and teachers. A description of the activities organized by Fundaler and the results of the surveys are given. One is a physician survey and the other is a patient survey. The latter shows the lack of patient knowledge of simple but useful methods for therapy and for assessment of their disease. Also, a large percentage of patients are fearful of using first-line asthma medications. The usefulness of the lectures and courses organized by Fundaler was also surveyed. The vast majority of individuals were satisfied with them, and were planning on attending future related events. Seventy eight percent of those surveyed stated that the knowledge of their disease improved, and 68% had a decrease in their fears. We feel that certain patients would benefit from more prolonged educational programs, with reinforcement of the acquired knowledge.

There are four asthma foundations in Latin America: the Argentine Asthma and Allergy Foundation (Fundaler), the Chilean Asthma Foundation, the Mexican Asthma Foundation, and the Peruvian Asthma Foundation. The activities and facilities provided by Fundaler, which are similar to those of the other foundations, are as follows:

- Patient education (1–4)
- Grants for research and specialization in allergy and immunology
- Library for physicians
- Epidemiologic studies
- Awards for scientific papers
- Immunology laboratory studies for certain groups of patients
- Free supplies of medication for patients that cannot otherwise afford them

The educational objectives are:
1. Awareness of early asthma symptoms.
2. Detecting risk factors.
3. Increasing self-management.
4. Decreasing asthma morbidity and mortality.
5. Facilitating the asthmatic patient's return to a normal social life.

Asthma education needs to be developed at different levels:
1. Patient and his/her family.
2. General practitioners.
3. Allied health professionals.
4. Teachers.
5. Informing the general public trough the media.

At all these levels, posters, handouts, videos, books, and booklets (5–7) can be used to facilitate education.

Patient and professional education conferences organized by Fundaler include the following:
- Orientation meetings for the asthmatic patient and his/her family: Ten have been organized between 1987 and 1994.
- Lectures for asthmatic patients and their parents: 181 have been given, with a total attendance of 5759.
- "Emergencies in Allergy and Immunology" courses for pediatricians, run in 1988 and 1989.
- Workshops for asthmatic patients and their parents in 1989, 1990, and 1991.

* Argentine Institute of Allergy and Immunology, Buenos Aires, Argentina.

- "Introduction to Allergy and Immunology" course for pharmacists, 1989.
- Updates in allergy and immunology for psychologists, physical therapists, pharmacists, teachers, and nurses.
- Drug allergy course for nurses, 1993.
- Lectures for patients at the Congreso de Alergia e Inmunologia del Cono Sur, Parana, 1990; Congreso Latinoamericano de Alergia e Inmunologia, Buenos Aires, 1991; Asma 91, Buenos Aires; Jornadas de Progresos en Alergia e Inmunologia, Buenos Aires, 1992.
- XV Congreso Argentino de Alergia e Inmunologia co-organized with the Asociacion Argentina de Alergia e Inmunologia, 1993.

Education Survey

We distributed a questionnaire to a group of patients attending our talks, inquiring whether they knew how to use a meter dose inhaler, a spacer device, and a peak flow meter. We also asked them whether they feared using a meter dose inhaler and/or corticosteroids. We compared the answers given by two groups of asthmatics: patients with severe disease (N = 26) and patients with mild and moderate disease (N = 104).

Do the patients really know how to use correctly the meter dose inhaler? and how many of them learn to use it properly? Drs. Greiding and Moreno investigated the correct use of the meter dose in-

Table 1. Characteristics of the education survey population.

Sex	
Males:	49%
Females:	51%

Age	
Under 10 years:	30.1%
10–20 years:	20.5%
21–50 years:	36.2%
Over 50 years:	10.9%
No response:	2.3%

Education level	
Elementary:	35.6%
High school:	26%
University:	19.8%
Teachers:	2.2%
No response:	16.4%

Table 2. Results concerning use of a meter dose inhaler.

Do you know how to use a meter dose inhaler?

Overall	
Yes:	45.8%
No:	43.8%
Not answered:	10.2%
Severe asthmatics	
Yes:	69.2%*
Mild or moderate:	
Yes:	46.1%*

*Difference statistically significant. RR (relative risk) = 2.26 (1.02–5.02), χ^2 test, Yates corrected (3.54, p = 0.05).

Table 3a. Knowledge of spacers.

Do you know what a spacer device is?

Yes:	14.4%
No:	78%
Not answered:	7.6%
Severe asthma	
Yes:	30.8%*
Mild or moderate:	
Yes:	6.8%*

*Difference statistically significant. RR = 3.20 (1.70–6.03), χ-square test (8.54, p = 0.003)

Table 3b. Knowledge of a peak flow meter.

Do you know what a peak flow meter is?

Yes:	6.2%
No:	84.2%
Not answered:	9.6%
Yes:	
Severe asthma:	26.9%*
Mild or moderate:	2.9%*

*Difference statiscally significant. RR = 4.53 (2.49–8.22), χ^2 test (13.81, p = 0.0004).

haler in a group of patients (n = 72). They used a *Vitalograph Aerosol Inhalation Monitor*, and they found that 12.5% used it correctly and that 87.5% used it incorrectly.

In the last group, after teaching them using the *Vitalograph Incentive Device*, 70% found the explanation helpful, and 30% did not find it helpful.

The following are the answers to a physician survey, done to assess what they felt was the most important topic in patient education:

1. Knowledge of *prevention* and appropriate *Treatment*: 52%

Table 4. Fear of meter dose inhalers.

Do you fear using meter dose inhalers?	
Yes:	48%
No:	40%
Not answered:	12%
Yes	
Severe asthma:	42.3%
Mild or moderate: Yes 52%	

Not statistically significant. RR = 0.63 (0.32–1.26), χ-square test (1.20, p = 0.27)

Table 5. Fear of corticosteroids.

Do you fear using corticosteroids?	
Yes:	68.5%
No:	24.7%
Not answered:	6.8%
Yes	
Severe asthma:	52%
Mild or moderate:	77%

Not statiscally significant. RR = 0.42 (0.21–0.83), χ-square (5.02, p = 0.025).

Table 6. Hospital admissions.

Have you ever been admitted to a hospital for a management of your asthma?	
Yes:	17.1%
No:	74%
Not answered:	8.9%
No. of hospital admissions	
1:	20.5%
1–3:	38.3%
3+:	38.3%
Not answered:	2.9%

Table 8. Type of physician treating the patients.

What kind of physician takes care of your disease?	
Allergist:	55.4%
Pulmonologist:	26.7%
Clinician:	21.4%
Pediatrician:	14.3%
Other:	5.3%
None:	7.1%

Table 7. The effect of the lecture.

After this lecture, do you have a better understanding of your disease?	
Yes:	78.6%
No:	8.9%
Not answered:	12.5%
Yes	
Severe asthma:	91%
Mild or moderate:	85%

Not statistically significant: RR = 1.62 (0.42–6.15), chi-square (0.15, p = 0.72).

Has it decreased your fears?	
Yes:	64.3%
No:	14.3%
Not answered:	21.4%
Yes	
Severe asthma:	86.9%
Mild or moderate:	75.3%

Not statistically significant: RR = 1.87 (0.61–5.68), chi-square (0.78, p = 0.37).

Do you plan to attend future lectures organized by Fundaler?	
Yes:	87.5%
No:	–
Not answered:	12.5%

2. Knowledge of *diagnosis* and appropriate *Treatment*: 9%
3. Fight *Fears* of *Allergies*: 3%
4. Usefulness of *meter dose inhalers*, and the different types: 1%
5. Teaching of *allied health* personnel: 1%
6. Teaching of *teachers*: –

Conclusions

We feel that appropriate patient education during an office visit is difficult due to the length of time that it entails. That is why Foundations, through courses, lectures and the media, can make up for this lack of information. Through our surveys we found that many patients are not aware of useful methods for appropriate therapy and assessment of their disease, and that a high percentage of patients are afraid to use certain medications. Overall, patients with severe asthma have more knowledge of their disease and are less afraid of medication, but this difference is not statistically significant. Also, in certain cases, the lectures are not enough to solve the lack of knowledge, bringing up the need for more supportive and prolonged educational programs with reinforcement of acquired knowledge.

Address for correspondence:

Natalio Salmun
Argentine Institute of Allergy and Immunology
Billinghurst 2565.3 A
(1425) Buenos Aires
Argentina

References

1. Strunck RC, Mascia AB, Lipkowitz MA, Wolf SI. Rehabilitation of a patient with asthma in the outpatient setting. *J Allergy Immunol* 3 1991; 87:601

2. Sheffer AL. Expert Panel on the Management of Asthma. *Guidelines for the Diagnosis and Management of Asthma.* NIH Publication 1991; 91:3042.

3. *Teach your patients about asthma: A Clinician's guide.* Publication 1992; 92:2737.

4. Parker S, Mellins RB, Song D. Asthma education: A national strategy. *Am Rev Respir Dis* 1989; 140:848.

5. Salmun N, Sanchez de la Vega W. *Orientacion para el Alergico.* Printed by Argentine National Congress. 1990: Fundaler, 1990.

6. Plaut TF. *Children with Asthma.* Pedipress Inc. 1993

7. Blessing-Moore J. Self-management programs for childhood asthma. *Clin Rev Allergy 3.* 1987; 5:195.

Changing Prevalence of Allergies Worldwide

Ann J Woolcock*, Jennifer K Peat*, Louise M Trevillion*

Keywords: Allergy, skin prick tests, asthma, hay fever, children, prevalence, worldwide

Allergy, defined as the presence of elevated levels of circulating IgE antibody specific for aeroallergens, is usually measured by skin prick tests. Few studies of the prevalence of allergy have been done but, in general, about 40 to 50% of young adults in most populations are allergic and only some of them have symptoms of asthma or hay fever (allergic rhinitis). There is evidence that the prevalence of both asthma (defined as a diagnosis by a doctor or as the presence of current symptoms) and hay fever are increasing in children and that this is occurring in all countries (where measurements that allow comparisons have been made). It is not known if the prevalence of asthma and hay fever are increasing in adults. Data from Australia show that the increase in symptoms is occurring within the allergic children in the community and that exposure to allergens of house dust mites, cats, and *Alternaria* is the biggest risk factor for the onset of asthma (defined as the presence of both symptoms and airway hyperresponsiveness). It seems likely that increased domestic allergen is one cause of the increase, but other factors associated with affluent and urban life styles must be postulated to account for this worldwide increase in allergic diseases. Current studies using standardized protocols will be of great help in comparing data from different populations, for observing changes with time, and for defining putative risk factors. However, there are now sufficient data to propose that infants living in affluent societies should be protected from domestic allergens and from maternal smoking.

Definitions

Allergy is defined as the presence of elevated levels of circulating IgE antibody specific for aeroallergens. An individual who is allergic may have symptoms of asthma, of rhinitis (often called hay fever), of eczema or may have no symptoms related to the allergic state. However, not all individuals with asthma, rhinitis or eczema are "allergic."

Asthma is defined as a disease of the airways that makes them prone to narrow too easily and too much to a variety of provoking stimuli (1). Rhinitis is defined as excessive nasal blocking, running, or sneezing when a common cold is not present. Allergic asthma and allergic rhinitis are defined as asthma or rhinitis in an individual who is allergic.

Prevalence is the percentage of individuals in a population with a particular condition. This can be "cumulative" (the condition present at any time) or "point" (condition present at the time of investigation). The cumulative prevalence of asthma is frequently estimated from answers to the question, "Have you ever been diagnosed as having asthma?"

Introduction

There are few data about the prevalence of allergy but the prevalence of asthma has been widely reported, especially for children. However, meaningful comparisons with time within and between populations are difficult because presently available results are from studies that have used nonstandardized methods. Prevalence data for rhinitis are also commonly reported but the definitions used in questionnaires vary widely. The prevalence of allergic asthma is rarely reported but sometimes it can be calculated from published data. This paper reviews what little is known about the prevalence of allergy and recent changes in the prevalence of asthma and hay fever.

Specific IgE

Specific IgE against common allergens can be measured using a RAST test or by undertaking skin prick tests (2, 3). If the skin prick test procedure includes the use of negative and positive controls

---

*   Institute of Respiratory Medicine, University of Sydney, NSW, Australia.

Table 1. Prevalence of allergy as measured by skin prick tests in populations of children and adults.

Country	Age group	Number	Size	% Positive	Reference
Australia	8–10	1217	> 2 mm	44	(8)
	8–10	380	> 4 mm	24	(9)
	18–88	891	> 4 mm	49	(10)
New Zealand	13	662	> 2 mm	44	(5)
England	7–8	392	> 2 mm	51	(11)
	7–11	311	> 3 mm	32	(12)
USA	5–65	1333	> Control	51	(13)
Papua New Guinea	18–65	743	> 4 mm	24	(14)
China	11–17	1515	> 2 mm	38	(15)

The age range of the populations studied is in years, the size indicates the mean wheal diameter considered by the authors to indicate a positive test. In these studies allergens tested included 8 to 14 common aeroallergens.

Table 2. Changes in prevalence of asthma and allergic rhinitis in populations studied with the same methods on two occasions.

Country	Study Year	No.	Age	Current Asthma	Diag. Asthma	Allergic Rhinitis#	Ref.
Australia	82	718	8–11	4.5	9.1	20.5	(16)
(Belmont)	92	873	8–11	11.9	37.7	34.0	(7)
New Zealand	75	715	12–18		26.2*	8.8 (82)	(17, (5))
	89	435	12–18		34.0*	21.3 (92)	(17, (18))
Wales	73	818	12		6.0		(19)
	88	965	12		12.0		(19)
USA	71–74	large	6–11		4.8		(20)
	76–80	27275	6–11		7.6		(20)
Finland	61	>38000	19	0.1			(21)
	89	>38000	19	1.8			(21)
France	68	8140	21		3.3		(22)
	82	10559	21		5.4		(22)
Tahiti	79	3870	16		11.5		(22)
	84	6731	13		14.3		(22)
Scotland	64	2510	8–13		4.1	3.2	(23)
	89	3403	8–13		10.2	11.9	(23)
Sweden	71	55393	17–20	1.9		4.4	(24)
	81	57150	17–20	2.8		8.4	(24)

year of study and reference given in brackets, *cumulative prevalence of asthma and/or wheeze.
Diag. asthma = positive answer to question "Have you (or your child) ever been diagnosed as having asthma?" Current asthma = asthma present at the time the subject (or parent) was questioned. Allergic rhinitis (hay fever) = symptoms of nasal blocking, running or sneezing other than with a common cold.

and standardized allergens, reliable data about the allergic status can be obtained. Skin prick tests are easier, cheaper, and less invasive than RAST test for epidemiological studies. The size of the wheal does not give a precise indication of the amount of specific IgE but wheals of 3 mm in diameter are reproducible (4). The greater the number of positive responses (5), the more likely the person is to have symptoms of asthma and, in the case of house dust mites, the larger the wheal size, the greater the risk of asthma (5, 6).

Table 1 shows the results of skin prick tests, performed in random populations of children and adults, in Australia, Papua New Guinea, and the USA, and in children in New Zealand, Indonesia, China, and England. Differences in the allergens tested, the techniques used, and the wheal sizes considered to be positive obviously influence the results shown. However, when 3 mm wheals in children and 4 mm wheals in adults are used to define the allergic state, about 40% of populations are allergic. The exception is the population in Papua New Guinea where the prevalence of allergy was lower. When a smaller wheal diameter is used as the criterion for positivity, about 50% of the population are allergic. Few studies have measured changes in the prevalence of allergy, as measured by skin prick tests, with time. In Australia, 8 to 10 year old children were studied in two towns (Belmont and Wagga Wagga) at a ten year interval. The prevalence of allergy increased slightly but not significantly in both towns (7). The results for Wagga Wagga are shown in Figure 1, where the prevalence of allergy increased only slightly but the large increase in symptoms (wheezing in the last year), AHR, and current asthma (defined as those children with both symptoms and AHR) occurred in the allergic rather than in the nonallergic children. Thus a greater proportion of allergic children had symptoms in 1992 than in 1982. The results for current asthma and hay fever for Belmont children are shown in Table 2.

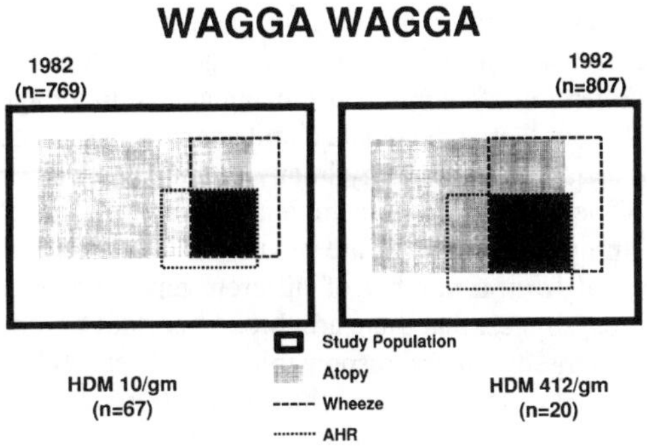

Asthma

Table 2 shows the prevalence of asthma, as measured by standardized questionnaire-based studies in children, adolescents, and young adults at intervals of at least five years. All studies show an increase in the prevalence of asthma — either "current asthma" (asthma present at the time of the study) or "doctor diagnosed asthma" (asthma at some time in the subject's life). There is no indication of the percentage of the subjects who were allergic and thus it is not known if there has been an increase in allergic asthma. However, in Australia about 88% of the children with current asthma were allergic on both occasions and a similar proportion of asthmatic children in New Zealand are allergic (5). In Australia and New Zealand, it appears that the increase in asthma has occurred within the allergic population. An example can be seen in Figure 1, where, in Wagga Wagga, there was a relatively small increase in the number of allergic children, but a greater percentage of them had recent wheeze, airway hyperresponsiveness, and current asthma in 1992.

WAGGA WAGGA

Figure 1. The relationship between percentages of children, aged 8 to 11 years, living in Wagga Wagga, Australia, with allergy defined by skin prick tests, symptoms of wheeze in the last 12 months, and airway hyperresponsiveness (AHR) in 1982 and 1992. Similar methods and questionnaires were used in both studies. There was little change in allergy but a large increase in symptoms and in AHR as well as in current asthma (defined as those children with both symptoms and AHR) in the allergic portion of the population. The numbers of house dust mites (*Dermatophagoides pterynissinus*) in household dust in the homes of children in this town are shown, and they also increased in this 10-year period.

Allergic Rhinitis

Table 2 also shows the prevalence of allergic rhinitis, as documented by questionnaire, in studies in Australia, New Zealand, Scotland, and Sweden. In all of the countries shown, it has been increasing. It is assumed that the majority of children whose parents say they have "hay fever" are, in fact, allergic. In Australia (7) and New Zealand (5) the percentage of children with nasal symptoms who were allergic was similar to that found for children with asthma (between 85 and 90%).

Discussion

Apart from the data shown in Table 2, there are a number of suggestions in the literature and in editorials, that the prevalence of asthma, rhinitis, and "allergies" has increased in recent years (25–28), but there are few data in the literature to support this commonly held belief. Our own studies from Australia suggest that the prevalence of allergy is not increasing and remains at about 40 to 50% of the population (depending on the age group and the size of the wheal considered positive) (7, 29). However, within the allergic population, an increasing number of subjects have symptoms of either asthma or hay fever. It is possible that the acquisition of allergy is occurring at a younger age (30), but there are no data about changes in the rate of acquisition of allergy in any population.

The reasons for the increase in symptoms of asthma and hay fever are unknown. Our data, obtained from a number of different environmental areas, suggest that there are three important groups of allergens that are responsible for asthma in children – house dust mites, the mold *Alternaria*, and cats. Large numbers of different populations are sensitive to pollens (grass, weed, and trees), but these allergens appear to be associated with hay fever and are less of a risk factor for persistent asthma (31, 32). Part of the increase in symptoms of asthma may result from higher levels of exposure to house dust mite and mold allergen as levels in houses increase, but it is likely that levels of cat and house dust mite allergen have been high in Australian and New Zealand homes for many years, and well above disease-inducing levels. It seems most unlikely that the increase in prevalence is the result of air pollution since the change has occurred in rural areas and the prevalence of passive smoking has decreased. It thus seems more likely that the observed increases are a result of other life-style changes, including diet (33). The task of identifying the factors responsible for this increase is large, since it is likely that a number of interacting factors are present.

Studies of the prevalence of asthma and allergy in adults are now being undertaken in Europe and a worldwide study of the prevalence in children is also starting (34). Hopefully, the allergic status, the environment of the children, and the putative risk factors (including diet) will be studied so that, in the future, it will be possible not only to describe the changes in allergic diseases with time and between populations, but also to know the risk factors that are responsible in different populations.

Our studies in Australia, supported by those of Sears in New Zealand, show that allergy is the biggest risk factor associated with the development of asthma in children. Furthermore, the early acquisition of allergy appears to be an added risk (30). Our studies show that those who become allergic after the age of 7 years have a greatly reduced risk of asthma compared to those already allergic at the age of 7 years (32). Australian and New Zealand studies show that allergy to house dust mites, cats, and *Alternaria* appear to be important risk factors for the development of asthma (9, 31). Our studies

also show that allergy or asthma in one or both parents is an added risk factor for the development of asthma (5, 6, 35). Thus we already know that in these affluent societies, action needs to be taken to reduce exposure to domestic allergens, particularly in infants who have allergic parents, but it seems unlikely that the prevalence of diseases associated with allergy will decrease without positive intervention studies.

Acknowledgments

These studies were supported by grants from the NHMRC of Australia, the Asthma Foundation of NSW and Allen and Hanburys Australia.

Address for correspondence:

Prof Ann J Woolcock
Institute of Respiratory Medicine
Royal Prince Alfred Hospital
Camperdown
NSW 2050
Australia

References

1. Woolcock AJ. Asthma. In: JF Murray, J Nadel (Eds) *Textbook of respiratory medicine*, 2nd edition. Philadelphia: Saunders, 1994: p. 1288.

2. Pepys J. Skin testing. *Br J Hosp Med* 1975; 14:412.

3. Herbert FA, Weimer N, Salkie ML. RAST and skin test screening in the investigation of asthma. *Ann Allergy* 1982; 49:311.

4. Dreborg S, Holgersson M, Nilsson G, Zetterstrom O. Dose response relationship of allergen, histamine, and histamine releasers in skin prick test and precision of the skin prick test method. *Allergy* 1987; 42:117.

5. Sears MR, Burrows B, Flannery EM, Herbison GP, Holdaway MD. Atopy in childhood. 1. Gender and allergen related risks for development of hay fever and asthma. *Clin Exp Allergy* 1993; 23:941.

6. Peat JK, Mellis CM, Leeder SR, Woolcock AJ. Asthma severity and morbidity: an epidemiological study of children and their parents living in Lismore in northern New South Wales. *Eur Resp J* 1994; (in press).

7. Peat JK, Toelle B, Haby MM, Gray L, Tovey E, Woolcock AJ. Evidence for a large increase in the prevalence of asthma in Australian children. *BMJ* 1994; (in press)

8. Hurry VM, Peat JK, Woolcock AJ. Prevalence of respiratory symptoms, bronchial hyperresponsiveness and atopy in school children living in the Villawood area of Sydney. *Aust NZ J Med* 1988; 18:745.

9. Peat JK, Salome CM, Woolcock AJ. Longitudinal changes in atopy during a 4-year period: Relation to bronchial hyperresponsiveness and respiratory symptoms in a population sample of Australian schoolchildren. *J Allergy Clin Immunol* 1990; 85:65.

10. Witt C, Stuckey MS, Woolcock AJ, Dawkins RL. Positive allergy prick tests associated with bronchial histamine responsiveness in an unselected population. *J Allergy Clin Immunol* 1986; 77:698.

11. Clough JB, Williams JD, Holgate ST. Effect of atopy on the natural history of symptoms, peak expiratory flow, and bronchial responsiveness in 7-and 8-year-old children with a cough and wheeze. *Am Rev Respir Dis* 1991; 143:755.

12. Clifford RD, Radford M, Howell JB, Holgate ST. Prevalence of atopy and range of bronchial response to methacholine in 7 and 11 year old schoolchildren. *Arch Dis Child* 1989; 64:1126.

13. Barbee RA, Kaltenborn W, Lebowitz MD, Burrows B. Longitudinal changes in allergen skin test reactivity in a community population sample. *J Allergy Clin Immunol* 1987; 79:16.

14. Woolcock AJ, Peat JK, Keena V, Smith D, Molloy C, Simpson A, Middleton P, Vallance P, Alpers M, Green W. Asthma and chronic airflow limitation in the highlands of Papua New Guinea: Low prevalence of asthma in the Asaro Valley. *Eur Respir J* 1989; 2:822.

15. Zhong NS, Chen RC, O-Yang M, Wu JY, Fu WX, Shi LJ. Bronchial hyperresponsiveness in young students of southern China: Relation to respiratory symptoms, diagnosed asthma, and risk factors. *Thorax* 1990; 45:860.

16. Britton WJ, Woolcock AJ, Peat JK, Sedgwick CJ, Lloyd DM, Leeder SR. Prevalence of bronchial hyperresponsiveness in children: The relationship between asthma and skin reactivity to allergens in two communities. *Int J Epidemiol* 1986; 15:202.

17. Shaw RA, Crane J, O'Donnell TV, Porteous LE, Coleman ED. Increasing asthma prevalence in a rural New Zealand adolescent population: 1975–1989. *Arch Dis Childhood* 1990; 65:1319.

18. Barry DMJ, Burr ML, Limb ES. Prevalence of asthma among 12 year old children in New Zealand and South Wales: A comparative survey. *Thorax* 1991; 46:405.

19. Burr ML, Butland BK, King S, Vaughan-Williams E. Changes in asthma prevalence: Two surveys 15 years apart. *Arch Dis Child* 1989; 64:1452.

20. Gergen PJ, Mullally DI, Evans R. National survey of prevalence of asthma among children in the United States, 1976 to 1980. *Pediatrics* 1988; 81:1.

21. Haahtela T, Lindohlm H, Bjorksten F, Koskinen S, Laitinen LA. Prevalence of asthma in Finnish young men. *BMJ* 1990; 301:266.

22. Perdrizet S, Neukirch F, Cooreman J, Liard R. Effects of long-term inhaled salbutamol therapy on the provocation of asthma by histamine. *Chest* 1987; 6:104S.

23. Ninan TK, Russell G. Respiratory symptoms and atopy in Aberdeen schoolchildren: evidence from two surveys 25 years apart. *BMJ* 1992; 304:873.

24. Aberg N. Asthma and allergic rhinitis in Swedish conscripts. *Clin Exp Allergy* 1989; 19:59.

25. Burney PG, Chinn S, Rona RJ. Has the prevalence of asthma increased in children? Evidence from the national study of health and growth 1973–86. *BMJ* 1990; 300:1306.

26. Robertson CF, Heycock E, Bishop J, Nolan T, Olinsky A, Phelan PD. Prevalence of asthma in Melbourne schoolchildren: Changes over 26 years. *BMJ* 1991; 302:1116.

27. Fleming DM, Crombie DL. Prevalence of asthma and hay fever in England and Wales. *BMJ* 1987; 294:279.

28. Britton J. Asthma's changing prevalence. *BMJ* 1992; 304:857.

29. Peat JK, Mellis CM. Has the prevalence of asthma in Australia and New Zealand increased? *Search* 1992; 23:252.

30. Van Asperen PP, Kemp AS, Mukhi A. Atopy in infancy predicts the severity of bronchial hyperresponsiveness in later childhood. *J Allergy Clin Immunol* 1990; 85:790.

31. Sears MR, Herbison GP, Holdaway MD, Hewitt CJ, Flannery EM, Silva PA. The relative risks of sensitivity to grass pollen, house dust mite and cat dander in the development of childhood asthma. *Clin Exp Allergy* 1989; 19:419.

32. Peat JK, Woolcock AJ. Sensitivity to common allergens: Relation to respiratory symptoms and bronchial hyperresponsiveness in children from three different climatic areas of Australia. *Clin Exp Allergy* 1991; 21:573.

33. Seaton A, Godden DJ, Brown K. Increase in asthma: A more toxic environment or a more susceptible population? *Thorax* 1994; 49:171.

34. Pearce N, Weiland S, Keil U, Langride P, Anderson HR, Stoachan D, Bauman A, Young L, Gluyas P, Ruffin D, Crane J, Beasley R. Self-reported prevalence of asthma symptoms in children in Australia, England, Germany and New Zealand: An international comparison using the ISAAC protocol. *Eur Respir J* 1993; 6:1455.

35. Peat JK, Salome CM, Woolcock, AJ. Factors associated with increased bronchial responsiveness in Australian adults and children. *Eur Respir J* 1992: 5: 921.

The Distribution of Total and Specific IgE in the European Community Respiratory Health Survey

Peter Burney*

Keywords: European Community Respiratory Health Survey, IgE

The ECRHS is a multicentre study, the coordination of which has been finanaced by the European Union. The aims of the study have been to measure (1) variation in the prevalence of asthma, asthma-like symptoms, and bronchial lability; (2) exposure to known and suspected risk factors for asthma, their association with asthma, and the extent to which they explain variations in asthma prevalence; and (3) variations in treatment for asthma. This paper describes the study briefly as well as preliminary data from 32 centres.

The European Community Respiratory Health Survey is a multicentre study with a common protocol. The surveys in each centre were conducted in two stages: The first stage was a screening survey to assess the prevalence of symptoms and diagnosis by age and sex, the second stage was a more detailed survey to assess risk factors and management. In the first stage, 1500 men and 1500 women aged 20–44 were selected from population of 150,000 total (minimum) defined by preexisting administrative boundaries; all were sent a revised version of the IUATLD questionnaire. In the second stage, 300 men and 300 women were selected at random from the stage I sample and were invited for testing. These subjects were given a more detailed questionnaire relating to symptoms, history, relevant exposures, and treatment, had lung-function tests including methacholine challenge, skin tests, and blood drawn for IgE; in some centres the men were asked for 24-hour specimens of urine. This paper reports on the results from the testing for IgE.

Blood was drawn from each subject into plain tubes and allowed to clot *either* overnight at 4°C *or* for 3–6 hours at room temperature; the serum was then separated and stored at –20°C until sent on dry ice to Pharmacia Diagnostics (Uppsala). All specimens were then analysed in the same laboratory using the CAP System. All samples were tested for total IgE and for specific IgE against *Der p* I, cat, timothy grass, and *Cladosporium*. In addition, the samples were tested in each centre for specific IgE against birch, *Parietaria*, or ragweed. This allergen was selected as the most relevant allergen for the centre.

This paper presents preliminary data on 32 centres. There are other centres from which data will be analysed, but at the time of writing the data have not been linked. In the present analysis, 30,246 subjects were identified from stage I, and there are 12,194 (40.3%) with IgE data. In 23 centres, we have information on why blood was not collected for IgE: Where data were missing, 21% refused, 15% were untraced, 4% had moved, and 1% were temporarily away, had an incorrect address, were unable to participate, or had died.

Because of the high number of missing values, we tested the effects of adjusting the data for these by assuming the missing values are the same as for people with known IgE values from the same centre who are of the same age group and gender and have the same symptoms in the screening questionnaire. The effect of this adjustment is to change the geometric mean total IgE level by less than 5% in almost all cases.

By contrast, the variation in the geometric mean total serum IgE adjusted for age and sex is over four-fold from the lowest recorded centre to the highest recorded centre, and the differences between the countries are highly significant. This is also true for the variation in specific IgE, though this is not distributed in the same way as the total IgE levels.

* Public Health Medicine, UMDS St Thomas's Hospital, London, UK.

We conclude that there are large variations in the geometric mean serum IgE levels between populations, that there are large variations in the prevalence of specific serum IgE antibodies between populations, and that these variations are not yet well explained.

Address for correspondence:

Public Health Medicine
UMDS St Thomas's Hospital
London SE1 7EH
UK

Impact of Air Pollution on Allergic Diseases: Clinical and Epidemiologic Studies

Johannes Ring*, Heidrun Behrendt*,**, Torsten Schäfer*, Dieter Vieluf*, Ursula Krämer**

Keywords: Pollution, allergy, atopic eczema, asthma, pollinosis, East Germany, West Germany, epidemiology

Allergic diseases have increased in prevalence during the last decades in many industrialized countries. The reasons for this increase are not known. Among other hypotheses, the possible role of environmental pollutants has received much public and scientific attention. Epidemiologic studies in Western countries have shown associations between allergic sensitization and air pollution in the outdoor and indoor environment. In multivariate analyses the following risk factors were significantly associated with development of atopic diseases: genetic factors (family history of atopy), allergen exposure (pets, house dust mites), exposure to pollutants from indoor (gas excluding vehicle exhaust, tobacco smoke) and outdoor (motor traffic) sources. In a comparative epidemiologic study between various regions in former Eastern and Western Germany immediately after the German reunification carried out in 1990, higher rates of upper respiratory tract infections and airway irritation were found in the highly polluted East German regions, while the prevalence rates of allergic rhinitis and allergic bronchial asthma were lower. Atopic eczema was higher in East Germany. The most striking difference between East and West German preschool-children with regard to allergological examinations was a 2–4 times increased total serum IgE level in East German children, independent of air pollution measured. At the same time, there was a higher rate of parasitic infestation in East German children. The total serum IgE level showed a significant positive correlation with the number of persons living in one apartment, in contrast to the prevalence of allergic sensitization. On analyzing these data, it becomes clear that different patterns of air pollution must be distinguished, namely type I (classical smog with SO_2 and particles) and type II (with NO_x and volatile organic compounds), the latter being associated with allergic sensitization. These epidemiologic findings must still be substantiated and further analyzed by experimental studies using *in vitro* and *in vivo* models.

Some studies have shown a modulatory effect of some pollutants on both IgE-production and mediator release. Furthermore, direct interactions between pollutants and allergen carriers must be considered. In addition, the well-known irritant effects of many pollutants on the skin and mucous membranes might play a role in aggravating allergic respiratory and skin diseases.

At present, the impact of pollution on allergic diseases can only be roughly estimated. Increased research efforts are needed to answer this question with any degree of certainty, and to draw practical conclusions for prevention and therapy.

Introduction

The prevalence of allergic diseases has increased in many countries of the world (9, 28) over the last decades. Studies from the United Kingdom, Sweden, Switzerland, and Japan have shown a dramatic increase in the prevalence of pollinosis from 1–3% to around 15% within the last three decades (9, 20, 28, 36). A twin study from Denmark showed an increase from 3% to 12% in the prevalence of atopic eczema between 1960 and 1980 (33). Little information is available regarding the prevalence of other allergic diseases such as food allergy, drug allergy, insect allergy, extrinsic alveolitis, allergic contact dermatitis, or urticaria (9).

The reasons for this increase in the prevalence of atopic diseases are not known. Among many hypotheses (Table 1), the possible role of environmental pollutants has received substantial public and scientific attention. The methods for serious scientific investigations in this area include:

---

* Universitätshautklinik und Allergie-Abteilung, Universitätskrankenhaus Eppendorf, Hamburg, Germany.
** Medizinisches Institut für Umwelthygiene, Universität Düsseldorf, Germany.

- Clinical observation
- Epidemiologic studies
- Experimental investigations, using both *in vitro* and *in vivo* models
- Standardized provocation procedures in selected patients in order to prove the clinical relevance of the observed findings.

In this paper we would like to focus on clinical and epidemiologic studies.

Table 1. Possible explanations of the increasing prevalence of allergy worldwide.

- Improved diagnostic tools
- Increased awareness
- Increased allergen exposure (quality, quantity)
- Decreased immune stimulation
- Improved standards of hygiene, fewer infections ("jungle hypothesis")
- Increasing age of mothers
- Decreasing number of children/family members
- Increasing social mobility ("allergy follows liberty")
- Environmental pollution

Clinical Observation

It is interesting that much more information is available on respiratory atopic diseases than on skin allergies. The question as to whether atopic eczema itself can be regarded as an allergic disease is still controversial. However, there is increasing evidence that exogenous environmental substances, such as aeroallergens or food allergens, play a role in exacerbation of skin lesions. Recently, not only IgE (8) but also the high affinity receptor for IgE has been described on the surface of epidermal Langerhans cells (5). By epicutaneous application of aeroallergens, eczematous skin lesions can be provoked in a procedure called an atopy patch test (23, 24).

In allergists' offices, an increasing number of patients suffering from suspected allergies to chemicals or environmental pollutants have been seen over the past few years. Many of these patients are suffering intensely from polysomatic complaints, without objective findings of allergic sensitization. We have suggested the term "eco-syndrome" for this group of patients (27), while others have called it "environmental illness," "allergy to the 20th century," or "multiple chemical sensitivity" etc. (25).

In the majority of these patients, psychosomatic interactions seems to play a major role; however, in a thorough investigation of 30 patients with "eco-syndrome" we found objective hypersensitivity reactions (both allergic and pseudo-allergic in origin) in placebo-controlled provocation tests (27). We have to bear in mind that our diagnostic tools for hypersensitivity to small chemicals are limited and that there may be false-negative test and provocation reactions hidden among patients classified as "psychosomatic" (10).

Irritant Effects of Pollutants

It has become clear that many pollutants exert irritant effects upon skin and mucous membranes, leading to aggravation of the symptoms of allergic respiratory or skin disease (19, 28).

In a recent study, Molfino et al. have shown that the inhalation of ozone may enhance the reactivity to allergen exposure in predisposed individuals (22).

Another entity about which we know relatively little, but which is of great concern, is the so-called "sick building syndrome," where unspecific symptoms like impairment of well-being and headache, but also irritation of the eyes and mucous membranes, erythematous skin eruptions, and itch have been described. The factors under discussion in the etiology of this entity include lack of ventilation and increased dryness of the air, together with possible allergen exposure from air-conditioners and humidifiers, as well as psychophysiological factors (12).

Many of these conditions may be influenced by the increased public awareness. However, the possible effect of pollutants on allergic sensitization, i. e., the development of allergic diseases, can not be studied in individual patients. Epidemiologic studies must be carried out.

Epidemiologic Studies

Many epidemiologic studies in different countries have found clear associations between the prevalence of respiratory diseases and air pollution (4, 7, 11, 13, 28). There is no doubt that high concentrations of such air pollutants as suspended particles, sulfur dioxide, ozone, etc., can be found in the air over regions with high prevalence rates

175

of atopic allergies. On the other hand, the air concentrations of some of these substances have shown a considerable decrease during the last decades, e. g., sulfur dioxide and particles in Japan or West Germany. Over the same time period, an epidemiologic study found an increasing prevalence of allergic rhinoconjunctivitis due to Japanese cedar pollen (20). The air concentration of car exhaust particles had also increased at the same time. The Japanese authors compared the prevalence of pollinosis in five different regions with low or high air concentrations of pollen or car exhaust particles, respectively. The highest incidence of cedar pollinosis was found in areas with cedar trees and a high traffic density (20).

Similarly high rates of allergic sensitization have been observed in other investigations in children living near (< 50 meters) roads with high traffic densities (4, 16).

Another air pollutant which can be associated with an increased prevalence of atopic diseases may be tobacco smoke (17, 31, 37). In a study performed in different regions of Bavaria, we found a significantly increased risk of atopic disease or atopic sensitization in children whose mothers had smoked during pregnancy or lactation (17, 31). In this study, we found a cumulative prevalence for atopic disease of 22.8% in preschool children (12% allergic rhinoconjunctivitis, 9.5% atopic eczema, 5% bronchial asthma) (17). We also found a rather high prevalence of positive patch tests (15.8%), with nickel being the most frequent allergen; this was significantly associated with piercing of the ears at an early age (28).

In a comparison between three areas with different degrees of air pollution as measured by SO_2 concentrations, the highest prevalence rates of atopic eczema as well as minimal variants of atopic eczema were found in the region with high pollution (Figure 1). While this difference was significant at the descriptive level, it was no longer significant when multivariate regression analysis was performed.

These experiences and findings led us to perform other epidemiologic studies in a heavily polluted area, namely in former Eastern Europe. As soon as the Iron Curtain had fallen, a comparative study among 2045 preschool children (5–6 years old) was performed in differently polluted areas of the former East and West Germany. The aim of this study was to monitor the effects of air pollution upon human health, especially on allergic sensitization and allergy formation. Based on doctor's diagnosis, the descriptive cumulative prevalence of respiratory atopic diseases was higher in the West than in the East (Figure 2). By contrast, the prevalence rates of upper respiratory tract infection or irritation were higher in East German towns (Figure 3).

The prevalence rates of atopic eczema were higher in East Germany than in West Germany, but there was a wide variation in prevalence between different study regions in West Germany (Schäfer, Ring, Behrendt et al.; in preparation).

The most striking difference between East and West in this study was that serum IgE levels were significantly higher in East Germany (geometric mean 51.4 kU/l) than in West Germany (geometric mean 20.3 kU/l) (Figure 4).

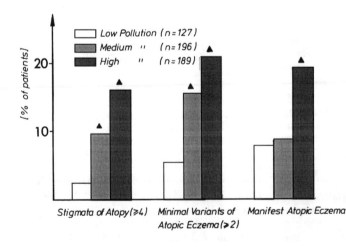

Figure 1. Cumulative prevalence of manifest atopic eczema and minimal variants of eczema in preschool children in areas of Bavaria with different degrees of air pollution.

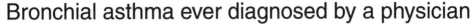

Bronchial asthma ever diagnosed by a physician

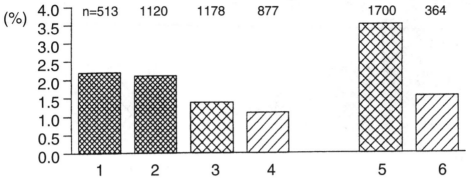

Hay fever ever diagnosed by a physician

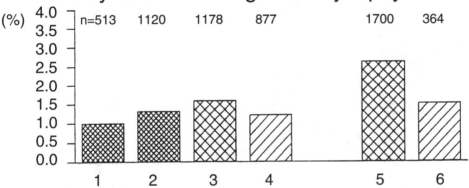

Eczema ever diagnosed by a physician

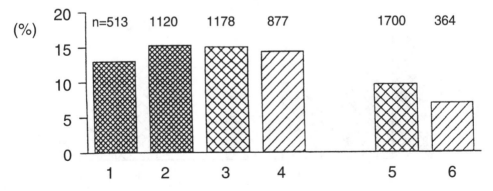

1 = Leipzig; 2= Halle; 3 = Magdeburg; 4 = Osterburg, Gardelegen, Salzwedel;
5 = Köln, Düsseldorf; 6 = Borken

Figure 2. Prevalence of allergic diseases (doctor's diagnosis) in preschool children living for at least 2 years at their place of residence in various towns in East (1–4) and West (5, 6) Germany (from 32).

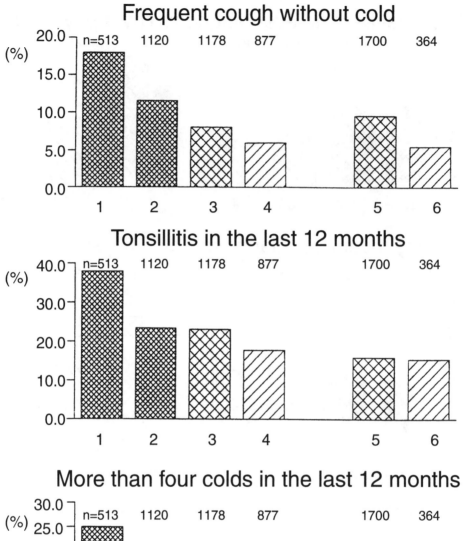

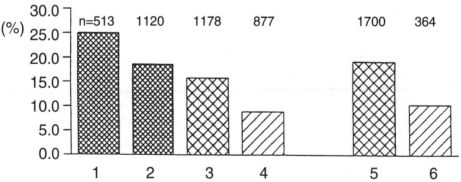

1 = Leipzig; 2= Halle; 3 = Magdeburg; 4 = Osterburg, Gardelegen, Salzwedel;
5 = Köln, Düsseldorf; 6 = Borken

Figure 3. Prevalence of infectious and irritant upper respiratory diseases in preschool children living for at least 2 years at their place of residence in various towns in East (1–4) and West (5, 6) Germany (from 32).

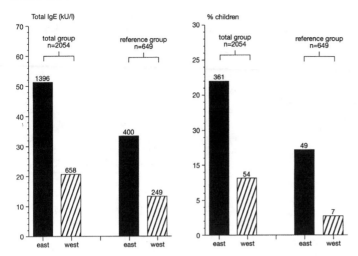

Figure 4. Geometric means of total serum IgE levels in preschool children in East and West Germany in 1991 (from 1).

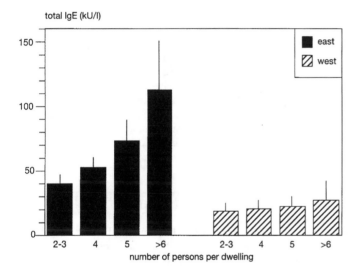

Figure 5. Influence of the number of persons per apartment on geometric means and upper 95% percentile of total serum IgE levels among preschool children in East (n = 1395) and West Germany (n = 655) in 1991 (from 1).

This difference persisted when children with positive allergy-related variables were excluded. The relative risk for East German children of developing elevated IgE (above 180 kU/l) was 2.7 (95% confidence interval: 2.08–3.45). The serum IgE levels were higher, the more persons were living within one apartment (Figure 5); at the same time, the prevalence of allergic sensitization decreased (1). Similar findings regarding reduced allergy prevalence rates with increasing numbers of family members have been reported by von Mutius et al. (21), who also reported decreased rates of allergic respiratory diseases in the East German city of Leipzig compared to the West German city

of Munich. Similarly reduced allergy rates were reported by Björksten et al. in Estland compared to Sweden (6).

In our study, the following factors were found to influence the total serum IgE levels in children: history of parasitic infection, number of persons per dwelling, passive smoking, and gender. It was found that the prevalence of parasitic infection was significantly higher in East German children than in West German children (1).

The results of this East/West German study were surprising in several ways, and in part totally against our earlier hypotheses. There were four main antinomies (i.e., obvious contradictory re-

Table 2. "Obvious antinomies" from the results of the epidemiologic study comparing East and West German preschool children with regard to prevalence of allergic diseases and allergic sensitization.

1. East: More air pollution	Less atopy
2. East: Less respiratory atopy	Equal or less eczema
3. East: High serum IgE	Less respiratory atopy
4. East: More family members, higher total IgE more parasitic infestations	Less specific IgE (?), less respiratory atopy

Table 3. The concept of various T helper cell subpopulations in the induction of parasite defense and allergic sensitization.

T lymphocytes			
T suppresser/ cytotoxic	T helper		
	Th1	Th2	
		Th2α	Th2β
Viral defense, tolerance	DTH, contact allergy	Parasite defense	Atopic allergy

sults hard to reconcile [Kant]; Table 2). If air pollution plays a role in the induction of allergy, one would expect a higher prevalence of atopic diseases in East Germany. There was also an interesting dissociation in the prevalence patterns between respiratory atopic disease (more frequent in West Germany) and atopic eczema (more frequent in East Germany) (32).

Obviously, the markedly elevated serum IgE levels are not associated with higher prevalence rates of atopic allergy, but may rather reflect a higher rate of parasitic infestation. This may also be reflected by the finding that IgE increases with the number of persons per apartment. One could speculate that parasite infections in the early years of life may be protective against allergies. This "jungle hypothesis" is based on studies from Ecuador, where high serum IgE levels went along with parasitic infections and low allergy rates (18).

How can we explain the protective effect of parasitic infections on the development of allergic sensitization? One might suggest a new model based on the concept of Th1 and Th2 cells, and postulate two subpopulations of Th2 cells: as Th2α (helpful in the defense against parasitic infections) and Th2β (inducing the sensitizing IgE formation against apathogenic environmental substances, and thus favoring allergic diseases (Table 3) (29).

Can we therefore safely state that air pollution has nothing to do with the development of allergic diseases? The answer to this question is clearly no! In the same East/West German epidemiology study, multivariate regression analysis showed significantly increased odds ratios for the development of atopic diseases or atopic sensitization when the children had been exposed to the following environmental agents: natural allergens (such as animal epithelia) and indoor (e. g., tobacco smoke, indoor gas without exhaust) or outdoor environmental pollutants (e. g., living near a road with high traffic density) (4).

The seemingly discrepant results may partly be explained by the fact that air pollution is not always the same as air pollution. As shown by Behrendt et al. (1, 4), at least two different types of air pollution have to be differentiated. The classical smog type (type I) with suspended particles, sulfur dioxide, etc., is still present in East Germany and other Eastern European countries. The modern smog type (type II) is characterized by high concentrations of nitrogen oxides and volatile organic compounds (VOC), possibly derived from car exhausts. It is becoming clearer that this type II of air pollution is the one associated with increased prevalence rates of atopic respiratory diseases. Atopic eczema may also be frequent in regions with high degrees of type I air pollution.

Experimental Investigations

The mechanisms by which pollutants may influence allergic reactions are poorly understood. There is no doubt that high concentrations of air pollutants can exert irritant effects upon skin and mucous membranes and thereby aggravate the symptoms of allergic respiratory and skin diseases (19, 35).

On the other hand, animal experiments have shown that various pollutants can have an adjuvant effect upon IgE-mediated sensitization in that animals are more easily sensitized to natural allergens when they were previously exposed to air pollutants such as diesel exhaust particles (20), tobacco smoke (37), SO_2 (26), and others (cited in 2, 28).

Some pollutants may modulate the effector phase of allergic reactions. This has been shown in various cell systems and for different pollutants, such as modulation of the degranulation or histamine release from basophils (3, 4). Pesticides such as polychlorinated biphenyls enhance eicosanoid production by granulocytes and platelets (24). Extracts from dust particles collected in highly polluted areas were able to increase the secretion of interleukin 8, prostaglandins, and oxygen radicals (4).

A totally new approach to studying the influence of air pollution upon allergic diseases came from experiments showing that pollen grains in polluted areas are highly loaded with particles (2, 4). *In vitro*, Behrendt et al. showed that after contact with pollutant particles, pollen grains show signs of activation, changes in the surface structure, and increased release of cytosolic allergenic proteins (2). Similar results were reported by the group from Vienna, showing that birch pollen in air-polluted regions expressed increased amounts of the major allergen Bet V 1 (15).

Conclusions

From all these clinical, experimental, and epidemiologic data it is clear that environmental pollutants can act at different levels and via complex interactions, both outside and inside to organism, to influence the induction, elicitation and maintenance of allergic reactions ("allergotoxicologic effects") (2).

At the moment, the relevance of these investigations for individual patients is not clear. So far, no single chemical has been proven to be responsible for the increasing number of atopic diseases in humans. However, there is increasing evidence that among several mixtures of pollutants, especially organic compounds, substances may be found with a great impact on IgE formation. The field of allergotoxicology is one of the most exciting research areas within experimental and clinical allergy in the 1990s.

Address for correspondence:

Prof Dr Dr J Ring
Universitätshautklinik
Martinistraße 52
D-20246 Hamburg
Germany

References

1. Behrendt H, Krämer U, Dolgner R, Hinrichs J., Willer H., Hagenbeck H, Schlipköter W. Elevated levels of total IgE in East German children: Atopy, parasites or pollutants? *Allergo J* 1993; 2:31–40.

2. Behrendt H, Friedrichs KH, Kainka-Stänicke F, Darsow U, Becker W, Tomingas R. Allergens and pollutants in the air: A complex interaction. In Ring J, Przybilla B (Eds) *New trends in allergy III*. Berlin: Springer, 1991, pp. 467–478.

3. Behrendt H, Becker WM, Friedrich KH, Darsow U, Tomingas R. Interaction between aeroallergens and airborne particulate matter. *Int Arch Allergy Immunol* 1992; 99:425–428.

4. Behrendt H, Friedrichs KH, Krämer U, Hitzfeld B, Becker WM, Ring J. The role of indoor and outdoor air pollution in allergic diseases. *This volume.*

5. Bieber T, De la Salle H, Wollenberg A, Hakimi J, Chizzonite R, Ring J, Hanau D, De la Salle C. Human Langerhans cells express the high affinity receptor for immunoglobin E (FcER1). *J Exp Med* 1992; 175:1285–1290.

6. Björkstén B. Genetic and environmental interaction in children. *This volume.*

7. Braun-Fahrländer C, Ackermann-Liebrich K, Schwartz J, Gnehm HP, Rutishauser M, Wanner HK. Air pollution and respiratory symptoms in preschool children. *Am Rev Resp Dis* 1992; 145:42–47.

8. Bruijnzeel-Koomen C, van Wichen L, Toostra J, Berrens W, Bruijnzeel P. The presence of IgE-molecules on epidermal Langerhans cells from patients with atopic dermatitis. *Arch Dermatol Res* 1986; 278:940–945.

9. Burr ML (Ed). *Epidemiology of allergic diseases.* Basel: Karger, 1993.

10. Bullinger M. Psychological effects of air pollution on healthy residents – a time- series approach. *J Environ Psychol* 1989; 9:103–118.

11. Dockery DW, Speicer FE, Frank E, Stram BO, Ware JH, Spengler JD, Ferris Jr BG. Effects of inhalable particles on respiratory health of children. *Am Rev Resp Dis* 1989; 139:587–594.

12. Finnegan MJ, Pickering CA, Burge PS. The sick building syndrome: Prevalence studies. *Br Med J* 1984; 283:1573.

13. Goren AI, Hellmann S. Prevalence of respiratory symptoms and diseaes in school-children living in a low polluted area in Israel. *Environ Res* 1988; 45:28–37.

14. Hitzfeld B, Friedrichs KH, Tomingas R, Behrendt H. Organic atmospheric dust extracts and their effects on functional parameters of human polymorphonuclear leukocytes. *J Aerosol Sci* 1992; 23 (Suppl 1):531–534.

15. Jilek A, Swoboda I, Breiteneder H, Fogy I, Ferreira F, Schmid E, Heberle-Bros E, Scheiner O, Rumpold H, Koller HT, Breitenbach M. Biological functions, isoforms, and environmental control in the Bet V 1 gene family. In Kraft D, Sehon A (Eds) *Molecular biology and immunology of allergens*. Boca Raton: CRC Press, 1993, pp. 39–46.

16. Krämer U, Behrendt H, Dolgner R, Kainka-Stänicke E, Oberbarnscheidt J, Sidaoui H, Schlipköter W. Auswirkung der Umweltbelastung auf allergologische Parameter bei 6-jährigen Kindern. Ergebnisse einer Pilotstudie im Rahmen der Luftreinhaltepläne von Nordrhein-Westfalen. In Ring J (Ed) *Epidemiologie allergischer Erkrankungen*. Munich: MMV Medizin, 1991, pp. 165–178.

17. Kunz B, Ring J, Dirschedl B, Przybilla B, Vieluf D, Greif A, Gries A, Huber HCh, Kapsner Th, Letzel H, Römmelt H, Michel R, Schotten K, Stickl H, Vogl-Vosswinckel E, Überla K. Innenraumluftbelastung und atopische Erkrankungen bei Kindern. In Ring J (Ed) *Epidemiologie allergischer Erkrankungen*. Munich: MMV Medizin, 1991, pp. 202–220.

18. Larrick JW, Buckley CE, Machamer CE, Schlagel GD, Yost JA, Blessign-Moore J, Jevy D. Does hyper-immunoglobulinemia-E protect tropical populations from allergic disease? *J Allergy Clin Immunol* 1983; 71:184–188.

19. Magnussen H, Jörres R, Wagner HM, von Nieding G. Relationship between the airway response to inhaled sulfur dioxide, isocapnic hyperventilation and histamine in asthmatic subjects. *Int Arch Occup Environ Health* 1990; 62: 485.

20. Miyamoto T, Takafuji S. Environment and Allergy. In Ring J, Przybilla B (Eds) *New trends in allergy III*. Berlin: Springer, 1991, pp. 459–468.

21. von Mutius E, Fritzsch C, Weiland SK, Röll G, Magnussen H. Prevalence of asthma and allergic disorders among children in united Germany: A descriptive comparison. *Br Med J* 1992; 305:1395–1399.

22. Molfino NA, Wright StC, Katz I, Tarlo S, Silverman F, McClean PA, Szalai JP, Raizenne M, Slutsky AS, Zamel N. Effect on low concentrations of ozone on inhaled allergen responses in asthmatic subjects. *Lancet* 1991; 338:199–203.

23. Platts-Mills TAE. Epidemiology of the relationship between exposure to indoor allergens and asthma. *Int Arch Allergy Immunol* 1991; 94:339–345.

24. Raulf M, König W. Induction of mediator generation in human inflammatory cells by polychlorinated biphenyles. In Ring J, Przybylla B (Eds) *New trends in allergy III*. Berlin: Springer, 1991, pp. 489–499.

25. Rest K (Ed). *Advancing the understanding of multiple chemical sensitivity*. Princeton: Princeton Scientific Publ, 1992.

26. Riedel F, Krämer M, Scheibenbogen C, Rieger CHL. Effects of SO_2 exposure on allergic sensitization in the guinea pig. *J Allergy Clin Immunol* 1988; 82:527–534.

27. Ring J; Vieluf D, Przybilla B, Gabriel G, Rad M v, Braun-Falco O. The "Clinical Ecology Syndrome" (Eco-Syndrome"):Psychology or allergy. In Ring J, Przybilla B (Eds) *New trends in allergy III*. Berlin: Springer, 1991, pp. 500–513.

28. Ring J (Ed). *Epidemiologie allergischer Erkrankungen*. Munich: MMV, 1991.

29. Ring J, Behrendt H. Allergy and IgE production: Role of infection and environmental pollution. Allergo J 1993; 2:27–30.

30. Rusnak C. The impact of pollution on allergic disease. *Allergy* 1994; 49:21–27.

31. Schäfer T, Dirschedl P, Przybilla B, Kunz B, Ring J, Greif A, Überla K. Maternal smoking (MS) and atopy manifestation (AM) in children are significantly correlated. *ACI News* 1991; Suppl 1:221(abstr).

32. Schlipköter HW, Krämer U, Behrendt H, Dolgner R, Stiller-Winkler R, Ring J, Willer HJ. Impact of air pollution on children's health. Results from Saxony-Anhalt and Saxony as compared to Northrhine-Westphalia. In *Health and ecological effects. Critical issues in the global environment. Air and waste management association*, Vol 5. Pittsburgh, 1992, IU-A 2103.

33. Schultz-Larsen F, Holm NV, Henningsen K. Atopic dermatitis. A genetic-epidemiologic study in a population based twin sample. *J Am Acad Dermatol* 1986; 15:487–494.

34. Vieluf D, Kunz B, Bieber T, Przybilla B, Ring J. "Atopy Patch Test" with aeroallergens in patients with atopic eczema. *Allergo J* 1993; 2:9–12.

35. Walsh PJ, Dudney CS, Copenhaven ED (Eds). *Indoor air quality*. Boston: CRC Press, 1983.

36. Wüthrich B. Epidemiology of the allergic diseases; are they really on the increase? *Int Arch Allergy Appl Immunol* 1989; 90:3–10.

37. Zetterström O, Osterman K, Machedo L, Johansson SGO. Another smoking hazard: raised IgE concentration and increased risk of occupational allergy. *Br Med J* 1981; 283:1215–1217.

Global Trends in the Treatment of Allergic Diseases

Romain Pauwels*

Keywords: Treatment, asthma, trend, international

The therapy of allergic diseases has changed considerably over the last years, due to the development of new treatment modalities, a better understanding of the pathogenesis of these diseases and large scale clinical trials. There has been a very significant increase in the total prescription and sales of medications for allergic diseases. The treatment of asthma has been influenced by the development of therapeutic guidelines. A WHO Study Group Report on a Global Strategy for Asthma Management presents a broad consensus of the currently recommended treatment. The actual prescription and sales figures show that there are still large differences in the therapy of asthma between countries, and that further efforts are needed to educate physicians about asthma treatment. International collaborative studies should be started to resolve some of the important treatment issues.

Introduction

The treatment of allergic diseases requires a considerable amount of resources in most countries (Figure 1). There has been a very significant growth in the treatment of allergic diseases over the last decades, for various reasons (Figure 2).

The economic and social burden of the treatment of allergic diseases has resulted in a need for better standardization and more rational treatment approaches. Various guidelines for treatment have been published (1–4). The recommended treatment strategies are based on a better understanding of the pathogenesis of the disease and on controlled therapeutic trials. A guideline for the treatment of rhinitis has also been developed recently (5).

WHO/NHLBI Report on a Global Strategy for Asthma Management

The World Health Organisation (WHO) has in collaboration with the National Heart, Lung and Blood Institute (NHLBI) of the US organized a workshop to develop "A Global Strategy for Asthma Management" (in press). The study report of this workshop will be published soon. A summary of the recommendations concerning the treatment of chronic asthma will be presented here as a touchstone for the current treatment of this disease in the world.

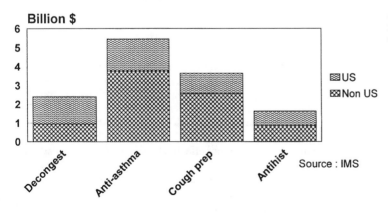

Figure 1. Global sales figures for the treatment of allergic diseases in 1993.

---

* Department of Respiratory Diseases, University Hospital, Ghent, Belgium.

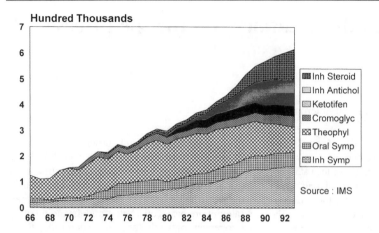

Hundred Thousands

Figure 2. Sales of anti-asthma drugs (in hundred thousands of units) in Belgium per year from 1966 to 1993.

Legend: Inh Steroid, Inh Antichol, Ketotifen, Cromoglyc, Theophyl, Oral Symp, Inh Symp

The treatment recommendations are based on the following premises:
– Asthma is a chronic inflammatory disorder of the airways. This inflammation causes recurrent episodes of symptoms, variable airflow limitation, and increased airway responsiveness. The most effective management is to prevent this inflammation by eliminating the causal factors.
– Asthma can be effectively controlled in most patients, although it cannot be cured.
– The goal of management is to achieve control of asthma, which is defined as:
  – Minimal (ideally no) chronic symptoms, including nocturnal symptoms
  – Minimal (infrequent) exacerbations
  – No emergency visits
  – Minimal (ideally no) need for p.r.n. (as needed) β_2-agonist
  – No limitations on activities, including exercise
  – PEF circadian variation of less than 20%
  – (Near) normal PEF
  – Minimal (or no) adverse effects of medication
– Any asthma more severe than mild, intermittent asthma is more effectively controlled by treatment to suppress and reverse the inflammation than by treatment only of acute bronchoconstriction and related symptoms.
– Effective control of asthma can be accomplished by a six-part asthma management program:
  – Educate patients to develop a partnership in asthma management.
  – Assess and monitor asthma severity with both symptom reports and, as far as possible, measurements of lung function.
  – Avoid or control asthma triggers.

– Establish individual medication plans for long-term management.
– Establish plans for managing exacerbations.
– Provide regular follow-up care.
– The choice of management should be guided by the severity of the patient's asthma, the benefits and the risks of each treatment, the cost-effectiveness, and the availability of the various forms of asthma treatment. Cultural preferences and differing health care systems need to be considered.
– A stepwise approach to pharmacologic therapy – in which the number and frequency of medications increase as the need for asthma therapy increases – is recommended. The aim is to accomplish the goals of therapy with the least possible medication.
– Although in many countries traditional methods of healing are used, their efficacy has not yet been established and their use can therefore not be recommended.

Route of Administration

Medications for asthma can be administered via different routes, including inhalation, orally (ingested) and parenterally (subcutaneous, intramuscular, or intravenous). The major advantage of delivering drugs directly into the airways via inhalation is that high concentrations can be delivered more effectively to the airways, and systemic side effects are avoided or minimized. Some of the drugs that are effective in asthma can only be used via inhalation because they are not absorbed when given orally. The onset of action of bronchodilators given via inhalation is substantially shorter than when administered orally.

Medications for Asthma

Controller Medications

Controller medications – medications used to achieve and maintain control of persistent asthma – include inhaled corticosteroids, systemic corticosteroids, sodium cromoglycate (cromolyn sodium), nedocromil sodium, sustained release theophylline, long-acting inhaled β_2-agonists, and possibly ketotifen, other oral antiallergics and experimental/other medications. Inhaled corticosteroids are at present the most effective controller medications.

Reliever Medications

Reliever medications – medications that act quickly to relieve bronchoconstriction and its accompanying acute symptoms – include short-acting inhaled β_2-agonists, systemic corticosteroids, inhaled anticholinergics, short-acting theophylline, and short-acting oral β_2-agonists.

Steps to Achieve and Maintain Control of Asthma

This section describes the steps of therapy appropriate for different levels for asthma severity. The presence of one or more features of clinical severity places a patient at the respective therapeutic step.

In the stepwise approach to therapy, progression to the next step is indicated when control is not achieved or is lost at the current step, and there is an assurance the patient is using the medication correctly. The frequent (e. g., more than three times a week) presence of such symptoms as cough, wheezing and dyspnea, and the increased use of short-acting bronchodilators, may indicate inadequate control of asthma. The presence of symptoms at night or early in the morning is an especially useful indicator. Increasing variability in PEF indicates inadequately controlled asthma and is often observed before a change in symptoms. Measurements of PEF and its variability are helpful in the initial assessment of asthma severity and in monitoring the initial treatment, assessing changes in severity, and preparing stepdowns in therapy.

The steps suggested here are guidelines only.

Specific medication plans should be tailored by the health care professional, depending on the availability of antiasthma medication, the conditions of the health care system, and individual patient circumstances.

Step 1. A patient has intermittent asthma if he or she experiences exacerbations (episodes of cough, wheezing or dyspnea) less than once a week over a period of at least 3 months and the exacerbations are brief, generally lasting only a few hours to a few days. Nocturnal asthma symptoms do not occur more than two times a month. In between exacerbations the patient is asymptomatic and has a completely normal lung function, i. e., a pretreatment baseline FEV_1 or PEF greater than 80% of predicted and personal best and PEF variability of less than 20%.

Intermittent asthma is not trivial. The severity of the asthma exacerbation may vary from patient to patient and from time to time. Such an exacerbation might even be life threatening, although this is extremely rare in patients with intermittent asthma. The low frequency of the exacerbations and the fact that in between exacerbations the patient has a completely normal lung function support the recommendations that no long-term treatment with a controller medication should be started. Rather, the exacerbations should be treated as such, depending on the severity of the exacerbations. Treatment includes medication as needed prior to exercise (inhaled β_2-agonist, cromoglycate, nedocromil) or to allergen exposure (sodium cromoglycate or nedocromil). Treatment of the exacerbation includes an inhaled short-acting β_2-agonist taken as needed to relieve the asthma symptoms. An inhaled anticholinergic, oral short-acting β_2-agonist, or short-acting theophylline may be considered as alternatives to inhaled short-acting β_2-agonists, although these alternatives have a slower onset of action and/or a higher risk for side effects. Occasionally, more severe or prolonged exacerbations may require a short course of oral corticosteroids.

If medication is required more than once a week over a 3-month period, the patient should be moved to the next step of care, regardless of PEF measurements. The same applies if the lung function in between exacerbations becomes abnormal.

Step 2. A patient has mild persistent asthma if he or she experiences exacerbations, persistent symptoms, and/or declines in lung function with sufficient frequency to warrant daily long-term therapy with controller medications. Mild persistent asthma is present: if the patient experiences exacerbations at least once a week but less than once a day over the lst 3 months and some of the exacerbations affect sleep and activity levels; and/or if the patient has chronic symptoms that require symptomatic treatment almost daily and experiences nocturnal asthma symptoms more than two times a month. The patient with mild persistent asthma has a pretreatment baseline PEF of more than 80% of predicted or personal best and PEF variability of 20–30%. Furthermore, cough variant asthma should be treated as mild persistent asthma.

Patients with mild persistent asthma require controller medication every day to achieve and maintain control of their asthma. The primary therapy for mild persistent asthma is regular use of anti-inflammatory medication taken on a daily basis. Treatment can be started with either inhaled corticosteroids, sodium cromoglycate, or nedocromil sodium. A spacer device and mouth washing after inhalation are recommended when using inhaled corticosteroids to reduce oropharyngeal side effects. Children are usually given an initial trial (4–6 weeks) of sodium cromoglycate. The suggested introductory dose of inhaled corticosteroids is 200–500 μg per day of beclomethasone diproprionate (BDP) or budesonide or equivalent.

Long-term treatment with sustained-release theophylline may be considered, but the need for monitoring of serum concentration levels may make this treatment less feasible. Inhaled short-acting β_2-agonist should be available to take as needed to relieve symptoms, but should not be taken more than three to four times a day.

If symptoms persist despite the initial dose of inhaled corticosteroids, and the health care professional is satisfied that the patient is using the medications correctly, the inhaled corticosteroids should be increased from 400 or 500 to 750 or 800 μg per day BDP or equivalent. A possible alternative to increasing the dose of inhaled corticosteroids, especially to control nocturnal symptoms, is the addition of a long-acting bronchodilator to a dose of at least 500 μg inhaled corticosteroids. The long-term efficacy of a combination of low-dose inhaled corticosteroids with a long-acting bronchodilator as compared to higher doses of inhaled corticosteroids remains to be studied.

If the patient's long-term therapy was initiated with sustained-release theophylline, sodium cromoglycate, or nedocromil sodium, and symptoms persist after 4 weeks of this initial treatment,

then inhaled corticosteroids should be introduced. The inhaled corticosteroids may be initiated either instead of or together with the other medication to allow an overlap period.

Step 3. Moderate persistent asthma is characterized by daily symptoms over a prolonged time or nocturnal asthma more than once a week. The patient with moderate persistent asthma has a pretreatment baseline PEF of more than 60% but less than 80% of predicted or personal best and PEF variability of 20–30%.

Patients with moderate persistent asthma require controller medication every day to achieve and maintain control of their asthma.

The dose of inhaled corticosteroids should be 800–2,000 μg beclomethasone dipropionate or equivalent a day. A spacer device with the inhaler is recommended to reduce oropharyngeal side effects and systemic absorption.

Long-acting bronchodilators in addition to the inhaled corticosteroids may also be considered, particularly to control nocturnal symptoms. Sustained-release theophylline, an oral slow-release β_2-agonist, or a long-acting inhaled β_2-agonist may be used. Theophylline serum concentrations should be monitored, with a general therapeutic range of 5–15 μg/ml.

A long-acting inhaled β_2-agonist may have a complementary effect to inhaled corticosteroids, although more data are necessary to establish the place of long-acting β-agonist in asthma therapy. The role of anticholinergics (ipratropium bromide) in long-term therapy is not well established, but an introduction of anticholinergics may be considered as an alternative for patients who experience such adverse effects as tachycardia or tremor from inhaled β-agonists.

Inhaled short-acting β-agonists should be available to take as needed to relieve symptoms, but should not be taken more than three to four times a day.

Step 4. A patient has severe persistent asthma if he or she experiences highly variable, continuous symptoms, and frequent nocturnal symptoms, has limited activities, and experiences severe exacerbations in spite of medications. The patient with severe persistent asthma has a pretreatment baseline PEF of less than 60% of predicted or personal best and PEF variability greater than 30%. Control of asthma as defined earlier may not be possible. In severe persistent asthma, the goal of therapy becomes achieving best possible results: the least symptoms, the least need for short-acting β-agonist, the best flow rates, the least circadian (night to day) variation, and the least side effects from medication.

Therapy usually requires multiple daily controller medications. Primary therapy includes inhaled corticosteroids at higher doses (more than 800–2,000 µg per day of beclomethasone diproprionate or equivalent).

A bronchodilator is recommended in addition to the inhaled corticosteroids, such as oral sustained-release theophylline or oral β2-agonist and/or a long-acting inhaled β2-agonist. An inhaled short-acting β2-agonist regularly scheduled once a day, usually upon arising, may also be considered. A trial of inhaled anticholinergic (ipratropium) may be considered, particularly for those patients who experience adverse effects from β2-agonist.

Inhaled short-acting β2-agonist should be available as needed up to three to four times a day to relieve symptoms.

Long-term oral corticosteroids should be used in the lowest possible dose (alternate or single daily dose after a 3- to 7-day burst). Persistent trials of high doses of inhaled corticosteroids administered with a spacer device should be made in an attempt to reduce oral corticosteroids. When patients are transferred from oral corticosteroids to high-dose inhaled corticosteroids, they should be monitored closely for evidence of adrenal insufficiency.

Stepdown: Reduction of maintenance therapy. Asthma is a variable disorder, and spontaneous and therapy-induced variations in severity occur. Especially anti-inflammatory therapy has been shown to reduce asthma severity over the long term. Once control of asthma is achieved and maintained for at least 3 months, a gradual stepwise reduction of the maintenance therapy should be tried in order to identify the minimum therapy require to maintain control. This will help reduce the risk of side effects and enhance patient adherence to the treatment plan. The therapy reduction should be done stepwise, following the reverse order of what has just been described with close monitoring of symptoms, clinical signs, and, as much as possible, lung function.

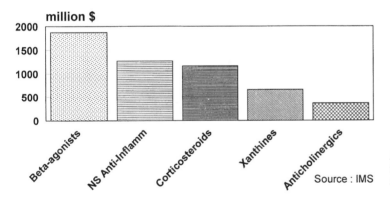

Figure 3. Global sales figures for different categories of anti-asthma therapy in 1993.

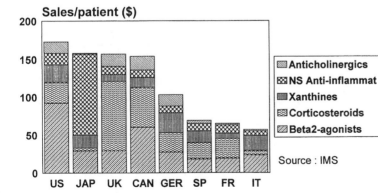

Figure 4. Sales figures for different categories of anti-asthma therapy in 1993 in selected countries.

187

Current Treatment of Asthma

The sales figures show that there is still a large difference between recommended treatment and actually prescribed and used anti-asthma treatment (Figures 3 and 4).

Bronchodilators form still the majority of the anti-asthma therapy, although clinical studies show the superior efficacy of anti-inflammatory therapy and many efforts have been made to educate physicians and patients. Large differences also exist between countries in the use of anti-asthma medications (Figure 4). The actual prescription and sales figures therefore show that there are still large differences in the therapy of asthma between countries and that further efforts are needed to educate physicians about asthma treatment. International collaborative studies should be started to resolve some of the important treatment issues.

Address for correspondence:

Romain Pauwels
Department of Respiratory Diseases
University Hospital
B-9000 Ghent
Belgium

References

1. British Thoracic Society, Research Unit of Royal College of Physicians, Kings Fund Centre, National Asthma Campaign. Guidelines for management of asthma in adults. I. Chronic persistent asthma. *Br Med J* 1990; 301:651–653.

2. Hargreave FE, Dolovich J, Newhouse MT. The assessment and treatment of asthma: A conference report. *J Allergy Clin Immunol* 1990; 85:1098–1111.

3. International Pediatric Consensus Group. Asthma: A followup statement from an international pediatric consensus group. *Arch Dis Childhood* 1992; 67:240–248.

4. National Heart, Lung and Blood Institute, National Institutes of Health. *International consensus report on diagnosis and treatment of asthma*. US Department of Health and Human Services, Public Health Service, National Institutes of Health, June 1992, pp. 1–72.

5. International Rhinitis Management Working Group. International consensus report on the diagnosis and management of rhinitis. *Allergy* 1994; 49 (Suppl 19):1–34.

Definition and Identification of Individuals at High Risk of Death Due to Asthma

Albert L Sheffer*

Keywords: Fatal asthma

Asthma-related fatalities have increased world-wide in the decade since 1980, and since 1990 no reduction in this death rate has occurred. Inadequate assessment of the severity of asthma and consequent inappropriate treatment are considered central to deaths due to asthma. Physiologic, epidemiologic, pathologic, pharmacologic and clinical factors all contribute to the recognition of fatality-prone asthma. Clinically, the most significant risk factors for death due to asthma include: hospital admission for asthma or multiple hospitalizations for asthma in the preceding 12 months; asthma that requires at least 3 categories of anti-asthma drugs; and a peak expiratory flow rate (PEFR) of < 100 L/min. Reduction in asthma fatalities requires not only early recognition of factors contributing to such events, but also an appreciation and reversal of those pathophysiologic mechanisms underlying life-threatening exacerbations. These include inflammatory changes in the airways leading to eosinophilic or neutrophilic infiltration, thickening of large and small airways, and blunting of the hypoxic response and perception of dyspnea. PEFR monitoring in asthma sufferers who exhibit some clinical risk factors may facilitate prompt identification of exacerbations. With appropriate intervention, death from asthma may be prevented.

Asthma fatalities are not just a recent observation, for such deaths were noted as early as 200 B.C. by Aretaeus of Cappadocia (1). Although descriptions over the centuries have been episodic, during the recent decade considerable concern has been expressed in this regard by the international medical community (2). As a consequence, national and international strategies have been developed to identify and treat asthma sufferers and to reduce fatalities. Most asthma deaths are preventable with prompt identification and early, effective treatment (3). Factors associated with increased risk of asthma-related death factors have been attributed to

characteristics of disease processes, and asthma management (4). In this paper, risk factors are categorized by epidemiologic, physiologic, pharmacologic, pathologic, and clinical parameters. Considerable attention has been directed previously to socioeconomic, psychologic, and clinical factors related to asthma deaths (4). With identification of pathophysiologic risk factors, a more definitive profile of the individual with fatality-prone asthma can be made.

Epidemiologic Factors

Asthma mortality increased world-wide in the decade after 1980, chiefly in the age ranges of 5–34 and > 50 years (1–4). The incidence of asthma-related deaths does not appear to be decreasing. At higher risk for asthma fatalities are patients of certain ethnic minorities; this has especially been documented among African-Americans (who had death rates five times higher than their white counterparts) and the Maoris (indigenous Polynesians) of New Zealand (2, 3). In the United States, those living in socioeconomically deprived areas are particularly susceptible to fatal asthma attacks (5). This may be due to the intense exposure to allergens and irritants in urban sites as well as inadequate access to medical care.

Physiologic Factors

The relationship of dyspnea and chemosensitivity to hypoxia and hypercapnia have been evaluated as contributory events in fatal asthma (7). Inves-

---
* Brigham and Women's Hospital, Department of Rheumatology and Immunology; and Harvard Medical School, Department of Medicine, Boston, MA, USA.

189

tigators noted that the mean hypoxic ventilatory response and airway occlusion pressure were reduced in patients with near-fatal asthma when compared to normal subjects and patients with asthma who had not experienced near-fatal attacks. The perception of dyspnea was also lower in patients with near fatal asthma than in normal subjects. Their lower hypoxic response was associated with a blunted perception of asthma. These results suggested to the authors that reduced chemosensitivity to hypoxia and blunted perception of dyspnea predisposes asthma patients to fatal attacks (7).

Three patterns of respiratory decompensation have been described in 34 patients who were intubated and mechanically ventilated for severe asthma. Group I experienced rapid deterioration between onset of symptoms and endotracheal intubation over a period of > 3 h; Group II developed a gradual respiratory failure over 9.2 ± 7.7 days; and Group III experienced an acute exacerbation during unstable asthma over 4.2 ± 3.5 days (8). It was felt by these authors that bronchodilation was central to the pathogenesis of sudden asphyxic asthma.

Pharmacologic Factors

The increasing mortality rate for asthmatic individuals has been related to anti-asthma therapy and bronchodilators particularly β_2-agonists such as Fenoterol (9). Analyses of such data were difficult because of confounding variables, such as disease severity, in that those with the more severe asthma were treated with Fenoterol rather than Salbutamol. Furthermore, assessment in a nested case control study conducted in Canada confined the relationship of asthma fatality to β_2-agonist abuse (10). In this assessment the authors defined an overall fatality rate of 9.6/10,000 asthmatic individuals per year. The risk of death in this study increased when 1.4 canisters or more a month of inhaled β_2-agonists were consumed. Although an association was documented, these studies do not causally relate the dispensing of large amounts of inhaled β_2-agonists to the risk of death due to asthma as a toxic effect of the pharmacologic agent or vehicles, or use of the agents. It has not been established whether the increased use of β_2-agonists con-

tributes to mortality or is merely a marker of severe disease (10).

Near-fatal asthma exacerbations have been shown to result from severe asphyxia rather than cardiac arrhythmias (11). This observation suggests that undertreatment, rather than overtreatment, contributes to increased asthma mortality (12).

Prescribed corticosteroids were only slightly associated with subsequent death, but more strongly associated with readmission. Prescribed psychotropic drugs were also associated with an increased risk of death (12).

Pathologic Factors

Severe asthma has been the subject of several assessments (13, 14). A recent study differentiated between slow onset and sudden onset fatal asthma exacerbations set was related to submucosal eosinophilia, as compared to mucosal eosinophils and submucosal neutrophils, whereas submucosal neutrophils predominated in sudden onset fatal asthma. Both these observations were statistically significant. Thus, submucosal correlation was significant in all cases, whereas the number of eosinophils in the airway correlated with the time interval between onset of asthma attack and death (13).

In one study (14) comparing the autopsy results of subjects with asthma who died of asthma (fatal asthma) to subjects with asthma who died of other causes (nonfatal asthma), and to subjects without asthma (controls), airway dimensions were measured in large and small airways. Airways were grouped by size using the basement membrane perimeter for comparison. All areas were expressed as areas/mm of basement membrane. In cartilaginous airways the cases of fatal asthma had greater ($p < 0.05$) total wall, inner wall, outer wall, smooth muscle, mucous gland, and cartilage areas than did control and nonfatal asthma cases ($p < 0.05$) in the small cartilage airways and membranous bronchioles (14). In the large membranous bronchioles (perimeter: 2–4 mm) the area of smooth muscle was greater in fatal and nonfatal asthma cases than in non-asthmatic control cases ($p < 0.05$), but there were no differences in smooth muscle area between the fatal and nonfatal asthma cases versus the control cases. Smooth muscle sheathing and epithelial disruption varied significantly between cases. There were no significant differences between the fatal and nonfatal asthma groups in large and small airways. The authors concluded that structural changes that may increase airway responsiveness occur in both large and small airways in fatal asthma, but they occur predominantly in the small airways in nonfatal cases of asthma. Thus, one interpretation of sudden death in asthma may relate to the structural changes in large and small airways. Furthermore, pulmonary functional changes consistent with large and small airway dysfunction may indicate a predisposition to airway hyper-responsiveness and, in turn, fatality-prone asthma (14).

Autopsy assessments demonstrate that the airway wall is thicker in cases of fatal asthma than in cases of either nonfatal asthma or normal subjects. The cases of fatal asthma in this investigation were all sudden onset, outpatient deaths, in patients who had not received mechanical ventilation. The patients had long histories of asthma, had previously been hospitalized from the asthma, often had frequent episodic attacks, and they had significant airflow impairment for sustained periods.

Thus, studies of altered airways may contribute to understanding airway dysfunction and in turn fatal asthma. The increased smooth muscle allows for greater shortening in response to a bronchoconstrictor stimulus, whereas the outer wall increase may allow uncoupling of the distending force of parenchymal recoil from the forces contributing to airway recovery. Mucous gland hypertrophy may contribute to excess mucus production, and increased inner wall thickness will accentuate the narrowing of the airway with muscle hypertrophy. Although the authors (14) concluded that the importance of such alterations has yet to be determined, it is clear that this is an area that would benefit from further investigation.

Clinical Factors

What are the markers for risk of asthma death? In one assessment of 39 asthma deaths that excluded patients who were prescribed Fenoterol (9, 12), a hospital admission in the past 12 months was the strongest marker of subsequent risk of death and a strong marker of subsequent risk of readmission. The risk of death increased with the number of previous admissions. Measurement of asthma severity provides clinicians with insights as to who is at increased risk of death due to asthma. A PEFR < 100 L/min carried a 2-fold risk of subsequent death or readmission, and a $pCO_2 > 45$ mm Hg was associated with an increased risk of death (12). It is therefore imperative to classify the disease severity; this was initially proposed by Rea (6) and developed in more detail in the NHLBI International Consensus for the Diagnosis and Management of Asthma. Clinical manifestations correlated with peak flow assessment were used to establish asthma severity. Identification of the individual at high risk of asthma-related death used additional criteria. Patients with severe asthma requiring three or more admissions/year and who have had a very severe asthma attack within the same year, are highly susceptible to fatal attacks of asthma (6). A history of previous life-threatening attacks provides a 3-fold risk of death when compared with individuals whose asthma is treated on an outpatient basis. A previous life-threatening attack has a 14-fold risk of death, whereas a previous hospital admission has a 7-fold increased risk (6).

Three markers of severity of chronic asthma were associated with an increased risk of death. A hospital admission for asthma in the previous 12 months was the most consistent indicator of fatal asthma (6); multiple hospital admissions for asthma in the previous year shows an even greater increased risk; and the chronic use of three or more categories of asthma drugs had an increased risk of asthma fatality in this study (6). Interestingly, oral corticosteroids had only a weak association with subsequent risk of death. In the acute exacerbation, a pCO_2 of > 45 mm Hg, and a PEFR of < 100 L/min are markers for increased risk. As markers of a severe attack, these findings are consistent with a life-threatening attack associated with asthma death (12).

Other clinical factors contributing to asthma mortality include inadequate assessment of asthma severity by both patients and clinicians; as a consequence, the patients are often under-treated (13). Such assessments should, therefore, include a definition of severity (mild, moderate or severe asthma) based on clinical symptoms and objective measurements of lung function. The latter are especially important because fatality-prone asthmatics are frequently poor perceivers of airflow limitation. A detailed evaluation of response to therapy should include a definition of the response to therapy (beneficial, no change, worse) in reference to clinical status as well as appraisal of lung function following a therapeutic trial.

Under-treatment – or more specifically, inappropriate treatment – is reflected in: infrequently-obtained pulmonary function assessment, reliance mainly on high-dosage frequently-administered bronchodilator therapy, and under-utilization of corticosteroid therapy to treat the underlying pathophysiologic mechanisms of fatal asthma, particularly inflammation (6). Other management characteristics contributing to risk factors for death included: discontinuity of medical care, and delays in seeking medical attention. Delays in seeking care were frequently related to the absence of a prepared written plan for treating acute asthma exacerbations as well as inadequate access to emergency medical care (6).

Asthma, as other chronic diseases, may produce psychological reactions. Attention has been focused on the role of depression in asthma morbidity and mortality, particularly in children, which may lead to increased risk of death from asthma. Although the information linking depression and increased death from asthma is derived from clinical reports, the association is striking. In a review of cases in which children died suddenly and unexpectedly of asthma, there is clinical evidence that the children had expressed despair, hopelessness, a wish to die, and other evidence of depression. Psychosocial problems that have been documented as associated with those at increased risk include alcohol abuse, documented depression, recent family loss and disruption, recent unemployment, and schizophrenia.

Patients who have experienced a life-threatening asthma exacerbation have been observed, on the whole, to deny that they are at risk of death. Following a near fatal exacerbation of asthma, they tend to either develop decompensating psychiatric disease and symptoms of extreme anxiety or develop even higher levels of denial. Some patients tend to minimize their symptoms and avoid access to health care.

Regardless of the possible physiologic and psychologic interactions that link anxiety, depression, and asthma fatality, it is evident that patients who have these psychological disruptions are at increased risk for death and require specific professional intervention.

Conclusion

To prevent asthma fatality it is critical to identify and eliminate, as much as possible, the factors contributing to the risk of death. Most asthma deaths are avoidable (12). There are several dimensions to identifying patients at high risk of asthma-related deaths (Tables 1 and 2). The greatest risk to the individual with asthma is complacency or underestimation of the severity of the disease on the part of the patient, the patient's family, and the physician.

This risk can be mitigated by appropriate identification of the high risk patient through careful

Table 1. Risk factors for asthma mortality.

Epidemiologic
– Age 5–34, > 50 years
– Ethnic minorities, e. g., African-Americans, Maoris
– Economically disadvantaged
– Inadequate access to medical care

Physiologic
– Low hypoxic response
– Blunted perception of asthma

Pathologic
– Increased submucosal eosinophilia > slow onset attack
– Increased submucosal neutrophilia > sudden onset attack
– Altered airway:
  – increased smooth muscle
  – mucous gland hypertrophy

Pharmacologic
– Increased use of β_2-agonist a month
– Use of > 1.4 canisters β_2-agonist a month

Clinical
– Hospital admission in past 12 months
– Recent discharge from hospital
– Severe asthma of prolonged duration
– Use of 3 or more categories of asthma drugs
– Persistent abnormal lung functions
– Variations in daily PEFR
– Lack of adherence to therapy
– Delay in seeking medical care
– Absence of written plan for managing attacks
– Inappropriate treatment – either daily therapy or managing attacks
– Psychosocial problems
– Depression
– Denial of asthma severity

Table 2. Clinical parameters of assessment indicating significant respiratory deterioration.

- $FEV_1 < 500\,ml$
- $PEFR < 120\,L/min$
  - $< 120\,L/min$ or 20% predicted
  - reduction of: FVC, FEV_1, or PEFR to half of normal
  - respiratory rate > 30/min
- Minimal or no response to bronchodilators at 1 h
- Moderate to severe dyspnea
- Pulse rate > 120/min
- *Pulsus paradoxus* (inspiratory decline > 18 mmHg)
- Wheezing, or "silent chest"
- Moderate to severe use of accessory muscles
- Paradoxic abdominal or diaphragmatic movement on inspiration

clinical assessment. This includes a careful history of asthma duration and medication use, measurement of symptoms, and objective measurement of lung function. Adequate identification begins the process of prescribing appropriate therapy, teaching skills to adhere to the therapy, and using PEFR to monitor the course of the disease and alert the patient where medical care is urgently required. Written management plans will enhance this process.

Thus, early recognition of factors contributing to risk of asthma-related death will help clinicians to intervene effectively. Careful clinical history continues to be paramount; objective measures are critical; and new insights in airway pathology will help prevent deaths.

Address for correspondence:

Albert L Sheffer, MD
Brigham and Women's Hospital
75 Francis Street
Boston, MA 02115–6195
USA

References

1. Sly RM. Mortality from asthma. *J Allergy Clin Immunol* 1989; 84:421.
2. Sears MR. Worldwide trends in asthma mortality. *Bull Int Union Tuberc Lung Dis* 1992; 66:79.
3. Strunk RC. Identification of the fatality-prone subject with asthma. *J Allergy Clin Immunol* 1989; 53:477.
4. Sears MR. Why are deaths from asthma increasing? *Eur J Respir Dis* 1986; 69:175.
5. Weiss KB, Wagener DK. Changing patterns of asthma mortality. Identifying target populations at high risk. *JAMA* 1990; 264:1683.
6. Rea HH, Scragg R, Jackson R, Beaglehole R, Fenwick J, Sutherland DC. A case-control study of deaths from asthma. *Thorax* 1986; 41:833.
7. Kikuchi Y, Okabe S, Tamura G, Hida W, Homma M, Shirato K, Takishima T. Chemosensitivity and perception of dyspnea in patients with a history of nearfatal asthma. *N Engl J Med* 1994; 330:1329.
8. Wasserfallen J-B, Schaller MD, Feihl F, Perret CH. Sudden asphyxic asthma: A distinct entity? *Am Rev Respir Dis* 1990; 142:108.
9. Pearce N, Crane J, Burgess C, Jackson R, Beasley R. Beta agonists and asthma mortality: *Déjà vu. Clin Exp Allergy* 1991; 21:401.
10. Suissa S, Ernst P, Boivin JF, Horwitz RI, Habbick B, Cockcroft D, Blais L, McNutt M, Buist S, Spitzer WO. A cohort analysis of excess mortality in asthma and the use of inhaled β-agonists. *Am J Respir Crit Care Med* 1994; 149:604.
11. Molfino NA, Nannini LJ, Martelli A, Slutsky AS. Respiratory arrest in near-fatal asthma. *N Engl J Med* 1991; 324:285.
12. Crane J, Pearce N, Burgess C, Woodman K, Robson B, Beasley R. Markers of risk of asthma death or readmission in the 12 months following a hospital admission for asthma. *Int J Epidemiol* 1992; 21:737.
13. Sur S, Crotty TB, Kephart GM, Hyma BA, Colby TV, Reed CE, Hunt LW, Gleich GJ. Sudden-onset fatal asthma: A distinct entity with few eosinophils and relatively more neutrophils in the airway submucosa? *Am Rev Respir Dis* 1993; 148:713.
14. Carroll N, Elliot J, Morton A, James A. The structure of large and small airways in nonfatal and fatal asthma. *Am Rev Respir Dis* 1993; 147:405.

The Role of Respiratory Infections as a Risk Factor in Asthma

William W Busse, James N Gern, Elliot C Dick*

Keywords: Asthma, respiratory infections, viruses

Respiratory infections can alter airway physiology. In patients with asthma, respiratory infections can cause an increase in wheezing, this association usually being seen in children over 2 years of age and in individuals with existing asthma. In infants, viral respiratory infections can cause wheezing. The most common respiratory virus causing this problem is respiratory syncytial virus. Furthermore, there are certain risk factors that make the child more prone to wheeze with respiratory infections. This is the focus of the following paper.

Introduction

Respiratory viruses play an important and varied role in asthma. For example, patients with existing asthma often have exacerbations of wheezing with a viral respiratory infection. These episodes are usually short in duration and resolve with either initiation of asthma therapy or escalation of current medications. However, in some patients, virus-induced episodes of asthma can be very severe and require hospitalization. In addition, children less than 5 years of age often have transient episodes of wheezing with viral respiratory infections. Although many of these children experience recurrent episodes of wheezing with repeat infections, current data suggest that these episodes resolve as the child grows older. Another area of considerable interest, for which there is little factual knowledge, is the possibility that viral respiratory infections may actually be an etiological event or cause asthma. Most commonly, this association is seen in adults who have a nonatopic background and develop asthma following a viral respiratory infection. Although this association has yet to be substantiated, it further underscores the importance of viral respiratory infections to asthma and influence on airway responsiveness.

Risk Factors for Wheezing in the Early Years of Life

Numerous investigators, including Henderson and colleagues at North Carolina (1), have shown that the relationship of viral organisms associated with respiratory infections and wheezing is age-dependent. In children of less than 1 year of age, respiratory syncytial virus (RSV) – and parainfluenza to a lesser degree – are the most important triggers of wheezing. As the child grows older, these particular viral infections appear to be less of a problem as a cause for wheezing. In patients 5 years and older, rhinovirus (RV) respiratory infections become the most common cause of a cold and the cause of increased asthma. In the adult population, RV remains an important factor in triggering asthma, but influenza virus and mycoplasma pneumoniae are also commonly associated with episodes of wheezing. Although other infectious agents are found to play a role in episodes of wheezing, these viral illnesses are the most common.

In children, lower respiratory tract infections are a very common occurrence. In a subpopulation of these patients, wheezing often accompanies these episodes. It has been well documented that RSV infections are the most common cause of these events during the first year of life. Furthermore, there is evidence that wheezing with a viral respiratory infection is often recurrent. This is particularly true during the first 5 years of life. An important area of investigation has been on the role that the initial episode of bronchiolitis with wheezing has as an etiological factor in asthma. Numerous publica-

*   University of Wisconsin Medical School, Madison, WI, USA.

tions in the 1970s and early 1980s suggested that an episode of bronchiolitis with wheezing was a harbinger, or predicator, to recurrent episodes of wheezing and possibly the development of asthma. For example, McConnochie and Roghmann (2) identified and followed patients who had been hospitalized for episode of RSV bronchiolitis. They found these individuals had an increased relative risk for current wheezing, exercise-associated wheezing and wheezing from colds. However, when re-examined at 13 years of age, children who had been hospitalized with RSV bronchiolitis were no more likely to have asthma symptoms than a control population.

This conclusion has been substantiated by others including John Price (3). He found that by 10 years of age, the prevalence of wheezing after acute viral bronchiolitis diminishes to the same as in a control population. Such observations indicate that although wheezing occurs with and following viral bronchiolitis, this does not appear to be a risk factor for the development of asthma.

Other risk factors for wheezing with viral respiratory infections have been identified and evaluated. Wright and colleagues (4) at the University of Arizona noted that children who were the offspring of smoking mothers were more likely to have wheezing than the children of nonsmoking mothers. This was particularly true when the mother smoked more than 20 cigarettes per day. The same investigators from the University of Arizona evaluated the role of lung function as a factor in the development of wheezing with respiratory infections. In an initial study, Martinez and colleagues (5) measured lung function very early in life and prior to the child's first viral respiratory infection. They found that boys were more likely to wheeze with viral respiratory infections than girls. Secondly, boys with smaller lung function were more prone to have wheezing when they developed a viral respiratory infection. This observation raised the possibility that lung function of the host was also a critical factor in determining whether wheezing occurred with a respiratory illness. As the child grew, lung function increased, and presumably this process of maturation diminished the probability for wheezing with infections.

Odds ratios for wheezing during lower respiratory infection were also assessed in light of the patient's parents and their history of respiratory infections as a child. Camilli and colleagues (6) found that if the parent of an offspring had a history of asthma or bronchiolitis, wheezing was more likely

to occur with a viral bronchiolitis during the first three years of life. As the child grew older, this became less of a problem.

Finally, Welliver and co-workers (7) measured the IgE immune response to viruses in children with an episode of bronchiolitis that required hospitalization. In an initial study, Welliver and colleagues (7) found that those children who produced IgE to the virus were more likely to have an obstructive airway component with their illness, i.e., wheeze. Furthermore, the level of IgE antibody produced to the virus was a good indicator as to whether the child would have subsequent episodes of wheezing 4 years post illness (8). When these patients were re-evaluated 10 years later, the IgE response to virus no longer appeared to be a risk factor for the appearance of asthma.

Therefore, host and environmental factors determine the patient's response to a viral respiratory infection and whether wheezing is likely to occur; these include gender, history of maternal smoking, propensity towards production of IgE antibody, and lung size. Furthermore, these risk factors appear to contribute to the outcome of wheezing only during the first decade of life.

Viral Respiratory Infection as a Precipitant of Asthma

Over the last 25 years, multiple prospective studies have shown that respiratory viruses – not bacteria – are important causes of wheezing in patients with existing asthma. The patient population profile in this setting is well illustrated in a recent study by Duff and colleagues (9). This group of investigators collected nasal washes from children who presented to the emergency room with acute wheezing. In children less than 2 years of age, wheezing was most likely to occur in association with an RSV infection. Evidence of allergy was uncommon in these children. When children greater than 2 years of age were seen in the emergency room with wheezing, the profile was quite different: First, RV was the virus most likely to be cultured; furthermore, the child with acute wheezing was more likely to have allergic disease than the less than 2-year-old counterpart. These observations suggest the possibility that viral respiratory infections in the older child act to accentuate existing pulmonary factors, i.e., existing allergic diseases, and that this action accentuation of underlying allergic inflammation promotes the expression of asthma.

The importance of viral respiratory infections as a precipitant for asthma has been rigorously evaluated by Johnston and associates at Southhampton (personal communication). They selected a group of 9–11 children for study. Clinical parameters for acute wheezing were closely monitored, and respiratory secretions were collected to detect viruses. To increase the sensitivity to detect viruses, they used a polymerized chain reaction (PCR) technique to analyze respiratory secretions. Here, RV emerged as the most commonly isolated virus and was found in approximately 80% of children with acute episodes of asthma. Thus, respiratory infections are an extremely common precipitant of wheezing, and RV is the predominant organism associated with this event.

We have further evaluated the relationship that underlying allergic disease assumes in the host's response to a viral respiratory infection. Thirty-one patients were experimentally infected with RV: 13 nonallergic subjects and 18 individuals with existing allergic disease. The frequency of colds was the same in both groups. However, the allergic subjects were more likely to have an increase in airway responsiveness during the cold. This observation raises the possibility that the viral effect on the airway is more likely to be expressed on lung function when the host is allergic. Thus, underlying allergic disease is a risk factor for altered lung function during a cold.

To further indicate the importance of a rhinovirus-allergic interaction, we evaluated the effect of an RV infection on the airway response to inhaled allergen (10). Prior to RV infection, 1 of 10 subjects had a late allergic response to inhaled allergen. At the time of the viral respiratory infection, the frequency of late allergic reactions to inhaled antigen increased to 8 out of 10 subjects. This increased propensity to a late allergic reaction was still noted 4 weeks following the infection. Thus, the allergic constituency of the subject may be a risk factor not only for the development of airway hyperresponsiveness with a cold, but also for the pattern of their airway response to allergen. In those subjects with existing allergic disease, the viral respiratory infection is more likely to promote the development of an inflammatory response, i.e., the late allergic response. This association may explain how existing allergic disease is a risk factor in the subject's response to a viral illness.

Summary

Viral respiratory infections are frequent occurrences for most people and are generally benign. However, in certain individuals, risk factors predispose them to wheezing with these infections. Many of these risk factors appear to be age-related, i.e., lung size, maternal smoking, and an episode of bronchiolitis as an infant. Others, such as underlying allergic disease, become more important as the patient ages. Not only are these risk factors important clinically, they likely hold clues to underlying mechanisms of asthma.

Acknowledgements

Supported by NIH Grants AI26609 and HL44098.

Address for correspondence:

Dr William W Busse
University of Wisconsin Hospital and Clinics
H6/360 CSC
600 Highland Avenue
Madison, WI 53792-3244
USA

References

1. Henderson FW, Clyde WA Jr, Collier AM, et al. The etiologic and epidemiologic spectrum of bronchiolitis in pediatric practice. *J Pediatr* 1979; 95:183.

2. McConnochie KM, Roughmann KJ. Parental smoking, presence of older siblings, and family history of asthma increase risk of bronchiolitis. *Am J Dis Child* 1986; 140:806.

3. Price JF. Acute and long-term effects of viral bronchiolitis in infancy. *Lung* 1990; Suppl:414.

4. Wright AL, Holberg C, Martinez FD, Taussig LM, Group Health Medical Associates. Relationship of parenteral smoking to wheezing and nonwheezing lower respiratory tract illnesses in infancy. *J Pediatr* 1991; 118:207.

5. Martinez FD, Morgan WJ, Wright AL, et al. Diminished lung function as a predisposing factor for wheezing respiratory illness in infants. *N Engl J Med* 1988; 319:1112.

6. Camilli AE, Holberg CJ, Wright AL, Taussig LM, and Group Health Medical Associates. Parenteral childhood respiratory illness and respiratory illness in their infants. *Pediatr Pulmonol* 1993; 16:275.

7. Welliver RC, Wong DT, Sun M, Middleton E Jr, Vaughan RS, Ogra PL. The development of respiratory syncytial virus-specific IgE and the release of histamine in nasopharyngeal secretions after infection. *N Engl J Med* 1981; 305:841.

8. Welliver RC, Sun M, Rijnaldo D, Ogra PL. Predictive value of respiratory syncytial virus-specific IgE responses for recurrent wheezing following bronchiolitis. *J Pediatr* 1986; 109:776.

9. Duff AL, Pomeranz ES, Gelber LE, Price GW, Farris H, Hayden FG, Platts- Mills TAE, Heymann PW. Risk factors for acute wheezing in infants and children: Viruses, passive smoke, and IgE antibodies to inhalant allergens. *Pediatrics* 1993; 92:535.

10. Lemanske RF Jr, Dick EC, Swenson CA, Vrtis RF, Busse WW. Rhinovirus upper respiratory infection increases airway hyperreactivity and late asthmatic reactions. *J Clin Invest* 1989, 83:1.

High Risk Asthmatics: Psychological Aspects

Rainer Richter*, Bernhard Dahme**

Keywords: Bronchial asthma, psychology, psychosomatic medicine, perception, dyspnea, anxiety, depression, high-risk, psychophysiology, personality, emotion

The treatment of bronchial asthma is usually guided by patients' perceptions of their symptoms. If patients cannot accurately judge their symptoms' severity, however, they may not be adequately treated. A review of the literature indicates that psychological factors have an effect on asthmatic symptoms and have a measurable influence on respiratory function in some asthmatics. Of asthmatic patients treated in general practice, more than half discriminate poorly between high and low peak flow values. If patients cannot accurately judge the severity of their symptoms, they are at risk for not being treated adequately. Poor discrimination was not linked to sex, age, or particular practices, but correlated with depression and anxiety. This has been demonstrated in clinical and experimental studies. High-risk patients with severe asthma show higher scores for depression and anxiety. We conclude from these findings that the consideration of psychological factors should be added to the medical management of asthma, and that the management of asthma should be based on objective lung function measurements as well as self-assessment of symptoms.

It is a well known fact, which has been shown repeatedly by both clinical evidence and empirical psychophysiological research, that physical stimuli – specific allergens, pollution, cold air – as well as psychological stimuli – repressed anger, madness, and specific conflicts – can provoke or maintain bronchial asthma. These stimuli can trigger asthmatic difficulties, but do not cause the asthmatic disease itself. The focus of this paper is on psychological factors which interact with other factors in provoking acute asthmatic attacks. It has been demonstrated in a number of experimental studies that changes in airway resistance in response to emotional stress can be reliably produced among asthmatics [1]. Recently, Isenberg et al. [2] again reviewed the literature on the relation between asthma, suggestion, and emotion, and proposed that these effects are mediated parasympathetically.

As an example of these relations, we will first present the data from a one year study of asthmatic patients in the emergency rooms of hospitals in Hamburg [3]. Within 48 hours after admission to emergency care, these patients were interviewed by a psychosomatic consultant, who weighted the different factors which preceded their asthmatic attack. As can be seen from Table 1, psychological factors were relevant in 60–70% of the asthmatic attacks.

Table 1. Precursors of an asthma attack (N = 30).

	Psychosomatic consultant	Physician	Weighted mean[1]
Respiratory viral infections	80%	87%	76.9%[2]
Specific antigens	47%	60%	46.7%[3]
Emotional stressors	67%	60%	60.3%[4]
Nonantigenic irritants (smoke, cold air, exercise, etc.)	47%	47%	62.3%[5]
Analgesics	7%	3%	10%[6]

[1]Maxwell (1936), McDermott and Cobb (1939), Rees (1956), Williams et al. (1958), Wright (1965), Kleeman (1967), Pearson (1968), Linser and Kleinsorge (1969), Teiramaa (1977), Stevenson et al. (1975). [2]N = 1339; [3]N = 1489; [4]N = 2249; [5]N = 177; [6]N = 34.

* Department of Child and Adolescent Psychiatry, Universitätskrankenhaus Hamburg-Eppendorf, Hamburg, Germany.
** Institute of Psychology, University of Hamburg, Germany.

It can also be seen that we found the well known factors such as allergens, cold air, and infections as well. Further, the data show that somatic and psychological stimuli occurred simultaneously in a number of cases. The weighted means of a number of studies asking the same question are also shown, and yield quite similar results.

Of course, the relative weighting of psychological and somatic factors in retrospective designs is difficult. These data, however, show the relevance of psychological factors in provoking asthmatic complaints, which in turn is the main reason for considering bronchial asthma as a classical psychosomatic disease. The following short case history illustrates this psychosomatic relationship:

On the day of the asthma attack, the 24 year old patient had a date with a former girlfriend. They had separated the previous year and met only sporadically. He felt that the relationship was over for him, but feared that his former girlfriend might still be in love with him. They had a date, he flirted with her, and they made love.

He had a bad conscience as they were sitting next to each other on the couch, and he realized that she was in love with him. He did not want to have anything to do with her feelings.

The situation preceding the attack: His girlfriend approached him, and he got the impression that she would start flirting again. He started to feel smothered and a need to defend himself. He asked her for an aspirin, because he had had a mild cold for two days. Shortly after taking the tablet he became acutely breathless and withdrew to another room. He did not feel comfortable being in the same room with her. Shortly afterwards he had to be admitted to the emergency room of a hospital.

Conclusion regarding the psychological factors: The patient put himself into a situation in which he felt smothered by the closeness of his former girl friend. He sent her away to bring him the tablet, which prevented the closeness for a short time. The asthma attack was elicited by aspirin intolerance, which he knew about, but forgot under these circumstances. This could be interpreted as a Freudian slip or some sort of self-destructive behavior, which is why we rated this attack as being linked to an analgesic and to an emotional factor. It is very interesting to look at how the young woman reacted to the withdrawal of the patient, because she apparently understood his non-verbal message: She accused him of being allergic to her. When he was interviewed about similar situations in his past he reported the very first asthmatic difficulties. He

was engaged without being sure of his feelings. When the family of his fiancee pushed for the marriage, he got a cold, took aspirin, and developed asthmatic difficulties for the first time.

There is one question which was raised in the early days of psychosomatic research: Is there a specific high risk personality structure in asthmatic patients? This question was followed by a great number of publications which tried to describe the specific personality profile of the asthmatic patient. A critical review (1) of all these studies shows that this specific personality profile does not exist. In some studies, however, small but significant differences between asthmatic patients and healthy people have been shown. This plausible criticism, mainly made by pneumologists, did not consider that these differences in personality could be the consequences of the long persisting, life threatening chronic disease. This means that group differences could reflect more or less successful coping with anxiety and dyspnea related to asthma. Indeed, positive correlations between the duration of illness and introversion and neuroticism have been reported (4).

Following these rather disappointing results, specific symptoms and complaints of asthma have become more interesting in the last ten years, especially the leading asthmatic symptom: dyspnea.

The acute asthmatic attack is characterized by airway obstruction. The asthmatic patient suffers, however, from breathlessness, tightness, and shortness of breath. Consistently dyspnea is defined by Comroe (5) as: "Difficult, labored, uncomfortable breathing, though it is not painful in the usual sense of the word. It is subjective and, like pain, it involves both perception of the sensation by the patient and his reaction to the sensation." In contrast to pain, the physiological components of dyspnea, namely the increase in airway resistance, can be measured directly and related to the subjective experience.

By investigating this relationship in a controlled experimental design, we found that the correlation between the physiological obstruction, as measured by airway resistance, and the degree of breathlessness is relatively weak. In the course of a diagnostic inhalation provocation test, we asked asthmatic patients to rate their current dyspnea. We could thus evaluate the clinical finding that some patients can estimate their bronchial airway resistance quite well, whereas others are rather poor raters. Some of them overestimate, while others underestimate their obstructions. Our data fit well to those of other research groups, who found, for example (6), that about 15% of patients undergoing an acute asthma attack induced by methacholine were unable to sense the presence of considerable airflow obstruction.

The question is now: Are these patients who can estimate their airway resistance well different from those who have a poor interoception, as this ability to perceive inner bodily functions is called?

Before answering this question we must return to the subjective symptoms which are related to dyspnea. What do patients mean when they report these unpleasant feelings, when they report "feeling breathless"? This question was investigated first by the research group of Kinsman at Denver University (7), who developed an asthma symptom checklist. We replicated these studies among German speakers: A factor analysis of a total of 77 typical subjective complaints, disturbances, subjective feelings, and bodily symptoms, reported by more than 300 asthmatic patients, yielded five dimensions of asthmatic breathlessness. The first dimension can be called nervous anxiety; in the American symptom checklist it is called panic-fear: We found that 83% of the patients reported anxious and nervous feelings during their asthmatic difficulties. Nearly 90% of the patients reported obstructive symptoms in a narrower sense. The third factor, which is well known to clinicians, is called anger/irritability: patients describe themselves as cross and/or impatient. The fourth factor describes the well known symptoms of hyperventilation: about 10% of all patients hyperventilated during their asthmatic attacks, which is in accordance with clinical knowledge. The last factor is "tiredness." Patients described themselves as tired, exhausted, and/or sluggish.

A comparison of asthmatic dyspnea with the dyspnea of patients suffering from chronic bronchitis revealed them to have quite different factorial structures (8). in this case, an independent panic-fear dimension was missing. One can therefore assume that this factorial structure of five dimensions is specific for asthmatic obstructive dyspnea.

Now we come back to the question of which patients have good and which patients have poor interoception of obstructive changes. To answer this question, we developed an experimental method where patients have to breath through different mesh resistors which are placed into the airflow for two breathing cycles.

The patient then has to decide whether he or she noticed a change in flow resistance and, if so, how strong the resistance was. We found that patients who have high anxiety scores on the symptom checklist felt a higher degree of dyspnea at the same added resistive load as patients with less anxiety. This difference between anxious and nonanxious patients is only significant for lower resistive loads. For higher resistances, anxiety obviously does not play such an important role as an intervening variable. Another important finding was that this correlation was obvious only for the perception of changes in bronchial airway resistance, not for the perception of external added resistive loads. Thus, the experimental technique of using external resisitive added loads which has been used for a long time in physiological research seems to be invalid for clinical research.

Patients who are nervous and anxious during their asthmatic difficulties overestimate the degree of their airway obstruction. This finding has been replicated in a number of perceptual experiments by other research groups and by our team as well. It must be emphasized that "anxious" or "nervous" does not mean a long lasting trait anxiety, but rather a short lasting, situational state anxiety, which is correlated with interoception. Of course, this does not mean there is a causal relationship: Some patients possibly estimate the degree of airway obstruction higher because their perception of very mild symptoms is influenced by marked anxiety. Other patients pay attention to their respiration with vigilance and anxiety, because they overestimate the real degree of the threatening airway obstruction. In any case, these patients are at risk: They call the ambulance more often and have to be treated more often in an emergency room than less anxious patients.

Our findings seem to support the results of Kinsman and his group, who showed a distinct relationship between psychological variables of symptom perception and coping strategies on the one hand, and clinical and somatic variables on the other hand. They proposed the concept of psychomaintainance of bronchial asthma (9). They were able to demonstrate, for example, that anxious patients take their medication much too often, and use their bronchodilator spray even when pulmonary functions are normal. On the other hand, there are patients who stay calm or even indifferent during their asthmatic difficulties, and who use their medication too rarely, even when pulmonary functions are impaired. Other results show that highly anxious patients, independently of their lung functions, are treated more often with steroids. As a consequence, it has been proposed by a Swedish group (10) that psychological status indicators should be included in respiratory symptom questionnaires.

The results concerning the correlation between psychological factors and somatic variables are not uniform, however. Kinsmans's findings have not be replicated in their entirety. This is perhaps due to a characteristic of most empirical studies: the asthmatic patient is usually looked on as an isolated research object, and not as a partner in an interpersonal relationship. The characteristics of the relationship between the asthmatic patient and persons close to him – partners, relatives, doctors, therapists – has not been the topic of empirical research in the past. However, when we look at the large number of clinical case studies which have been published in the psychosomatic literature in the last 100 years, we can see a rather specific conflict in which the asthmatic patient is involved. This specific conflict could be described as an ambivalence between simultaneous wishes for independence and dependency. The short case study in this paper provides a fairly good example of this conflict: The patient's wishes for closeness and his fear of becoming dependent were in conflict, which he was not able to resolve on a interactional, i. e., psychological, level. The asthmatic attack, however, helped him to get out of this entanglement. This ambivalence conflict between closeness and distance is very well known to the doctor on night duty, when he is called around four o'clock in the morning to a wheezing and suffering asthmatic patient, and is criticized aggressively by the patient for coming so late and for prescribing the wrong medication. From a scientific viewpoint one could have doubts about the validity of casuistic findings. Empirical social science, however, can be accused of leaving out these components of the two-person relationship and of not having specific and suitable psychological methods to describe and analyze the relationships between the doctor and his patient scientifically.

There are some empirical hints that this scientific approach could be fruitful, especially for bronchial asthma. Asthmatic children, for example, show a distinct improvement immediately after hospitalization. For a long time, allergists, as well as psychotherapists, used this well-known clinical experience to support their own hypotheses: Specific allergens are absent in the hospital, or, the symptom-stimulating influence of parents and siblings is absent in the hospital. Systematic studies support the psychosomatic hypotheses: Hospitalized asthmatic children with a proven house mite

allergy improved immediately when the parents and siblings were removed from the household and replaced by a nurse. All those children for whom the authors predicted an improvement after the so-called parentectomy indeed remained free of symptoms during the separation from their parents. The importance of the interpersonal relationship can be shown even in psychophysiological experiments: It is known that asthmatic patients do not generally react to psychological stressors with an increase of their airway resistance (11). They only react with a mild but significant bronchoconstriction when they are confronted with unconscious personal conflicts. The relevant themes are illustrated by the following typical situation: The asthmatic patient first feels aggressive towards a close relative or friend, against whom he means to defend himself. The desire to distance himself and the simultaneous inability to show adequate aggressive behavior is in conflict with the desire to be protected and sheltered. Only in situations when these conflicts are touched on does the asthmatic patient show the physiological response. Of course, these findings do not answer the question of whether these specific interpersonal conflicts are the cause or the consequence of a chronic disease. There is important empirical evidence that some of these psychological characteristics are the consequence, not the cause of the chronic disease.

Evaluating the role of psychological factors may be critically important in some asthmatic patients. In some studies (13), patients who saw themselves as having severe asthma and in great danger of dying had more depressive symptoms than others. Depression can seriously hamper asthma management and may be a factor in untimely death. Patients have to develop their own practical knowledge about symptoms and should be able to recognize severe episodes. This practical knowledge is similar to that of expert clinicians, although it is based on different sources of information (e. g., body sensations and associated sequelae).

This is the reason why educational programs, psychological intervention, and physical exercises have been developed and evaluated in a number of countries. The information given in these "Asthma schools", as they were developed in Sweden (12) as well as in other European countries, includes elementary anatomy and physiology, and how to prevent asthma attacks. Self-treatment is taught in the form of breathing control, relaxation, physical exercise, inhalation techniques, and early drug treatment. Another aim of the school is to give the patients the opportunity to meet other people who are suffering from the same disease. They often have a great need to discuss problems relating to the disease, and can often help each other (sometimes with the assistance of a teacher or psychotherapist) to solve problems, and to manage the asthma in a better way. This requires both the continuous objective measurement of lung functions, and the use of self-assessment diaries to evaluate symptoms and treatment.

Acknowledgment

This study was supported by the Deutsche Forschungsgemeinschaft (Ri 448–2).

Address for correspondence:

Prof Dr Rainer Richter
Universitätskrankenhaus Eppendorf
Pavillon 67
D-20246 Hamburg
Germany

References

1. Schüffel W, Herrmann JM, Dahme B, Richter R. Asthma bronchiale. In Uexküll T (Ed) *Lehrbuch der Psychosomatischen Medizin,* 4th Ed. Munich: Urban & Schwarzenberg, 1990, pp. 745–760.

2. Isenberg SA, Lehrer PM, Hochron S. The effects of suggestion and emotional arousal on pulmonary function in asthma: A review and a hypothesis regarding vagal mediation. *Psychosom Med* 1992; 192–216.

3. Oppermann M, Leplow B, Dahme B, Richter R. Identifikation von Auslösebedingungen für einen unmittelbar zurückliegenden schweren Asthmaanfall. *Prax Psychother Psychosom* 1991; 148–159.

4. Meyer AE, Weitemeyer W. Zur Frage krankheitsdependenter Neurotisierung. Psychometrisch-varianzanalytische Untersuchungen an Männern mit Asthma bronchiale, Lungentuberkulose oder mit Herzvitien. *Arch Psychiatr Z Ges Neurol* 1967; 21–29.

5. Comroe I. Some theories on the mechanism of dyspnea. In Howell JB, Campbell E: *Breathlessness.* Oxford: Blackwell Scientific Publication, 1966.

6. Rubinfeld AR, Pain MCF. Perception of asthma. *Lancet* 1976; 882–884.

7. Kinsman, RA, Luparello TJ, O'Banion K et al. Multidimensional analysis of subjective symptomatology of asthma. *Psychosom Med* 1977; 102–119.

8. Dahme B, König R, Nußbaum B, Richter R. Haben Asthmatiker Defizite in der Symptomwahrnehmung? Quasi-experimentelle und experimentelle Befunde zur Interozeption der Atemwegsobstruktion. *Psychother Psychosom Med Psychol* 1991; 41:490–499.

9. Kinsman RA, Dirks JF, Schraa JC. Psychomaintenance in asthma. Personal styles affecting medical management. *Respir Ther* 1981; 39–46.

10. Janson C., Bjoernsson E, Hetta I, Boman G. Anxiety and depression in relation to respiratory symptoms and asthma. *Amer J Respir Crit Med* 149, 1994; 930–934.

11. Richter R. Auslösung und Unterhaltung des Asthma durch psychologische Faktoren. In Schultze-Werninghaus G, Debelic M (Eds) *Asthma.* Berlin: Springer, 1988, pp. 190–201.

12. Ringsberg KC, Wiklund L, Wilhelmsen L. Education of adult patients at an "asthma school": effects on quality of life, knowledge and need for nursing. *Eur Resp J* 1990; 33–37.

13.. Janson-Bjerklie S, Ferketich S, Benner P, Becker G. Clinical markers of asthma severity and risk: importance of subjective as well as objective factors. *Heart Lung* 1992; 265–272.

Management Strategies for the "High-Risk" Asthmatic

Jon Miles, Wendyl D'Souza, Carl Burgess, Richard Beasley*

Keywords: Asthma management, high-risk patients

"High-risk" asthmatic patients represent a small but important group that requires special medical attention if a significant impact is to be made on morbidity and mortality from asthma. This review briefly outlines a management strategy whereby high-risk asthmatic patients are identified and provided with a simple system of self-assessment and treatment.

Identification of the "High-Risk" Asthmatic

The first priority is to develop a clinical profile of the asthmatic patient who is at an increased risk of a severe attack, leading to either a hospital admission or a fatal outcome. Particularly useful markers of risk include a history of a previous life-threatening attack, a recent hospital admission or emergency room visit for asthma, psychosocial problems

and discontinuity of general practice care (1, 2) (Table 1). These risk factors can be considered to fall broadly into two categories: the former reflecting the presence of severe disease, and the latter those that may lead to problems associated with the utilisation of medical care.

Probably the best way to recognise those patients at greater risk is to identify those who have had a recent hospital admission. Amongst these patients, the marker particularly associated with an increased risk of death is a previous life-threatening attack (i. e., a previous ICU admission for asthma).

Recognition of Clinical Circumstances Associated with Fatal Asthma

The next priority is to recognise the factors associated with a life-threatening attack of asthma. Investigations of the clinical circumstances of death from asthma have consistently identified several factors relating to either the long-term management or the treatment of the acute attack (3–6) (Table 2). Problems associated with long-term management include a lack of appreciation by both the patient and/or the doctor of the patient's chronic asthma severity, the inadequate long-term use of inhaled corticosteroids, and discontinuity of general practice care with the failure to attend a general practitioner between attacks.

Similar problems have been identified with the treatment of severe asthma attacks, in particular the inability of the patient, family, or doctor to recognise the severity of the fatal attack, and overreliance on inhaled bronchodilator treatment without addi-

Table 1. Identification of the high risk asthmatic: Factors associated with an increased risk of death*.

	Relative risk of death
A. Patients with asthma	
Hospital admission in last year	16.0
One or more emergency room visits in last year	8.5
Three or more asthma medications prescribed	3.0
B. Patients with severe asthma**	
Previous life-threatening attack	3.8
Psychosocial problems	3.5

* Derived from Rea et al. (1)
** Patients with a recent hospital admission for asthma

---

*   Department of Medicine, Wellington School of Medicine, Wellington South, New Zealand.

Table 2. Clinical circumstances associated with death from asthma.

A. Long term:
   – Lack of appreciation of chronic asthma severity and risk of death
   – Poor compliance with management
   – Discontinuity of medical care
   – Underutilisation of inhaled corticosteroids

B. Fatal attack:
   – Delay in seeking medical help
   – Inability to recognise the severity of the attack
   – Over-reliance on bronchodilator therapy
   – Insufficient systemic steroid use
   – Lack of written guidelines for management

Table 3. The basic principles of self-management for the high risk asthmatic.

1. Requirement for the objective assessment of asthma severity with the educated interpretation of key symptoms and peak flow recordings.
2. The use of regular inhaled corticosteroids and intermittent beta agonists for the long term treatment of asthma; the use of systemic corticosteroids, high dose inhaled beta agonists, oxygen therapy and medical review for severe asthma.
3. The integration of self-assessment and self-management with written guidelines for both the long-term treatment of asthma and the treatment of acute severe asthma.

tional therapy. These factors have been considered to be particularly important in leading to delay in seeking medical help despite the development of a life-threatening asthma attack.

Post-mortem studies have illustrated the importance of the inflammatory process in fatal asthma, with extensive mucous plugging causing widespread occlusion of airways (7, 8). These pathological observations may explain the unresponsiveness of patients to the self-administration of high doses of inhaled beta agonist therapy in life-threatening asthma and reinforce the importance of also administering systemic corticosteroids in this clinical situation.

Management Strategies

By considering these circumstances associated with fatal asthma, it is now possible to devise management strategies that can potentially overcome many of the problems encountered. If one accepts that the most important factor contributing to a fatal outcome is the inability of the patient to recognise worsening asthma and make the appropriate therapeutic response, the logical management strategy would be to develop a system of self-assessment and self-management for the patient to follow, in accordance with predetermined written guidelines. Support for this approach is also strengthened with the knowledge that the majority of asthma attacks occur in the community and are self-managed by patients without immediate consultation with their general practitioner. Thus, if an

impact is to be made on morbidity and mortality from asthma, a pre-arranged system of assessment and management needs to be established for high-risk patients. The basic principles of such a system of self-management are outlined in Table 3.

Fundamental to the success of the strategy of asthma self-management is the ability of the patient to recognise changes in asthma control. This requires the objective assessment of asthma severity through the educated interpretation of key symptoms and measurements of lung function. The development of nocturnal wakening is recognised to be a good marker of unstable asthma, whereas the poor response to the increased use of inhaled β agonist therapy is an important marker of a severe attack requiring medical treatment (9, 10). Domiciliary measurements of peak expiratory flow, with values expressed as a percentage of normal predicted or previous best achieved recordings, are crucial if the patient is to successfully recognise the degree of airflow obstruction. Peak flow monitoring should form the framework of any system of self-assessment, being of particular importance in the severe asthmatic, as they have been shown to have the worst perception of asthma severity (11, 12).

The requirement for regular inhaled corticosteroids and the use of inhaled β agonist drugs as required for relief of symptoms is recognised as the basis of long-term treatment of the high-risk asthmatic (9, 13). Similarly, the administration of oxygen, high-dose inhaled β agonists and systemic corticosteroids, together with medical review are accepted as the essential features of the treatment of the high-risk asthmatic experiencing a severe attack (9, 13).

Asthma Self-Management Plans

A number of systems of asthma self-management have been developed (9, 13–19), based on the basic principles outlined above, but varying with respect to the amount of detail they provide, the specific drug treatment recommended at each stage, and the level of decrease in peak flow or severity of symptoms chosen for the different therapeutic responses recommended. One such self-management plan integrating many of the features of the different self-management systems developed for use by high-risk asthmatics is outlined in Table 4.

In many respects the first two stages can be considered to provide guidelines for the long-term management of asthma. In particular, the instructions to vary the dose of inhaled corticosteroid treatment in a stepwise manner in accordance with changes in asthma severity represents one practical method whereby the recommendations for the long-term treatment of chronic persistent asthma in adults can be implemented (9, 13). The third and fourth stages provide guidelines for the treatment of severe asthma, with intensive treatment started by the patient in an attempt to prevent the development of a life-threatening attack. Thus, self-management plans represent one way in which the recommendations for acute severe and chronic persistent asthma can be brought together within the framework of one system.

As the requirements of individual asthmatic patients may vary considerably, no single plan is likely to be suitable for every patient. Thus, features such as the precise level (or range of levels) of peak flow (whether pre- or postbronchodilator) at which patients are advised to modify therapy or seek medical assistance, have not been clearly established. A flexible approach is required – for example, patients who have recurrent precipitous attacks, occurring against a background of apparently stable asthma, may require modification of their plan so that each stage is set at a higher level, particularly for self-referral to hospital. Some additional resources such as the availability of oxygen in the patient's home, and a nebuliser to administer high doses of β agonist may also be recommended. The provision of a syringe preloaded with adrenaline for subcutaneous injection may need to be considered. However, it should be emphasised that these therapeutic measures are to be undertaken while medical attention is urgently being sought and are not a substitute for medical assessment. All patients with previous life-threatening asthma should have direct access to an acute medical ward at their local hospital, even if this requires prior arrangement with the Ambulance Service. The existence of such facilities has not only been shown to reduce the number of fatal asthma attacks, but it also provides a degree of continuity of care for the patient (20, 21).

Other Considerations

It is beyond the scope of this review to discuss in detail the numerous other issues that need to be considered as part of the management strategy for the poorly controlled asthmatic. Some of these issues are documented in Table 5. While the relative contribution of some of these factors to high-risk asthma are uncertain and may vary in importance

Table 4. Self-management plan for the high risk asthmatic: What to do and when.

Step	Peak Flow	Symptoms	Action
1	80–100% best	Intermittent/few	Continue regular inhaled corticosteroid; inhaled beta agonist for relief of symptoms; +/– oral theophylline
2	60–80% best	Waking at night with asthma or coughing	Increase the dose of inhaled cortico-steroid
3	40–60% best	Increasing breathlessness or poor response to bronchodilator	Start oral corticosteroids and contact a doctor
4	<40% best	Severe attack	Self-administer high dose inhaled beta agonist, continuous oxygen therapy; call emergency doctor or ambulance urgently

The peak flow values recommended for each stage can be altered in accordance with physician preference and the asthmatic patient's individual needs. At all stages, take inhaled bronchodilator for relief of symptoms.

Table 5. Other considerations in the high risk asthmatic.

– Allergen avoidance
– Allergic bronchopulmonary aspergillosis
– Aspirin (NSAID) sensitivity
– Compliance
– Diet – preservatives
– Gastro-oesophageal reflux
– Inhaler delivery systems
– Psychological factors
– Sinusitis/rhinitis
– Smoking

between individuals, they should be considered in the overall management.

The importance of allergen exposure in the dynamics of severe asthma deserves special recognition. Patients with severe brittle asthma possess a greater degree of atopy when measured by either skin-prick test or allergen-specific IgE (22). Environmental allergen exposure may result in increasing disease severity (23), and exposure to allergens has been identified as a predisposing factor for acute asthma attacks with respiratory arrest (24). As a result, it is mandatory to quantify atopic status in high-risk patients with a view to exploring the feasibility of implementing allergen avoidance strategies.

Address for correspondence:

Prof Richard Beasley
Department of Medicine
Wellington School of Medicine
PO Box 7343
Wellington South
New Zealand

References

1. Rea HH, Scragg R, Jackson R, Beaglehole R, Fenwick J, Sutherland DC. A case control study of deaths from asthma. *Thorax* 1986; 41:833–9.

2. Crane J, Pearce NE, Burgess C, Woodman K, Robson B, Beasley R. Markers of risk of asthma death or readmission in the 12 months following a hospital admission for asthma. *Int J Epidemiol* 1992; 21:737–44.

3. Macdonald JB, Seaton A, Williams DA. Asthma deaths in Cardiff 1963–74: 90 deaths outside hospital. *Br Med J* 1976; iii:1493–1495.

4. British Thoracic Association. Death from asthma in two regions of England. *Br Med J* 1982; 285:1251–1255.

5. Rea HH, Sears MR, Beaglehole R et al. Lessons from the national asthma mortality study: circumstances surrounding death. *NZ Med J* 1987; 100:10–13.

6. Sears MR, Rea HH. Patients at risk for dying of asthma: New Zealand experience. *J Allergy Clin Immunol* 1987; 80:477–81.

7. Huber HL, Koessler KK. The pathology of bronchial asthma. *Arch Int Med* 1922; 30:689–760.

8. Houston JC, de Navasquez S, Trounce JR. A clinical and pathological study of fatal cases of status asthmaticus. *Thorax* 1953; 8:207–13.

9. Lenfant C. *International Consensus Report on Diagnosis and Management of Asthma.* National Heart, Lung and Blood Institute, National Institute of Health. US Department of Health and Human Services, Bethesda, USA 1992.

10. Windom HH, Burgess CD, Crane J, Pearce N, Kwong T, Beasley R. The self-administration of inhaled β agonist drugs during severe asthma. *NZ Med J* 1990; 103:205–207.

11. Rubinfield AR, Pain MCF. Perception of asthma. *Lancet* 1975; 2:822–824.

12. Burdon JGW, Juniper EF, Killian KJ, Hargreave FE, Campbell EJM. The perception of breathlessness in asthma. *Am Rev Respir Dis* 1982; 126:825–828.

13. British Thoracic Society, Research Unit of the Royal College of Physicians, Kings Fund Centre, National Asthma Campaign, The Royal College of General Practitioners, the General Practitioners in Asthma Group, the British Association of Accident and Emergency Medicine, and the British Paediatric Respiratory Group. Guidelines on the management of asthma in adults. *Thorax* 1993; (Suppl):S1–S24.

14. Beasley R, Cushley M, Holgate ST. A self-management plan in the treatment of adult asthma. *Thorax* 1989; 44:200–204.

15. Charlton I, Charlton G, Broomfield J, Mullee MA. Evaluation of peak flow and symptoms only self-management plans for control of asthma in general practice. *Br Med J* 1990; 301:1355–1359.

16. D'Souza W, Crane J, Burgess C et al. Community-based asthma care: trial of a 'credit card' asthma self-management plan in a New Zealand Maori community. *Eur Resp J* 1994 (in press).

17. Muhlhauser I, Richter B, Kraut D, Weske G, Worth H, Berger M. Evaluation of a structured treatment and teaching programme on asthma. *J Int Med* 1991; 230:157–164.

18. Mayo PH, Richman J, Harris W. Results of a program to reduce admissions for adult asthma. *Ann Int Med* 1990; 112:864–871.

19. Ruffin RE, Latimer K, Schembri DA. Longitudinal study of near fatal asthma. *Chest* 1991; 99:77–83.

20. Crompton GK, Grant IWB. Edinburgh emergency asthma admission service. *Br Med J* 1975; 4:680–682.

21. Barriot P, Riou B. Prevention of fatal asthma. *Chest* 1987; 92:460–6.

22. Miles JF, Cayton RM, Ayres JG. Atopic status in patients with brittle and non-brittle asthma: A case-control study. *Am Rev Respir Dis* 1994; 149:A245.

23. Pollart SM, Chapman MD, Fiocco GP et al. Epidemiology of acute asthma: IgE antibodies to common inhalant allergens as a risk factor for emergency room visits. *J Allergy Clin Immunol* 1989; 83:875–82.

24. O'Hollaren MT, Yunginger JW, Offord KP et al. Exposure to aeroallergen as a possible precipitating factor in respiratory arrest in young patients with asthma. *N Engl J Med* 1991; 324:359–63.

Steroid-Resistant Asthma

P Chanez, A Des Roches, FB Michel, P Godard, J Bousquet*

Keywords: Asthma, steroid resistance

Although severe asthmatics only represent a small group of patients, they are at high risk. The responsiveness to glucocorticosteroids (GS) is highly variable in severe asthmatics. In most patients with an acute exacerbation, the airways obstruction can be reversed by high doses of GS. However, a large heterogeneity exists in patients with persistent asthma. Among GS-dependent asthmatics, some need oral GS to maintain control of their disease but have normal pulmonary functions, whereas others cannot improve their FEV_1 over 70% despite oral GS. GS-resistant asthmatics are also heterogeneous, and no firm definition has been accepted. A better clinical characterization of severe asthma is needed before biological studies are carried out. Several defects have been proposed or identified for explaining GS-dependent asthma. They include accelerated plasma cortisol clearance, variable pharmacokinetics of GS molecules, monocyte or T-cell defects, and GS receptor abnormalities.

Introduction

Asthma is a common disease throughout the world, but patients with severe asthma only represent a small group that should be identified since they are at high risk of developing life-threatening exacerbations. This group of patients appears to be highly heterogeneous in terms of clinical and biological characteristics as well as in terms of their responsiveness to glucocorticosteroids (GS). GS are the most potent drugs used in the treatment of asthma, and the only drugs that have been shown unequivocally to reduce bronchial inflammation. Although use of the inhaled route is favored, in some case the asthma can still not be controlled using high doses of inhaled GS, and requires treatment with oral or parenteral GS (1).

Long term administration of oral GS is likely to induce side effects, thus: (1) the mechanisms of GS resistance or GS dependence must be better understood; (2) the minimal dose required to control asthma must be determined, and this dose needs to be adapted to the variability of asthma; and (3) the use of alternative anti-inflammatory treatments is also of great importance.

Clinical Characteristics of Steroid-Resistant Asthma

Resistance to High Dose GS in Patients with Unstable or Acute Asthma

In acute asthma, parenteral or oral GS have been used successfully, but the dose of GS and the duration of the treatment are not perfectly characterized. Some studies have examined the dose-response curve of GS (2–5) but more studies are needed to fully characterize the dose and duration of GS needed. The data available indicate that 10–15 mg/kg of hydrocortisone or its equivalent is effective therapy in acutely ill asthmatic adults (6), but the percentage of patients who show an improvement is unknown. In a study of 45 unstable asthmatics with FEV_1 under 70% of predicted values, Chanez et al. (unpublished data) found that 95% of them showed a reversibility of the FEV_1 of over 15% after 10 days of methylprednisolone IV (120 mg daily). The two patients who failed to respond to this dose had the most severe asthma (Aas score 5). All patients with an Aas score of 1–3 had normal pulmonary function after treatment (FEV_1 80% of predicted values). This study shows that very few unstable asthmatics fail to respond to a high dose of GS administered for a sufficient time.

* Clinique des Maladies Respiratoires, Hopital Arnaud de Villeneuve, Montpellier, France.

Characteristics of GS-Dependent Asthmatics

Although the use of high dose inhaled steroids and long-acting β_2-agonists has significantly reduced the number of patients requiring oral steroids (GS-dependent asthmatics), a relatively small group of patients requiring continuous administration of oral GS to control their asthma still exists. Such patients appear to be heterogeneous in terms of their GS needs and the variability of the airflow obstruction (7). These patients can be assigned to several broad groups (Chanez et al., unpublished data):

- Patients with a normal or subnormal pulmonary function requiring high doses of inhaled GS (2 mg or equivalent BDP daily) and small doses of oral GS (5–20 mg daily) to prevent acute exacerbations or asthma instability,
- Patients with abnormal pulmonary function (FEV$_1$ under 65% of predicted values) who require high doses of inhaled GS and who need variable doses of oral GS to improve FEV$_1$,
- Patients with an abnormal pulmonary function (FEV$_1$ under 65% of predicted values) who require high doses of inhaled GS and who usually need high doses of oral GS to prevent acute exacerbations or asthma instability, but in whom oral GS do not improve significantly basal FEV$_1$.

GS-dependent asthmatics who receive an optimal oral GS regimen should be followed for a period of several months to a year to evaluate the baseline pulmonary function and PEFR variability (8). Three different patterns of peak flow diurnal variability can be observed:

- A few patients have a PEFR variability under 10% throughout the year.
- Most patients present wide variations in PEFR variability, ranging from 5% to over 50%.
- A few other patients always present a PEFR variability of over 15%.

GS-dependent asthmatics represent a high risk group for severe exacerbations and the occurrence of iatrogenic disease.

The reasons for the prolonged need for oral GS in patients receiving high doses of inhaled GS and long-acting β_2-agonists are still unclear. In some cases a direct cause can be demonstrated (e. g., patients suffering from bronchopulmonary aspergillosis), but often GS-dependent patients are indistinguishable from GS-responsive asthmatics (although they tend to be older and more often to be nonallergic). It has been shown that many GS-

dependent patients with persistent asthma have permanent CT-scan abnormalities, whereas those with brittle asthma do not (9). These findings suggest that some GS-dependent asthmatics may have increased remodeling of the airways (10), leading to an irreversible component of the airways obstruction.

GS have different anti-inflammatory activities and pharmacokinetics, and are deposited in lung to different extents (22). Thus, a given molecule may be more effective than others in certain patients. It was observed that betamethasone has a greater effect on bronchial obstruction than prednisolone, probably because of its longer biological half-life (11). However, betamethasone appears to elicit more side effects than GS with shorter half-lives. In another study, Chanez et al. (unpublished) were unable to find any difference in FEV$_1$, PEFR, or PEFR diurnal variability in patients treated serially with prednisone, prednisolone, or methylprednisolone.

The prevalence of GS-dependent asthma is very low, probably under 3% of all asthmatics, as shown recently by an epidemiologic study carried out in France.

Characteristics and Heterogeneity of GS-Resistant Asthmatics

There is a very small but still significant subset of asthmatics who may not respond favorably to oral GS. In 1968, Schwartz et al. (12) were among the first to describe patients who did not improve when treated with more than 15 mg cortisol daily. In 1981, Carmichael et al. (13) described a GS-resistant asthma population defined by an increase in FEV$_1$ of less than 15% after 7 days on an daily oral dose of 20 mg prednisolone. However, the definition of GS resistance is still highly variable. Many studies have tried to define it by using various doses and durations of GS treatment (14–19). The highest dose of GS used to define GS-resistant patients was reported by Kamada, who administered a mean dose of 70 mg of IV prednisolone for at least 10 days (20). Thus, whether a higher GS dose or a longer period of treatment may reverse the resistance in a larger number of patients has not been studied (Table 1).

The definition of GS resistance therefore needs to be improved, and it is often difficult to differentiate patients who are GS dependent from those

Table 1. Characteristics of patients ascribed to corticosteroid resistance.

		No. of patients	Age	FEV^1 pre-GS (% predicted)	Treatment pre-GS	GS treatment				Definition of GS resistance
						GS	route	dose	duration	
Carmichael	1981	116	adults	< 60%		prednisolone	oral	20 g	7 days	CR: FEV^1 increase < 15% CS: FEV^1 increase > 30%
Corrigan	1991	37	adults	< 70%	ICS ± oral GS	prednisolone	oral	20+40 mg	7+7 days	CR: FEV^1 pre-β_2 < 30% CS: FEV^1 pre-β_2 > 30%
Lane	1991	17	adults	50–60%*		prednisolone	oral	40 mg	14 days	CR: FEV^1 increase < 15% CS: FEV^1 increase > 30%
Alvarez	1992	17	adults	< 60%	oral GS	prednisolone	oral	> 40 mg	14 days	pre-β_2 morning FEV^1 < 60%
Kamada	1992	30	children		ICS ± oral GS	prednisone	oral	> 20–200 mg	variable	CR: morning FEV^1 increase < 15%
Sher	1994	29	adults	< 70%		prednisone	oral	2 × 20 mg	7 days	CS: morning FEV^1 increase > 30% CR: morning FEV^1 increase < 15%

GS, glucocorticosteroid; CR, GS-reststant asthma; CS, GS-sensitive asthma; ICS, inhaled corticosteroids.
* Mean value.

210

who are GS resistant. One could propose defining GS-resistant asthmatics as:

- Patients who are unstable according to the proposals of the International Consensus of Asthma (1) and/or who have persistent impairment of the pulmonary function (FEV_1 under 65% of predicted values) despite prolonged treatment with high doses of oral steroids. The duration and the dose of GS should, however, be defined. Premenstrual asthma represents a special form of GS-resistant asthma in which patients present life-threatening exacerbations resistant to high doses of systemic GS just before the menses (21).
- And/or patients who improve under alternative anti-inflammatory treatment such as methotrexate, dapsone, chloroquine, cyclosporin, or IVIG. However, to assess a steroid-sparing treatment accurately, the baseline pulmonary function of the patients should be established reliably over several months to eliminate weekly spontaneous variations (8).

The prevalence of GS-resistant asthma is even lower than that of GS-dependent asthma, but these patients are at very high risk of hospitalizations and death.

GS-dependent or resistant asthmatics are therefore highly heterogeneous, and a better clinical characterization is needed before biological studies are carried out.

Biological Characteristics of GS-Resistant Asthma

To cause their effects, GS interact with their receptors (GR), transcription factors that recognize specific genomic sequences, namely glucocorticoid responsive elements (GRE). The transcription of genes occurs in association with other transcription factors such as Fos, Jun, and CREB. These combinatorial associations – differing according to the differentiation and/or activation state of the cell – may therefore fine-tune the induction or repression of genes.

Biological studies were started very soon after the individualization of GS-resistant asthma, although GS resistance is still far from clearly defined. Several defects have been proposed or identified (14). They include accelerated plasma cortisol clearance (12), variable pharmacokinetics of GS molecules (22), monocyte (23, 24) or T-cell defects (17, 25), possibly abnormal survival of eosinophils in the airways related to cytokine responsiveness to steroids (26), and GS receptor (GR) abnormalities (18).

Monocyte Defects in GS-Resistant Asthmatics

Glucocorticoids act on the many functions of macrophages, mainly by modulating the production of inflammatory mediators such as cytokines, phospholipid-derived mediators, proteases, and oxygen metabolites (27).

Several studies have found that patients with GS-resistant asthma had impaired mononuclear phagocyte functions (23, 28). The effects of monocytes from asthmatics on granulocytes differ according to the clinical effects of GS. A 3 kDa neutrophil priming activity derived from peripheral blood monocytes is suppressed by GS treatment of monocytes derived from individuals with GS-sensitive but not GS-resistant asthma (29). These results suggest that monocytes of GS-resistant asthmatics can increase the inflammatory potential of neutrophils and that they are hyperactive, as indicated by the increased cytokine production and enhanced expression of activation markers, despite the presence of GS (24). On the other hand, the release of cytokines by LPS-stimulated monocytes was inhibited in a similar fashion in GS-sensitive and GS-resistant asthmatics (15). Different results were observed by Vecchiarelli et al. (30), who found that LPS-induced TNF secretion was reduced in blood monocytes obtained from GS-sensitive asthmatics after a course of treatment with prednisolone, whereas monocytes from GS-resistant asthmatics released the same amount of TNF before and during treatment.

Glucocorticosteroid Receptor (GR)

One of the most likely explanations for GS resistance is a qualitative or quantitative defect in GR. However, the effects of GR on monocytes were shown to be similar in patients sensitive or resistant to GS (29), and Vachier et al. (31) found that GR mRNA levels before GS treatment were similar in asthmatics and normal subjects. On the other hand, Sher et al. have recently found that in most cases of GS-resistant asthma there is a functional hyporesponsiveness of the GR on T cells (but not on other peripheral blood cells), whereas a small number of such patients show a reduction in GR numbers (18).

It is possible that GS treatment may reduce the function or number of GR. Sher et al., studying a small number of subjects, did not confirm this hypothesis when patients received oral GS (18), whereas Vachier et al. found that high dose parenteral GS reduced GR mRNA levels on monocytes in all patients treated (31).

Address for correspondence:

Jean Bousquet, MD
Clinique des Maladies Respiratoires
Hôpital Arnaud de Villeneuve
F-34295 Montpellier Cedex 5
France

References

1. International Consensus Report on Diagnosis and Management of Asthma. International Asthma Management Project. *Allergy* 1992; 47:1–61.

2. Britton M, Collins J, Brown D, Fairhurst N, Lambert R. High dose corticosteroids in severe acute asthma. *Br Med J* 1976; 2:73–74.

3. Tanaka RM, Santiago SM, Kuhn GJ, Williams RE, Klaustermeyer WB. Intravenous methylprednisolone in adults in status asthmaticus. Comparison of two dosages. *Chest* 1982; 82:438–440.

4. Haskell RJ, Wong BM, Hansen JE. A double-blind, randomized clinical trial of methylprednisolone in status asthmaticus. *Arch Intern Med* 1983; 143:1324–1327.

5. Ratto D, Alfaro C, Sipsey J, Glovsky MM, Sharma OP. Are intravenous corticosteroids required in status asthmaticus? *JAMA* 1988; 260:527–529.

6. McFadden E Jr. Dosages of corticosteroids in asthma. *Am Rev Respir Dis* 1993;147:1306–1310.

7. Dykewicz MS, Greenberger PA, Patterson R, Halwig JM. Natural history of asthma in patients requiring long-term systemic corticosteroids. *Arch Intern Med* 1986; 146:2369–2372.

8. Klaustermeyer WB, Garb KS, Santiago SM, Kinney JL. Variability of pulmonary function tests in stable corticosteroid dependent asthma patients. *Allergy Proc* 1991; 12:255–259.

9. Paganin F, Trussard V, Seneterre E, et al. Chest radiography and high resolution computed tomography of the lungs in asthma. *Am Rev Respir Dis* 1992; 146:1084–1087.

10. Bousquet J, Chanez P, Lacoste JY, et al. Asthma: a disease remodeling the airways. *Allergy* 1992; 47:3–11.

11. Grandordy B, Belmatoug N, Morelle A, De-Lauture D, Marsac J. Effect of betamethasone on airway obstruction and bronchial response to salbutamol in prednisolone resistant asthma. *Thorax* 1987; 42:65–71.

12. Schwartz H, Lowell F, Melby J. Steroid resistance in bronchial asthma. *Ann Intern Med* 1968; 69:493–499.

13. Carmichael J, Paterson IC, Diaz P, Crompton GK, Kay AB, Grant IW. Corticosteroid resistance in chronic asthma. *Br Med J Clin Res* 1981; 282:1419–1422.

14. Cypcar D, Busse WW. Steroid-resistant asthma. *J Allergy Clin Immunol* 1993; 92:362–372.

15. Lane SJ, Wilkinson JR, Cochrane GM, Lee TH, Arm JP. Differential *in vitro* regulation by glucocorticoids of monocyte-derived cytokine generation in glucocorticoid-resistant bronchial asthma. *Am Rev Respir Dis* 1993; 147:690–696.

16. Alvarez J, Surs W, Leung DY, Ikle D, Gelfand EW, Szefler SJ. Steroid-resistant asthma: Immunologic and pharmacologic features. *J Allergy Clin Immunol* 1992; 89:714–721.

17. Corrigan CJ, Brown PH, Barnes NC, et al. Glucocorticoid resistance in chronic asthma. Glucocorticoid pharmacokinetics, glucocorticoid receptor characteristics, and inhibition of peripheral blood T cell proliferation by glucocorticoids *in vitro. Am Rev Respir Dis* 1991; 144:1016–1025.

18. Sher E, Leung D, Surs W, et al. Steroid resistant asthma. Cellular mechanisms contributing to inadequate response to glucocorticoid therapy. *J Clin Invest* 1994; 93:33–39.

19. Woolcock AJ. Steroid resistant asthma: What is the clinical definition? *Eur Respir J* 1993; 6:743–747.

20. Kamada AK, Leung DY, Gleason MC, Hill MR, Szefler SJ. High-dose systemic glucocorticoid therapy in the treatment of severe asthma: A case of resistance and patterns of response. *J Allergy Clin Immunol* 1992; 90:685–687.

21. Perrin B, Bousquet J, Michel F, et al. Severe premenstrual asthma. *Lancet* 1988; ii:843–844.

22. Szefler SJ. Measuring the response to glucocorticoids. *J Allergy Clin Immunol* 1990; 85:985–987.

23. Kay AB, Diaz P, Carmicheal J, Grant IW. Corticosteroid-resistant chronic asthma and monocyte complement receptors. *Clin Exp Immunol* 1981; 44:576–580.

24. Wilkinson JR, Lane SJ, Lee TH. Effects of corticosteroids on cytokine generation and expression of activation antigens by monocytes in bronchial asthma. *Int Arch Allergy Appl Immunol* 1991; 94:220–221.

25. Corrigan CJ, Brown PH, Barnes NC, Tsai JJ, Frew AJ, Kay AB. Glucocorticoid resistance in chronic asthma. Peripheral blood T lymphocyte activation and comparison of the T lymphocyte inhibitory effects of glucocorticoids and cyclosporin A. *Am Rev Respir Dis* 1991; 144:1026–1032.

26. Wallen N, Kita H, Weiler D, Gleich GJ. Glucocorticoids inhibit cytokine-mediated eosinophil survival. *J Immunol* 1991; 147:3490–3495.

27. Russo-Marie F. Macrophages and the glucocorticoids. *J Neuroimmunol* 1992; 40:281–286.

28. Poznansky MC, Gordon AC, Grant IW, Wyllie AH. A cellular abnormality in glucocorticoid resistant asthma. *Clin Exp Immunol* 1985; 61:135–142.

29. Lane SJ, Lee TH. Glucocorticoid receptor characteristics in monocytes of patients with corticosteroid-resistant bronchial asthma. *Am Rev Respir Dis* 1991; 143:1020–1024.

30. Vecchiarelli A, Siracusa A, Cenci E, Puliti M, Abbritti G. Effect of corticosteroid treatment on interleukin-1 and tumour necrosis factor secretion by monocytes from subjects with asthma. *Clin Exp Allergy* 1992; 22:365–370.

31. Vachier I, Roux S, Altieri E, et al. Influence of glucocorticoids on mRNA GR expression in blood monocytes from asthmatic patients. *Am J Respir Crit Care Med* 1994; 149:A720.

Peptide Handling by the Immune System

Gerard F Hoyne*,**, Timothy Bourne*, Nanna M Kristensen*, Charlotte Hetzel*, Jonathan R Lamb**

Keywords: Antigen presentation, epitopes, immunotherapy, MHC, peptides, T cells

Antigen-specific T cells play an important role in the induction and regulation of a range of immunologically based diseases in man such as allergy and autoimmunity. In this review we examine some of the recent developments which have become central in shaping our view of how T cells recognise and respond to foreign and self antigens. In addition, we discuss the mechanisms by which antigenic peptides have been used to modulate the response of antigen-specific T cells *in vivo*. The results of these latter studies imply a potential application for peptide ligands in immune intervention.

T lymphocytes play a central role in the immune response to foreign antigens. They provide signals both for the induction of antibody synthesis and for the direction of isotype switching. They are also involved in controlling inflammatory responses and killing infected cells. Unlike B-cell receptors (antibodies), which recognise whole proteins, antigen-specific receptors on T cells (TCR) recognise processed peptides complexed to molecules encoded by the major histocompatibility complex (MHC) expressed on the surface of antigen presenting cells (APC). Two types of MHC molecules have been identified: class I MHC molecules which are expressed on all somatic cells, and class II MHC molecules which are restricted in their distribution to professional APCs such as dendritic cells, macrophages and B cells. Dendritic cells constitutively express very high levels of class II MHC molecules on their surface while expression on B cells and macrophages is usually low but is inducible under the influence of the cytokines IL-4 and IFN-γ respectively.

MHC Molecules: Structure and Function

In recent years there have been major advances in our knowledge of the physico-chemical nature of MHC-peptide complexes. This has been facilitated by a variety of structural studies, including analysis of peptide binding to isolated MHC molecules *in vitro* (1, 2), investigation of the cell biology of antigen processing (3) and resolution of the crystal structure of both class I and class II MHC molecules (4–7). Within a population of individuals MHC molecules are highly polymorphic and allelic variants arise due to amino acid substitutions within the floor and walls of the peptide binding site. Naturally processed peptides eluted from class I MHC molecules are usually 8 or 9 amino acids in length (8–10) and bind in an extended conformation along the groove (5, 11, 12). Analysis of the three-dimensional structure of various class I MHC molecules of murine and human origin has revealed that there are usually 2 allele-specific pockets per MHC molecule, which provide the important anchor sites that stabilise peptide binding (5, 6, 10–12). These pockets also determine the allelic specificity since they accommodate only a limited number of amino acids (9). The peptide binding site of class I MHC molecules has closed ends, which acts as another structural characteristic that limits the peptides that are able to bind (4, 5). Recently, it was reported that longer peptides (11–13 amino acids) could be accommodated in class I MHC molecules provided that the anchor-specific residues were present within the peptide sequence (13). Longer peptides were attached at the ends of the peptide groove and the extra sequences bulged out-

*   Department of Biology, Imperial College of Science, Technology and Medicine, London.
** Department of Immunology, St. Mary's Hospital Medical School, Imperial College of Science, Technology and Medicine, London.

wards from the middle displaying a larger accessible surface.

Sequencing of naturally processed peptides isolated from either human or murine class II MHC molecules has demonstrated that, in general, their lengths range between 13 and 17 amino acids (14, 15). In contrast to the previously eluted class I MHC peptides, the class II derived peptides have ragged N- and C-terminal ends (14, 15). From these observations it was predicted that the structure of MHC class II molecules would differ from their class I counterparts in that one or both ends of the antigen combining site would be open (14) and this has been confirmed by analysis of their crystal structures (4, 7). The structure of HLA-DR1 (B1*0101) complexed with the influenza virus haemagglutinin peptide HA 306–318 has now been reported and has provided details of the peptide binding site of class II molecules (16). It appears that HLA-DR1 has one deep pocket which accommodates tyrosine at position 308 in the peptide and contributes to the allelic specificity of peptide binding. The peptide binds in an extended conformation with a twist in the middle and contacts the groove along its entire length. A second shallower pocket was also identified which presumably could accommodate a large number of amino acid residues. These structural studies have supported previous hypotheses concerning the presence of allele-specific motifs in class II MHC binding peptides (14, 17).

Antigen Processing

Newly synthesised class I and class II MHC molecules bind peptides derived from distinct intracellular compartments. Peptides originating from antigens proteolytically degraded within the cytosol are transported into the lumen of the endoplasmic reticulum (ER) where they bind to nascent class I molecules. Exogenous antigens on the other hand are taken up by endocytosis and processed within lysosomes or acidified endosomes. Nascent class II molecules leave the ER complexed to the invariant chain molecule which is thought to act as a chaperone to target the class II MHC molecules to the lysosomal compartments involved in antigen processing (18–20). Once inside the lysosome the invariant chain is cleaved away by protease enzymes allowing exogenously-derived peptides to bind to the nascent MHC class II molecules. Newly formed peptide/MHC complexes are then transported to the cell surface where they are surveyed by passing T cells.

There are two largely distinct types of T cells which respond to peptide/MHC complexes. In general, CD8[+] cytotoxic T cells recognise peptides presented in association with class I MHC molecules and are especially effective in eliminating target cells whose biosynthetic machinery has been overcome by virus. In contrast, CD4[+] T cells respond to peptides presented on class II MHC molecules and in particular, provide help to antigen-specific B cells for the production of antibodies.

TCR Recognition of Peptide/MHC Complexes

Zinkernagel and Doherty first demonstrated the importance of MHC molecules in T-cell recognition of foreign antigens (21). However, it was almost a decade later before the molecular nature of TCR ligands was determined. Although it was reported in 1982 that T cells could respond to synthetic peptides derived from a foreign antigen (22) it was several years before it was demonstrated that synthetic peptides corresponding to immunogenic epitopes from foreign antigens could in fact bind to MHC molecules in vitro and that these complexes would activate T cells (1, 23–26). Studies on T-cell epitope mapping with different antigens established that, for a given protein antigen, there were usually only a limited number of immunogenic epitopes available to the immune system (27). Binding studies on isolated MHC molecules revealed that the half-life of defined peptide/MHC complexes is extremely long and is facilitated by the presence of anchor residues within the peptide (26).

Altered Peptide Ligands

It has been reported that peptide analogues based on known immunogenic T-cell epitopes which maintain the necessary MHC binding sites but have altered TCR contact residues may alter the effector response of T cells both in vitro and in vivo. De Magistris et al. (28) demonstrated that peptide analogues may act as TCR antagonists and prevent

T-cell activation, but that the recognition of these modified ligands failed to induce anergy (as described in the final section of this paper). Similarly, an altered peptide ligand for haemoglobin-specific murine T-cell clones has been identified that is able to uncouple proliferation from IL-4 secretion (29). This work was extended and revealed that another altered peptide ligand could induce long term clonal anergy in T cells representative of the Th1 functional subset (30). TCR antagonists which uncouple proliferation from cytotoxic responses also appear to exist for CD8$^+$ T cells (31). More recently, peptide analogues have also proved useful in studying the mechanisms involved in positive and negative selection of thymocytes (32, 33). More information needs to be collected on the mechanisms of action of altered peptide ligands in selecting specific T-cell effector function in view of their potential use as immunotherapeutic agents in the treatment of immunologically-based disease.

Peptides as Therapeutic Agents

T cells potentiate a range of autoimmune and allergic diseases in man. Strategies aimed at specifically controlling the effector response of disease-associated T cells are likely to provide long term clinical improvement. Many of the major allergens of the house dust mite (HDM) *Dermatophagoides pteronyssinus* have now been characterised at the molecular level and this has facilitated a highly detailed analysis of their recognition by CD4$^+$ T cells. Human CD4$^+$ T-cell clones reactive with the two major allergens *Der p* I and *Der p* II have been isolated and the epitopes they recognise have been characterised (34). Allergen-specific T cells from atopic individuals show a "Th2-dominant" cytokine secretion profile, with an overproduction of IL-4 and IL-5, while those from non-allergic patients display an IL-2/IFN-γ-secreting, "Th1-like" profile (reviewed in 35).

T-cell activation requires the delivery of two distinct sets of signals. The first consists of signals transduced through the TCR assembly following recognition of the peptide/MHC complex, whereas the second is mediated by the interaction between costimulatory molecules and their ligands. At present, the most well-defined second signal is the binding of the B7 ligand family expressed on APCs to CTLA-4 and CD28 on the T cell which triggers secondary messenger pathways. The delivery of both sets of signals appears to synergise mitogenic messages directed to the nucleus, resulting in transcriptional activation of the IL-2 gene and subsequent secretion of protein. Recognition of the peptide/MHC complexes on the APCs by T cells in the absence of costimulatory signals leads to a state of unresponsiveness termed clonal anergy (36). *In vitro* studies have shown that exposing human CD4$^+$ T-cell clones to high doses of peptide ligand or superantigens in the presence or absence of APCs results in a long lived state of anergy (37, 38). Collectively these studies point to the possibility that antigen-reactive T cells are susceptible to immune modulation.

Studies in animal models have shown that the response of antigen-reactive T cells may be modulated *in vivo*. Administering antigens either orally, by inhalation or intravenously are all effective in inducing a state of long-term unresponsiveness (39–41). Like the *in vitro* models for clonal anergy, T cells from tolerant animals fail to either secrete IL-2 or proliferate upon reactivation and antibody responses in tolerant mice are diminished. The results of our studies demonstrate that inhalation or feeding of peptides containing immunogenic epitopes from the *Der p* I allergen in naive mice may specifically inhibit responses to the intact antigen (42, 43). The induction of tolerance spread to all *Der p* I-specific T cells since those recognising other determinants on the antigen were also inhibited. These findings suggest that clonal anergy is not the only mechanism involved in down-regulating T-cell responses, since anergy should presumably only affect T cells specific for the epitope used for treatment. It is possible that infectious tolerance, perhaps mediated by a shift in the cytokine profiles or the induction of regulatory cells, may contribute to the observed non-responsiveness. This approach is not unique to the regulation of HDM-specific responses and peptide based therapies have also been used successfully to modulate responses in mice to other foreign proteins including autoantigens (44–47).

Summary

Our knowledge of the molecular basis of T-cell recognition of foreign antigens has advanced dramatically in recent years. Both *in vitro* and *in vivo* studies have demonstrated that peptide antigens may be used not only to activate but also to downregulate the responses of antigen-reactive T cells. Peptide analogues which may act as TCR antagonists or partial agonists may also prove effective in the regulation of selected effector functions of T cells. However, the potential of this new class of ligands remains to be resolved but perhaps further study may prove them to be effective reagents for immunotherapy.

Acknowledgements

This work was supported by grants from The Wellcome Trust and the Medical Research Council, U.K.

Address for correspondence:

Dr Gerard Hoyne
Department of Biology
Imperial College of Science
Technology and Medicine
Prince Consort Road
London, SW7 2BB
UK

References

1. Babbitt BP, Allen PM, Matsueda G, Haber E, Unanue ER. Binding of immunogenic peptides to Ia histocompatibility molecules. *Nature* 1985; 317:359.

2. Schumacher TNM, Heemels M-T, Neefjes JJ, Kast WM, Melief CJM, Ploegh HL. Direct binding of peptide to empty MHC class I molecules on intact cells and *in vitro*. *Cell* 1990; 62:563.

3. Brodsky FM, Guargliardi LE. The cell biology of processing and presentation. *Annu Rev Immunol* 1991; 9:707.

4. Bjorkman P, Saper M, Samaraoui B, Bennett W, Strominger J, Wiley D. Structure of the human Class I histocompatibility antigen, HLA-A2. *Nature* 1987; 329:506.

5. Fremont DH, Matsumura M, Stura EA, Peterson PA, Wilson IA. Crystal structure of two viral peptides in complex with murine MHC class I H2K^b. *Science* 1992; 257:919.

6. Young ACM, Zhang W, Sacchettini JC, Nathenson SG. The three dimensional structure of H2Db at a 2.4 Å resolution: Implications for antigen-determinant selection. *Cell* 1994; 76:39.

7. Brown JH, Jardetzky TS, Gorga JC, Urban RG, Strominger JL, Wiley DC. 3-Dimensional structure of the human histocompatibility antigen HLA-DR1. *Nature* 1993; 364:33.

8. Van Bleek GM, Nathenson SG. Isolation of an endogenously processed immunodominant viral peptide from the class I H-K^b molecule. *Nature* 1990; 348:213.

9. Falk K, Rotzschke O, Stevanovic S, Jung G, Rammensee HG. Allele-specific motifs revealed by sequencing of self-peptides eluted from MHC molecules. *Nature* 1991; 351:290.

10. Madden DR, Garboczi DN, Wiley DC. The antigenic identity of peptide-MHC complexes: A comparison of the conformation of five viral peptides presented by HLA-A2. *Cell* 1993; 75:693.

11. Matsamura M, Fremont DH, Peterson PA, Wilson IA. Emerging principles for the recognition of peptide antigens by MHC class I molecules. *Science* 1992; 257:927.

12. Madden DR, Gorga JC, Strominger JL, Wiley DC. The structure of HLA-B27 reveals a nonamer self-peptides bound in an extended conformation. *Nature* 1991; 353:321.

13. Guo H-C, Jartedsky TS, Garret TPJ, Lane WS, Strominger JL, Wiley DC. Different length peptides bind to HLA-Aw68 similarly at their ends but bulge out in the middle. *Nature* 1992; 360:364.

14. Rudensky AY, Preston-Hulburt P, Hong S-C, Barlow A, Janeway JCA. Sequence analysis of peptides bound to MHC class II molecules. *Nature* 1991; 353:622.

15. Rudensky AY, Preston-Hurlburt P, Al-Ramadi BK, Rothbard J, Janeway CAJ. Truncation variants of peptides isolated from MHC class II molecules suggests sequence motifs. *Nature* 1992; 359:429.

16. Stern LJ, Brown, JH, Jardetsky TS, Gorga JC, Urban RG, Strominger JL, Wiley DC. Crystal structure of the human class II MHC protein HLA-DR1 complexed with an influenza virus peptide. *Nature* 1994; 368:215.

17. Sette A, Buus S, Appella E, Smith JA, Chesnut R, Miles C, Colon SM, Grey HM. Prediction of major histocompatibility complex binding regions of protein antigens by sequence pattern analysis. *Proc Natl Acad Sci USA* 1989; 86:3296.

18. Lotteau V, Teyton L, Peleraux A, Nilsson T, Karlsson L, Schmid SL, Quaranta V, Peterson PA. Intracellular transport of class II MHC molecules directed by invariant chain. *Nature* 1990; 348:600.

19. Teyton L, O'Sullivan D, Dickson PW, Lotteau V, Sette A, Fink P, Peterson PA. Invariant chain distinguishes between the exogenous and endogenous antigen presentation pathways. *Nature* 1990; 348:39.

20. Gaugliardi LE, Koppelman B, Blum JS, Marks MS,

Cresswell P, Brodsky FM. Co-localization of molecules involved in antigen processing and presentation in an early endocytic compartment. *Nature* 1990; 343:133.

21. Zinkernagel RM, Doherty PC. Restriction of *in vitro* T cell mediated cytotoxicity in lymphocytic choriomeningitis within a syngeneic or semiallogeneic system. *Nature* 1974; 248:701.

22. Lamb JR, Eckels DD, Lake P, Woody JN, Green N. Human T cell clones recognize chemically synthesized peptides of influenza haemagglutinin. *Nature* 1982; 300:66.

23. Townsend ARM, Rothbard J, Gotch F, Bahadur G, Wraith D, McMichael AJ. The epitopes of influenza nucleoprotein recognized by cytotoxic T lymphocytes can be defined by short synthetic peptides. *Cell* 1986; 44:959.

24. Buus S, Sette A, Colon SM, Miles C, Grey HM. The relation between major histocompatibility complex (MHC) restriction and the capacity of Ia to bind immunogenic peptides. *Science* 1987; 235:1353.

25. Guillet JG, Lai MZ, Briner TJ, Buus S, Sette A, Grey HM, Smith JA, Gefter ML. Immunological self, nonself discrimination. *Science* 1987; 235:865.

26. Sette A, Buus S, Colon S, Smith JA, Miles C, Grey HM. Structural characteristics of an antigen required for its interaction with Ia and recognition by T cells. *Nature* 1987; 328:395.

27. Roy S, Scherer MT, Briner TJ, Smith JA, Gefter ML. Murine MHC polymorphism and T cell specificities. *Science* 1989; 244:572.

28. De Magistris MT, Alexander J, Coggeshall M, Altman A, Gaeta FCA, Grey HM, Sette A. Antigen analog-major histocompatibility complexes act as antagonists of the T cell receptor. *Cell* 1992; 68:625.

29. Evavold BD, Allen PM. Separation of IL-4 production from Th cell proliferation by an altered TcR ligand. *Science* 1991; 252:1308.

30. Sloan-Lancaster J, Evavold BD, Allen PM. Induction of T-cell anergy by altered T cell receptor ligand on live antigen presenting cells. *Nature* 1993; 363:156.

31. Jameson SC, Carbone FR, M.J. B. Clone-specific T cell receptor antagonists of major histocompatibility complex class I-restricted cytotoxic T cells. *J Exp Med* 1993; 177:1541.

32. Hogquist KA, Jameson SC, Heath WR, Howard JL, Bevan MJ, Carbone FR. T cell receptor antagonist peptides induce positive selection. *Cell* 1994; 76:17.

33. Ashton-Rickardt PG, Bandeira A, Delaney JR, Van KAer L, Pircher H-P, Zinkernagel RM, Tonegawa S. Evidence for a differential avidity model of T cell selection in the thymus. *Cell* 1994; 76:651.

34. O'Hehir RE, Hoyne GF, Thomas WR, Lamb JR. House dust mite allergy. From epitopes to immunotherapy. *Eur J Clin Invest* 1993; 23:763.

35. Romagnani S. Lymphokine production by human T cells in disease states *Annu Rev Immunol* 1994; 12:227.

36. Schwartz RH. A cell culture model for T lymphocyte clonal anergy. *Science* 1990; 248:1349.

37. Lamb JR, Skidmore BJ, Green N, Chiller JM, Feldmann M. Induction of tolerance in influenza virus-immune T lymphocyte clones with synthetic peptides of influenza haemagglutinin. *J Exp Med* 1983; 157:1434.

38. O'Hehir RE, Lamb JR. Induction of specific clonal anergy in human T lymphocytes by *Staphylococcus aureus* enterotoxins. *Proc Natl Acad Sci USA* 1990; 87:8884.

39. Tomasi T. Oral tolerance. *Transplantation* 1981; 29:353.

40. Sedgwick JD, Holt PG. Induction of IgE-isotype specific tolerance by passive antigenic stimulation of the respiratory mucosa. *Immunology* 1983; 50:625.

41. Gammon G, Sercarz E. How some T cells escape tolerance induction. *Nature* 1989; 342:183.

42. Hoyne GF, O'Hehir RE, Wraith DC, Thomas WR, Lamb JR. Inhibition of T cell and antibody responses to the major house dust mite allergen in naive and sensitized mice. *J Exp Med* 1993; 178:1783.

43. Hoyne GF, Callow MG, Kuo M-C, Thomas WR. Inhibition of T cell responses by feeding peptides containing major and cryptic epitopes. Studies with the *Der p* I allergen. 1994 (in press).

44. Wraith DC, Smilek DE, Mitchell DJ, Steinman L, McDevitt HO. Antigen recognition in autoimmune encephalomyelitis and the potential for peptide mediated immunotherapy. *Cell* 1989; 59:247.

45. Metzler B, Wraith DC. Inhibition of experimental autoimmune encephalomyelitis by inhalation of but not oral administration of the encephalitogenic peptide: Influence of MHC binding affinity. *Int Immunol* 1993; 5:1159.

46. Clayton JP, Gammon GM, Ando DG, Kono DH, Hood L, Sercarz EE. Peptide-specific prevention of experimental allergic encephalomyelitis. Neonatal tolerance induced to the dominant T cell determinant of myelin basic protein. *J Exp Med* 1989; 169:1681.

47. Briner TJ, Kuo M-C, Rogers BR, Keeting K, Fleishell ML, O'Brien MM, Bollinger BK, Craig S, Greenstein JL. Inhibition of allergen-specific murine T cell responses after subcutaneous injection of T cell epitope-containing peptide. *Proc Natl Acad Sci USA* 1993; 90.

Clinical Use of Synthetic Peptides: Peptide of Grass Pollen and Other Allergens

WM Becker, A Petersen, A Bufe, G Schramm, M Schlaak*

Keywords: *Phleum pratense*, grass pollen allergens, isoallergen, *Phl p* Va, *Phl p* Vb, *Phl p* VI, B-cell epitope

The current issues in grass-pollen allergy are prevention and therapy. In connection with immunotherapy, a controversy has broken out about the proper clinical use of natural or recombinant/synthetic allergens. In order to reconcile conflicting opinions, we have to broaden our knowledge about the chemical structure of allergens and their relation to the human immune system. A special feature of grass-pollen allergens is their interspecies cross-reactivity. Comparison of the structure of cross-reactive grass group V (a) allergens demonstrates a mean dissimilarity of 20%. A further manifestation of structural dissimilarities are the isoallergens. Studying the allergens of timothy grass pollen in more detail, we find that isoallergens are formed on the gene level. Moreover, in the grass group I allergen, *Phl p* I, we can demonstrate a hugh number of posttranslational modifications. Testing patients' IgE on the N-terminal and C-terminal fragments of *Phl p* Va presenting different B-cell epitopes, we detect an individual reaction pattern. Before attempting to solve the problems of immunotherapy with a small number of recombinant or synthetic allergens, we must elucidate the structural diversity of allergens within the context of the human immune system.

Introduction

Grass pollens are the main source of outdoor allergens and are found throughout the entire world. The flowering, i.e., pollination, season of the different grasses includes nearly the whole vegetation period. The consequence is a continuous exposure of the organism to a low dose of pollen and a continuous stimulus of the immune system by antigens released from particulate pollens. Clearance of these pollens from the body, especially of their biologically active components and of their related antigens, is an active process of the organism and ultimately of the immune system. The danger of the pollens does not lie directly in their antigens, but in their potential to trigger an overwhelming immune response activating a defense reaction that may get out of hand and become injurious. With dysregulation of the immune system caused by grass pollen, there is hardly a chance of avoiding contact. Normally, the immune system of any particular population has adapted to such a stimulus over periods of thousands of years through evolutionary balance. At first glance, this is also valid for grass pollen; but the growing number of grass-pollen allergic people in the last 10 years indicates a disturbance of the balance of the naturally developed system. In our attempt to understand this phenomenon scientific discussion has centered on some causes of a speculative nature: increasing environmental pollution and changes in the life style (1).

Today, grass-pollen allergy does not present a diagnostic problem; rather, in the present and immediate future the research issues are prevention and therapy. One way to solve these problems is the elucidation of the pathomechanism of type I allergy on a molecular level, with emphasis on the clarification of the structure of allergenic components. The key to understanding the pathomechanism is not to be found in the chemical structure alone, but more likely within the context of the immune system. On the molecular level, chemical structure and the immune system come together in the B- and T-cell epitopes. Therefore, the identification and characterization of B- and T-cell epitopes represents an important step in elucidating the problem of IgE regulation. This will help to solve the controversy about the proper clinical use of natural or recombinant allergens.

*   Forschungsinstitut Borstel, Borstel, Germany

Cross-reactivity and Diversity of Grass-Pollen Allergens

When investigating the molecular structure of grass pollen allergens, the potential for generation of artifacts must be kept in mind. Extracts made up with Coca's solution or similar water-based buffers have been shown to be an authentic allergen source *in vitro*. These extracts consist of a great number of components – proteins as well as glycoproteins – but only a minority of them are reactive to IgE. A special feature of grass-pollen allergens of different species is their high degree of cross-reactivity. The

Table 1. Characterized grass pollen allergens.

Allergen source	Allergen	Molecular weight (kDa)	pI	Sequence data	References
Sweet vernal grass (*Anthoxanthum odoratum*)	*Ant o* I	34	–	P	4
Bermuda grass (*Cynodon dactylon*)	*Cyn d* I	32	6.2	P	5, 6
Cock's foot (*Dactylis glomerata*)	*Dac g* I	32	6.4	P	7
	Dag g II	11		C	8
	Dac g V	25,28	4.9	P	9–11
Meadow fescue (*Festuca elatior*)	*Fes e* I	34			4
Rye-grass (*Lolium perenne*)	*Lol p* I	34	5.9	C	12–16
	Lol p II	11	5.2	C	12, 17
	Lol p III	11	9.2	C	12, 18
	Lol p IV	57	9.9	P	13, 19
	Lol p V	25,28	4.9	C	11
	Lop p IX; Ib (V?)	28		C?	20
	Lol p X	12			21
	Lop p XI	18	5.0–6.0	C	22
Timothy grass (*Phleum pratense*)	*Phl p* I	34	5.8	C	23*
	Phl p II	10 – 12		C	24
	Phl p III	10 – 12		C	24
	Phl p IV	54	9.5		25, 26
	Phl p V	29,31	4.8	C	3, 27–28,**
	Phl p VI	11	5.2, 5.4	C	29***
	profilin	14		C	30
Meadow grass (*Poa pratensis*)	*Poa p* I	34	5.9, 6.4	P	4, 31
	Poa p V	26,28	4.8	P	11
	Poa p IX	29	9.1	C	32, 33
Velvet grass (*Holcus Lanatus*)	*Hol l* I	34	5.0–5.5	C	****
	Hol l V	30	4.9–6.2	C	*****

* A. Petersen: EMBL Nucleotide sequence data library accession number: Z27090 (Phl p I)
** A. Bufe: X70942 (Phl p Va), Z27083 (Phl p Vb)
*** A. Petersen: Z27082 (Phl p VI)
**** G. Schramm: Z27084 (Hol l I)
***** G. Schramm submitted
pI = Isoelectric point, sequence data: P = partial, C = complete

abundance of information has been simplified through the introduction of group nomenclature (2). This system is based on structural and immunological homologies.

However, such nomenclature involves the risk of excess streamlining and not doing justice to individual findings of important differences. This can be demonstrated above by the *Phl p* Va/*Phl p* Vb paradigm, where components dissimilar in structure are put together. The cross-reactivity of different grass pollen allergens is experimentally shown in a Western blot analysis by monospecific IgE which was affinity purified on recombinant *Phl p* Va (3). However, a comparison of deduced primary structures of grass group Va allergens shows a dissimilarity of 20%. This range of dissimilarities would be likely to be found in other grass groups.

A list of identified, characterized, and cloned grass-pollen allergens is depicted in Table 1 (4–33). Of course, as far as completeness is concerned, the table is out of date the moment it is written. From an analytical point of view, the impressive number of allergenic components describes only the tip of the iceberg because on the molecular level most of the allergenic components comprise a multitude of isoallergens. Whether this diversity in the chemical structure is of biological/immunological consequence is an open question. But this problem is closely connected with the question of the proper clinical use of cloned and synthetic allergenic peptides. Moreover, the discussion of this question is influenced by the desire for simple solutions to solve diagnostic and therapy problems with only a small number of representative allergens.

By studying timothy grass pollen allergens – natural and recombinant ones – on a molecular level and investigating their immunochemical interaction with the organism we hope to answer the following questions:

1. What is the spectrum of timothy grass-pollen allergens and what is their relationship between each other? Are isoallergens a product of posttranslational modifications or programed on a genetic level?
2. What is the B-cell epitope pattern? Are allergen fragments biologically active?
3. Are recombinant allergens really valid surrogates of natural allergens?

Timothy Grass Pollen Allergens, Their Relationship Amongst Themselves, and Genetic and Posttranslational Modifications of Their Isoallergens

On the basis of a hundred individual binding patterns we identified grass group V (*Phl p* Va, *Phl p* Vb), grass group VI (*Phl p* VI) and grass group IV (*Phl p* IV) as major allergens and grass group I (*Phl p* I) as an intermediate allergen. Only through antisera in 2D electrophoresis were we able to localize *Phl p* II/III and profilin, which – in contrast to our findings – are described by others as prominent allergens (24, 26). By studying *Phl p* V, *Phl p* I, and *Phl p* VI, we include the most important allergens of timothy grass pollen in our analysis. In investigations of grass group V allergens by 2D electrophoresis immunoblot followed by N-terminal sequencing, we identified two isoforms *Phl p* Va and *Phl p* Vb, which differed by 40% in molecular weights and in their N-terminal structure. Moreover, the respective isoforms are each representatives of at least four isoallergens (34). Consequently, the question arises as to whether these isoforms are similar molecules in the sense that the larger one is a precursor of the smaller one, or whether they are similar but independent molecules. The last supposition was supported by the reactivity of the different monoclonal antibodies: where MoAb Bo1 reacts with both isoforms, whereas MoAb Bo9 reacts exclusively to *Phl p* Vb and MoAb BG6 only to *Phl p* Va. The conclusion is that the two isoforms share one epitope but differ in at least two. Moreover, degradation experiments with the two isoforms by Glu C resulted in different fragments that were far from being identical (35). These findings highlight the structural independence of the two isoforms. Cloning these allergens reveals deduced primary structures which have 70% identity and 80% homology. Nevertheless, when looking at the *Phl p* Va and *Phl p* Vb alignment, there are striking differences in the primary structure. Furthermore, these structures are encoded by two different genes. Interestingly, in sweet velvet grass *(Holcus lanatus)*, grass group V is only expressed as the *Phl p* Vb analogue (G. Schramm; manuscript in preparation). The final decision whether these allergens are functionally similar or not can be made only by B- and T-cell epitope mapping and by elucidating the biological function of these allergens in the plant.

Whereas *Phl p* Va and *Phl p* Vb are pure proteins, *Phl p* I has been identified as a glycoprotein (23). It consists of at least five isoallergens that vary slightly in their molecular weights between 37 kDa to 33 kDa (23). Comparing the N-termini of these isoallergens with the 35 kDa components as a point of reference, there is one amino acid exchange in position 18 with respect to the 37 kDa isoallergen, but four exchanges in positions 2, 12, 13, 15 with respect to the 33 kDa isoallergen.

It is noteworthy that a posttranslational modified proline, namely, a 4-hydroxyprolinewas found throughout at in positions 5 and 8 in all isoallergens. In position 9, a technically caused blank indicates a glycan binding site. This was verified by the deduced structure of a cloned *Phl p* I as asparagine residue, which was confirmed by a typical glycosylation site motif N-X-T. Analyzing the proline/hydroxyproline content of the natural *Phl p* I, we determined a content of 9 proline and 8 hydroxyproline residues. After the cloning of *Phl p* I, the deduced primary amino acid structure was available, demonstrating seven cysteine residues. These residues pose the problem of correct folding of the recombinant-produced allergen with respect to the natural allergen. Furthermore, immunoscreening for phosphorylated amino acids led to a positive reaction with phophorylserin (Petersen, manuscript submitted).

At 13 kDa, *Phl p* VI the smallest major allergen of timothy grass pollen, consisting of at least of three isoallergens (29). The N-termini of these isoallergens are similar to *Phl p* Vb/*Phl p* Va innercore sequences. The difference of two isoallergens found in spot 1 (pI 5.2) lies in a shift of two positions at the starting point of the N-terminus sequence. The third isoallergen is found in spot 2 (pI 5.4), showing an identical N-terminus to the one isoallergen in spot 1. The idea that these components are split products of *Phl p* Vb has to be rejected because no reactivity to *Phl p* V specific MoAbs can be observed. This view is supported by cloning experiments of these allergens which identified independent genes coding for *Phl p* VI isoallergens. The deduced primary structure shows identical elements of *Phl p* Vb and *Phl p* Va united in this structure. It is of interest that on immobilized recombinant *Phl p* VI, affinity-purified patients' IgE is reactive with *Phl p* Va and *Phl p* Vb (Petersen, manuscript submitted).

Timothy grass pollen by itself consists of a complex source of allergens representing immunochemically different clusters of similar, but distinct components, the heterogeneity of which is already organized at the gene level. This is true for the group V and group VI allergens. Moreover, there are strong hints at posttranslational modifications of *Phl p* I. These modifications could increase the structural variety and its possible immunological role.

Properties of *Phl p* Va Fragments

The clinical usefulness of synthetic grass-pollen peptides has only recently begun to be investigated. We started with the identification of IgE-reactive epitopes on *Phl p* Va using genetically engineered fragments. We were able to show that the N-terminal and the C-terminal fragments, representing a little more than half of the intact molecule, carry different IgE-reactive epitopes using affinity purified IgE antibodies in inhibition experiments (3). The question arises as to whether patients react to these epitopes generally or individually.

When testing 11 grass-pollen-allergic patients, we found patients reacting with the N-terminal and C-terminal fragments with equal intensity, whereas other patients responded more strongly to the C-terminus than to the N-terminus (3). Therefore, the intensity of reaction to the N- and C-terminal fragments must be individually regulated. This finding is an interesting aspect that should be borne in mind when designing new drugs for immunotherapy. Monitoring the development of IgE reactions – and their relative intensities – to special epitopes could be a new approach to calculating the clinical outcome of an immunotherapy.

Investigation of the biological activity of the N- and C-terminal fragments in a histamine release test showed that the N-terminal fragment of *Phl p* Va has a ten times higher activity than the intact molecule, whereas the C-terminal fragment reacts five times lower. Using analogue fragments of *Phleum p* Vb, we found the C-terminus to be more active than the N-terminus (Bufe et al., submitted).

By constructing a great number of fragments of *Hol l p* Vb in combination with predictions of antigenic sites according to Hopp-Woods and Chou and Fasman, we were able to localize IgE-reactive epitopes between amino acid numbers 19 to 27 and 175 to 181; the peptide sequences near the N-terminus are $A^{19}TTDEQKLL^{27}$ and near the C-terminus $I^{175}KESTGG^{181}$ (G. Schramm, manuscript in preparation). These common IgE-reactive epitopes were identified in *Phl p* Va, *Phl p* Vb, *Poa p* IX, *Lol p* Va, *Lop p* Vb and the N-terminal epitope in *Phl p* VI (Bufe et al., submitted).

Conclusion

Research needs a vision. The vision in allergen characterization is the molecular cloning of allergens, the use of the genetic engineering technology, and the recombinant preparation of tailored protein drugs for immunotherapy. Modern technology is very efficient in elucidating structures of allergens and in providing allergens for epitope mapping representing active compounds.

But doubts emerge whether recombinant allergens expressed in *E. coli* could really be the tailored surrogates for the natural allergens. These doubts are connected with the great number of similar but genetically independent allergenic grass pollen peptides. Doubts are connected with posttranslationally modifications of the natural allergen in comparison with the recombinant product. There are at least 16 posttranslational modifiable amino acids (36). In *Phl p* I we found three certain kinds of modification and two probable ones. We have in fact no experience about how the lack of such modifications – a typical feature of recombinant allergens – influences the biological handling of these defective components by the organism. The consequence of these findings should be a critical sequence analysis of original material guided by the deduced structure of the recombinant component. This laborious task has to be undertaken to overcome obstacles of recombinant or synthetic produced allergens and to avoid a disappointment in the proper clinical use of these components.

Address for correspondence:

Dr Wolf-M Becker
Forschungsinstitut Borstel
Parkallee 35
D-23845 Borstel
Germany

References

1. Wüthrich B. Zur Häufigkeit der Pollenallergie in der Schweiz. In J Ring (Ed) *Epidemiologie allergischer Erkrankungen: Nehmen Allergien zu?* Munich: MMV, Medizin-Verlag, 1991, 119.

2. Marsh DG, Goodfriend L, King TP, Löwenstein H, Platts-Mills TAE. Allergen nomenclature. *Int Arch Allergy Appl Immunol 1988;* 85:194.

3. Bufe A, Becker W-M, Schramm G, Petersen A, Mamat U, Schlaak M. Major allergen *Phl p* Va (timothy grass) bears at least two different IgE reactive epitopes. *J Allergy Clin Immunol*, 1994; 94: 173.

4. Esch RE, Klapper DG. Isolation and characterization of a major cross-reactive grass group I allergenic determinant. *Mol Immunol* 1989; 26:557.

5. Matthiesen F, Schumacher M, Løwenstein H. Characterization of the major allergen of *Cynodon dactylon* (Bermuda grass) pollen, *Cyn d* I. *J Allergy Clin Immunol* 1991; 88:763.

6. Smith PM, Singh MB, Knox RB. Characterization and cloning of the major allergen of Bermuda grass, *Cyn d* I. In D Kraft, A Sehon (Eds) *Molecular biology and immunology of allergens*. Boca Raton: CRC Press, 1993, 157.

7. Mecheri S, Peltre G, David B. Purification and characterization of a major allergen from *Dactylis gomerata* pollen: The Ag Dg 1. *Int Archs Allergy Appl Immunol* 1985; 78:283.

8. Roberts AM, Bevan LJ, Flora PS, Jepson I, Walker MR. Nucleotide sequence of cDNA encoding the group II allergen of Cocksfoot/Orchard grass *(Dactylis glomerata)*, *Dac g* II. *Allergy* 1993; 48:615

9. Ree R van, Clemens JGJ, Aalbers M, Stapel SO, Aalberse RC. Characterization with monoclonal and polyclonal antibodies of a new major allergen from grass pollen in the group I molecular weight range. *J Allergy Clin Immunol* 1989; 83:144.

10. Walsh DJ, Matthews JA, Denmeade R, Maxwell P, Davidson M, Walker MR. Monoclonal antibodies to proteins from cocksfoot grass *(Dactylis glomerata)* pollen: Isolation and N-terminal sequences of a major allergen. *Int Arch Allergy Appl Immunol* 1990; 91:419.

11. Klynser S, Welinder K, Løwenstein H, Matthiesen F. Group V allergens in grass pollens – IV. Similarities in aminoacid composition and NH_2-terminal sequence of group V allergens from *Lolium perenne*, *Poa pratensis* and *Dactylis glomerata*. *Clin Exp Allergy* 1992; 22:491.

12. Marsh DG. Allergens and the genetics of allergy. In M Sela (Ed) *The antigens, vol. 3*. New York: Academic Press, 1975, 271.

13. Howlett BJ, Clarke AE. Role of carbohydrate as an antigenic determinant of glycoprotein from rye-grass

(*Lolium perenne*) pollen. *Biochem J* 1981; 197:695.

14. Cottam GP, Moran DM, Standring R. Physiochemical and immunochemical characterization of allergenic proteins from rye grass (*Lolium perenne*) pollen prepared by a rapid and efficient purification. *Method Biochem J* 1986; 234:305.

15. Perez, M, Ishioka, GY, Walker, LE, Chesnut, RW. cDNA cloning and immunological characterization of the rye grass allergen *Lol p* I. *J Biol Chem* 1990; 265:16210.

16. Griffith IJ, Smith PM, Pollock J, Theerakulpisut P, Avjioglu A, Davies S, Hough T, Singh MB, Simpson RT, Ward LD, Knox RB. Cloning and sequencing of *Lot p* I, the major allergenic protein of rye-grass pollen. *FEBS Lett* 1991; 279:210.

17. Ansari AA, Shenbagamurthi P, Marsh DG. Complete amino acid sequence of a *Lolium perenne* (perennial rye grass) pollen allergen, *Lol p* II. *J Biol Chem* 1989; 264:11181.

18. Ansari AA, Shenbagamurthi P, Marsh DG. Complete primary structure of a *Lolium perenne* (perennial rye grass) pollen allergen, *Lol p* III: Comparison with known *Lol p* I and *Lol p* II sequences. *Biochem* 1989; 28:8665.

19. Ekramoddoullah AKM, Kisil FT, Sehon AH. Immunochemical characterization of a high molecular weight basic allergen (HMBA) of rye grass (*Lolium perenne*) pollen. *Mol Immunol* 1983; 20:465.

20. Singh MB, Hough T, Theerakulpisut P, Avjioglu A, Davies S, Smith PM, Taylor P, Simpson RJ, Ward LD, McCluskey J, Puy R, Knox RB. Isolation of cDNA encoding a newly identified major allergenic protein of rye-grass pollen: Intracellular targeting to the amyloplast. *Proc Natl Acad Sci USA* 1991; 88:1384.

21. Ekramoddoullah AKM, Kisil FT, Sehon AH. Allergenic cross reactivity of cytorchrom c from Kentucky Blue grass and perennial ryegrass pollens. *Mol Immunol* 1982; 19:1527.

22. van Ree R. *Specificity of grass pollen allergens.* Amsterdam, Thesis, 1994.

23. Petersen A, Becker W-M, Schlaak M. Characterization of grass group I allergens in timothy grass pollen. *J Allergy Clin Immunol* 1993; 92:789.

24. Dolecek C, Vrtala S, Laffer S, Steinberger P, Kraft D, Scheiner O, Valenta R. Molecular characterization of *Phl p* II, a major timothy grass (*Phleum pratense*) pollen allergen. *FEBS* 1993; 335:299.

25. Løwenstein H. Isolation and partial characterization of three allergens of timothy pollen. *Allergy* 1978; 33:30.

26. Haavik S, Paulsen BS, Wold JK. Glycoprotein allergens in pollen of timothy. II. Isolation and characterization of a basic glycoprotein allergen. *Int Archs Allergy Appl Immunol* 1985; 78:260.

27. Matthiesen F, Løwenstein H. Group V allergens in grass pollens – I. Purification and characterization of the group V allergen from *Phleum pratense* pollen, *Phl p* V. *Clin Exp Allergy* 1991; 21:297.

28. Vrtala S, Sperr WR, Reimitzer I, van Ree R, Laffer S, Müller W-D, Valent P, Lechner K, Rumpold H, Kraft D, Scheiner O, Valenta R. cDNA cloning of a major allergen from timothy grass (*Phleum pratense*) pollen: Characterization of the recombinant *Phl p* V allergen. *J Immunol* 1993; 151; 4773.

29. Petersen A, Bufe A, Schramm G, Schlaak M, Becker W-M. Studies on the major allergen *Phl p* VI on the protein and cDNA level. *J Allergy Clin Immunol* 1994; 93:206.

30. Valenta R, Duchene D, Sperr WR, Valent P, Vrtala S, Hirschwehr R, Ferreira F, Kraft D, Scheiner O. Profilin represents a novel plant pan-allergen. In D Kraft, A Sehon (Eds) *Molecular biology and immunology of allergens.* Boca Raton: CRC Press, 1993, 47.

31. Lin Z, Ekramoddoullah AKM, Kisil FT, Hebert J, Mourad W. Isolation and characterization of *Poa p* I allergens of Kentucky bluegrass pollen with murine monoclonal anti-*Lol p* I antibody. *Int Arch Allergy Appl Immun* 1988; 87:294.

32. Mohapatra SS, Hill R, Astwood J, Ekramoddoullah AKM, Olsen E, Silvanovich A, Hattom T, Kisil FT, Sehon AH. Isolation and characterization of a cDNA clone encoding an IgE-binding protein from Kentucky bluegrass (*poa pratensis*) pollen. *Int Arch Allergy Appl Immunol* 1990; 91:362.

33. Silvanovich A, Astwood J, Zhang L, Olsen E, Kisil F, Sehon A, Mohapatra S, Hill R. Nucleotide sequence analysis of three cDNAs coding for *Poa p* IX isoallergens of Kentucky bluegrass pollen. *J Biochem Chem* 1991; 266:1204.

34. Petersen A, Becker W-M, Schlaak M. Characterization of isoforms of the major allergen *Phl p* V by two-dimensional immunoblotting and microsequencing. *Int Arch Allergy Immunol* 1992; 98:105.

35. Petersen A, Becker W-M, Schlaak M. Structural investigations of isoforms of the major allergen *Phl p* V by fingerprinting and microsequencing. *Clin Exp Allergy* 1994; 24:250.

36. Arnstein HRV, Cox RA. Protein biosynthesis. In D Rickwood (Ed) *In focus Oxford.* New York, Tokyo: IRL Press, 1992, 72

Diagnostic and Therapeutic Concepts Based on Recombinant Allergens

Rudolf Valenta*, Christiane Dolecek*, Günther Menz**, Ursula Schönheit-Kenn**, Markus Susani***, Hans Grönlund****, Dietrich Kraft*

Keywords: Type I allergy, recombinant allergens, diagnosis, therapy

The number of recombinant allergens produced in heterologous expression systems increases continuously. The current contribution briefly summarizes successful methods to obtain recombinant allergens that behave similarly to their natural counterparts and describes *in vitro* and *in vivo* assays to check the immunological properties of recombinant allergens. Using two bacterially expressed birch pollen allergens, *Bet v* I and birch profilin (*Bet v* II), the usefulness of recombinant allergens is illustrated. It is demonstrated that specific allergograms for individual allergic patients can be determined which may form the basis for improved and specific immunotherapy. Concepts for specific immunotherapy of Type I allergy based on the use of recombinant allergens are finally discussed.

1. Preparation of messenger RNA from the allergen source (pollen, mites, moulds)

↓

2. Reverse transcription of mRNA into cDNA

↓

3. Insertion of cDNA into expression systems (lambda gt11, lambda ZAP)

↓

4. Plating of the cDNA library and transfer of induced proteins to nitrocellulose filters

↓

5. IgE-immunodetection of clones expressing recombinant allergens

↓

6. Sequence analysis and further manipulation of the allergen encoding cDNA.

Figure 1. Antibody screening of cDNAs coding for allergens.

Isolation and Expression of cDNAs Coding for Allergens

Comparing different methods for the isolation of recombinant allergens, the screening of cDNA libraries prepared from RNA of the respective allergen source with serum IgE from allergic patients proved to be a successful technique (1, 2). The construction and IgE-screening of an expression cDNA library, mostly done in phage lambda gt11 (3) or lambda ZAP (4), is briefly outlined in Figure 1. The use of serum IgE from allergic patients to isolate phage clones ensures that cDNAs are obtained which most closely mimic natural allergens. If DNA probes are used for screening instead or PCR techniques are applied it is not unlikely that cDNAs will be isolated which bind IgE less effi-

ciently (5). This can be either due to the fact that isoallergenic variants of the respective allergens are isolated which may bind IgE less efficiently (5) or because during PCR amplification nucleotide exchanges lead to changes within the allergen encoding cDNA, subsequently changing the conformation and/or epitopes of the expressed allergen.

In the case of tree and grass pollen allergens, recombinant molecules were produced that bound IgE efficiently and which compared closely with their natural counterparts (6–12). Mite and animal dander allergens were apparently more difficult to express, which might be due to intrinsic properties of the allergens (13, 14) and also to the more complex composition of the molecules, e.g., consisting of different chains, as is the case with *Fel d* I (15). However, the increasing number of recombinant al-

* Institute of General and Experimental Pathology, AKH, University of Vienna, Austria.
** Hochgebirgsklinik Davos Wolfgang, Davos, Switzerland.
*** ABS (Advanced Biological Systems), Academy of Sciences, Salzburg, Austria.
****Pharmacia, Uppsala, Sweden.

lergens which are currently being characterized in many laboratories promises that within a reasonable period of time most relevant allergens can be produced as recombinant molecules and made available for diagnostic and therapeutic purposes (16).

In Vitro Immunological Characterization of Recombinant Allergens

The production of recombinant allergens first aims to obtain molecules which closely resemble their natural counterparts. Recombinant allergens should therefore be compared with natural allergens regarding their IgE-binding capacity (8, 9, 17), and whether they behave similarly in cellular assays such basophil histamine release (18) and T-cell proliferation (19). To further study the *in vivo* effects of recombinant allergens, animal models have to be established (20, 21), and finally recombinant allergens might be evaluated by skin testing in allergic patients (22, 23). The evaluation of the therapeutic potency of recombinant allergens and their modifications requires careful testing in experimental animal models.

IgE-Binding Capacity of Recombinant Allergens

In several studies, the IgE-binding capacity of recombinant allergens was investigated. It has been demonstrated that a small panel of recombinant tree (8) and grass pollen allergens (24) could be successfully used to diagnose pollen allergy in a representative number of patients. Recombinant tree pollen allergens (*Bet v* I and *Bet v* II) were meanwhile evaluated in commercial assay systems (25). It was shown that recombinant *Bet v* I bound a surprisingly high proportion of birch pollen specific IgE, and by using a combination of both recombinant allergens a high percentage of tree pollen allergic patients could be diagnosed (25).

It was further shown that single recombinant grass pollen allergens such as *Phl p* V (10) and *Poa p* IX (26) or combinations of a few recombinant grass pollen allergens (27) bound a high proportion of grass pollen specific IgE. Although many allergens occur as a multitude of isoallergenic variants, it was demonstrated that IgE binding against such isovariants could be successfully blocked by preadsorption of patient sera with a single recombinant isoform (10, 12). It was further shown that recombinant pollen allergens share IgE epitopes with homologous pollen allergens, as well as with homologous allergens in plant derived food (9, 28–31). It is therefore likely that due to structural similarities among relevant allergens only a few representative recombinant allergens may be sufficient for diagnostic and therapeutic purposes (32).

Cellular Assays for the Characterization of Recombinant Allergens

In addition to the antibody binding capacity, the effects of recombinant allergens on immune cells have to be demonstrated. The basophil histamine release allows us to study whether recombinant allergens are able to trigger allergic effector reactions without *in vivo* testing. Several studies have demonstrated that recombinant allergens are capable of inducing dose dependent and specific histamine release from patients' basophils (9, 18, 17). In addition. recombinant allergens have been successfully used to induce proliferation of T cells and T-cell clones which had been selected with natural allergens (19). In the case of T cells and antibodies, for example, it has been suggested that on the monoclonal level (T-cell clones, monoclonal antibodies) the immune system is capable to distinguish isoforms of allergens and homologous allergens from different sources. It appears therefore to be of importance to also investigate T-cell reactivity at the precursor frequency level and, in case of antibody reactivity, to estimate the sum of a polyclonal antibody response against a given recombinant allergen. Those recombinant allergens against which a high percentage of specific T cells responds and which bind a high proportion of specific IgE may be good candidates to redirect the allergic immune response.

In Vivo Characterization of Recombinant Allergens

Induction of IgE Responses in Animals Using Recombinant Allergens

It has been demonstrated in earlier studies that low dose injection of antigens together with aluminum hydroxide induces IgE antibodies in animals (33, 34). Using this technique, specific IgE antibodies could be induced against recombinant tree pollen and grass pollen allergens in mice (20). IgE antibodies of the allergic mice displayed extensive cross-reactivity with the natural allergens and homologous allergens, as is observed in allergic patients (20). A similar immunization protocol was successfully used to induce specific IgE antibodies in rhesus monkeys, which after injection showed similar type I allergy symptoms to allergic patients (21). Type I allergy induced in rodents or primates based on Al(OH)$_3$ injected recombinant allergens may provide well defined models for the *in vivo* study of specific IgE regulation, and is mandatory for testing the effects of therapeutic agents before they are used in patients.

Skin Testing of Patients With Recombinant Allergens

Skin testing of allergic patient represents a very sensitive and inexpensive method for the diagnosis of type I allergy. Currently, skin test solutions are crude extracts prepared from natural allergen sources such as pollen, animal pelts, mites, and fungi. Depending on the starting material used for the preparation of the test solutions, allergens will be more or less well represented. Although the skin test solutions can be checked for their allergen content using monoclonal antibodies or reference preparations, some extracts, in particular those made of fruits and vegetables, lack important allergens, and in the case of most test extracts minor allergens are less well represented.

Recombinant allergens may be extremely useful as reference preparations, and when used for skin testing may allow the specific sensitization pattern of patients to be determined (allergogram). Although some recombinant allergens have already been successfully used for skin testing, each recombinant allergen needs to be tested in a representative number of patients and non-allergic control individuals. At present, more recombinant allergens need to be isolated and characterized to set up screening tests for certain allergies. Screening tests still have to be done with natural extracts, whereas specific diagnosis can benefit from the use of recombinant allergens. The example below illustrates how the sensitization pattern (allergogram) of tree pollen allergic patients can be determined by using recombinant allergens.

Example: Specific Diagnosis of Tree Pollen Allergy With Recombinant *Bet v* I and Recombinant *Bet v* II (Birch Profilin) – The Allergogram

Extracts which are currently used for *in vitro* and *in vivo* diagnosis of birch pollen allergy contain a number of components, proteins and carbohydrates, as is shown in Figure 2. The Coomassie stained gel of a birch pollen extract shows numerous bands ranging between 10 and 100 kDa molecular weight. If a patient is tested using such an extract, any reactivity with any component can lead to a positive result, without providing detailed

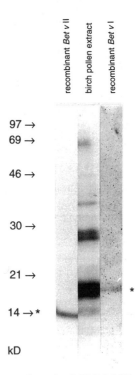

Figure 2. Coomassie stained SDS-PAGE containing natural birch pollen extract and purified recombinant *Bet v* I and *Bet v* II. Natural birch pollen extracts contain a number of components ranging between 10 and 90 kD. Bacterially expressed *Bet v* I and *Bet v* II migrate at comparable molecular weights to their natural counterparts (indicated by asterisks).

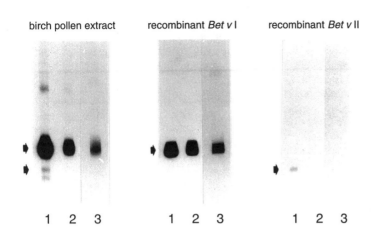

birch pollen extract   recombinant *Bet v* I   recombinant *Bet v* II

1 2 3   1 2 3   1 2 3

Figure 3. IgE-reactivity of tree pollen allergic individuals with nitrocellulose blotted natural and recombinant birch pollen allergens. Three tree pollen allergic individuals were selected according to case history, RAST and conventional skin testing. The patients sera were tested for IgE-reactivity with natural birch pollen extract, recombinant *Bet v* I and recombinant *Bet v* II.

NaCl: negative control
Histamine: positive control
ALK: commercial skin test solution (birch)
B: recombinant *Bet v* I
P: recombinant *Bet v* II = birch profilin

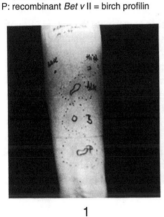
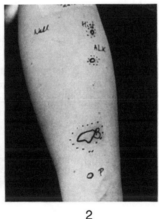
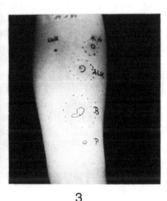

1   2   3

Figure 4. Skin prick testing of three tree pollen allergic patients with natural and recombinant birch pollen allergens. The tree pollen allergic patients shown in Figure 3 were skin prick tested with commercial skin-prick solutions (ALK, Horsholm, Denmark), histamine (positive control), saline (negative control) and recombinant *Bet v* I and *Bet v* II, respectively.

knowledge about what allergens the patient is sensitized to. If immunotherapy is then done with the same extract, the patient will receive injections containing a number of components against which he is not allergic, and desired components might be not present in the extract. The situation in the case of birch pollen allergy is less complicated because almost 95% of the patients show IgE reactivity against the major birch pollen allergen *Bet v* I. This migrates at 17 kDa molecular weight, and is also present in large amounts in birch pollen extracts. It should, however, be pointed out that diagnosis and treatment with extracts which are not composed according to the patient's sensitization pattern (allergogram) can not be regarded as satisfactory and need to be improved.

Figure 3 shows the IgE-binding pattern of three birch pollen allergic patients with nitrocellulose blotted natural and recombinant birch pollen allergens. Although a multitude of bands is present in the natural birch pollen extract, the patients showed binding only to distinct bands of 17 kD, representing *Bet v* I, and with a 14 kD band, representing birch profilin. The natural extract, however, does not allow a precise diagnosis of which allergens the patients are allergic to. When the same patients are tested with recombinant *Bet v* I and recombinant birch profilin (*Bet v* II) it is possible to precisely diagnose that patients 1–3 show IgE reactivity with *Bet v* I and that patient 1 is also allergic to *Bet v* II. As shown in Figure 4, the *in vitro* result is confirmed by a skin test performed with a commercial natural birch pollen extract and the recombinant allergens. From the example it becomes evident that optimal diagnosis may start with natural diagnostic extracts in an initial screening procedure to determine the allergen sources against which a patient is sensitized, followed by precise determination of the allergens against which a patient is sensitized using recombinant allergens. The correct choice of the recombinant allergens will, however, require a detailed knowledge of the distribution of certain allergens and their homologous proteins in different allergen sources. *Bet v* I homologous allergens can be found in pollen of related trees belonging to the Fagales order such as alder, hazel, or hornbeam (35, 36, 37, 5, 38), and in plant derived food such as apples and hazelnuts (28, 31). The knowledge of the distribution of *Bet v* I homologous allergens will then help to explain allergic cross-reactivities with sources other than birch pollen. In the case of IgE reactivity against profilin, extensive cross-reactivities with profilins from many unrelated sources, including grasses, weeds, fruits, and vegetables, can be expected (reviewed in 39).

Concepts for Specific Therapy of Type I Allergy Using Recombinant Allergens

Concerning therapy of type I allergy, the example shown above indicates that immunotherapy, which has been a standard therapy since 1911 (40), could be significantly improved by the use of recombinant allergens. Specific therapy has to be based on the accurate determination of the sensitization pattern of allergic individuals. Injection of non-allergenic components or allergens against which a patient is not sensitized should be avoided by ac-

curate determination of the patients individual allergogram and treatment with highly pure recombinant allergens. Concepts for specific immunotherapy with recombinant allergens are outlined briefly in the following paragraphs.

Immunotherapy With Complete Recombinant Allergens or Allergen Derived Epitopes

Purified recombinant allergens might be used together with current adjuvants and modification procedures such as natural allergens. However, before a certain recombinant allergen is used for immunotherapy an allergogram should be determined for each patient which defines exactly the targets for IgE antibodies in the individual patients. In addition, we believe that those recombinant allergens against which a high titer of specific IgE is produced should be selected for immunotherapy. It can reasonably be expected that one prerequisite for a decrease in allergic symptoms is a decrease in specific IgE antibodies. Using recombinant allergens, it is possible to estimate the percentage of IgE directed against defined allergens, which may then help to select the most relevant allergens for therapeutic purposes (27).

Whether immunotherapy can be substantially improved by application of T-cell or B-cell epitopes derived from complete allergens still needs to be resolved. Theoretically, a therapy based on T-cell epitopes or B-cell epitopes representing haptens, and which thus are not anaphylactogenic, might improve current forms of immunotherapy, but extensive studies in animal models need to be done beforehand.

Passive Therapy by Saturation of Mast Cells and Basophils with Allergen Derived Haptens

For the reduction of allergic symptoms, passive therapeutic approaches may be considered besides active immunomodulation. One possibility is to define IgE epitopes which represent haptens that bind IgE but cannot cross-link mast cell- and basophil-bound IgE. In principle it might be expected that B-cell epitopes would be less diverse than T-cell epitopes, and it might be feasible to dissect IgE haptens which can be used to saturate mast cell- and basophil-bound IgE, thus preventing release of mediators. Subsequent stimulation with the complete allergen might then be ineffective to trigger release of mediators. Since membrane-bound IgE is thought to be long lived, the blocking effects might be long lasting. Haptens derived from complete allergens could perhaps be used locally in the conjunctiva, nose, and lung. First studies with an immunodominant IgE hapten derived from the major grass pollen allergen *Phl p* I showed that a recombinant fragment did not trigger histamine release from basophils of most *Phl p* I allergic patients (41), and encourage the pursuit of this line.

Use of Allergen-Specific Antibodies that Compete With IgE Antibodies

In the case of some allergens, such as the major birch pollen allergen *Bet v* I, IgE epitopes could not yet be defined. It was, however, shown that mouse monoclonal antibodies and human monoclonal antibodies could efficiently compete with the binding of IgE antibodies to *Bet v* I and inhibited *Bet v* I induced basophil degranulation (42). Antibodies which compete with patients' IgE binding might be used, such as the haptens described above for a local therapy to inhibit allergic effector reactions. For a reduction of the immunogenicity of such antibodies, humanization or truncation to Fab fragments might be considered. Using RNA from the lymphocytes as a starting material and immunoglobulin specific primers, heavy and light chain fragments could be amplified and expressed in *E. coli* expression systems as blocking Fab fragments (43, 44, 45).

Acknowledgments

This study was supported by grant S06703 of the Austrian Science Foundation.

Address for correspondence:

Rudolf Valenta, MD
Institute of General and Experimental Pathology, AKH, University of Vienna
Währingergürtel 18–20
A-1090 Vienna

References

1. Baldo BA, Donovan GR. The structural basis of allergenicity: recombinant DNA-based strategies for the study of allergens. *Allergy* 1988; 43: 81.

2. Breitenbach M, Valenta R, Breiteneder H, Pettenburger K, Scheiner O, Rumpold H, Kraft D. Introduction to cDNA-cloning of plant allergens. In Sehon AH, Kraft D, Kunkel G (Eds) *Epitopes of atopic allergens.* Brussels: UCB Institute of Allergy, 1990, pp. 57.

3. Huynh TV, Young RA, Davis RW. Constructing and screening cDNA libraries in lgt 10 and lgt 11. In Glover DM (Ed) *DNA cloning, a practical approach*, vol. I. Oxford: IRL Press, 1985.

4. Short JM, Fernandez JM, Sorge JA, Huse WD. l ZAP: A bacteriophage l expression vector with *in vivo* excision properties. *Nucl Acids Res* 1988; 16:7583.

5. Breiteneder H, Ferreira F, Hoffmann-Sommergruber K, Ebner C, Breitenbach M, Kraft D, Scheiner O. Four recombinant isoforms of *Cor a* I, the major allergen of hazel pollen, show different IgE binding properties. *Eur J Biochem* 1993; 212:355.

6. Breiteneder H, Pettenburger K, Bito A, Valenta R, Kraft D, Rumpold H, Scheiner O, Breitenbach M. The gene coding for the major birch pollen allergen, *Bet v* I, is highly homologous to a pea disease resistance response gene. *EMBO J* 1989; 8:1935.

7. Valenta R, Duchêne M, Pettenburger K, Sillaber C, Valent P, Bettelheim P, Breitenbach M, Rumpold H, Kraft D, Scheiner O. Identification of profilin as a novel pollen allergen; IgE autoreactivity in sensitized individuals. *Science* 1991; 253:557.

8. Valenta R, Duchêne M, Vrtala S, Birkner T, Ebner C, Hirschwehr R, Breitenbach M, Rumpold H, Scheiner O, Kraft D. Recombinant allergens for immunoblot diagnosis of tree-pollen allergy. *J Allergy Clin Immunol* 1991; 88:889.

9. Valenta R, Duchêne M, Ebner C, Valent P, Sillaber C, Deviller P, Ferreira F, Tejkl M, Edelmann H, Kraft D, Scheiner O. Profilins constitute a novel family of functional plant pan-allergens. *J Exp Med* 1992; 175:377.

10. Vrtala S, Sperr WR, Reimitzer I, van Ree R, Laffer S, Müller WD, Valent P, Lechner K, Rumpold H, Kraft D, Scheiner O, Valenta R. cDNA cloning of a major allergen from timothy grass (*Phleum pratense*) pollen; characterization of the recombinant *Phl p* V allergen. *J Immunol* 1993; 151:4773.

11. Dolecek C, Vrtala S, Laffer S, Steinberger P, Kraft D, Scheiner O, Valenta R. Molecular characterization of *Phl p* II, a major timothy grass (*Phleum pratense*) pollen allergen. *FEBS Lett* 1993; 335:299.

12. Laffer S, Valenta R, Reimitzer I, Vrtala S, vanRee R, Mannhalter C, Kraft D, Scheiner O, Duchêne M. cDNA cloning and expression of the major allergen *Phl p* I of timothy grass (*Phleum pratense*); recombinant *Phl p* I inhibits IgE-binding to multiple group I isoallergens from eight grass species. *J Allergy Clin Immunol* 1994; (in press).

13. Chua KY, Stewart GA, Thomas WR, Simpson RJ, Dilworth RJ, Plozza TM, Turner KJ. Sequence anal-

ysis of cDNA coding for a major house dust mite allergen, *Der p* I. *J Exp Med* 1988; 167:175.

14. Chua KY, Kehal PK, Thomas WR, Vaughan PR, Macreadie IG. High-frequency binding of IgE to the *Der p* allergen expressed in yeast. *J Allergy Clin Immunol* 1992; 89:95.

15. Morgenstern JP, Griffith IJ, Brauer AW, Rogers BL, Bond JF, Chapman MD, Kuo MC. Amino acid sequence of *Fel d* I, the major allergen of the domestic cat: protein sequence analysis and cDNA cloning. *Proc Natl Acad Sci USA* 1991; 88:9690.

16. Scheiner O, Bohle B, Breitenbach M, Breiteneder H, Duchêne M, Ebner C, Ferreira F, Hoffmann-Sommergruber K, Pettenburger K, Rumpold H, Steiner R, Tejkl M, Valenta R, Kraft D. Recombinant allergens: Production and possible clinical implications. In Godard P, Bousquet J, Michel FB (Eds) *Advances in allergology and clinical immunology.* Carnforth, Park Ridge: Parthenon Publishing Group, 1992, pp. 115.

17. Ferreira F, Hoffmann-Sommergruber K, Breiteneder H, Pettenburger K, Ebner C, Sommergruber W, Steiner R, Bohle B, Sperr WR, Valent P, Kungl AJ, Breitenbach M, Kraft D, Scheiner O. Purification and characterization of recombinant *Bet v* I, the major birch pollen allergen. *J Biol Chem* 1993; 268:19574.

18. Valenta R, Sperr WR, Ferreira F, Valent P, Sillaber C, Tejkl M, Duchêne M, Ebner C, Lechner K, Kraft D, Scheiner O. Induction of specific histamine release from basophils with purified natural and recombinant birch pollen allergens. *J Allergy Clin Immunol* 1993; 91:88.

19. Ebner C, Ferreira F, Szephalusi Z, Jilek A, Valenta R, Parronchi P, Maggi E, Romagnani S, Scheiner O, Kraft D. Identification of multiple T-cell epitopes on *Bet v* I, the major birch pollen allergen. *J Immunol* 1993; 3:1047.

20. Vrtala S, Ferreira F, Stocker B, Kraft D, Scheiner O, Valenta R. Generation of tree pollen allergic mice with recombinant allergens. [abstract] *Allergy* 1993; 48:53.

21. Ferreira F, Valenta R, Mayer P, Liehl E, Sperr WR, Valent P, Ebner C, Scheiner O, Kraft D. Induction of Type I allergy in rhesus monkeys with recombinant allergens. [abstract] *Allergy* 1993; 48:53.

22. Moser M, Crameri R, Menz G, Schneider T, Dudler T, Virchow C, Gmachl M, Blaser K, Suter M. Cloning and expression of recombinant *Aspergillus fumigatus* allergen I/a (r*Asp f* I/a) with IgE binding and Type I skin test activity. *J Immunol* 1992; 149:454.

23. Moser M, Crameri R, Brust E, Suter M, Menz G. Diagnostic value of recombinant aspergillus fumigatus allergen I/a for skin testing and serology. *J Allergy Clin Immunol* 1994; (in press).

24. Valenta R, Vrtala S, Ebner C, Kraft D, Scheiner O. Diagnosis of grass pollen allergy with recombinant timothy grass (*Phleum pratense*) pollen allergens. *Int Arch Allergy Immunol* 1992; 97:287.

25. Zimmermann K, Kober A, Grönlund H, Yman L. IgE antibodies against native birch pollen allergens and recombinant allergens (*Bet v* I and Profilin) measured by Pharmacia CAP system. *ACI News* 1994; [abstract] Suppl. 2; 493.

26. Yang M, Olsen E, Dolovich J, Sehon AH, Mohapatra SS. Immunologic characterization of a recombinant kentucky bluegrass (*Poa pratensis*) allergenic peptide. *J Allergy Clin Immunol* 1991; 87:1096.

27. Laffer S, Vrtala S, Duchêne M, vanRee R, Kraft D, Scheiner O, Valenta R. IgE-binding capacity of recombinant timothy grass (*Phleum pratense*) pollen allergens. *J Allergy Clin Immunol* 1994; (in press).

28. Ebner C, Birkner T, Valenta R, Rumpold H, Breitenbach M, Scheiner O, Kraft D. Common epitopes of birch pollen and apples: studies by Western and Northern blot. *J Allergy Clin Immunol* 1991; 88:588.

29. Vallier P, Dechamp C, Valenta R, Vial O, Deviller P. Purification and characterization of an allergen from celery immunochemically related to an allergen in several other plant species. Identification as a profilin. *Clin Exp Allergy* 1992; 22:774.

30. vanRee R, Voitenko V, Van Leeuwen WA, Aalberse RC. Profilin is a cross-reactive allergen in pollen and vegetable foods. *Int Arch Allergy Immunol* 1992; 98:97.

31. Hirschwehr R, Valenta R, Ebner C, Ferreira F, Sperr WR, Valent P, Rohac M, Rumpold H, Scheiner O, Kraft D. Identification of common allergenic structures in hazel pollen and hazelnuts: a possible explanation for sensitivity to hazelnuts in tree pollen allergic patients. *J Allergy Clin Immunol* 1992; 90:927.

32. Valenta R, Duchêne M, Vrtala S, Ball T, Ferreira F, Laffer S, Hirschwehr R, Ebner C, Sperr W, Valent P, Kraft D, Scheiner O. Recombinant allergens as candidates for immunotherapy of Type I allergic diseases. In Ginsberg HS, Brown F, Chanock RM, Lerner RM (Eds) *Vaccines 93.* Cold Spring Harbor Laboratory Press, 1993, pp. 37.

33. Levine BB, Vaz NM. Effect of combinations of inbred strain, antigen and reagin production in the mouse. *Int Arch Allergy Immunol* 1970; 39:156.

34. Lehrer SB, Vaughan JH, Tan EM. Adjuvant activity of the histamine-sensitizing factor of Bordetella pertussis in different strains of mice. *Int Arch Allergy Immunol* 1975; 49:796.

35. Rohac M, Birkner T, Reimitzer I, Bohle B, Steiner R, Breitenbach M, Kraft D, Scheiner O, Gabl F, Rumpold H. The immunological relationship of epitopes on major tree pollen allergens. *Mol Immunol* 1991; 28:897.

36. Valenta R, Breiteneder H, Pettenburger K, Breitenbach M, Rumpold H, Kraft D, Scheiner O. Homology of the major birch pollen allergen, *Bet v* I, with the

major pollen allergens of alder, hazel, and hornbeam at the nucleic acid level as determined by cross-hybridization. *J Allergy Clin Immunol* 1990; 87:677.

37. Breiteneder H, Ferreira F, Reikerstorfer A, Duchêne M, Valenta R, Hoffmann-Sommergruber K, Ebner C, Breitenbach M, Scheiner O. Complementary DNA cloning and expression in *Escherichia coli* of *Aln g* I, the major allergen in pollen of alder (*Alnus glutinosa*). *J Allergy Clin Immunol* 1992; 90:909.

38. Larsen JN, Stroman P, Ipsen H. PCR based cloning and sequencing of isogenes encoding the tree pollen major allergen *Car b* I from *Carpinus betulus*, hornbeam. *Mol Immunol* 1992; 29:703.

39. Valenta R, Duchêne M, Vrtala S, Valent P, sillaber C, Ferreira F, Tejkl M, Hirschwehr R, Ebner C, Kraft D, Scheiner O. Profilin, a novel plant pan-allergen. *Int Arch Allergy Immunol* 1992; 99:271.

40. Noon, L. Prophylactic inoculation for hay-fever. *Lancet* 1911; 1:1572.

41. Ball T, Vrtala S, Sperr WR, Valent P, Scheiner O,

Kraft D, Valenta R. Isolation of an immunodominant IgE-hapten from an epitope expression cDNA library; dissection of the allergic effector reaction. *J Biol Chem* 1994 (in press).

42. Lebeque SJ, Denepoux S, Pin JJ, Ho S, Rousset F, Banchereau J. Generation and characterization of human anti-*Bet v* I monoclonal antibodies derived from allergic patients. *ACI News* 1994; [abstract] Suppl 2:88.

43. Huse WD, Sastry L, Iverson SA, Kang AS, Alting-Mees M, Burton DR, Benkovic SJ, Lerner RA. Generation of a large combinatorial library of the immunoglobulin repertoire in phage lambda. *Science* 1989; 246:1275.

44. Hoogenboom HR, Marks JD, Griffiths AD, Winter G. Building antibodies from their genes. *Immunol Reviews* 1992; 130:41.

45. Plückthun A. Mono- and bivalent antibody fragments produced in *Escherichia coli*: Engineering, folding and antigen binding. *Immunol Reviews* 1992; 130:151.

Initial Clinical Experiences with Allergen Peptides

Philip S Norman, Lawrence M Lichtenstein*

Keywords: Immunotherapy, peptides, allergens

Respiratory allergies have usually been considered as immediate IgE antibody mediated responses, but attention is now turning to inflammatory responses that appear to be initiated by T cells. These cells respond to peptide fragments from allergens presented in combination with HLA class II molecules. Although classic immunotherapy with allergen extracts downregulates these T cell responses, more efficient and safe methods are being sought. Peptides of relatively short chain length that contain epitopes for protein allergen molecules can, if presented without costimulatory signals, downregulate T cell responses in rodents, producing a state of anergy. The first of these to reach a clinical trial in human disease is a combination of two synthesized 27 member peptides based on the structure of Chain 1 of the principle allergen of cat hair and dander, *Fel d* 1. Early safety studies indicate that these peptides infrequently interact with human IgE antibodies to *Fel d* 1.

Immunotherapy by repeated subcutaneous injections of increasing doses of crude extracts of allergens redirects allergic immunologic responses. At first IgE antibodies increase, but then they decline slowly. Serum IgG antibodies rise markedly, and secretory antibodies increase modestly. Serum IgG and secretory IgA and IgG antibodies can block *in vitro* antigen stimulated mediator release by IgE antibody sensitized mast cells and basophils (1). After immunotherapy, allergic subjects show reduced immediate responses to allergen challenges to the nasal or bronchial mucosa (2).

Patients receiving immunotherapy also have a reduction of several antigen driven *in vitro* activities attributable to T cells. Furthermore, after immunotherapy, late phase responses to allergen challenges, by both clinical observations and measurements of local mediator release, are reduced (3). The potential role of downregulation of T cell activity in the immunologic management of allergic conditions is therefore being studied in man. The information obtained could lead to improvements in immunotherapy that would lessen the risk of allergic reactions to parenterally administered allergens and improve efficacy.

The recognition that the level of IgE antibody depends on T cell regulation leads to consideration of how to alter or downregulate T cell stimulation of the B cells that synthesize antibody. This is reinforced by the realization that the T cells that appear to play a direct role in allergic inflammation are probably the same CD4+ cells. Downregulation of these cells could at the same time reduce IgE synthesis and limit inflammatory responses to allergens.

T and B cells recognize different epitopes on the same protein. T cell responses to foreign proteins depend on T cell receptors that respond to peptidic fragments of the antigen associated with products of MHC expressed on the surface of accessory cells, i.e., antigen presenting cells (APC). The responses of CD4+ cells are class II MHC restricted and several examples of specific human class II alleles controlling IgE responses to specific allergenic proteins have been described (4).

The identification of T cell epitopes on allergens is now progressing rapidly. A number of major allergens have been cloned, sequenced and expressed. These include proteins from honey bee venom, cat, ragweed, rye grass, and the house dust mites, *D. pteronyssinus* and *D. farinae*. Knowing the full peptide sequence of an allergen allows the synthesis of a series of overlapping peptides or generation of a series of deletion mutants that can be used as test materials for T-cell stimulation.

Induction of tolerance (anergy) of T cells has been studied extensively *in vitro* and *in vivo*. This type of tolerance is to be distinguished from clonal deletion in the thymus. The T cells survive but their reactivity is downregulated. Of greatest interest therapeutically is tolerization of T cells with peptides derived from disease producing antigens. Such tolerization may be achieved *in vitro* by ex-

* Johns Hopkins Asthma and Allergy Center, Johns Hopkins University School of Medicine, Baltimore, MD, USA.

posure of T cells to peptide fragments bound to class II MHC molecules without costimulatory activity from APC (5). Tolerization of two clones of T cells from a D. *pteronyssinus* sensitive patient was also achieved *in vitro* by exposing them to high concentrations of the clone specific peptide in the absence of APC. During such exposure, however, there was considerable production of IL-2, IL-4, and IFN-γ. Subsequent cultures of tolerized cells with APC and peptide showed inhibition of IL-4 production while still producing IFN-γ (6). To quote the authors: "This information may be relevant in the design of immunomodulatory agents for potential use in the treatment of allergic or autoimmune diseases."

Preliminary study of T cell lines from patients with ragweed allergy shows that a degree of T cell tolerance can be induced *in vivo* by standard immunotherapy. The T cell lines were grown in the presence of ragweed allergen *Amb a* 1, along with IL-2 and IL-4, rested and then restimulated by allergen in the presence of irradiated mononuclear cells as APC. Cell lines from untreated patients regularly showed proliferation, whereas lines from patients receiving ragweed extract immunotherapy showed much less proliferation. In some cell lines there was no proliferation post treatment. Furthermore, production of IL-2, IL-3, and IL-4 during restimulation was reduced in the treated individuals (7). These results confirm that T cell anergy can be induced in man.

In vivo tolerization with peptides or proteins depends on administration in such a way as to preclude a costimulatory signal. This has been done in mouse strains susceptible to autoimmune encephalomyelitis (EAE) induced by immunization with myelin basic protein (MBP) in complete Freund's adjuvant (CFA). Intraperitoneal administration of either intact MBP or synthetic peptides (Ac 1–11 and 35–47) which correspond to the major immunodominant epitopes emulsified in incomplete Freund's adjuvant (IFA) tolerizes the animal to subsequent induction of EAE by immunization. More relevant to eventual therapeutic use is that animals can be immunized for EAE and at the first sign of disease be given the tolerizing regimen. The progression and severity of disease are blocked. Such treatment either before or after immunization induces anergy in proliferative, antigen-specific T cells (8).

A murine model for tolerance to an antigen important in human allergic disease, i.e., the principle allergen of cat hair and dander, *Fel d* 1, has been developed. The two peptide chains of this allergen (chains 1 and 2) have been cloned, sequenced and expressed (9). Mapping of the human T-cell epitopes for *Fel d* 1 has demonstrated that the majority of the T cell response is specific for a broad area of the protein contained within two 27 member peptides, IPC-1 and IPC-2, from *Fel d* 1 chain 1 (a 70 member peptide). Injections of IPC-2 subcutaneously were given before an immunizing dose of IPC-2 in CFA. IPC-2 specific production of IL-2, IL-4, and IFN-γ was decreased in the peptide tolerized animals in comparison with saline treated controls. In animals with a preexisting immune response induced by *Fel d* 1 in IFA, IPC-2 subcutaneously resulted in tolerization of T cells as evidenced by decreased IL-2 production when spleen cells were cultured with IPC-2. In another experiment, a combination of IPC-1 and IPC-2 produced as complete tolerance to subsequent immunization with chain 1 as did chain 1 itself (10). These results indicate that tolerance can be achieved without administering all possible T cell epitopes.

Indeed, tolerance to an allergen such as ragweed pollen that contains several allergenic proteins may be possible without epitopes from each protein. We showed many years ago that immunization with a single purified protein from ragweed, *Amb a* 1, would induce as useful a clinical tolerance as treatment with the whole extract containing many proteins (11).

Successful induction of tolerance to allergens in man depends on the development of peptides that do not interact with antibodies and thereby trigger immediate allergic responses. A survey of sera from cat sensitive humans has found no detectable interactions of IPC-1 or IPC-2 with IgE antibodies. A mix of these two peptides has therefore been proposed for human use. The goal would be achievement of T cell tolerance and the consequent downregulation of inflammatory responses on natural exposure to cats. Eventual decline of IgE antibodies to *Fel d* 1 might also be seen. Administration of potentially efficacious amounts of these substances has been started in cat sensitive patients. In a preliminary safety study 19 cat sensitive patients underwent intradermal tests with each peptide in concentrations up to 1500 mg/mL without an allergic response. Sixteen patients were started on increasing weekly doses of the two peptides given separately subcutaneously. Doses were 7.5, 75, 250, 750, and 1500 mg of each, the final dose being 500 nmol. In comparison, cat extract equivalent to

2.5 nmol *Fel d* 1 is the usual maximum tolerated dose for immunotherapy. The treatment was well tolerated. One asthmatic patient noted asthma after allergen skin testing and after the first injection and dropped out. After the 750 mg dose another asthmatic patient had an asthma attack at 6 hours and hives at 11 hours. A subsequent 250 mg dose was well tolerated. By ELISA, 2 patients developed low titers of IgE to peptides, but had had no allergic reaction to treatment. There was no change in IgE or IgG antibody titer to *Fel d* 1 (12). The relative safety and low antigenicity of AllerVax cat peptides have encouraged the initiation of several controlled studies of efficacy using either a cat room challenge model or bronchial provocation with cat extract. Dose per injection ranges from 7.5 to 750 mg in as many as four subcutaneous injections given a week apart.

Address for correspondence:

Philip S Norman
Johns Hopkins Asthma and Allergy Center
at the Francis Scott Key Medical Center
Allergy and Clinical Immunology Division
5501 Hopkins Bayview Circle
Baltimore, MD 21224-6801
USA

References

1. Norman PS. Immunotherapy for nasal allergy. *J Allergy Clin Immunol* 1988; 81:992–996.
2. Creticos PS, Marsh DG, Proud D, et al. Responses to ragweed-pollen nasal challenge before and after immunotherapy. *J Allergy Clin Immunol* 1989; 84(2):197–205.
3. Iliopoulos O, Proud D, Adkinson NF Jr. et al. Effects of immunotherapy on the early, late and rechallenge nasal reaction to provocation with allergen: Changes in inflammatory mediators and cells. *J Allergy Clin Immunol* 1991; 87:855–866.
4. Huang S-K, Marsh DG. Genetics of allergy. *Ann Allergy* 1993; 70:347–358.
5. OHehir RE, Garman RD, Greenstein JL, Lamb JR. The specificity and regulation of T-cell responsiveness to allergens. *Annu Rev Immunol* 1991; 9:67–95.
6. OHehir RE, Yssel H, Verma S, de Vries JE, Spits H, Lamb JR. Clonal analysis of differential lymphokine production in peptide and superantigen induced T cell anergy. *Int Immunol* 1991; 3:819–826.
7. Greenstein JL, Morgenstern JP, LaRaia J, et al. Ragweed immunotherapy decreases T cell reactivity to recombinant Amb a I. *J Allergy Clin Immunol* 1992; 89:322.
8. Gaur A, Wiers B, Liu A, Rothbard J, Fathman CG. Amelioration of autoimmune encephalomyelitis by myelin basic protein synthetic peptide-induced anergy. *Science* 1992; 258:1491–1494.
9. Morgenstern JP, Griggith IJ, Brauer AW, et al. Determination of the amino acid sequence of *Fel d* I, the major allergen of the domestic cat: Protein sequence analysis and cDNA cloning. *Proc Natl Acad Sci USA* 1991; 88:9690–9696.
10. Briner TJ, Kuo M-C, Keating KM, Rogers BL. Peripheral T-cell tolerance induced in naive and primed mice by subcutaneous injection of peptides from the major cat allergen *Fel d* I. *Proc Natl Acad Sci USA* 1993; 90:7608–7612.
11. Norman PS, Winkenwerder WL, Lichtenstein LM. Immunotherapy of hay fever with ragweed antigen E: Comparisons with whole pollen extract and placebos. *J Allergy* 1968; 42(2):93–108.
12. Norman PS, Ohman JL, Long AA, et al. Early clinical experience with T cell reactive peptides from cat allergen *Fel d* 1. *J Allergy Clin Immunol* 1994; 93:231 (Abstract).

Structure and Molecular Biology of Interleukin-5

Colin J Sanderson, Stéphane Karlen*

Keywords: Interleukin-5, eosinophils, IL-5 promoter, transgenic mice, IL-5 structure, IL-5 receptor, IL-2 promoter, IL-5 gene structure

Interleukin-5 (IL-5) is a disulfide-linked homodimer glycoprotein produced by T lymphocytes. The crystal structure of IL-5 has been determined. It is similar to the structure of other cytokines and most closely resembles IL-4 and GM-CSF. The monomer form of IL-5 consists of a bundle of four α-helices with two overconnecting loops. The dimer structure forms an elongated ellipsoidal disk, made up of two domains about a twofold axis. The two monomers are held together with two sulfide bridges connecting Cys44 of one molecule with Cys86 of the other. Only the IL-5 dimer is biologically active. The C-terminal domain appears to bind the α-chain of the receptor, and the N-terminal part of the protein seems to be involved in the interaction with the β-chain. IL-5 is produced by T cells and is often co-expressed with IL-4 after treatment with antigen, mitogen, or phorbol ester. After IL-2 treatment, however, only IL-5 mRNA can be detected, suggesting that IL-5 expression can be independently regulated. Corticosteroids were shown to inhibit IL-5 transcription, whereas progesterone and testosterone induce IL-5 transcription. The development of a transient assay in which the regulation of the IL-5 gene could be studied is therefore necessary to understand the complex mechanisms of IL-5 gene expression. By introducing the luciferase gene into the IL-5 genomic sequence, IL-5 promoter activity can be detected after treatment with a combination of phorbol myristate acetate and cyclic AMP, therefore providing a system in which IL-5 transcription can be monitored.

Introduction

Interleukin-5 (IL-5) is produced by T lymphocytes as a glycoprotein with an M_r of 40,000–45,000, and is unusual among the T-cell-produced cytokines in being a disulfide-linked homodimer. It is the most highly conserved member of a group of evolutionarily related cytokines, including also IL-3, IL-4, and granulocyte/macrophage colony stimulating factor (GM-CSF), which are closely linked on human chromosome 5.

There are two intriguing aspects of these dual biological activities of IL-5. Firstly, although there is a well-known association between eosinophilia and IgE levels, IL-5 does not appear to be involved in the IgE response, where IL-4 is the major controlling cytokine. Secondly, although the activity on murine B cells *in vitro* is well characterized (see below), hIL-5 is not active in assays on human B cells analogous to those used in the mouse system.

The role of IL-5 in eosinophilia, coupled with a better understanding of the part played by eosinophils in the development of tissue damage in chronic allergy, suggests that IL-5 will be a major target for a new generation of anti-allergy drugs.

Protein Structure

IL-5 is unusual among the T-cell-produced cytokines in being a disulfide-linked homodimeric glycoprotein which is highly homologous between species (Figure 1), with cross reactivity of the protein across a variety of mammalian species. Studies with mouse IL-5 indicate that the monomer has no biological activity and has no inhibitory activity, suggesting that it does not form high affinity interactions with the IL-5 receptor (1). The dimer exists in an antiparallel (head to tail) configuration (1–3).

Mature human IL-5 monomer comprises 115 amino acids (M_r of 12,000, and 24,000 for the dimer). The secreted material has a M_r of 40,000–45,000, and so nearly half the native material consists of carbohydrate. Human IL-5 has one N-linked carbohydrate chain at position Asn28, and one O-linked carbohydrate at position Thr3 (2).

* Institute for Child Health Research, Perth, Western Australia.

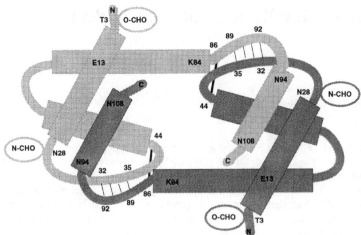

Figure 1. Diagram based on the crystal structure (7) of hIL-5 showing the main structural features. One monomer is shown in light gray and the other in dark gray. Helices are indicated A-D, and A'-D', respectively, starting at the N terminus (N). The disulfide bridges connecting cysteines at positions 44 and 86 are shown as black lines. The interactions between anti-parallel β-sheets are shown by fine black lines (residues 32–35 and 89–92). The attachment positions of O-linked carbohydrate (O-CHO) attached to residue 3 and N-linked carbohydrate (N-CHO) attached to residue 28 are indicated (5).

Mouse IL-5 has an additional N-linked carbohydrate at Asn55 (4); this site does not exist in hIL-5. The potential N-linked site at Asn71 is apparently not glycosylated in either species. Deglycosylated IL-5 has been reported to have full (5) activity or increased activity (6) *in vitro*.

The crystal structure of human IL-5 (7) shows it to be similar to the structures of other cytokines. It most closely resembles IL-4 and GM-CSF, which consist of a bundle of four a-helices (A, B, C, D from the N-terminus) with two overconnecting loops. The dimer structure of IL-5 forms an elongated ellipsoidal disk, made up of two domains about a twofold axis (Figure 1). Remarkably, each domain is made up of three helices from one monomer (A, B, C) and one helix (D') from the other. The two monomers are held together by two sulfide bridges connecting Cys44 of one molecule with Cys86 of the other. In addition residues 32 to 35 form an anti-parallel β-sheet with residues 89 to 92 of the other monomer. A large proportion of the monomer surface is at the interface of the two monomers. It is possible that the lack of biological activity in the monomer results from instability due to exposure of hydrophilic residues normally concealed in the dimer.

Il-5 Receptor Interaction

There is an area of sequence similarity, determined using Dayhoff mutation indices, at the C-terminal region of a number of different cytokines, including IL-5 (8). This region lies in helix D of IL-5, IL-4, and GM-CSF. Making use of the 100-fold lower specific activity of hIL-5 when tested in a mouse assay system, a series of human-mouse hybrid IL-5 molecules were constructed and tested for biological activity and receptor displacement. The C-terminal third of the molecule was found to determine the species specificity (9). This region contains eight residues which differ between human and mouse, two at the end of the C helix, three in the D helix, and the remaining three in the C-terminal tail. Determination of the residue(s) involved in species specificity will locate the region of interaction with the α-chain of the receptor more accurately. Despite the twofold symmetry of the IL-5 dimer, which suggests two potential binding sites for the receptor, the α-chain of the receptor appears to bind to IL-5 in a 1:1 ratio (10).

Experiments with GM-CSF suggest that the β-chain may bind in the region of residue 21 (11), and a series of mouse-human GM-CSF hybrids identified residue 20 as important in the interaction with the β-chain. Furthermore, a hybrid in which the N-terminal region of GM-CSF was substituted by the analogous region from IL-5 showed strong biological activity. This very elegant approach demonstrated that IL-5 uses the same β-receptor subunit as GM-CSF, and implies an interaction between the β-chain and the N-terminal region of the cytokine molecule (12). A comparison of the structure of IL-5 and GM-CSF suggests that the interaction site between IL-5 and the β-chain in the complex is Glu13 (13).

Gene Structure and Expression

Sequence information is available for both the human and mouse genomic genes (14, 15). There appears to be only a single copy of the gene per haploid genome. The coding sequence of the IL-5 gene forms four exons. The introns show areas of similarity between the mouse and human sequences, although the mouse has a considerable amount of sequence (including repeat sequences) which is not present in the human gene. Interestingly, the mouse gene includes a 738-base-pair segment in the 3'-untranslated region which is not present in the human gene. Each of the exons contains the codons for an exact number of amino acids, and in each case begins with GT and ends in AG. These features of the gene structure are also shared by IL-3, IL-4, and GM-CSF. All four cytokine genes are located in tandem on chromosome 5 in man (16–18) and on chromosome 11 in the mouse (19). Although there is no overall sequence homology, at either the nucleotide or amino acid level, between any of these four cytokines, the localization and structural similarities suggest a common evolutionary origin (8). In addition, they are all produced by T cells and show an overlap in some of their biological activities; thus they may be regarded as members of a gene family.

In T cells, transcription is induced by antigen, mitogens, and phorbol esters, and occurs for about 24 h before the gene becomes silent again (20). Studies with T cell clones *in vitro* indicate that IL-4 and IL-5 are often co-expressed in clones designated Th2 (21). However, anti-CD3 induces the expression of IL-4, IL-5, and GM-CSF mRNA in mouse T cells, whereas treatment with IL-2 induced IL-5 mRNA expression but did not induce detectable IL-4 or GM-CSF (22). The fact that eosinophilia can occur without increases in other leukocytes suggests an independent control for IL-5 expression, while the association between high levels of IgE antibody and eosinophilia suggests coordinate expression of IL-4 and IL-5 in these cases.

Corticosteroids inhibit IL-5 production both *in vivo* (23) and *in vitro* (24, 25). This may be an important mechanism of corticosteroid activity in asthma. Both progesterone and testosterone induce IL-5 transcription, which can be inhibited by dexamethasone but not by cyclosporine (25). These observations suggest complex mechanisms of IL-5 gene expression which are not yet understood. The fact that lymphocytes from the CD2-IL-5 trans-

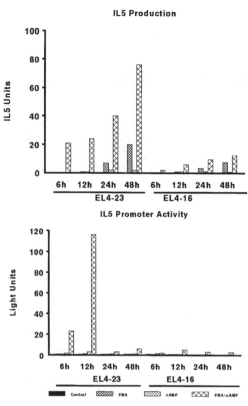

Figure 2. Production of IL-5 and activity of the IL-5 promoter in two sublines of EL4. The construct containing the luciferase gene inserted into the IL-5 genomic sequence was electroporated into EL4 cells. 24 h later, cells were stimulated with PMA (10 ng/ml), cAMP (1 mM) and a combination of the two. At different times after stimulation cells were harvested: the supernatant was tested for IL-5 production (top panel) and the cell pellet for luciferase activity (bottom panel).

genic mice produced high levels of IL-5 when stimulated with concanavalin A (26) suggested that the transgene did carry the sequences for normal inducible expression in T cells. The 10 kb fragment of mouse DNA used to produce these transgenic mice was therefore a good starting point for studying the expression of IL-5 *in vitro*. The luciferase reporter gene was inserted into the IL-5 genomic sequence, upstream of the cap site, without deleting any of the genomic sequences (Figure 2). This construct was electroporated into two subclones of mouse EL4 lymphoma cells. 24 h after electroporation, the cells were stimulated with phorbol myristate acetate (PMA) and cyclic AMP (cAMP) and combinations of the two.

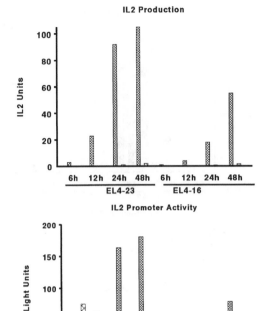

Figure 3. Production of IL-2 and activity of the IL-2 promoter in two sublines of EL4. A construct containing 600 bp of the human IL-2 promoter linked to the luciferase gene was electroporated into EL4 cells and analyzed as described in Figure 3. The supernatant was tested for IL-2 production (top panel) and the cell pellet for luciferase activity (bottom panel).

Expression of the reporter gene was monitored at different times. 12 h after stimulation with a combination of PMA and cAMP, expression from the IL-5 promoter in EL4–23 cells was at his highest (Figure 3). However, PMA and cAMP alone were shown to have almost no effect on promoter activity. In EL4–16, a subclone which produces only low level of IL-5, very low promoter activity was observed. Both EL4–23 and EL4–16 express IL-2 (Figure 4). 48 h after stimulation, high expression from the IL-2 promoter was observed in cells stimulated with PMA. This stimulation was partially inhibited when cAMP was used in combination with PMA. In contrast, stimulation of the IL-2 promoter with PMA alone was almost ineffective 6 h after addition of the activator, and promoter activity could be observed only in the presence of both PMA and cAMP.

cAMP has been involved in the regulation of IL-5 gene expression by acting synergistically with PMA (27). Although both activators were necessary for efficient production of IL-5, incubation with PMA alone was sufficient (Figure 3). In a transient assay, however, incubation with PMA alone led to no detectable IL-5 promoter activity, whereas expression from the IL-5 promoter was considerably increased 6–12 h after addition of both PMA and cAMP, before dropping again to background levels. These observations suggested that cAMP in combination with PMA is required for early promoter activity.

The stimulatory effect of cAMP during early transcription does not seem to be restricted to IL-5. Although cAMP has been shown to have a strong inhibitory effect on IL-2 production (27, 28), we observed that the activity of the IL-2 promoter was first increased in the presence of both PMA and cAMP (Figure 4). Only later after stimulation (12–24 h) could the inhibitory effect of cAMP be seen on PMA-induced IL-2 promoter activity.

The mechanisms of cAMP actions are unknown. cAMP acts probably via activation of the protein kinase A pathway and has been shown to affect the binding of several transcription factors, including NF-kB (28). In the context of IL-5 transcription, it could be envisaged that cAMP modifies the binding of a repressor and therefore activates transcription from the IL-5 promoter.

Address for correspondence:

Colin J Sanderson
ICHR
GPO Box 855
West Perth WA 6872
Australia

References

1. McKenzie ANJ, Ely B, Sanderson CJ. Mutated interleukin-5 monomers are biologically inactive. *Mol Immunol* 1991; 28:155.

2. Minamitake Y, Kodama S, Katayama T, Adachi H, Tanaka S, Tsujimoto M. Structure of recombinant human interleukin 5 produced by Chinese hamster ovary cells. *J Biochem Tokyo* 1990; 107:292.

3. Proudfoot AE, Davies JG, Turcatti G, Wingfield PT. Human interleukin-5 expressed in *Escherichia coli*: Assignment of the disulfide bridges of the purified unglycosylated protein. *FEBS Lett* 1991; 283:61.

4. Kodama S, Endo T, Tsujimoto M, Kobata A. Characterization of recombinant murine interleukin 5 expressed in Chinese hamster ovary cells. *Glycobiology* 1992; 2:419.

5. Tominaga A, Takahashi T, Kikuchi Y, Mita S, Noami S, Harada N, Yamaguchi N, Takatsu K. Role of carbohydrate moiety of IL5: Effect of tunicamycin on the glycosyation of IL5 and the biologic activity of deglycosylated IL5. *J Immunol* 1990; 144:1345.

6. Kodama S, Tsujimoto M, Tsuruoka N, Sugo T, Endo T, Kobata A. Role of sugar chains in the *in-vitro* activity of recombinant human interleukin-5. *Eur J Biochem* 1993; 211:903.

7. Milburn M, Hassell AM, Lambert MH, Jordan SR, Proudfoot AEI, Grabar P, Wells TNC. A novel dimer configuration revealed by the crystal structure at 2.4Å resolution of human interleukin-5. *Nature* 1993; 363:172.

8. Sanderson CJ, Campbell HD, Young IG. Molecular and cellular biology of eosinophil differentiation factor (interleukin-5) and its effects on human and mouse B cells. *Immunol Rev* 1988; 102:29.

9. McKenzie ANJ, Barry SC, Strath M, Sanderson CJ. Structure-function analysis of interleukin-5 utilizing mouse/human chimeric molecules. *EMBO J* 1991; 10:1193.

10. Devos R, Guisez Y, Cornelis S, Verhee A, Van der Heyden J, Manneberg M, Lahm H-W, Fiers W, Tavernier J, Plaetinck G. Recombinant soluble human interleukin-5 (hIL-5) receptor molecules. Cross-linking and stoichiometry of binding to IL-5. *J Biol Chem* 1993; 268:6581.

11. Lopez AF, Shannon MF, Hercus T, Nicola NA, Camareri B, Dottore M, Layton MJ, Eglinton L, Vadas MA. Residue 21 of human granulocyte-macrophage colony-stimulating factor is critical for biological activity and for high but not low afinity binding. *EMBO J* 1992; 11:(in press).

12. Scanafelt AB, Miyajima A, Kitamura T, Kastelelein RA. The amino-terminal helix of GM-CSF and IL-5 governs high affinity binding to their receptors. *EMBO J* 1991; 10:4105.

13. Lopez AF, Elliott MJ, Woodcock J, Vadas MA. GM-CSF, IL-3 and IL-5: Cross-competition on human haemopoietic cells. *Immunol Today* 1992; 13:495.

14. Campbell HD, Tucker WQ, Hort Y, Martinson ME, Mayo G, Clutterbuck EJ, Sanderson CJ, Young IG. Molecular cloning, nucleotide sequence, and expression of the gene encoding human eosinophil differentiation factor (interleukin 5). *Proc Natl Acad Sci USA* 1987; 84:6629.

15. Campbell HD, Sanderson CJ, Wang Y, Hort Y, Martinson ME, Tucker WQ, Stellwagen A, Strath M, Young IG. Isolation, structure and expression of cDNA and genomic clones for murine eosinophil differentiation factor. Comparison with other eosinophilopoietic lymphokines and identity with interleukin-5. *Eur J Biochem* 1988; 174:345.

16. Sutherland GR, Baker E, Callen DF, Campbell HD, Young IG, Sanderson CJ, Garson OM, Lopez AF, Vadas MA. Interleukin-5 is at 5q31 and is deleted in the 5q- syndrome. *Blood* 1988; 71:1150.

17. van-Leeuwen BH, Martinson ME, Webb GC, Young IG. Molecular organization of the cytokine gene cluster, involving the human IL-3, IL-4, IL-5, and GM-CSF genes, on human chromosome. *Blood* 1989; 73:1142.

18. Chandrasekharappa SC, Rebelsky MS, Firak TA, Le Beau MM, Westbrook CA. A long-range restriction map of the interleukin-4 and interleukin-5 linkage group on chromosome 5. *Genomics* 1990; 6:94.

19. Lee JS, Campbell HD, Kozak CA, Young IG. The IL-4 and IL-5 genes are closely linked and are part of a cytokine gene cluster on mouse chromosome 11. *Somat Cell Genet* 1989; 15:143.

20. Tominaga A, Matsumoto M, Harada N, Takahashi T, Kikuchi Y, Takatsu K. Molecular properties and regulation of mRNA expression for murine T cell-replacing factor/IL-5. *J Immunol* 1988; 140:1175.

21. Coffman RL, Seymour BWP, Lebman DA, Hiraki DD, Christiansen JA, Shrader B, Cherwinski HM, Savelkoul HFJ, Finkelman FD, Bond MW, Mosmann TR. The role of helper T cell products in mouse B cell differentiation and isotype regulation. *Immunol Rev* 1988; 102:5.

22. Bohjanen PR, Okajima M, Hodes RJ. Differential regulation of interleukin 4 and interleukin 5 gene expression: a comparison of T-cell gene induction by anti-CD3 antibody or by exogenous lymphokines. *Proc Natl Acad Sci USA* 1990; 87:5283.

23. Corrigan CJ, Haczku A, Gemou-Engesaeth V, Doi S, Kikuchi Y, Takatsu K, Durham SR, Kay AB. CD4 T-lymphocyte activation in asthma is accompanied by increased serum concentrations of interleukin-5: Effect of glucocorticoid therapy. *Am Rev Respir Dis* 1993; 147:540.

24. Rolfe FG, Hughes JM, Armour CL, Sewell WA. Inhibition of interleukin-5 gene expression by dexamethasone. *Immunology* 1992; 77:494.

25. Wang Y, Campbell HD, Young IG. Sex hormones and dexamethasone modulate interleukin-5 gene expression in T lymphocytes. *J Steroid Biochem Mol Biol* 1993; 44:203.

26. Dent LA, Strath M, Mellor AL, Sanderson CJ. Eosinophilia in transgenic mice expressing interleukin 5. *J Exp Med* 1990; 172:1425.

27. Lee HJ, Koyano-Nakawaga N, Naito Y, Nishida J, Arai N, Arai KI, Yokota T. cAMP activates the IL-5 promoter synergistically with phorbol phorbol ester through the signaling pathway involving proteine kinase A in mouse thymoma line EL-4. *J Immunol* 1993; 151:6135.

28. Chen D, Rothenberg E. Interleukin 2 transcription factors as molecular targets of cAMP inhibition: Delayed inhibition kinetics and combinatorial transcription roles. *J Exp Med* 1994; 179:931.

Interleukin-5 (IL-5) Receptors: Structure and Function

Kiyoshi Takatsu, Satoshi Takaki, Takuya Katagiri, Yasumichi Hitoshi, Yuji Kikuchi*

Keywords: IL-5, IL-5 receptor, signaling, proto-oncogene, tyrosine phosphorylation, Btk, JAK kinase

Interleukin-5 (IL-5) regulates the production and function of B cells, eosinophils, and basophils. The IL-5 receptor (IL-5R) consists of two distinct membrane proteins, α and β. The α chain (IL-5Rα) specifically binds IL-5. The β chain (βc) is indispensable for signal transduction and common to receptors for IL-5, IL-3, and granulocyte-macrophage colony-stimulating factor (GM-CSF). IL-5 stimulation results in the rapid tyrosine phosphorylation of βc and proteins containing *Src*-homology 2 (SH2) and/or SH3 domains such as phosphatidyl-inositol-3 (PI-3) kinase, Shc, Vav and HS1. IL-5 stimulation significantly activated Bruton's tyrosine kinase (Btk) and enhanced the tyrosine phosphorylation of Lyn and JAK2 protein tyrosine kinases. Both the cytoplasmic domain of βc and the membrane proximal proline-rich sequence of the cytoplasmic domain of IL-5Rα were found to be essential for the IL-5-induced proliferative response, expression of nuclear proto-oncogenes such as c-*jun*, c-*fos*, and c-*myc*, and tyrosine phosphorylation of cellular proteins. Analysis using chimeric receptors with the extracellular domain of IL-5Rα and the cytoplasmic domain of the βc suggested that dimerization of the cytoplasmic domain of the bc may be important in activating the IL-5R complex and transducing intracellular signaling.

Introduction

Interleukin-5 (IL-5) is a cytokine that regulates the production and function of B cells, eosinophils, and basophils (1–4). The IL-5 receptor (IL-5R) consists of two distinct membrane proteins, α and β. IL-5Rα alone specifically binds IL-5, but with low affinity (5, 6). While the β chain does not bind IL-5 by itself, it is required not only for high-affinity binding, but is also essential for IL-5 signal transduction (7–11). The β chain is common to receptors for IL-3 and granulocyte-macrophage colony-stimulating factor (GM-CSF) (12–16) and is called as βc. As IL-5, IL-3, and GM-CSF display a variety of overlapping actions for production and activation of eosinophils (4), βc shared by these three cytokine receptors provides the molecular basis for the functional redundancy of these cytokines. The extracellular domain of IL-5Rα and the βc are similar among members of the cytokine receptor superfamily. The α chain has a short cytoplasmic domain (~55 amino acid residues) with a short amino acid sequence (2, 5). The βc has a relatively large cytoplasmic domain (~440 amino acid residues) as compared to those of the α chain (12). The cytoplasmic domains of both the α chain and the βc have no homology with signaling molecules such as kinases, phosphatases, nucleotide binding proteins, or *src* homology domains.

Growth factors trigger proliferation of cells when they bind to their specific receptors. Receptors complexed with ligand provide signals that are transmitted through cascades of biochemical reactions. Phosphorylation of tyrosine residues on signal-transducing molecules is essential for activation of a signaling pathway. Several tyrosine-phosphorylated effector molecules for growth control have been identified on growth factor receptors. These effector molecules are phospholipase Cγ (PLC-γ), phosphatidylinositol-3 (PI-3) kinase, and Ras-associated GTPase-activating protein (GAP) (17–19), which contain *Src*-homology 2 (SH2) and/or *Src*-homology 3 (SH3) domains. The former binds to phosphorylated tyrosine on the protein and the latter is suggested to be responsible for the targeting of signaling molecules to specific subcellular locations. Although tyrosine phosphorylation of cellular proteins has been reported in various cytokine/cytokine receptor systems, we have little information on the PTKs involved in cytokine signaling, except that IL-2R β chain is associated with p56 ^{lck} (20). Recent studies have also shown that some cytokine receptors form receptor dimers by means of ligand binding. The dimerization of the receptor molecule, which has a large cytoplasmic

* Department of Immunology, Institute of Medical Science, University of Tokyo, Japan.

domain, may be a common mechanism for activation of and signal transduction through cytokine receptors (21).

IL-5, IL-3, and GM-CSF have been shown to induce a rapid tyrosine phosphorylation of cellular proteins (22, 23) and transcription of nuclear proto-oncogenes. Issues remaining to be resolved include how many receptor subunits the high-affinity IL-5R is composed of, and how the IL-5R complex activates the signal transduction machinery in the cell interior. Here we will show that IL-5Rα, together with βc, is essential for cell proliferation and tyrosine phosphorylation of cellular proteins in response to IL-5. We also demonstrate that IL-5 stimulation induces rapid tyrosine phosphorylation of βc and proteins containing one or two SH2 and/or SH3 domains, and enhances Bruton's tyrosine kinase (Btk) activity. We will also discuss the critical role of the membrane proximal proline-rich region in the induction of c-*fos*, c-*jun*, and c-*myc*, and tyrosine phosphorylation of cellular proteins.

Results

Cytoplasmic Regions Rich in Proline Residues of IL-5Rα Are Indispensable for the Interaction with βc for Signaling

A murine IL-3-dependent cell line, FDC-P1, intrinsically expresses βc. FDC-P1 transfectants (FDC-5R) expressing the wild type IL-5Rα, but not the mutant IL-5Rα (FDC-5RαΔcyto), which lacks the entire cytoplasmic domain, become responsive to IL-5 (11). These results indicate that the cytoplasmic region of IL-5Rα is indispensable for IL-5-mediated growth signal transduction. To identify the regions of the cytoplasmic domain of IL-5Rα which are critical for signaling, we created four different mutant cDNAs of IL-5Rα each of which had a deletion of 6 amino acid residues in its cytoplasmic domain (Figure 1A). DC1 and DC2 had a deletion in the region rich in proline residues and a deletion in the region adjacent to the proline-rich region, respectively. DC3 and DC4 had deletions in the carboxy-terminal region that is unique to IL-5Rα. Regardless of the cytoplasmic deletions, all four different transfectants expressed similar levels of IL-5Rα on their cell surfaces detected by anti-IL-5Rα mAb and expressed high-affinity IL-5-binding sites with K_d values equivalent to those of transfectants expressing the wild type IL-5Rα (24). These results indicate that mutations induced in the cytoplasmic domain of IL-5Rα do not affect the interactions of IL-5Rα with IL-5 or the βc, thereby facilitating reconstitution of the high-affinity IL-5R. As shown in Figure 2, DC3 and DC4 transfectants proliferated well upon stimulation with IL-5 in a dose dependent manner. In contrast, DC1 transfectants did not respond to IL-5. DC2 transfectants proliferated only with high concentrations of IL-5 in the culture. These results indicate that the region rich in proline residues, in the cytoplasmic domain of IL-5Rα, is essential for IL-5-mediated growth signal transduction. It is also clear that the proximal region, downstream from

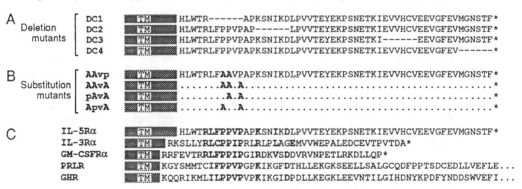

Figure 1. Cytoplasmic domains of the mutant mIL-5Rα used in this study. All mutants of IL-5Rα have the wild type extracellular domain. *(A)* Deletion mutants; bars represent deleted amino acid residues. *(B)* Substitution mutants; amino acid residues indicated by bold letters have been replaced with alanine. Dots represent the same amino acid residues as these of the wild type mIL-5Rα. *(C)* Comparison of the amino acid sequence of cytoplasmic domains of murine IL-5Rα, IL-3Rα, GM-CSFRα, prolactin receptor (PRLR), and growth hormone receptor (GHR). Conserved and related amino acid residues were indicated by bold letters. Shaded boxes with "TM" represent the transmembrane portion.

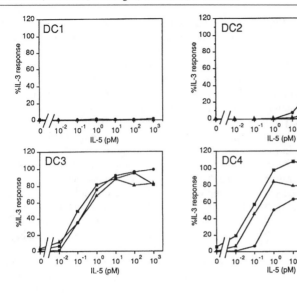

Figure 2. Proliferation of FDC-P1 transfectants expressing the deletion mutants of IL-5Rα. Transfectants were incubated for 48 h in the presence of various concentrations of IL-5 and incorporated [³H]thymidine was measured. The results were expressed as the percentage of [³H]thymidine incorporation in the same cells incubated with 100 units/ml of IL-3.

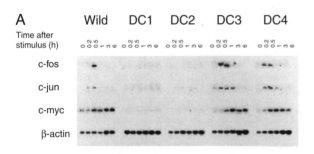

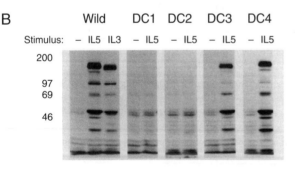

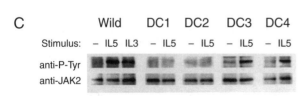

Figure 3. IL-5-induced cellular responses in FDC-P1 transfectants expressing the IL-5R α deletion mutants. *(A)* Induction of early response proto-oncogenes. Cytokine-starved cells were stimulated with 2 nM IL-5 for the indicated times (0, 0.2, 0.5, 1, 3, 6 h). Total RNA (10 µg) was separated through 1% agarose gel and transferred onto a nylon membrane. The membranes were hybridized with radiolabeled DNA probes, washed, and analyzed using a BAS-2000 Bio-Image analyzer. *(B)* Tyrosine phosphorylation of cellular proteins. Cytokine-depleted cells were either unstimulated (–) or stimulated with 2 nM of IL-5 (IL5) for 5 min. Transfectants expressing the wild type IL-5Rα were also stimulated with 2000 U/ml of IL-3 (IL3). Cell lysates (equivalent to 1×10^6 cells/lane) were separated by SDS-8% PAGE and immunoblotted with the monoclonal anti-PY mAb. *(C)* Tyrosine phosphorylation of JAK2 protein tyrosine kinase. Cell lysates, prepared as described above, were incubated with anti-serum against JAK2 and the immune complexes were precipitated. Protein samples were subjected to SDS 7.5% PAGE and transferred to PVDF membranes. The membranes were immunoblotted with anti-PY mAb and phosphorylated proteins were identified (upper). The same membranes were immunoblotted with anti-serum against JAK2 (lower).

the proline-rich area, is important, though not essential.

Induction of nuclear proto-oncogene expression has been clearly established to be critical for cytokine signal transduction. We examined the induction of c-*fos*, c-*jun*, and c-*myc* transcripts by Northern blot analysis in response to IL-5. In the wild type IL-5Rα transfectants, expression of c-*fos*, c-*jun*, and c-*myc* proto-oncogene mRNA was rapidly induced upon stimulation with IL-5 (Figure 3A). Increased levels of expression of these proto-oncogenes were also observed in DC3 and DC4 transfectants and were comparable to those observed in transfectants of the wild type IL-5Rα. In contrast, the above proto-oncogene expression were not induced in DC1 transfectants in response to stimulation with IL-5. In DC2 transfectants, induction of these proto-oncogenes was initially weak, but became significant with prolonged membrane exposure (data not shown). We observed the induction of c-*fos*, c-*jun*, and c-*myc* mRNA upon stimulation with IL-3, and the levels of expression of these proto-oncogenes were nearly the same in all four deletion mutant transfectants (data not shown).

We have shown that IL-5 induces rapid tyrosine phosphorylation of at least five distinct cellular proteins in the IL-5-dependent early B cell line T88-M (23). We also analyzed protein-tyrosine phosphorylations in the transfectants. In the wild type IL-5Rα transfectants, several tyrosine-phosphorylated cellular proteins (130–140, 120, 95, 70, 55, 50, 42 kDa) were also observed within 10 min of stimulation with IL-5 (Figure 3B). Their phosphorylation patterns were essentially the same as those induced by IL-3. A tyrosine-phosphorylated protein with 130 to 140 kDa over a period of 20 min following stimulation was shown to be βc by immunoprecipitation with anti-βc mAb followed by Western blotting with anti-phosphotyrosine (PY) mAb (Satoh et al. submitted). No phosphorylated cellular proteins were detected in DC1 and DC2 transfectants following IL-5 stimulation (Figure 3B), while IL-3 stimulation induced comparable levels of tyrosine phosphorylation of cellular proteins in all four deletion mutant transfectants (data not shown). In DC3 and DC4 transfectants, similar sets of cellular proteins were phosphorylated in response to IL-5 stimulation.

It has been reported that IL-3 stimulation results in rapid and specific tyrosine phosphorylation of JAK2 protein-tyrosine kinase in IL-3-dependent cells (25). We therefore investigated tyrosine phosphorylation of JAK2 in mutant IL-5Rα transfec-

tants. As shown in Figure 3C, JAK2 kinase was tyrosine phosphorylated upon stimulation of the wild type IL-5Rα transfectants with both IL-5 and IL-3. In DC3 and DC4 transfectants, IL-5 stimulation resulted in marked tyrosine phosphorylation of JAK2. In DC1 and DC2 transfectants, however, tyrosine phosphorylation of JAK2 was barely detectable following IL-5 stimulation.

Identification of Critical Amino Acid Residues in the Cytoplasmic Region Rich in Proline Residues by Substitution Analysis

To identify the critical amino acid residues in the cytoplasmic region of IL-5Rα, we made IL-5Rα mutants with a single amino acid substitution: alanine replacement of Arg^{349}, Phe^{351}, Pro^{353}, Pro^{355}, Lys^{358}, or Asp^{363}. The transfectants were tested for IL-5-induced proliferation and the comparative proliferative responses to those of wild type IL-5Rα transfectants. Next, we generated mutants (Figure 1B). Transfectants of IL-5Rα mutants in which alanine was substituted for two or three proline residues expressed high-affinity IL-5 binding sites and K_d values nearly the same as those of transfectants expressing the wild type IL-5R. Substitution of Pro^{352} and Pro^{353} for Ala (AAvp mutant), or Pro^{353} and Pro^{355} for Ala (pAvA mutant), resulted in transfectants showing a proliferative response to IL-5. Substitution of Pro^{352} and Pro^{355} for Ala (ApvA mutant) lead to a slightly impaired proliferative response to IL-5. Substitution of all three proline residues for Ala (AAvA) resulted in a complete loss of IL-5-induced proliferation (24). These results indicate that the existence, in IL-5Rα, of one of these three proline residues is adequate for IL-5 signal transduction. In addition, Pro^{352} and Pro^{355}, in the proline-rich region, appear to have a more critical function in the cytoplasmic domain of IL-5Rα than does Pro^{353}.

Chimeric Molecules of IL-5Rα with the βc Can Transduce IL-5 Signals

In addition to growth factor receptors having intrinsic tyrosine kinase activity, some cytokine receptors, such as growth hormone receptor, gp130 of IL-6R, and GM-CSFR, are activated by forming receptor dimers (21, 26). As described above, all functions of the cytoplasmic domain of IL-5Rα in signal transduction depend on the short-stretch proline-rich region. It is likely, therefore, that IL-

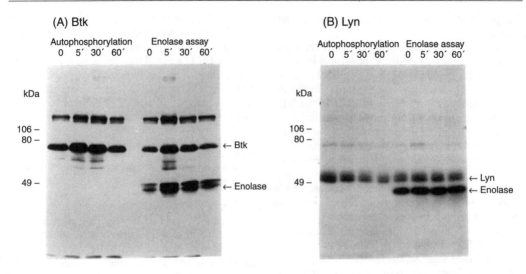

Figure 4. Time-courses of Btk *(A)* and Lyn *(B)* kinase activities in IL-5-stimulated Y16 cells. Y16 cells were stimulated with mIL-5 for 0, 5, 30, or 60 min. Cells were lysed and immunoprecipitated with anti-Btk or anti-Lyn antibodies. Immune complexes were subjected to SDS-PAGE analysis on 8% polyacrylamide gels. Kinase assays were conducted as described, and kinase activity was detected by autoradiography. *(A)* Autophosphorylation and enolase phosphorylation resulting from anti-Btk immune-complex kinase assay were revealed by autoradiography. The positions to which Btk and enolase migrated are indicated, and marker proteins are given in κDa. *(B)* Autophosphorylation and enolase phosphorylation, resulting from the immune-complex kinase activity of immunoprecipitates using anti-Lyn antibodies, were detected by autoradiography. The position of Lyn and enolase migrated are indicated and marker proteins are given in κDa.

5Rα may only amplify dimerization, resulting in transduction of an IL-5-mediated growth signal that is mediated through its proline-rich cytoplasmic regions. To evaluate this hypothesis, we generated chimeric receptor molecules consisting of the extracellular domain of IL-5Rα with the cytoplasmic domain of the βc. Two chimeric receptors with transmembrane portions from IL-5Rα (ααβ mutant) or βc (αββ mutant) were generated. FDC-P1 transfectants of these two chimeric receptors were capable of proliferating in response to IL-5. Expressions of c-*fos*, c-*jun*, and c-*myc* transcripts were also induced by IL-5 stimulation. In addition, a set of cellular proteins were tyrosine-phosphorylated upon stimulation with IL-5. These intracellular changes, induced by IL-5 stimulation, appeared to be weak in the chimeric receptor transfectants as compared to that in the wild type IL-5Rα transfectant. The patterns of proto-oncogene and tyrosine phosphorylation were, however, similar to these observed in transfectants of the wild type IL-5Rα. The growth-related signals for IL-5, including induction of proto-oncogene expression and tyrosine phosphorylation of cellular

proteins, appeared to be transduced by dimerization (multimerization) of the cytoplasmic domain of the βc without the cytoplasmic domain of IL-5Rα.

IL-5 Stimulation Induces Tyrosine-Phosphorylation of βc and Cellular Proteins Containing One or Two SH2 and/or SH3 Domains

We then investigated IL-5-induced tyrosine phosphorylations of PLC-γ, GAP, PI-3 kinase, Shc, p95[Vav], and p75[HSI], all of which contain SH2 and/or SH3 domains. Immunoprecipitation followed by immunoblot analysis of cell lysates of IL-5-stimulated Y16 cells, using polyclonal or monoclonal antibodies specific for each of the above proteins, revealed that Y16 cells expressed all of these molecules. The cell lysates of IL-5-stimulated Y16 cells immunoprecipitated with anti-PI-3 kinase antibody, followed by immunoblotting with anti-PY mAb, revealing that marked tyrosine-phosphorylation of PI-3 kinase had occurred in response to IL-5 stimulation. In contrast, no bands corresponding to tyrosine-phosphorylated PLC-γ or GAP were detected, under similar assay conditions, by immunoprecipitation with antibodies specific for each protein, regardless of how long the cells were stimulated with IL-5 (1–30 min). No tyrosine-phosphorylated protein bands were observed even when the samples were immunoprecipitated with anti-PY mAbs and then immunoblotted with anti-PLC-γ or anti-GAP antibodies. Intriguingly, Vav, Shc, and HS1 proteins were tyrosine-phosphorylated within 5 min of being stimulated with IL-5 but had disappeared by 30 min after IL-5 stimulation. No tyrosine-phosphorylation of any of these SH2/SH3-containing proteins was observed in IL-5-stimulated FDC-5RαΔcyto.

Bruton's Tyrosine Kinase, Btk, is Activated Upon IL-5 Stimulation

Bruton's tyrosine kinase (Btk), a B-cell specific cytosolic tyrosine kinase, was recently cloned and identified as the molecule involved in X-linked human agammaglobulinemia (XLA) (27, 28). A single conserved residue within the amino terminal unique region of Btk was shown to be mutated in XID mice (29, 30), the B cells of which, but not eosinophils, showed impaired responsiveness to IL-5 (31). Lyn kinase was reported to be associated with B-cell antigen receptors and to play roles in B-cell development, and has also been suggested to be associated with the signaling cascade mediated by IL-3R and GM-CSFR in myeloid cell lines. Thus, we examined the effects of IL-5 on kinase activities for Btk and Lyn. Cell lysates were immunoprecipitated with anti-Btk and anti-Lyn antibodies, and each of the immunoprecipitates was used for an *in vitro* kinase assay. We monitored kinase activities by autophosphorylation of each kinase and the phosphorylation of enolase, an exogenously added substrate. As shown in Figure 4A, significantly enhanced Btk kinase activity (two to three times higher than that of unstimulated controls) was detected in anti-Btk immunoprecipitates of Y16 cells stimulated with IL-5 for 5–20 min by

both the autophosphorylation and the enolase assay. In contrast, no significant enhancement of either Lyn (Figure 4B) kinase activity was detected under the conditions employed. No enhancement of Btk activity was detected in IL-5-stimulated FDC-5RαΔcyto (data not shown).

Discussion

We described four major observations in this study:
1. The cytoplasmic domain of IL-5Rα is indispensable, together with βc, for IL-5-mediated growth signaling. In particular, the membrane proximal proline-rich sequences and the adjacent downstream proline-rich region are essential and important. These two regions are well conserved among IL-5Rα, IL-3Rα, and GM-CSFRα, prolactin and growth hormone receptors.
2. Induction of nuclear proto-oncogene expression and rapid tyrosine phosphorylation of cellular proteins, in particular signal transducing molecules having SH2 and/or SH3 domains such as PI-3 kinase, Shc, Vav, and HS1, are indispensable for IL-5-mediated signaling.
3. The activities of B-cell specific Bruton's tyrosine kinase (Btk) and JAK2 kinase are significantly enhanced after IL-5 stimulation.
4. One of the proline residues in the well-conserved cytoplasmic region common to IL-5R, IL-3R, and GM-CSFR (from Leu^{350} to Pro^{355} in mIL-5Rα) must be maintained to interact with the βc for signal transduction. Taking account of the critical cytoplasmic region of the βc, we would like to propose a schematic model, illustrated in Figure 5.

The interactions between proline-rich sequences in various proteins and the SH3 domains of adapter proteins have attracted considerable attention as possible mediators of intracellular signal transduction through growth factor receptors (32). Proline residues in the critical region of IL-5Rα may contribute to the flexibility of its cytoplasmic domain, which is important for signal transduction, or may be important for the interaction with a certain intracellular signaling protein(s) without an SH3 domain. However, we must consider the possibility that Pro^{357} in IL-5Rα, which is not conserved in IL-3Rα and GM-CSFRα, might have affected our

247

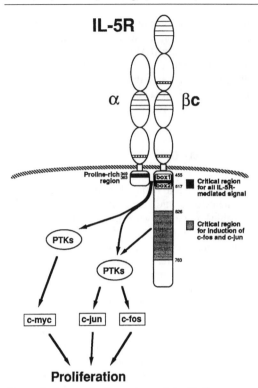

Figure 5. Schematic illustrations of the IL-5 receptor-complex.

results. Further study is required to explore the function of the proline-rich residues of IL-5Rα, IL-3Rα, and GM-^{CS}FRα.

To identify protein tyrosine kinases (PTKs) associated with IL-5R, we immunoprecipitated IL-5R using anti-βc mAb or anti-IL-5Rα mAb from cell lysates of IL-5-stimulated Y16 cells, and carried out an immune complex kinase assay. We could not detect any tyrosine-kinase activity in the immunoprecipitates in any conditions so far tested. Recent studies by many investigators have revealed the essential roles of the JAK family of protein-tyrosine kinases in signal transduction through cytokine receptors (25). It has been reported that the JAK family kinases induce tyrosine phosphorylation of ~91-kDa cellular transcription factors, as well as their translocation into the nucleus, upon stimulation with IFNs or IL-6. We demonstrated that JAK2 kinase was rapidly tyrosine-phosphorylated upon IL-5 stimulation in an IL-5-dependent early B cell line, Y16. Treatment of human basophils with IL-5 was reported to induce tyrosine phosphorylation and activation of DNA

binding proteins that recognize the IFN-γ response region (33). It is likely, therefore, that JAK2 tyrosine kinase may have important functions in the activation of transcription factors in IL-5-mediated signal transduction. The IL-5 signal transduction pathway via JAK2 kinase also appears to require the cytoplasmic proline-rich sequence of IL-5Rα.

Results obtained using chimeric receptors, between IL-5Rα and the βc, indicated that dimerization of the cytoplasmic domain of the βc leads to the ability to transduce growth signal without the cytoplasmic domain of IL-5Rα. Considered together with observation that the cytoplasmic proline-rich residues of IL-5Rα are essential, two models of the activation of the IL-5R complex can be postulated. In one model, IL-5 binding to IL-5Rα together with the βc results in multimerization of receptor subunits and dimerization (multimerization) of the cytoplasmic domain of the βc. The proline-rich regions of the cytoplasmic domain of IL-5Rα interact directly or indirectly with the βc, and this interaction is also essential for either dimerization or conformational changes in the cytoplasmic domain of the βc. In the other model, the proline-rich sequences of IL-5Rα interact with a certain intracellular protein(s) and thereby activate signaling molecules downstream together with the cytoplasmic domain of the βc. At present, we have no definite evidence supporting either of these models. Deletions in the carboxy-terminal region of the cytoplasmic domain of IL-5Rα (DC3 or DC4) did not affect growth signal transduction ability. The carboxy-terminal regions of the α chains of IL-5R, IL-3R, and GM-CSFR are different from each other. As only these regions are diversified among the three cytokine receptor complexes, they may contribute to the transduction of ligand specific signals. IL-5 induces not only proliferation but also differentiation of B cells and eosinophils as well. We are interested in clarifying the signal transduction pathways of mutant IL-5Rα, especially DC3, DC4, and chimeric receptors, in the differentiation of B cells.

In conclusion, we have presented evidence for the involvement of multiple families of signal-transducing molecules, such as Vav, Shc, HS1, and PI-3 kinase, and cytoplasmic PTKs such as Btk and JAK2, in IL-5-mediated signaling pathways. We would like to particulary emphasize the involvement of Btk and HS1 in the IL-5-mediated signaling pathways. These data may provide important clues for clarifying the precise role of each molecule in the development, proliferation, and differentiation of hematopoietic cells. We should also clarify the unique signaling pathway which appears to be associated with IL-5R complexes, as well as elucidating differences in IL-5-mediated signal transduction between cell proliferation and differentiation.

Acknowledgments

We wish to thank Drs. Akira Tominaga, Masamichi Koike, Ken-ichi Yamamura, Fumiya Imamura, Satoshi Satoh, Hiroko Kanazawa, Masashi Shiiba, Shin Yonehara, and Atsushi Miyajima for providing reagents used in this study, technical assistance, and valuable suggestions. This study was supported in part by Grant-in-Aid for Scientific Research and for Special Project Research, Cancer Bioscience, from the Ministry of Education, Science and Culture of Japan; by Special Coordination Funds for Promoting Science and Technology of the Science and Technology Agency, Japan; by the Mochida Memorial Foundation for Medical and Pharmaceutical Research; and by a Research Grant from the Uehara Memorial Foundation.

Address for correspondence:

Kiyoshi Takatsu
Department of Immunology
Institute of Medical Science
University of Tokyo
4-6-1 Minato-ku
Tokyo 108
Japan

References

1. Takatsu K. Interleukin-5 Receptor. *Curr Opin Immunol* 1992; 3:299.

2. Takatsu K, Takai S, Hitoshi Y. Interleukin 5 and its receptor system: Implications in the immune response and inflammation. *Adv Immunol* 1994; (in press).

3. Tominaga A, Takaki S, Koyama N, Katoh S, Matsumoto R, Migita M, Hitoshi Y, Hosoya Y, Yamauchi S, Kanai Y, Miyazaki J, Usuku G, Yamamura K, K Takatsu. Transgenic mice expressing a B cell growth and differentiation factor gene (interleukin 5) develop eosinophilia and autoantibody production. *J Exp Med* 1991; 173:429.

4. Sanderson CJ. Interleukin-5, eosinophils, and disease. *Blood* 1992; 79:3101.

5. Takaki S, Tominaga A, Hitoshi Y, Mita, S, Sonoda E, Yamaguchi N, Takatsu K. Molecular cloning and expression of the murine interleukin-5 receptor. *EMBO J* 1990; 9:4367.

6. Devos P, Plaetinck G, der Heyden JV, Cornelis S, Vandekerckhove J, Fiers W, Tavernier J. Molecular basis of a high affinity murine interleukin-5 receptor. *EMBO J* 1991; 10:2133.

7. Murata Y, Takaki S, Migita M, Kikuchi Y, Tominaga A, Takatsu K. Molecular cloning and expression of the human interleukin-5 receptor. *J Exp Med* 1992; 175:341.

8. Takaki S, Mita S, Kitamura T, Yonehara S, Tominaga A, Yamaguchi N, Miyajima A, Takatsu K. Identification of the second subunit of the murine interleukin 5 receptor: Interleukin-3 receptor-like protein, AIC2B is a component of the high affinity interleukin-5 receptor *EMBO J* 1991; 10:2833.

9. Mita S, Takaki S, Hitoshi Y, Rolinck AG, Tominaga A, Yamaguchi N, Takatsu K. Molecular characterization of the β chain of the interleukin 5 (IL-5)receptors. *Int Immunol* 1991; 3:665.

10. Tavernier J, Devos R, Cornelis S, Tuypens T, Van der Heyden J, Fiers W, Plaetinck G. A human high affinity interleukin-5 receptor (IL5R) is composed of an IL5-specific α chain and a β chain shared with the receptor for GM-CSF. *Cell* 1991; 66:1175.

11. Takaki S, Murata Y, Kitamura T, Miyajima A, Tominaga A, Takatsu K. Reconstitution of the functional receptors for murine and human interleukin 5. *J Exp Med* 1993; 177:1523.

12. Miyajima A, Kitamura T, Harada N, Yokota T, Arai K. Cytokine receptors and signal transduction. *Annu Rev Immunol* 1992; 10:295.

13. Hara T, Miyajima A. Two distinct functional high affinity receptors for mouse interleukin-3 (IL-3). *EMBO J* 1992; 11:1875.

14. Park LS, Martin U, Sorensen R, Luhr S, Morrissey PJ, Cosman D, Larsen A. Cloning of the low-affinity murine granulocyte-macrophage colony-stimulating factor receptor and reconstitution of a high-affinity receptor complex. *Proc Natl Acad Sci USA* 1992; 89:4295.

15. Hayashida K, Kitamura T, Gorman DM, Arai K-I, Yokota T, Miyajima A. Molecular cloning of a second subunit of the receptor for human granulocyte-macrophage colony-stimulating factor (GM-CSF): Reconstitution of a high-affinity GM-CSF receptor. *Proc Natl Acad Sci USA* 1990; 87:9655

16. Kitamura T, Sato N, Arai K, Miyajima A. Expression cloning of the human IL-3 receptor cDNA reveals a shared β subunit for human IL-3 and GM-CSF receptors. *Cell* 1991; 66:1165.

17. Koch CA, Anderson D, Moran MF, Ellis C, Pawson T. SH2 and SH3 domains: Elements that control in-

teractions of cytoplasmic signaling proteins. *Science* 1991; 252:668.

18. Bar-Sagi D, Rotin D, Batzer A, Mandiyan V, Schlessinger J. SH3 domains direct cellular localization of signaling molecules. *Cell* 1993; 74:83.

19. Stahl N, Yancopoulos GD. The alphas, betas and kinases of cytokine receptor complexes. *Cell* 1993; 74:587.

20. Hatakeyama M, Kono T, Kobayashi N, Kawahara A, Levin SD, Perlmutter RM, Taniguchi T. Interaction of the IL-2 receptor with the src-family kinase p56[lck]: Identification of novel intermolecular association. *Science* 1991; 252:1523.

21. Kishimoto T, Akira S, Taga T. Cytokine and signal transduction. *Cell* 1994; 76:253.

22. Sakamaki K, Miyajima I, Kitamura T, Miyajima A. Critical cytoplasmic domains of the common β subunit of the human GM-CSF, IL-3 and IL-5 receptor for growth signal transduction and tyrosine phosphorylation. *EMBO J* 1993; 11:3541.

23. Murata Y. Yamaguchi N, Hitoshi Y, Tominaga A, Takatsu K. Interleukin 5 and interleukin 3 induce serine and tyrosine phosphorylation of several cellular proteins in an interleukin 5-dependent cell line. *Biochem Biophys Res Commun* 1990; 173:1102.

24. Takaki S, Kanazawa H, Shiiba M, Takatsu K. Critical region of the cytoplasmic domain of IL-5Rα in the tyrosine phosphorylation and proto-oncogene expression. Mol Cell Biol 1994; (in press).

25. Ihle JN, Witthuhn BA, Quelle FW, Yamamoto K, Thierfelder WE, Kreider B, Silvenoinen O. Signaling by the cytokine receptor superfamily: JAKs and STATs. *TIBS* 1994; 19:222.

26. Murakami M, Hibi M, Nakagawa N, Nakagawa T, Yasukawa K, Yamanishi K, Taga T, Kishimoto T. IL-6-induced homodimerization of gp 130 and associated activation of a tyrosine kinase. *Science* 1993; 260:1808.

27. Tsukada S, Saffran DC, Rawlings DJ, Parolini O, Allen RC, Klisak I, Sparkes RS, Kubagawa H, Mohandas T, Quan S, Belmont JW, Cooper MD, Conley ME, Witte O N. Deficient expression of a B cell cytoplasmic tyrosine kinase in human X-linked agammaglobulinemia. *Cell* 199; 72:279.

28. Vetrie D, Vorechovsky I, Sideras P, Holland J, Davies A, Flinter F, Hammarstrom L, Kinnon C, Levinsky R, Bobrow M, Smith CIE, Bentley DR. The gene involved in X-linked agammaglobulinaemia is a member of the src family of protein-tyrosine kinases. *Nature* 1993; 361:226–233.

29. Rawlings D, Saffran DC, Tsukada S, Largaespada DA, Grimaldi JC, Cohen L, Mohr RN, Bazan JF, Howard M, Copeland NG, Jenkins NA, Witte ON. Mutation of unique region of Bruton's tyrosine kinase in immunodeficient Xid mice. *Science* 1993; 261:358.

30. Thomas JD, Sideras P, Smith CIE, Vorechovsky I, Chapman V, Paul WE. Colocalization of X-linked agammaglobulinemia and X-linked immunodeficiency genes. *Science* 1993; 261:355.

31. Hitoshi Y.Sonoda E, Kikuchi Y, Yonehara S, Nakauchi H, Takatsu K. Interleukin-5 receptor positive B cells, but not eosinophils are functionally and numerically influenced in the mice carried with X-linked immunedeficiency. *Int Immunol* 1993; 5:1183.

32. Ren R, Mayer BJ, Cicchetti P, Baltimore D. Identification of a ten-amino acid proline-rich SH3 binding site. *Science* 1993; 259:1157.

33. Larner AC, David M, Feldman GM, Igarashi K, Hackett RH, Webb DSA, Sweitzer SM, Petricoin III EF, Finbloom DS. Tyrosine phosphorylation of DNA binding proteins by multiple cytokines. *Science* 1993; 261:1730.

250

The Role of IL-5 and other Cytokines in Allergic Pulmonary Eosinophilia in the Mouse

Ted T Kung, Dawn Stelts, Jackie A Zurcher, Arthur S Watnick, Howard Jones, Peter J Mauser, Xiomara Fernandez, Shelby Umland, William Kreutner, Richard W Chapman, Robert W Egan*

Keywords: Eosinophil, interleukin 5, interleukin 4, γ-interferon, asthma, steroids, hyperreactivity

Following allergic challenge, eosinophils are formed from precursor cells in the bone marrow in response to various cytokines and accumulate in the lung during pulmonary inflammation. We have investigated eosinophil accumulation in the lung tissue and lung lavage fluid of ovalbumin-sensitized, aerosol-challenged B6D mice at various times after the ovalbumin challenge. During this IgE-based allergic response, the eosinophil levels in various tissue compartments followed the temporal changes that would be anticipated. In response to allergic challenge, bone marrow eosinophils increased slightly from a baseline of 200,000/femur, then plummeted as they were released into the circulation in excess of the ability of the marrow to replenish them. Meanwhile, blood levels increased dramatically within hours, lung tissue levels increased within a day, and lung lavage levels peaked in 2 days. Within 2 weeks, these changes resolved spontaneously.

Accumulation of eosinophils in the lung and in the lavage was inhibited by acute treatment with steroids or antibodies to IL-5. Both betamethasone and a neutralizing anti-IL-5 antibody inhibited eosinophil release from the bone marrow. An antibody to IL-4 or IFN-γ itself also dramatically inhibited allergic eosinophilia when added during the sensitization period by preventing antigen-specific IgE accumulation. Using the same protocol for sensitization and challenge, W/W^v mice that are mast cell deficient did not produce as significant a pulmonary eosinophilia in response to the aerosol ovalbumin challenge. Hence, the mast cell as well as the T lymphocyte is a critical component of this response.

Introduction

Although the most observable feature in asthma is the bronchoconstriction associated with an acute "asthmatic attack," this really results from an ongoing inflammatory disorder. Some aspects of the chronic pulmonary inflammation (1) are edema, decreased mucocilliary clearance, epithelial damage with the ensuing neuronal hyperresponsiveness, and bronchoalveolar eosinophilia. Therefore, when treating asthma, it is important to address the chronic inflammation that underlies the hyperreactivity, rather than just the acute bronchospastic episodes.

Eosinophils are the major cells infiltrating into the lung during pulmonary inflammation. They develop from precursors in the bone marrow in response to a variety of cytokines, including interleukin 5 (IL-5), and are stored in the bone marrow for release in response to a stimulus. Once released, they move rapidly through the circulation and become tissue cells. Eosinophils are almost nonexistent in normal lung, but they accumulate in very large numbers in the lungs during asthma. They possess a full complement of lipid metabolizing pathways (2). Their secretory granules also contain a series of highly cytolytic enzymes and proteins that can destroy the epithelium and are detected in the lungs during asthma (3). Furthermore, the role of the eosinophil in immune surveillance is somewhat limited compared to that of neutrophils, macrophages, or lymphocytes, so it should be possible to inhibit the actions of eosinophils without causing severe immunosuppressive effects.

Using a mouse model, we have investigated the effects of steroids, IL-5, and other cytokines on allergic eosinophilia. Eosinophil levels have been measured in the appropriate tissues to establish the mechanism of action of these agents, and mast cell deficient mice have been studied to determine the endogenous source of the relevant cytokines.

---

*   Allergy and Immunology Department, Schering-Plough Research Institute, Kenilworth, NJ, USA.

Results and Discussion

Tissue Distribution of Eosinophils in the Allergic Mouse

B6D2F1/J mice were sensitized by an intraperitoneal injection of 0.5 ml of alum-precipitated antigen containing 8 μg of ovalbumin (OVA) adsorbed to 2 mg of aluminum hydroxide (alum) gel in saline vehicle. A booster injection of this alum-OVA mixture was given 5 days later. Non-sensitized control animals received alum gel only. Twelve days after immunization, the mice were exposed to antigen bronchoprovocation. For the antigen challenge, the mice were placed in a Plexiglas chamber and exposed to aerosolized OVA (0.5%) for 1 h in both the morning and the afternoon of a single day. At various times after antigen bronchoprovocation, the animals were sacrificed by CO_2 asphyxiation, and then bronchoalveolar lavage (BAL) fluid, blood, bone marrow aspirate, and lung tissue were collected. Total cell numbers were counted with a standard hemocytometer. Smears of BAL cells were made by cytocentrifuging 100 μl of BAL fluid at 150×g for 10 minutes. The blood samples were obtained by cardiac puncture and the numbers of leukocytes and differential counts were determined using standard hematological procedures. For the histological evaluation of pulmonary tissue, the lungs were removed, fixed with 10% phosphate-buffered formalin, embedded in paraffin, sectioned at 5 μm thickness, and stained with hematoxylin and eosin.

During the allergic response in this mouse model, the levels of eosinophils in the various tissue compartments underwent the changes that would be anticipated (Figure 1). Bone marrow eosinophils were measured in the femur where they originated and were stored for release into the circulation on demand (upper left panel). Prior to challenge, there was a baseline level of approximately 200,000 eosinophils per femur. Following stimulation, they increased somewhat, and then plummeted as they were released into the circulation in excess of the ability of the marrow to regenerate new eosinophils. There may have been something of an overshoot at day 4 as resynthesis caught up, then they largely returned to normal by day 6. There were virtually no eosinophils in the blood prior to challenge (upper right panel) The level increased dramatically within hours after challenge, dropped off as they were assimilated by the tissue, and again

resolved spontaneously. There were very few eosinophils in the lung prior to challenge (lower left panel). Accumulation in the lung lagged behind the appearance in the blood by several hours, as expected. Within a day, they reached a maximum then dropped off gradually. To get into the lavage, eosinophils must travel through the tissue to the luminal surface, so the peak of lavage eosinophils lagged behind the appearance in the tissue, apparently by about a day (lower right panel). The peak was transient between days 2 and 3, then the levels declined to normal within 2 weeks, very similar to the tissue itself.

Inhibition of BAL Eosinophilia in the Mouse

Steroids should block pulmonary eosinophilia (4), and so we examined the effects of betamethasone, prednisolone, and hydrocortisone on the cell content of BAL from sensitized challenged mice. These drugs were administered orally 2 h prior to the OVA challenge, and the BAL was collected and analyzed 24 h later. There was a dose-dependent inhibition of total cell and eosinophil infiltration in each instance. The ED_{50} for betamethasone was 0.2 mg/kg, for prednisolone 4.3 mg/kg, and for hydrocortisone 8.5 mg/kg.

The role of IL-5 in murine pulmonary eosinophilia was also studied. IL-5 can enhance eosinophil production and survival (5), so depletion of IL-5 should selectively suppress eosinophil levels in animal models. Antibodies have been used to accomplish this (6, 7). The antibody that was used most extensively is from the TRFK-5 hybridoma line, which secretes a rat IgG_1 isotype that neutralizes recombinant murine IL-5. As an isotype control antibody, we used a rat IgG_1 isotype from GL113 cells. This antibody was raised against bacterial β-galactosidase and should have no mammalian biology. Using the standard protocol, the antibody was administered by i.p. injection 2 h prior to the OVA challenge. In each paradigm, the mice were challenged with OVA (Figure 2). The unsensitized mice did not respond with BAL eosinophilia. In contrast, the sensitized mice produced a BAL eosinophilia of 5×10^5 eosinophils/ml, about 50% of the total cells. The TRFK-5 antibody at 0.1 and 1 mg/kg inhibited the eosinophilia > 95%. At 0.01 mg/kg, it had no effect. As a control, the GL113 antibody that should have no effect was inactive at 1 mg/kg. Therefore, specific depletion of

IL-5 can totally inhibit lavage eosinophilia in the allergic mouse.

The effects of a series of other cytokine-based treatments on eosinophil accumulation in this model have also been assessed (Table 1). In addition to the TRFK-5 antibody against murine IL-5, we also evaluated 39D10, a rat monoclonal an-

tibody raised against human IL-5. Administered 2 h prior to the OVA challenge, 39D10 inhibited the pulmonary eosinophilia to the same extent as the TRFK-5 antibody, but with about 10 times less potency. We evaluated the role of IL-4 in this model using 11B11, a rat monoclonal antibody against murine IL-4. As opposed to IL-5, which crosses

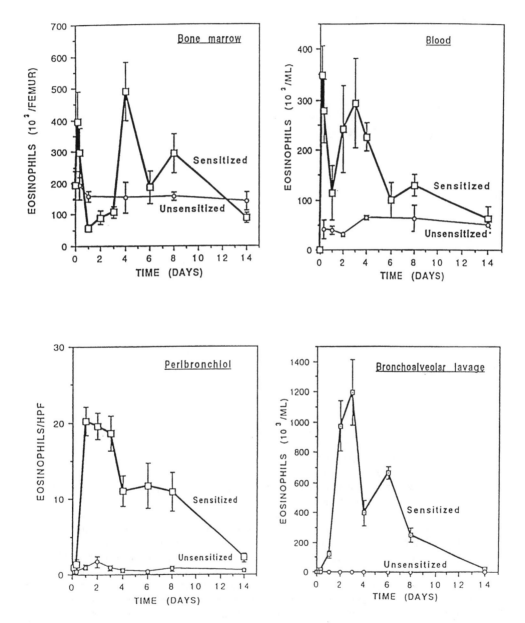

Figure 1. Eosinophil levels in various tissues after challenging OVA sensitized mice.

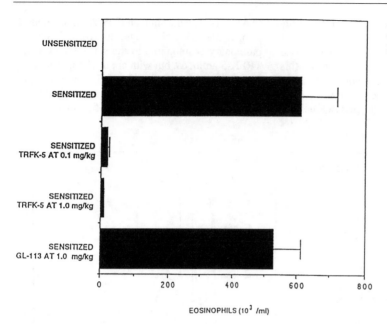

Figure 2. The effect of anti-IL-5 on mouse BAL eosinophilia following OVA challenge.

Table 1. The effects of cytokine antibodies and IFN-γ on eosinophil accumulation.

Cytokine inhibited	Antibody	Protocol	Dose	% Inhibition
IL-5	TRFK-5	−2 h	0.1 mg/kg	80
IL-5	39D10	−2 h	1.0 mg/kg	74
IL-4	11B11	3×/week during sensitization	40.0 mg/kg	95
IL-4	11B11	−2 h	40.0 mg/kg	36
IFN-γ	XMG 1.2	3×/week during sensitization	40.0 mg/kg	0
IFN-γ directly	NONE	3×/week during sensitization	0.4 mg/kg	74

species very nicely (5), IL-4 and IFN-γ are very species specific (8, 9), so we used only murine reagents. 11B11 blocked eosinophilia and also the increases in IgE when administered during sensitization at 40 mg/kg. It was as if the animals were not sensitized and, therefore, did not respond. In contrast, when the 11B11 was administered once 2 h prior to the OVA challenge, there was a marginal and not dose-dependent effect on eosinophil accumulation. IFN-γ itself administered during sensitization also blocked eosinophil accumulation, probably by redirecting T-cell maturation away from the Th2 type, thereby suppressing IL-4 levels. IFN-γ did not inhibit when administered just prior to the challenge. An antibody to IFN-γ had no effect. Therefore, eosinophil accumulation in this mouse model can be inhibited by blocking eosinophil maturation using IL-5-based technology or by inhibiting IgE synthesis using IL-4 or IFN-γ-based technology.

Mechanism of Inhibition of BAL Eosinophilia

To investigate the mechanisms by which betamethasone and the TRFK-5 antibody inhibited pulmonary eosinophilia, we measured the changes in eosinophil levels in the bone marrow, blood, lung tissue, and BAL in drug-treated compared to untreated sensitized challenged mice. Eosinophil measurements were conducted 24 h after the OVA challenge. The mice were treated orally with 0.5 mg/kg of betamethasone either 1 h or 1 and 24 h

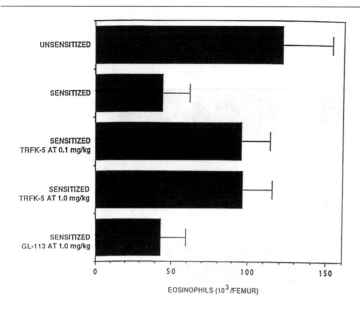

Figure 3. The effect of anti-IL-5 on mouse bone marrow eosinophil levels following OVA challenge.

prior to the OVA challenge (data not shown). There were no noticeable eosinophils in the BAL prior to challenge; they increased, as expected, 24 h after the challenge. This increase was blocked to baseline by both betamethasone treatments. The steroid was inhibiting at the level of the bone marrow. The drop in eosinophils noted in the challenged animals at 24 h did not occur when the steroid was present. In other words, the bone marrow did not respond by releasing its store of eosinophils so they, of course, never accumulated in the lung.

Much as with the steroid, we have also examined the effects of neutralizing IL-5 on marrow eosinophils (Figure 3). The results are fundamentally the same as with the betamethasone. In the sensitized and challenged mice, there was a decrease in bone marrow eosinophils 24 h after the OVA challenge. This was largely blocked by the IL-5 antibody, but not by the GL113 antibody. Some studies that we have conducted in blood and tissue suggest that the IL-5 antibody may be having an effect on activation of eosinophils as well as on release of eosinophils.

Mast Cell Involvement in BAL Eosinophilia

It appears that eosinophilia is IL-5 based, but what is the source of the IL-5? Th2 lymphocytes and mast cells are two reasonable candidates. To address this question, we used a mast cell deficient mouse, the W/W^v (10), and a protocol very similar to the model described above. To make our point conclusively, it was necessary to reconstitute the

W/W^v animals with mast cells from the W/W$^+$ mouse, the normal congenic littermate.

Bone marrow cells were collected from femurs and tibias of W/W$^+$ mice with Hanks' balanced salt solution containing 10% fetal bovine serum. To obtain mast cells from mice, the bone marrow cells were cultured in RPMI 1640 containing 10% concentrated conditioned medium and 10% fetal calf serum. In the third week, 1 ng of rmIL-3 (R&D, Minneapolis, MN) was added to the medium. After 3 weeks, 90% of the viable cells were mast cells. 10^7 of the mast cells suspended in 0.2 ml of phosphate-buffered saline were transferred intravenously into the tail vein of each W/W^v recipient. Animals were sensitized with OVA 42 days after the adoptive transfer with W/W$^+$ bone marrow derived mast cells.

When unsensitized W/W$^+$ mice were challenged with OVA, they did not respond with pulmonary eosinophilia that could be detected in the BAL (Figure 4). On the other hand, they did respond when they were both sensitized and challenged. The mast cell deficient W/W^v mice did respond compared to the unsensitized controls. However, this increase was not statistically significant, although it seemed real, and may have been due to lymphocytic sources of IL-5. On the other hand, the mast cell reconstituted W/W^v mice developed a much more profound eosinophilia, under the same experimental conditions. Hence, the mast cell appears to be involved in eosinophil accumulation in the W/W^v mouse.

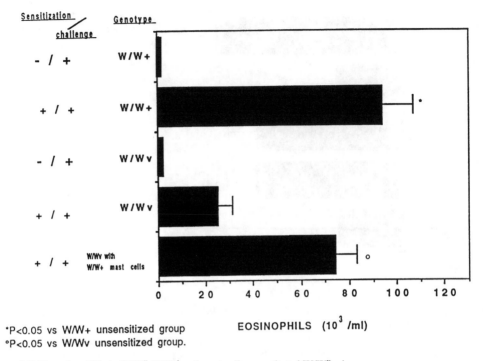

*P<0.05 vs W/W+ unsensitized group
°P<0.05 vs W/Wv unsensitized group.

EOSINOPHILS (10^3 /ml)

Figure 4. BAL eosinophilia in W/W^v, W/W$^+$ and mast cell reconstituted W/W^v mice.

To summarize, in many ways, this allergic mouse model is consistent with what is seen in human pulmonary inflammation. Following allergic challenge, the distribution of eosinophils in the various tissue compartments followed the temporal changes that would be expected, culminating in tissue and BAL eosinophilia. Using BAL eosinophilia as a quantitative readout, we found that steroids, anti-IL-5 antibodies, anti-IL-4 antibodies, and IFN-γ block pulmonary eosinophilia by various mechanisms. Lastly, the W/W^v mouse that is mast cell deficient did not respond significantly to antigen challenge with pulmonary eosinophilia, until it was reconstituted with purified bone marrow mast cells from its congenic littermate, implicating a role for mast cell products, possibly IL-5, in eosinophil recruitment.

Acknowledgments

We thank Mrs. Virginia Citarella and Mrs. Teresa Ruhnke for typing this manuscript and Dr. Michael Minnicozzi for his assistance in preparing the manuscript.

Address for correspondence:

Robert W Egan
Schering-Plough Research Institute
2015 Galloping Hill Road
Kenilworth, NJ 07033
USA

References

1. Arm JP, Lee TH. The pathobiology of bronchial asthma. *Adv Immunol* 1992; 51:323–382.

2. Owen WF, Soberman RJ, Yoshimoto T, Sheffer AL, Lewis RA, Austen KF. Synthesis and release of leukotrienes C4 by human eosinophils. *J Immunol* 1987; 138:532–538.

3. Jones DG. The eosinophil. *J Comp Pathol* 1993; 108:317–335.

4. Bass DA. Eosinopenia. In: Mahmoud SSF, Austen KF (Eds) *The eosinophil in health and disease*. New York: Grune and Stratton, 1980, pp. 275–291.

5. McKenzie ANJ, Sanderson CJ. Interleukin 5. In: Kishimoto T (Ed) *Interleukins: Molecular biology and immunology*. Basel: Karger, 1992, pp. 135–152.

6. Gulbenkian AR, Egan RW, Fernandez X, Jones H, Kreutner W, Kung T, Payvandi F, Sullivan L, Zurcher JA, Watnick AS. Interleukin-5 modulates eosinophil accumulation in allergic guinea pig lung. *Am Rev Respir Dis* 1992; 146:263–265.

7. Mauser PJ, Pitman A, Witt A, Fernandez X, Zurcher JA, Kung T, Jones H, Watnick AS, Egan RW, Kreutner W, Adams GK. Inhibitory effect of the TRFK-5 anti-IL-5 antibody in a guinea pig model of asthma. *Am Rev Respir Dis* 1993; 148:1623–1627.

8. Mosmann TR, Yokota T, Kastelein R, Zurawski S, Arai N, Takeb Y. Species specificity of T cell stimulating activities of IL-2 and BSF-1 (IL-4); comparison of normal and recombinant mouse and human IL-2 and BSF-1 (IL-4). *J Immunol* 1987; 138:1813–1816.

9. Farrar MA, Schreiber RD. The molecular cell biology of interferon-γ and its receptor. *Annu Rev Immunol* 1993; 11:571–611.

10. Kitamura Y, Go S, Hatanaka K. Decrease of mast cells in W/W^v mice and their increase by bone marrow transplantation. *Blood* 1978; 52:447–452.

The Role of Interleukin-5 (IL-5) in the Pathogenesis of Asthma

Chris J Corrigan, A Barry Kay*

Keywords: Asthma, pathogenesis, interleukin-5, T-lymphocyte, eosinophil

Asthma is thought to be an inflammatory disease of the bronchial mucosa characterised by an accumulation of T cells and eosinophils. Products of eosinophils have been implicated in causing the bronchial mucosal damage in asthma which is thought to underlie the clinical features (variable airways obstruction and bronchial hyperresponsiveness). Interleukin-5 is particularly implicated in asthma pathogenesis because of its specific effects in enhancing eosinophil survival, maturation, hyperadherence, activation and local accumulation. A consideration of these eosinophil-specific properties of IL-5 provides some explanation for the specific accumulation of these cells in the asthmatic bronchial mucosa. The activated CD4 T cell is the principal physiological source of IL-5 in asthmatic inflammation. There is now considerable evidence in support of the hypothesis that activated CD4 T cells in the asthmatic airway secrete IL-5, and that the amount of this secretion regulates eosinophil recruitment and, thereby, disease severity. Therapy of asthma with glucocorticoids is associated with reduced secretion of IL-5, which may be a principal mechanism of the anti-asthma effect of these drugs. Alternative drugs which inhibit the secretion of IL-5 or its action on eosinophils may form useful alternatives to glucocorticoids for asthma therapy.

Structure of Interleukin-5 (IL-5) and its Receptor

The cDNA molecule encoding human IL-5 has been cloned and sequenced. It encodes a mature polypeptide of 115 amino acids, with an additional 22 amino acid leader sequence. The polypeptide contains 2 potential N-linked glycosylation sites and 3 cysteine residues. The apparent molecular weight of human recombinant IL-5 produced in mammalian cells ranges from 45 to 60 kDa, resulting predominantly from the variable degree of glycosylation. The active IL-5 molecule exists as a disulphide-linked homodimer. Dimerisation is effected by cross-linking of 2 conserved cysteine residues in an anti-parallel arrangement; the monomer is biologically inactive. Solving of the crystal structure of IL-5 (1) has revealed a 2 domain arrangement, with each domain similar to the "cytokine fold" found in other cytokines such as GM-CSF, M-CSF, IL-2, IL-4, and hormones such as growth hormone. Both paired chains of the dimer contribute to this structure, which explains why the monomer is biologically inactive. The genes encoding human IL-5, IL-3 and GM-CSF are clustered on the long arm of chromosome 5 along with the genes encoding IL-4, M-CSF and the M-CSF receptor (c-fms).

Freshly isolated human eosinophils express a single, high-affinity (K_d 170–300 pM) IL-5 receptor. This receptor is a heterodimer composed of 2 polypeptide chains, α and β. The cDNA sequences for both membrane-bound and soluble forms of the IL-5 receptor α-chain have been isolated from human peripheral blood eosinophils (2), although the presence of the soluble α-chain, a potential physiological inhibitor of IL-5 activity, has not yet been described in human biological fluids. The β-chain of the IL-5 receptor is identical to the β-chains of the receptors for IL-3 and GM-CSF (3). Although the α-chain alone binds IL-5 with comparable affinity to the native dimeric receptor, both chains are necessary, at least in some transfected cell lines, for transmission of a proliferation signal (3, 4).

Cellular Sources of IL-5

Activated T cells, particularly CD4 T cells of the Th2 phenotype, are the major physiological source

* Department of Allergy and Clinical Immunology, National Heart and Lung Institute, London, England.

of IL-5 (5). In addition, expression of mRNA encoding IL-5 has been described in tryptase-positive mast cells and eosinophils in the nasal mucosa of patients with allergen-induced rhinitis (6), and in eosinophils in the bronchoalveolar lavage fluid of patients with atopic asthma (7). Although secretion of IL-5 protein by these granulocytes has not yet been clearly demonstrated *in vivo*, the possibility that IL-5 may be secreted in inflammatory processes by cells other than T cells remains substantial.

Activities of IL-5 *In Vitro* and *In Vivo*

Whereas eosinophil differentiation is influenced, at least *in vitro*, by IL-3, IL-5 and GM-CSF, only IL-5 specifically exerts its actions on cells of the eosinophil/basophil lineage, whereas IL-3 and GM-CSF exert a broad array of biological activities on many different cell types. There is now good evidence that IL-5 is the single most important regulator of eosinophil numbers during inflammatory processes *in vivo*, both through its effects in enhancing the growth and differentiation of committed eosinophil precursor cells (8) and through its prolongation of the viability of mature eosinophils (9). In addition, the pro-inflammatory effector functions of mature eosinophils are selectively enhanced by prior exposure to IL-5 (10). Striking demonstrations of the role of IL-5 in regulating eosinophil numbers have been provided by experiments on animals. Transgenic mice constitutively expressing the murine IL-5 gene linked to the CD2 promoter (11) had greatly increased numbers of eosinophils in their peripheral blood as well as in many organs including lymphoid organs, lungs and liver. In spite of this, these animals were apparently healthy, sounding a note of caution regarding the possible role of IL-5 in disease as distinct from the regulation of eosinophil numbers and tissue infiltration. Anti-IL-5 antibodies have also been shown to block the development of the eosinophilic responses which accompany many infectious processes, for example helminthic infection in mice (12).

In addition to its activities on eosinophils, IL-5 also induces the growth and differentiation of human basophils (13), which share with eosinophils a common precursor cell. The existence of possible effects of IL-5 on human B-cell function

in vitro remains controversial, since different results have been obtained with different systems. These discrepancies may be related to the fact that the time course of responsiveness of activated B-cells to IL-5 differs with different stimuli.

Role of IL-5 in Asthma Pathogenesis

Asthma is a disease characterized clinically by reversible obstruction of the airways, or bronchi, and bronchial non-specific hyperresponsiveness. It is now widely accepted that chronic inflammation of the bronchial mucosal lining plays a fundamental role in the genesis of these clinical manifestations.

The most striking feature of the histopathology of asthma is the intense infiltration of the bronchial mucosa with eosinophils, macrophages and lymphocytes (14). In fact, the disease has many histopathological features of a chronic, cell-mediated immune response. The eosinophil appears to be a key cell in producing injury to the bronchial mucosa (15). This in turn is believed to result in bronchial obstruction and irritability, although the precise mechanisms by which this occurs are not clear. Immunocytochemical studies of bronchial biopsies taken from patients with asthma (16–19) have shown that activated (CD25[+]) T cells can be detected in the bronchial mucosa, and that their numbers can be correlated both with the numbers of local activated eosinophils and with disease severity.

One problem with asthma pathogenesis is the mechanism by which eosinophils preferentially accumulate in the inflamed mucosa. Local expression of IL-5 may play a fundamental role in this process by selectively enhancing eosinophil differentiation and survival. In addition, IL-5 is also selectively chemotactic for eosinophils (20), although only weakly so as compared with established (but non-specific) eosinophil chemoattractants such as platelet-activating factor, and primes eosinophils for an enhanced chemotactic response to these chemoattractants (21).

Another way in which IL-5 may bring about eosinophil accumulation in asthma is by selectively promoting the emigration of these cells into the bronchial mucosa through the vascular endothelium. Leucocyte adhesion molecules probably play a role in selective eosinophil migration. Three major families of adhesion molecules have been defined as being involved in leucocyte migration: (i) the immunoglobulin superfamily, including ICAM-1, VCAM-1 and PECAM; (ii) the integrins, including LFA-1, Mac-1 and VLA-4; (iii) the selectins, including E-selectin, P-selectin and L-selectin. Leucocyte migration is initiated by an interaction between receptors on the cell surface with their ligands on the surface of vascular endothelial cells. Selectins mediate the initial weak tethering of leucocytes to the endothelial wall. Eosinophils can bind to endothelium using all three selectins, with no apparent differences between these cells and neutrophils. Integrins such as LFA-1 and Mac-1, also on the leucocyte surface, mediate firm adhesion and transmigration by binding to immunoglobulin-like molecules such as ICAM-1 and VCAM-1 on the endothelium (22). Eosinophils appear to be unique, however, in that IL-3 and IL-5 upregulate eosinophil, but not neutrophil, adhesion to unstimulated endothelial cells (23). This observation offers another possible explanation for the selective recruitment of eosinophils observed in asthmatic inflammation.

CD4 T cells are clearly an important source of IL-5. The possible role of IL-5 in enhancing eosinophil survival, maturation, hyperadherence, activation and local accumulation has been discussed above (8–10, 23). These observations emphasise the fact that local secretion of IL-5 by activated CD4 T cells (and perhaps other cells including eosinophils themselves) may play a substantial role in effecting the *selective* accumulation and activation of eosinophils in tissues.

There is now substantial evidence consistent with the hypothesis that activated CD4 T cells in patients with asthma secrete IL-5 which in turn regulates local eosinophil recruitment and thereby disease severity. Activated CD4, but not CD8 T cells were detected in the peripheral blood of patients with severe asthma as compared with controls (24), and their numbers were reduced following glucocorticoid therapy of the asthmatics to a degree which correlated with the degree of clinical improvement. In addition, elevated serum concentrations of IL-5 were also detected in a proportion of the asthmatics, but not in non-asthmatic controls, and again concentrations were reduced in association with glucocorticoid therapy. Preferential activation of memory CD4 T cells in the bronchoalveolar lavage (BAL) fluid of mild atopic asthmatics was observed to correlate with asthma symptoms and bronchial hyperresponsiveness (25).

Cultured peripheral blood CD4 and CD8 T cells from both atopic and non-atopic asthmatics were shown spontaneously to secrete factors which prolonged the life of eosinophils *in vitro* to an extent which correlated with the numbers of peripheral blood eosinophils in the same subjects (26); antibody neutralization experiments suggested that this activity was attributable partly to GM-CSF and partly to IL-5. T cells purified from the peripheral blood of non-atopic asthmatics spontaneously secreted elevated quantities of IL-5 but not IL-4 as compared with normal controls, whereas those from atopic asthmatics secreted elevated quantities of IL-5 and IL-4 (27).

Measurement of cytokines *in vivo* is problematical because of their low concentrations, rapid metabolism and unquantifiable degree of dilution. Furthermore, "physiological" concentrations of cytokines have in general not been defined, and so it is often unknown whether a specific assay, such as ELISA, is sufficiently sensitive. One alternative to the direct measurement of cytokines is the detection of their mRNA using the technique of *in situ* hybridization with cytokine-specific cRNA probes or riboprobes. Although this is not a strictly quantitative technique, and with the proviso that mRNA synthesis does not necessarily equate with secretion of the corresponding protein, it does have the advantage that it can localize the secretion of cytokines within cells and tissues. Using this technique it was demonstrated that IL-5 mRNA was elaborated by cells in bronchial biopsies from a majority of mild asthmatics but not normal controls (28). The amount of mRNA correlated broadly with the numbers of activated T-LC and eosinophils in biopsies from the same subjects. In another study (29), it was shown that significantly elevated percentages of bronchoalveolar lavage cells expressed mRNA encoding IL-2, IL-3, IL-4, IL-5 and GM-CSF but not IFN-γ in mild atopic asthmatics as compared with non-atopic normal controls. Separation of CD2$^+$ T cells from the remainder of the BAL cells showed that the majority (>90%) of the cells expressing IL-5 and IL-4 mRNA were T cells. Over a broad range of asthma severity, the percentages of BAL fluid cells from atopic asthmatics expressing mRNA encoding IL-5, IL-4, IL-3 and GM-CSF, but not IL-2 and IFN-γ, could be correlated with the severity of asthma symptoms and bronchial hyperresponsiveness (30). In a double-blind, parallel group study, therapy of mild atopic asthmatics with oral prednisolone, but not placebo, resulted in clinical improvement associated with a reduction in the percentages of BAL fluid cells expressing IL-5 and IL-4 and an increase of those expressing IFN-γ (31). Allergen challenge of sensitized atopic asthmatics was associated with increased numbers of activated T cells and eosinophils and increased expression of mRNA encoding IL-5 and GM-CSF in the bronchial mucosa (32).

Conclusion

Taken together, these studies provide overwhelming evidence in support of the general hypothesis that, in asthma, activated CD4 T cells secrete cytokines, particularly IL-5, which are relevant to the accumulation and activation of eosinophils in the bronchial mucosa, and that glucocorticoids exert their anti-asthma effect at least partly by reducing the synthesis of IL-5 by these cells. They also suggest that antagonism of the activity of IL-5, in addition to inhibition of its secretion, may form a useful therapeutic approach to the therapy of asthma and allergic diseases. One *caveat* to this proposition is the observation that the receptors for IL-3 and GM-CSF share common β-chains with that for IL-5, raising the possibility that these cytokines might in part substitute for the functions of IL-5 if the activities of the latter were ablated therapeutically.

Acknowledgment

Funded by a Clinician Scientist Fellowship awarded to Dr Corrigan by the Medical Research Council (UK).

Address for correspondence:

A Barry Kay MD PhD
Department of Allergy and Clinical Immunology
National Heart and Lung Institute
Dovehouse Street
London SW3 6LY
UK

References

1. Milburn MV, Hassell AM, Lambert MH, Jordan SR, Proudfoot AE, Graber P, Wells TNC. A novel dimer configuration revealed by the crystal structure at 2.4A resolution of human interleukin-5. *Nature* 1993; 363:172.

2. Murata Y, Takaki S, Migita M, Kikuchi Y, Tominaga A, Takatsu K. Molecular cloning and expression of the human interleukin-5 receptor. *J Exp Med* 1992; 175:341.

3. Takaki S, Murata Y, Kitamura T, Miyajima A, Tominaga A, Takatsu K. Reconstitution of the functional receptors for murine and human interleukin-5. *J Exp Med* 1993; 177:1523.

4. Sakamaki K, Miyajima I, Kitamura T, Miyajima A. Critical cytoplasmic domains of the common b subunit of the human GM-CSF, IL-3 and IL-5 receptors for growth signal transduction and tyrosine phosphorylation.

5. Mosmann TR, Coffman RL. Th1 and Th2 cells: different patterns of lymphokine secretion lead to different functional properties. *Annu Rev Immunol* 1989; 7:145.

6. Sun Y, Durham SR, Barkans J, Masuyama K, Jacobson M, Rak S, Lowhagen O, Moqbel R, Kay AB, Hamid QA. T cells are the principal source of interleukin-5 mRNA in allergen-induced rhinitis. *Am J Resp Cell Mol Biol* 1993; 9:356.

7. Broide DH, Paine MM, Firestein GS. Eosinophils express interleukin-5 and granulocyte/macrophage colony-stimulating factor mRNA at sites of allergic inflammation in asthmatics. *J Clin Invest* 1992; 90:1414.

8. Clutterbuck EJ, Sanderson CJ. Human eosinophil haematopoiesis studied *in vitro* by means of murine eosinophil differentiation factor (IL-5): Production of functionally active eosinophils from normal human bone marrow. *Blood* 1988; 71:646.

9. Rothenberg ME, Petersen J, Stevens RL, Silberstein DS, McKenzie DT, Austen KF, Owen WF. IL-5 dependent conversion of normodense human eosinophils to the hypodense phenotype uses 3T3 fibroblasts for enhanced viability, accelerated hypodensity and sustained antibody-dependent cytotoxicity. *J Immunol* 1989; 143:2311.

10. Lopez AF, Sanderson CJ, Gamble JR, Campbell HD, Young IG, Vadas MA. Recombinant human interleukin-5 is a selective activator of eosinophil function. *J Exp Med* 1988; 167:219.

11. Dent LA, Strath M, Mellor AL, Sanderson CJ. Eosinophilia in transgenic mice expressing interleukin-5. *J Exp Med* 1990; 172:1425.

12. Coffman RL, Seymour BWP, Hudak S, Jackson J, Rennick D. Antibody to interleukin-5 inhibits hel-

minth-induced eosinophilia in mice. *Science* 1989; 245:308.

13. Denburg JA. Basophil and mast cell lineages *in vitro* and *in vivo*. *Blood* 1992; 79:846.

14. Dunnill MS, Massarella GR, Anderson JA. A comparison of the quantitative anatomy of the bronchi in normal subjects, in status asthmaticus, in chronic bronchitis and in emphysema. *Thorax* 1969; 24:176.

15. Filley WV, Holley KE, Kephart GM, Gleich GJ. Identification by immunofluorescence of eosinophil granule major basic protein in lung tissues of patients with bronchial asthma. *Lancet* 1982; ii:11.

16. Azzawi M, Bradley B, Jeffery PK, Frew AJ, Wardlaw AJ, Knowles G, Assoufi B, Collins JV, Durham SR, Kay AB. Identification of activated T lymphocytes and eosinophils in bronchial biopsies in stable atopic asthma. *Am Rev Respir Dis* 1990; 142:1410.

17. Bradley BL, Azzawi M, Assoufi B, Jacobson M, Collins JV, Irani A, Schwartz LB, Durham SR, Jeffery PK, Kay AB. Eosinophils, T-lymphocytes, mast cells, neutrophils and macrophages in bronchial biopsies from atopic asthmatics: Comparison with atopic non-asthma and normal controls and relationship to bronchial hyperresponsiveness. *J Allergy Clin Immunol* 1991; 88:661.

18. Bentley AM, Maestrelli P, Saetta M, Fabbri LM, Robinson DR, Bradley BL, Jeffery PK, Durham SR, Kay AB. Activated T-lymphocytes and eosinophils in the bronchial mucosa in isocyanate-induced asthma. *J Allergy Clin Immunol* 1992; 89:821.

19. Bentley AM, Menz G, Storz C, Robinson DR, Bradley B, Jeffery PK, Durham SR, Kay AB. Identification of T-lymphocytes, macrophages and activated eosinophils in the bronchial mucosa in intrinsic asthma: relationship to symptoms and bronchial responsiveness. *Am Rev Respir Dis* 1992; 146:500.

20. Wang JM, Rambaldi A, Biondi A, Chen ZG, Sanderson CJ, Mantovani A. Recombinant human interleukin-5 is a selective eosinophil chemoattractant. *Eur J Immunol* 1989; 19:701.

21. Sehmi R, Wardlaw AJ, Cromwell O, Kurihara K, Waltmann P, Kay AB. Interleukin-5 selectively enhances the chemotactic response of eosinophils obtained from normal but not eosinophilic subjects. *Blood* 1992; 79:2952.

22. Kyan-Aung U, Haskard DO, Poston RN, Thornhill MH, Lee TH. Endothelial leukocyte adhesion molecule 1 and intercellular adhesion molecule 1 mediate adhesion of eosinophils to endothelial cells *in vitro* and are expressed by endothelium in allergic cutaneous inflammation *in vivo*. *J Immunol* 1991; 146:521.

23. Walsh GM, Hartnell A, Wardlaw AJ, Kurihara K, Sanderson CJ, Kay AB. IL-5 enhances the *in vitro* adhesion of human eosinophils, but not neutrophils, in a leucocyte integrin (CD11/CD18)-dependent manner. *Immunology* 1990; 71:258.

24. Corrigan CJ, Haczku A, Gemou-Engesaeth V, Doi S, Kikuchi Y, Takatsu K, Durham SR, Kay AB. CD4 T-lymphocyte activation in asthma is accompanied by increased concentrations of interleukin-5: Effect of glucocorticoid therapy. *Am Rev Respir Dis* 1993; 147:540.

25. Robinson DS, Bentley AM, Hartnell A, Kay AB, Durham SR. Activated memory T helper cells in broncoalveolar lavage from atopic asthmatics. Relationship to asthma symptoms, lung function and bronchial responsiveness. *Thorax* 1993; 48:26.

26. Walker C, Virchow J-C, Bruijnzeel PLB, Blaser K. T cell subsets and their soluble products regulate eosinophilia in allergic and non-allergic asthma. *J Immunol* 1991; 146:1829.

27. Walker C, Bode E, Boer L, Hansel TT, Blaser K, Virchow J-C. Allergic and non-allergic asthmatics have distinct patterns of T cell activation and cytokine production in peripheral blood and bronchoalveolar lavage. *Am Rev Respir Dis* 1992; 146:109.

28. Hamid Q, Azzawi M, Ying S, Moqbel R, Wardlaw AJ, Corrigan CJ, Bradley B, Durham SR, Collins JV, Jeffery PK, Quint DJ, Kay AB. Expression of mRNA for interleukin-5 in mucosal bronchial biopsies from asthma. *J Clin Invest* 1991; 87:1541.

29. Robinson DS, Hamid Q, Ying S, Tsicopoulos A, Barkans J, Bentley AM, Corrigan C, Durham SR, Kay AB. Evidence for a predominant "Th2-type" bronchoalveolar lavage T-lymphocyte population in atopic asthma. *N Engl J Med* 1992; 326:298.

30. Robinson DS, Ying S, Bentley AM, Meng Q, North J, Durham SR, Kay AB. Relationships among numbers of bronchoalveolar lavage cells expressing messenger ribonucleic acid for cytokines, asthma symptoms, and airway methacholine responsiveness in atopic asthma. *J Allergy Clin Immunol* 1993; 92:397.

31. Robinson DS, Hamid Q, Ying S, Bentley AM, Assoufi B, North J, Meng Q, Durham SR, Kay AB. Prednisolone treatment in asthma is associated with modulation of bronchoalveolar lavage cell interleukin-4, interleukin-5 and interferon-gamma cytokine gene expression. *Am Rev Respir Dis* 1993; 148:420.

32. Bentley AM, Meng Q, Robinson DS, Hamid Q, Kay AB, Durham SR. Increases in activated T-lymphocytes, eosinophils and cytokine messenger RNA for IL-5 and GM-CSF in bronchial biopsies after allergen inhalation challenge in atopic asthmatics. *Am J Resp Cell Mol Biol* 1993; 8:35.

Food Allergy in Adults with Atopic Dermatitis: A Guide to Diagnosis*

Frederike de Maat-Bleeker, Carla Bruijnzeel-Koomen**

Keywords: Food allergy, adults, atopic dermatitis

Atopic dermatitis in childhood is often related to sensitization to milk, egg, peanut and fish, which occurs in the vulnerable period of the first year of life, when the mucosa of the gut is still easily permeable. At a later age, sensitization to inhalants, and especially to birch and mugwort pollens, accounts for simultaneous sensitization to food allergens of vegetable origin. This cross-sensitivity is often widespread, but of the many positive skin tests probably only a few are of clinical importance.
Oral food challenges may help to distinguish between relevant and irrelevant positive skin tests. Guidelines to select food items for oral challenges are discussed. Six patients were observed in whom cow's milk allergy first became apparent in adolescence. Strong positive skin tests and high specific IgE levels, especially for casein, were found. Elimination of dairy products was reasonably successful. Analysis of the data from 45 patients receiving hospital treatment for severe atopic dermatitis showed a high prevalence of pollen allergy. Sensitization to a selected panel of food allergens was found in 21 patients and was almost exclusively seen in the pollen-positive group. In these patients, who were mainly sensitized to vegetable food, the results of open challenge were often negative and the results of diets unrewarding.

Atopic dermatitis is a disease with a multifactorial etiology. Atopy may be defined as the genetic predisposition of the immune system to react inappropriately, with marked IgE production, to otherwise harmless environmental antigens (inhalants, foods). Atopy is probably the main causative factor in atopic dermatitis, but other non-allergenic environmental factors may influence pathogenesis (1). The sensitivity of the skin to these non-allergenic factors is called *hyper-reactivity*. Factors that may aggravate the disease and play a role in its maintenance are numerous: cutaneous infections and irritants, climatic factors, or emotional and physical stress.

The complex pathogenesis makes it difficult to judge the relative importance of inhalant and food allergens in modulating the expression of the disease, both in terms of their capacity to act as triggers and in terms of the benefit that interventions, such as house dust-mite avoidance or elimination diets, may have. Patients with atopic dermatitis differ from those with asthma and hay fever in having higher total IgE levels that tend to parallel the extent and severity of the disease. They have a higher frequency of positive immediate skin tests to food, and higher levels of food-specific IgE (2). A fairly significant number of patients experience food-induced hypersensitivity reactions of immediate onset, both localized and generalized (1). However, the results of diets are disappointing with regard to the course of the chronic skin lesions in atopic dermatitis, especially in the case of adults. Nevertheless, the question of whether food allergens do play a role in the pathogenesis of the skin lesions remains intriguing.

Development of Food Allergy in Relation to Age

The role of food allergy has been best studied in infancy, the most important food allergens in childhood being egg, cow's milk, peanut, fish, wheat, and soy bean. According to Sampson, almost 60% of children with severe atopic dermatitis have positive food-challenges to one or two of these foods (3). Sensitization to these potent allergens occurs mainly in the vulnerable period of the first year of life, when the mucosa of the gut is still easily permeable and devoid of defense mechanisms like endogenous IgA production. With in-

* Presented on the occasion of the 75th Anniversary of Dermatology (June 1994) in Utrecht University.
** Department of Dermatology – Allergology, University Hospital Utrecht, Utrecht, The Netherlands.

263

creased maturity of the gut barrier, egg and cow's milk allergy tend – though not always – to disappear (4–6). Fish and especially peanut allergy often remain a life-long problem (5, 7).

When the atopic subject gets older and sensitization to common inhalants, especially birch and mugwort pollen, comes into effect, there is an ever increasing possibility of simultaneous sensitization to food allergens of vegetable origin that share epitopes with the previously mentioned allergens. This cross-sensitivity is often widespread, and may account for a multitude of positive skin tests to vegetable food (only a few of which are usually of clinical relevance). In the acute, often generalized, food allergic reactions (urticaria, anaphylaxis) that can occur in patients sensitized to birch and mugwort pollen, but who do not have atopic dermatitis, a careful clinical history, knowledge of the characteristic sensitization patterns, insight into food preparation habits and knowledge of the components of prepacked food are usually sufficient to pinpoint the relevant positive skin test. However, patients with atopic dermatitis clearly find it very difficult to judge how much which food allergens influence the severity of their disease, thus creating a greater desire for challenge tests. Apart from being time-consuming, these challenge tests have other flaws. Food allergy has a variable expression, and the symptoms depend on the amount of food eaten, the way it was prepared, the presence or absence of a combination with alcohol, and physical exercise. So the causative food may not induce a reaction if it is not eaten under exactly the right circumstances (1). Furthermore, it is not clear whether only one or repeated challenges are necessary to provoke this chronic allergic disease.

Considering the drawbacks of challenge tests, a careful selection of food items that are most likely to be of influence is an absolute prerequisite to obtain a positive challenge test. In our opinion, this selection must be done according to certain basic principles: taking a detailed clinical food history, performing skin tests with and specific IgE measurements for a careful chosen panel of food allergens, and making a neatly arranged (preferably one page) overview of these data.

The Clinical Food History

The clinical food history includes more then the question of whether the patient noticed ill-effects of food on his skin disease. It also involves obtaining information about any acute local or generalized symptoms caused by a large panel of food items, as well as their influence on itchiness or worsening of atopic dermatitis. The patient history should be structured in order to get a clear impression of the number of and the relationship between the offending food items. The first important division is judging the effects of (a) food of animal origin, and (b) food of vegetable origin.

Relevant Food of Animal Origin. Questions should be asked about occurrence of symptoms after consumption of the milk, egg, fish, meat, poultry and seafood (such as crustaceans).

Food of Vegetable Origin. Several categories should be discussed with the patient:
– nuts and seeds,
– fruits and vegetables (arranged in groups according to botanical family),
– herbs and spices,
– grain products,
– drinks, such as wine, beer, tea, cola.

Panel of Food Items for Testing

The panel of food items for skin tests and specific IgE measurements should include:
1. *The well-known food allergens* of both animal and vegetable origin:
   – cow's milk*, egg*, fish*, meat, seafood (shrimp)
   – peanut*, soy*, wheat* (*the well-known food allergens in childhood!)
   – the classic "para-pollen" allergens: nuts, apple, celery and potato.
2. *More items of those food families showing extensive cross-sensitivity*: Papilonaceae, Umbelliferae, Solanaceae, in order to obtain a more clear view on their clinical importance.
3. *Food items that may serve as "alimentary alternatives"*: For example, fruit not belonging to the Rosaceae (citrus, banana, grape, melon, etc.); maize, rice, buckwheat to use in case of wheat allergy; herbs and spices not belonging to the Umbelliferous plant family. In the case of widespread vegetable food sensitivity, at least one edible variant of the different botanical families (Compositae, Liliaceae, Cruciferae, Chenopodiaceae) should be tested. The selection should be based on the usual diet. Special atten-

tion to food habits is necessary in dealing with patients from other cultures.

4. *The food items the patient regards as (possibly) harmful.*

Table 1. Clinical symptoms in six adult patients with cow's milk allergy (5 females, 1 male; mean age of onset 26 years).

Clinical symptom	Frequency
Worsening of atopic eczema	6
Oral allergy	6
Urticaria, angioedema	6
Vomiting, diarrhea	2
Rhinitis, asthma	2
Anaphylaxis	3
Atopy: positive skin tests to common inhalants	6
"Complex" food allergy (>3 items positive)	5

An Overview

The synopsis should comprise the results of history taking, as well as the results of skin tests and specific IgE measurements. Finally, the overview can serve to record the effects of oral challenge tests.

Food of Animal Origin

Interestingly, cow's milk can still be an important causative allergen in adult patients and sometimes even a recently acquired cow's milk allergy is seen clinically. Since 1989 we have observed six patients (five females, one male) with atopic dermatitis, whose signs of cow's milk allergy became apparent for the first time in adolescence (8). All six had been able to tolerate cow's milk in childhood, without any apparent influence on their usually mild atopic dermatitis. However, between the ages of 20 and 30 years these patients became aware of adverse effects of cow's milk. Apart from worsening of atopic dermatitis, consumption of cow's milk caused oral pruritus, swelling of lips and tongue, urticaria and angioedema, vomiting,

Table 2. Skin test results in six adult patients with cow's milk allergy (5 females, 1 male; mean age of onset: 26 year).

Patient no.	Whole cow's milk*	Casein**	α-Lactalbumin***	β-Lactoglobulin***
1	+	+++	−	−
2	++	+++	+	+
3	+	+++	−	−
4	n.d.	+	+	−
5	++	+++	−	++
6	n.d.	++	−	−

* Prick test according to Diephuis (patients 1, 3) and Bencard (patients 2, 5).
** Scratch patch test with Na-caseinate powder in saline.
*** Prick test ARTU Biologicals NV, Lelystad.
n.d. = not done.

Table 3. Serological tests in six adult patients with cow's milk allergy (kU/l in Pharmacia CAP system; 5 females, 1 male; mean age of onset 26 years).

Patient no.	Total IgE	Specific IgE (CAP classes)			
		Whole cow's milk	Casein	α-Lactalbumin	β-Lactoglobulin
1	663	56 (V)	73 (V)	<0.35	<0.35
2	18168	92 (V)	>100 (VI)	58 (V)	80 (V)
3	9256	99 (V)	>100 (VI)	RAST 3+	RAST 1+
4	18774	n.d.	91 (V)	9 (III)	1.5 (II)
5	96	0.7 (II)	0.9 (II)	<0.35	<0.35
6	4464	20 (IV)	80 (V)	<0.35	<0.35

n.d. = not done.
RAST = Radio Allergosorbent Test carried out by the Central Laboratory of the Red Cross Blood Transfusion Service, Amsterdam.

265

diarrhea, rhinitis and asthma and (in three of them) signs of anaphylaxis (Table 1).

All six were atopic as judged by positive skin tests to common inhalants; in five, multiple positive skin tests were found to other food allergens, mainly of vegetable origin. All six had positive skin tests and/or high specific IgE for whole cow's milk. Skin prick tests with Na-caseinate powder and commercially obtained extracts of β-lactoglobulin and α-lactalbumin revealed positive reactions to casein protein and generally much weaker or negative reactions to whey proteins (Table 2). Five had high specific IgE levels to casein (class V-VI in Pharmacia CAP system). One had a rather low level, but in all six the casein antibody level exceeded the levels for α-lactalbumin and β-lactoglobulin (Table 3). The data suggest that in this "late-onset" cow's milk allergy the main sensitizing protein is casein, and that casein-containing food items are probably the most hazardous for these patients. Elimination diets proved reasonably successful in controlling both the acute symptoms and the atopic dermatitis.

Onset of cow's milk allergy in adult life as well as the predominant sensitization to casein has been described by others (9–12).

Food of Vegetable Origin

Our impression that birch and/or mugwort pollen sensitization and the consequent multi-sensitization to vegetable food is seen especially in patients with severe atopic dermatitis was confirmed by analyzing the data from 45 patients receiving in-hospital treatment for their eczema (13). Taking into account CAP values > 3 kU/l, 62% of these patients were sensitized to grass pollen, 47% to birch, and 17% to mugwort pollen. Sensitization to food was found in 21 patients (46%), and was almost exclusively seen in the "pollen-positive" group (Table 4). In the patients with "isolated" grass pollen allergy, raised specific IgE values for food were found in only four subjects: three were sensitized to food of animal origin, and only one was sensitized to food of vegetable origin. This is in agreement with the well-known fact that sensitization to food of vegetable origin is related to birch and mugwort pollen allergies.

The prevalence of atopic disease, and especially of pollen allergy, is increasing, probably because of atmospheric pollution (14, 15). Pollutants damage the epithelium of the respiratory tract, thus increas-

Table 4. Pollen and food allergy in 45 patients with a severe form of atopic dermatitis (a CAP value of 3 kU/l serum is used to discriminate between positive and negative patients).

Category	No.	%	Category	No.	%
Pollen +	28	62	Pollen –	17	38
Grass	28	62			
Birch	21	47			
Mugwort	7	17			
Food* +	19	70	Food* +	2	12

* Egg, cow's milk, peanut, hazelnut, potato, wheat, celery, soy.

ing its permeability to allergens. In animal studies, suspended particles (aerosols) such as those present in diesel exhaust may act as adjuvant in promoting the IgE response. Hay fever in the UK has increased 4-fold over the past 30 years (16).

The increased prevalence of pollen allergy, and the consequent multi-sensitization to food of vegetable origin, may account for the increasing number of patients we see with difficult to treat forms of atopic dermatitis. However, it is not quite clear whether we should regard this "pollen-related" food allergy as merely a sign of the broader expression of atopy, that only serves as an explanation for the frequently mentioned oral allergy symptoms, or whether we must consider vegetable food allergy to be a real cause in the pathogenesis of the atopic dermatitis. Results of open (bulk) challenge tests at the end of a period of hospital observation were disappointing (often negative), and the results of diets were unrewarding, even when we selected the food items for challenge tests carefully and according to the guidelines mentioned above.

The debate is still not settled. Did we select the right food items, and did we create the desired conditions for our challenge tests? Or should we have serious doubts about the influence of vegetable food allergens on atopic dermatitis.

Tryptase and in particular ECP (eosinophil cationic protein) measurements have been described as potentially useful parameters for monitoring the effects of oral food challenges, especially in atopic dermatitis, and might help to distinguish between relevant and irrelevant positive skin tests and RASTs for food allergens (17, 18).

Though of great interest, food allergy as a cause of atopic dermatitis in adult patients remains a controversial subject.

Address for correspondence:

Frederike de Maat-Bleeker
Department of Dermatology – Allergology
University Hospital Utrecht
Heidelberglaan 100
NL-3508 GA Utrecht
The Netherlands

References

1. Atherton DJ. Diet and atopic eczema. *Clin Allergy* 1988; 18:215–228.

2. Hanifin JM. Basic and clinical aspects of atopic dermatitis. *Ann Allergy* 1984; 52(6):386–393.

3. Sampson HA. Immediate hypersensitivity reactions to foods: Blinded food challenges in children with atopic dermatitis. *Ann Allergy* 1986; 57(3):209–212.

4. Bahna SL, Heiner DC. *Allergies to milk.* Grüne and Stratton, 1980.

5. Dannaeus A, Inganäs M. Follow-up study of children with food allergy. Clinical course in relation to serum IgE and IgE antibody levels to milk, egg and fish. *Clin Allergy* 1981; 11:533–539.

6. Koers WJ, Van der Elst AMC, Van Dijk AG, Berrens L. Cow's milk allergy in an adult patient. *Ann Allergy* 1986; 56(3):267–269.

7. Allan Bock S, Atkins FM. The natural history of peanut allergy. *J Allergy Clin Immunol* 1989; 83:900–904.

8. Maat-Bleeker F de, Koers WJ, Heide S van der. Late onset cow's milk allergy in atopic dermatitis. *Allergy* 1992; 47(12):250.

9. Paganelli R, Sgambato F et al. Cow's milk hypersensitivity in an elderly woman: Clinical and immunological findings. *Ann Allergy* 1986; 56(6):480–483.

10. Olalde S, Bensabat Z et al. Allergy to cow's milk with onset in adult life. *Ann Allergy* 1989; 62(3):185 a–185 b.

11. Stöger P, Wüthrich B. Type I allergy to cow milk proteins in adults. *Int Arch All Immunol* 1993; 102:399–407.

12. Jessberger B, Rakoski J. Kuhmilch Allergie beim Erwachsenen *Allergologie* 1991; 14(4):133–136.

13. Bruijn J. *Inventarisatie van het uitgevoerde onderzoeksprotocol bij patienten met constitutioneel eczeem tijdens klinische behandeling. Een retrospectief onderzoek.* Utrecht, 1993.

14. Wüthrich B. Epidemiology of the allergic diseases: Are they really on the increase? *Int Arch Allergy Appl Immunol* 1989; 90:3–10.

15. Bousquet J, Burney P. Evidence for an increase in atopic disease and possible causes. *Clin Exp Allergy* 1993; 23(6):484–492.

16. Varney V. Hayfever in the United Kingdom (Allergy Practice Forum). *Clin Exp Allergy* 1991; 21:757–762.

17. Ohtsuka T, Matsumaru S et al. Timecourse of plasma histamine and tryptase following food challenges in children with suspected food allergy. *Ann Allergy* 1993; 71:139–146.

18. Wahn U, Niggeman B, Kleinau I, Beyer K. Monitoring of inflammation during challenge tests in children. *Allergy* 1993; 48 (Suppl 17):107–109.

New Controversial Techniques in the Diagnosis of Food Hypersensitivity

Carsten Bindslev-Jensen*,**, Tine K Hansen**, Astrid Norgaard**, Helle Vestergaard**, Lars K Poulsen***

Keywords: Food hypersensitivity, review, double-blind method, skin tests, IgE measurement, diagnosis, basophils, diagnostic procedures

Any new diagnostic test should be validated according to standard procedures, and it must be validated against the outcome of DBPCFC. A "controversial test" in this respect may mean any test used in food hypersensitivity, since most of these tests are not thoroughly validated. A full validation program for a new test should include data enabling the customer to answer the following questions: (1) Can the test diagnose the parameter in question with sufficient specificity and precision? (2) Are abnormal values of the parameter associated with clinical disease, and has an age- and sex-related normal range been established? (3) Can other conditions (pathological or physiological) give rise to values outside the normal range?

Introduction

The diagnosis of food hypersensitivity must rely entirely on the outcome of double-blind, placebo-controlled food-challenges (DBPCFC) (1). When properly performed, DBPCFC is the only confirmatory test in children and adults; in infants, however, open challenges controlled by trained personnel may be sufficient. A flowchart for controlled diagnosis of nontoxic adverse reactions to foods (food hypersensitivity) is presented in Table 1.

In many clinical situations, doctors (and patients) find this procedure difficult to perform, time-consuming, and potentially dangerous, and therefore try to base the diagnosis on case history supported by one or more allergy tests, i.e., skin prick test (SPT), measurement of specific IgE ("RAST"), or other more or less well-documented techniques.

The commercial market for these diagnostic tests for *in vivo* or *in vitro* determination of food hypersensitivity is enormous, and it is therefore not surprising that a vast variety of more or less serious companies have launched such tests. It is, however, worthwhile to bear in mind that doctors are restricted by the International Code of Ethics, which, for example, in Denmark means that a doctor may only use justifiable methods and tools in the diagnosis and treatment of patients.

Criteria for Justifiable Methods and Tools

1. Can the test diagnose the parameter in question with sufficient specificity and precision?
   Data for technical validation of the test should be available to the customer – a claim rarely fulfilled even in the best investigated tests such as some of the RASTs.
2. Are abnormal values of the parameter associated with clinical disease, and has an age- and sex-related normal range been established?
   Since no single diagnostic test exists in allergology, the above claim cannot be thoroughly fulfilled in food hypersensitivity.
3. Can other conditions (pathological or physiological) give rise to values outside the normal range?
   This criterion is particularly important in multiple allergy and in patients in pharmacotherapy, where drugs may interfere with the test (e.g.,

* Department of Dermatology I, Odense University Hospital, Odense, Denmark.
** Food Allergy Unit TTA 7523, National University Hospital, Copenhagen, Denmark.
*** Laboratory for Medical Allergology TTA 7542, National University Hospital, Copenhagen, Denmark.

Table 1. Flowchart for diagnosis of nontoxic adverse reactions to foods.

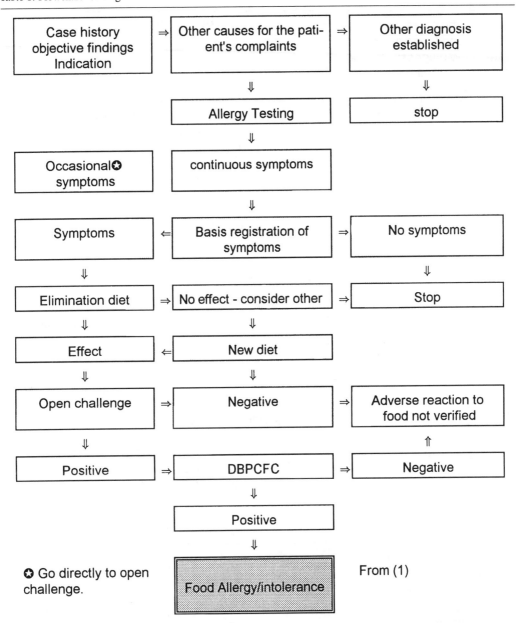

RAST in atopic dermatitis patients or SPT in patients taking antihistamines).

In food hypersensitivity, any new test *must* be validated against "the gold standard", i.e., DBPCFC instead of against the most used test – the market leader – in the field (1, 2).

Many of the tests claim to be able to detect hypersensitivity against many different foods, but data must be available on every single food – every single allergen is unique and must be evaluated as such (3). As an example, it is impossible to deduct anything on basophil histamine release performance in cow's milk allergy from data on allergy to

Table 2. Classification of diagnostic tests.

Tests which has been validated and found to be useful in the diagnosis of food hypersensitivity **Category I**	Skin Prick Test Specific IgE (RAST®)
Tests which has not been thoroughly validated **Category II**	Basophil Histamine Release Gut permeability tests Intragastric provocation (IPEC) Patch tests Histamine release from gut mast cells T-cells and subsets New tests for specific IgE in serum specific IgE in other body fluids IgE-complexes IgG-complexes complement (or split products) Other mediators: Tryptase Histamine in body fluids ECP IgG subsets cytokines blood-xylose All kinds of "alternative methods" e.g. "Bi-digital O-ring dysfunction localization method" diagnostic acupuncture "sublingual challenge test" ALCAT-test and many others
Tests which has been validated and found **not** to be useful in the diagnosis of food hypersensitivity **Category III**	serum-IgG

cod fish; in the first case, the sensitivity of the test when using a commercial extract is low, whereas in the latter a very high sensitivity is obtained (4, 5).

For most of the commercial tests on the market today, the above criteria cannot be met, although the amount and quality of documentation varies greatly. Based on documentation, the tests may be divided into three groups (Table 2).

In Category I, only SPT with validated extracts

and the original Phadebas RAST® are placed. Both tests has been used in numerous studies using DBPCFC technique and in both children and adults (1, 6–10). In most papers (reviewed in (3)), these two tests have demonstrated a sufficiently high sensitivity and specificity to justify their use in daily clinical practice. This is at least true for the most common allergens, though data are lacking on the more rare allergens.

One of the major problems with SPT and RAST is the lack of standardized extracts used in the tests; in some cases allergenic activity is somehow lost during the processing of the allergen, thus rendering fresh, unprocessed foods more convenient at least for SPT (11). It is worthwhile to bear in mind that the overall performance of a test depends on several parameters (Table 3), and both SPT and RAST may be greatly improved by ascertaining allergen quality by standardization and by increasing the knowledge on the degree and clinical significance of cross-reactivity between botanically related foods. An example of how botanical cross-reactivity interfere with diagnosis is Bernhisel-Broadbent's study (12) on peanut-allergic children, the majority of whom also demonstrated positive SPT to botanically related (cross-reacting) foods such as soybean, greenbean, or pea. By DBPCFC, however, clinical cross-reactivity proved to be very rare.

Table 3. Determinants for a diagnostic test.

Technical performance
Allergen quality
Patient sample (quality)
Cross-reactivity
Economics

Even in optimal cases, neither SPT nor RAST are "plus-minus" tests capable of dividing a population into a positive group (those with the clinical disease) and a negative group (those without the clinical disease). Interpretation of a test should therefore be cautious in order to avoid false conclusions.

Innumerable tests are available in Category II. There are several reasons for a test not being sufficiently investigated. One reason is that the test is new and under investigation and therefore not thoroughly validated, whereas in fact the manufacturer may not be interested in having the test validated. The latter is true for many of the "alternative tests," where the person offering the test often try to make a living off it (13, 14).

The new tests for specific IgE are listed in Category II. The reason for this is that in some cases the tests are new (Pharmacia CAP® or Ciba Corning Magic Lite®) and in other cases that only few data are available on a tests (e. g., FAST®) (15, 16). When launching a new IgE test, comparative studies against the market leader – in this case Phadebas RAST® – are often used and the quality of the new test calculated on the basis of correlation to this "reference test." As previously mentioned, such a procedure is insufficient to truly validate a diagnostic test, especially because of the unstandardized allergen extracts used in the IgE tests. As an example, two new techniques (Phadezym® and FAST®) were compared to Phadebas in patients with suspected food allergy (case history but no DBPCFC) and found to be much less sensitive in diagnosing allergies towards vegetables (16). The validity of such a finding is unknown since at least 50% of case histories of food hypersensitivity even in obvious cases are ruled out by DBPCFC, (1, 17–20), and the low number of positive findings with the new techniques might reflect the true clinically allergic patients – a statement that can be verified only by using DBPCFC as the true diagnosis. In this connection it is important to emphasize that also the gold standard has its limitations and drawbacks, as reviewed by David (21).

Another unsolved problem with some of the new tests for IgE is their improved chemical sensitivity, i. e., their ability to detect smaller amounts of specific IgE than Phadebas RAST®. Since no data are available on the correlation between chemical sensitivity and clinical sensitivity, we may face even greater problems in the future when trying to ascertain a clinical disease by measuring specific IgE. Finally, it is very difficult to compare the various assays for specific IgE, as reviewed in (22).

Measurements of specific IgE directly at mast cells in other body fluids (23, 24) or in feces (25) are interesting, but more data are needed.

Histamine release from blood basophils has long been regarded as being only a research tool, considering the time-consuming cell preparation technique needed, but recently a new whole-blood based technique (HRT) has been launched (26, 27). In comparative studies from our own group, we investigated this new technique (HRT) and compared it to SPT and RAST in selected groups of food allergic patients, verified by DBPCFC (5, 11, 28). As is the case with SPT, the HRT is very dependent on the quality of the allergen used for stimulation of histamine release: When using a commercial extract in SPT or HRT in egg- or milk-allergic patients, sensitivity was low, but increased to 80–90% when fresh, unprocessed egg, or milk were used as stimulants (11). In this case, the outcome of the tests were very dependent on the allergen quality, whereas in another study on allergy to hazel nut in birch-pollen patients, HRT were superior to SPT (sensitivity 86% and 43%) even when the same allergen extract was used for SPT and HRT (28). The place for HRT has not been established yet, but since fresh, unprocessed foods may be used in the test, it may prove useful in cases of suspected reactions to the more uncommon foods, outside the classical, better investigated foods, such as milk, egg, peanut, fish or wheat.

Measurement of gut permeability with various probes to establish a diagnosis of food hypersensitivity especially with intestinal symptoms has so far been disappointing, especially since the specificity of this test is seemingly too low. In a study on patients with cow's milk allergy, Jalonen (29) found identical increase in lactulose/mannitol ratio in patients developing skin symptoms during challenge and those developing gastro-intestinal symptoms.

The concept of measuring the events taking place directly in the target organ has been used in the asthma disease for several years. The same concept was tried by Ring et al. (30), who made prick tests directly in the gastric mucosa via an endoscope. The authors obtained high sensitivity and specificity in their study, which, however, was lacking in blinded applications; furthermore, their patients were not controlled by DBPCFC. When we repeated the experiment in a double-blind protocol with appropriate controls (31), the test was found to have a low specificity, and we concluded that the test offered no major advantages over SPT.

Measurement of other mediators in serum or other body fluids may in the future improve diagnosis, but presently insufficient data are available on, e.g., ECP, cytokines or mast cell tryptase. Regarding tryptase and food hypersensitivity, so far it has only been found in increased amounts in the sera of patients dying in food anaphylaxis (32).

On the alternative market, all kinds of unproven techniques and tests are abundant and usually totally escape official control. Only rarely are the results of these tests published in papers covered by the normal databases (14). One exception is the paper on "Omura's Bi-digital O-ring dysfunction localization method," from which the following statement is taken (33):

"By critically evaluating exceptions which may lead to false diagnosis, as well as by improving the currently-used applied kinesiology diagnostic method, the author was able to develop the 'Thumb-Index Finger Bi-Digital O-ring Diagnostic Method' using the Applied Kinesiology Dysfunction Localization Principle. By combining with clinically useful organ representation points in acupuncture medicine it has become possible to make early diagnosis of most of the internal organs, with an average diagnostic accuracy of over 85%, without knowing the patient's history or using any instruments."

Such results exceeds what most doctors may hope to achieve; on the other hand, such "investigations" do not fulfill the above-mentioned criteria and should of course be validated accordingly.

The ALCAT test launched for non-IgE-mediated food hypersensitivity measures changes in white cell diameter after challenge with foods in vitro. Only three papers are available for MEDLINE (17.05.94), one of which discourages the use of the test based on lack of reproducibility, whereas the two others do not fulfill the criteria mentioned earlier, so more investigations are needed – or at least need to be published: Since many trials with a negative outcome are never published, there is the risk of a tendency towards overestimation of the capability of a test which should be borne in mind.

In conclusion, any new diagnostic test should be validated according to standard procedures, and must be validated against the outcome of DBPCFC. The concept of a "controversial test" may relate to any test used in food hypersensitivity since most of these tests are not thoroughly validated.

Address for correspondence:

Carsten Bindslev-Jensen, MD, Ph D, D SC
Department of Dermatology I
Odense University Hospital
JB Winsløwsvej
DK 5000 Odense C
Denmark

References

1. Bindslev-Jensen C, Bjorksten B. Diagnostic procedures. Chapter III in C Ortolani and C Bruinjzel-Koomen (Eds) *Position paper on adverse reactions to food. Allergy Eur J Allergy Clin Immunol* 1994, in press.

2. Metcalfe DD, Sampson HA. Workshop on experimental methodology for clinical studies of adverse reactions to foods and food additives. *J Allergy Clin Immunol* 1990; 86:421–442.

3. Bindslev-Jensen C, Skov P, Madsen F, Poulsen LK. Food allergy and food intolerance – What is the difference? *Ann Allergy* 1994; 72:317–320.

4. Norgaard A, Bindslev-Jensen C. Egg and milk allergy in adults. Diagnosis and characterization. *Allergy* 1992; 47:503–509.

5. Hansen TK, Bindslev-Jensen C. Codfish allergy in adults. Identification and diagnosis. *Allergy* 1992; 47:610–617.

6. Burks AW, Sampson HA. Diagnostic approaches to the patient with suspected food allergies. *J Pediatr* 1992; 121:S64–S71.

7. Bock SA, Sampson HA, Atkins FM, Zeiger RS, Lehrer S, Sachs M, Bush RK, Metcalfe DD. Double-blind, placebo-controlled food challenge (DBPCFC) as an office procedure: a manual. *J Allergy Clin Immunol* 1988; 82:986–997.

8. Sampson HA. Comparative study of commercial food antigen extracts for the diagnosis of food hypersensitivity. *J Allergy Clin Immunol* 1988; 82:718–726.

9. Bindslev-Jensen C. Respiratory reactions induced by food challenges in adults. *Ped Allergy Immunol* 1992; 3:201–206.

10. American Academy of Allergy and Immunology Committee on Adverse Reactions to Foods. *Adverse reactions to foods*. National Institutes of Health., publ 84–2442, 1984.

11. Norgaard A, Skov PS, Bindslev-Jensen C. Egg and milk allergy in adults: Comparison between fresh foods and commercial allergen extracts in skin prick test and histamine release from basophils. *Clin Exp Allergy* 1992; 22:940–947.

12. Bernhisel Broadbent J, Sampson HA. Cross-allergenicity in the legume botanical family in children with food hypersensitivity. *J Allergy Clin Immunol* 1989; 83:435–440.

13. Clinical ecology. Executive Committee of the American Academy of Allergy and Immunology. *J Allergy Clin Immunol* 1986; 78:269–271.

14. American Academy of Allergy: Position statements – Controversial techniques. *J Allergy Clin Immunol* 1981; 67:333–338.

15. Marinkovich VA. Evaluation of a multiple food specific IgE antibody test. *Clin Exp Allergy* 1992; 22:804.

16. Moneret Vautrin DA, Gueant JL, Abdel Ghani A, Maria Y, Nicolas JP. Comparative evaluation between two immunoenzymatic techniques (FAST and Phadezym) and the Phadebas RAST in food allergy. *Allergy* 1990; 45:104–108.

17. Sampson HA, Metcalfe DD. Food allergies. *JAMA* 1992; 268:2840–2844.

18. Metcalfe DD. Diagnostic procedures for immunologically-mediated food sensitivity. *Nutr Rev* 1984; 42:92–97.

19. Atkins FM, Steinberg SS, Metcalfe DD. Evaluation of immediate adverse reactions to foods in adult patients. I. Correlation of demographic, laboratory, and prick skin test data with response to controlled oral food challenge. *J Allergy Clin Immunol* 1985; 75:348–355.

20. Atkins FM, Steinberg SS, Metcalfe DD. Evaluation of immediate adverse reactions to foods in adult patients. II. A detailed analysis of reaction patterns during oral food challenge. *J Allergy Clin Immunol* 1985; 75:356–363.

21. David TJ. Hazards of challenge tests in atopic dermatitis. *Allergy* 1989; 44 (Suppl 9):101–107.

22. Lockey RF, Lichtenstein LM, Bloch KJ, Kaliner M, Zweimann B, Rachelefsky G, Anderson JA. Position statement. The use of *in vitro* tests for IgE antibody in the specific diagnosis of IgE-mediated disorders and in the formulation of allergen immunotherapy. *J Allergy Clin Immunol* 1992; 90:263–267.

23. Baenkler HW, Lux G. Antigen-induced histamine release from duodenal biopsy in gastrointestinal food allergy. *Ann Allergy* 1989; 62:449–452.

24. Nolte H, Schiotz PO, Kruse A, Stahl Skov P. Comparison of intestinal mast cell and basophil histamine release in children with food allergic reactions. *Allergy* 1989; 44:554–565.

25. Sasai K, Furukawa S, Sugawara T, Kaneko K, Baba M, Yabuta K. IgE levels in faecal extracts of patients with food allergy. *Allergy* 1992; 47:594–598.

26. Nolte H. The clinical utility of basophil histamine release. *Allergy Proc* 1993; 14:251–254.

27. Kleine Tebbe J, Werfel S, Roedsgaard D, Nolte H, Skov PS, Wahn U, Kunkel G. Comparison of fiberglass-based histamine assay with a conventional automated fluorometric histamine assay, case history, skin prick test, and specific serum IgE in patients with milk and egg allergic reactions. *Allergy* 1993; 48:49–53.

28. Bindslev-Jensen C, Vibits A, Skov P, Weeke B. Oral allergy syndrome: The effect of astemizole. *Allergy* 1991; 46:610–613.

29. Jalonen T. Identical intestinal permeability changes in children with different clinical manifestations of cow's milk allergy. *J Allergy Clin Immunol* 1991; 88:737–742.

30. Reimann HJ, Ring J, Ultsch B, Wendt P. Intragastral provocation under endoscopic control (IPEC) in food allergy: Mast cell and histamine changes in gastric mucosa. *Clin Allergy* 1985; 15:195–202.

31. Bindslev-Jensen C, Norgaard A, Ladefoged K, Hyl-

lander E, Poulsen L. On the diagnosis of food allergy in adults. In E Przysbilla, J Ring (Eds) *New trends in allergy III*. Berlin: Springer Verlag, 1992, 243–246.

32. Yunginger JW, Nelson DR, Squillace DL, Jones RT, Holley KE, Hyma BA, Biedrzycki L, Sweeney KG, Sturner WQ, Schwartz LB. Laboratory investigation of deaths due to anaphylaxis. *J Forensic Sci* 1991; 36:857–865.

33. Omura Y. New simple early diagnostic methods using Omura's "Bi-Digital O-Ring Dysfunction Localization Method" and acupuncture organ representation points, and their applications to the "drug & food compatibility test" for individual organs and to auricular diagnosis of internal organs – part I. *Acupunct Electrother Res* 1981; 6:239–254.

Use of Interferon in Allergic Disease and its Possible Use in Food Allergy

Joseph A Bellanti*, Yung-Hao Pung**

Keywords: Cytokines, cytokine cascade, interferons, interleukins, allergic diseases, atopic dermatitis (AD), natural killer (NK) cells, hyper-IgE syndrome (HIES), IgE regulation, T-helper cells, IL-4 mutant protein, interferon therapy

The regulation of IgE responses by cytokines is of critical importance in our understanding of the pathogenesis of human allergic diseases. It is now established that a polarization of T-helper cells into Th1 cells responsible for cellular immunity and Th2 cells responsible for antibody synthesis is under the control of specific cytokines. The absence of IL-4 and the presence of IL-12 favors the induction of the Th1 subset. The presence of IL-4 favors the induction of Th2 subsets. IFN-γ produced by natural killer (NK) cells or Th1 cells and INF-α exert an inhibitory or suppressive effect on B-cell differentiation and particularly on IgE production. This knowledge has provided a basis for the use of the cytokines, specifically the interferons, in the treatment of allergic diseases. The present study describes the results of treatment of three patients with AD and one with HIES with INF-γ and/or IFN-α. Two of the three patients with AD had significant food allergy that was found to aggravate the clinical condition. The results of these studies suggest a beneficial effect on improving the activity of the allergic disease and suggests that the combined use of IFN-γ and IFN-α may offer additional therapeutic benefit.

Introduction

In recent years, the pathogenesis of human allergic diseases has been elucidated by the rapid progress in our understanding of the regulation of human IgE synthesis (1–14). It is now generally accepted that T-cells play a pivotal role in the elaboration of IgE responses. Although formally a balance between T-helper and T-suppressor activities was considered a primary determinant of IgE synthesis, more recent studies indicate that a polarization exists between Th1 and Th2 subsets and that the modulation of IgE synthesis by these cells through the effects of cytokines appear to be of critical importance (15). This knowledge has encouraged new therapeutic interventions in the treatment of allergic diseases. This presentation briefly reviews our current understanding of the cytokine cascade involved in IgE regulation, some clinical observations on the treatment of patients with atopic dermatitis and food hypersensitivity together with projections for future use of cytokines in the treatment of allergic diseases.

Cytokines

Cytokines are molecules produced by cells of the immune system directly involved in the immunologic communication network (16). At least 13 major types of interleukins are now recognized, each affecting a variety of target cells, several factors affecting growth and differentiation of hematopoietic tissues, and three major types of interferons. Several other cytokines involved in inflammation have also been described, e. g., tumor necrosis factor-α (TNF-α). For simplicity's sake, the cytokines may be grouped according to their biologic function(s) into four major categories: (1) the interferons, (2) the hematopoietic growth factors, (3) interleukins and immunostimulants, and (4) anti-inflammatory cytokines (Table 1).

* Department of Pediatrics, International Center for Interdisciplinary Studies of Immunology, Georgetown University School of Medicine, Washington, DC, USA.
** Departments of Pediatrics and Microbiology-Immunology, International Center for Interdisciplinary Studies of Immunology, Georgetown University School of Medicine, Washington, DC, USA.

Table 1. Types of cytokines.

Type	Cytokine
Interferons	IFN-α IFN-β IFN-γ
Hematopoietic growth factors	GM-CSF, G-CSF Erythropoietin (EPO) IL-3, IL-1, IL-6
Interleukins acting as immuno-stimulants or anticancer adjuvants	IL-1, IL-2, IL-4, IL-6 IL-12, TNF-α
Anti-inflammatory cytokines	TNF binding protein (TBP) IL-4, IL-10 Transforming growth factor β (TGF-β) IL-1 receptor antagonist (IL-1Ra), IL-13

Concept of Cytokine Cascade

It is becoming increasingly apparent that the mode of action of the cytokines is quite complex, and that these molecules do not act in isolation; rather, the cytokines act in various sets of interacting sequences or cascades, resulting in targeted cellular responses. The responses to cytokines may result in proliferation or differentiation, and at times may be suppressive or inhibitory. Moreover, following the interaction of a cytokine with a target cell, the production of other cytokines may be seen during the interaction.

The most primordial of immune responses is that associated with the initial antigen-phagocytic cell interaction (Figure 1). Following the introduction of antigen to a host and its interaction with cells of the mononuclear phagocyte system (MPS) and its subsequent processing, there is the synthesis of interferon-α (INF-α). INF-α together with antigen provides a signal for the synthesis of small amounts of interleukin-1 (IL-1) by the MPS. Then selection and activation of T lymphocytes occur through their T-cell receptor (TCR), the expression of receptors for interleukin-2 (IL-2), and the synthesis of

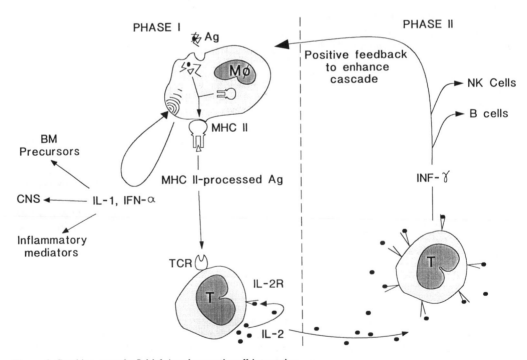

Figure 1. Cytokine cascade: Initial Ag-phagocytic cell interaction.

IL-2, resulting in expansion of T-lymphocyte populations. This completes phase I of this cytokine cascade. In addition, the production of IL-1 leads to the proliferation of bone marrow precursors, the stimulation of certain hypothalamic and pituitary functions, e. g., fever, and the production of a wide variety of inflammatory mediators including cell adhesion molecules, prostaglandins, cytokines, and platelet-activating factor.

Under the influence of IL-2, antigen-sensitized T lymphocytes are then stimulated to produce interferon-γ (IFN-γ), which begins phase II of this cytokine cascade and which is responsible for the stimulation of a wide variety of cellular functions including the stimulation of natural killer (NK) cells and B cells as well as the stimulation of class-II molecule expression on the cells of the MPS and other antigen presenting cells. This includes a positive feedback on the MPS with additional produc-

Table 2. Immunoregulatory effect of cytokines on IgE synthesis.

Induces or upregulates	Inhibits or suppresses
Interleukin-4	Interferon-γ
Interleukin-5	Interferion-α
Interleukin-6	Tumor necrosis factor-β
Interleukin-13	Transforming growth factor-β
Tumor necrosis factor-α	Interleukin 8
	Prostaglandin E$_2$
	PAF-acether
	Vasoactive intestinal peptide
	Somatostatin

tion of IL-1 in large quantity, which in turn stimulates the production of more IL-2 and IFN-γ. The continued production of IFN-γ and the stimulation of immunologic processes are thought to contribute significantly to the perpetuation of immunologic mechanisms of tissue injury, resulting in the chronicity of many chronic infectious diseases and autoimmune diseases.

Regulation of Human IgE Responses

It is now generally accepted that the induction of IgE synthesis in human B cells requires at least two signals (17–19): The first signal is delivered by IL-4, which induces Ig heavy-chain gene switching to the epsilon locus (17, 18); the second signal can be triggered by a number of B-cell activators such as EBV infection, hydrocortisone, or actual physical contact between T and B cells delivered through cognate and noncognate interactions (16, 19).

A number of cytokines and mediators have been found to modulate IL-4-induced IgE synthesis (Table 2). IL-4, IL-5 and IL-6, and IL-13 and TNF-α may enhance IgE synthesis. In contrast, a number of cytokines inhibit or suppress IgE synthesis. These include IFN-γ, IFN-α, tumor necrosis factor-β, transforming growth factor-β, interleukin-8, and a number of mast cell mediators and neuropeptides (Table 2).

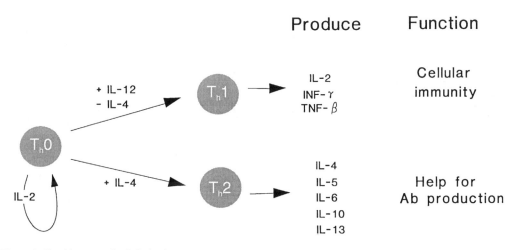

Figure 2. Cytokine cascade: Polarization.

Polarization into Th1 and Th2 Cells

More recently, a better understanding of the role of the uncommitted CD4⁺IL-2-producing T cells (Th0 cells) has been gained, as shown schematically in Figure 2. This scheme illustrates the polarization of immune responses into two subsets of T-helper cells, Th1 and Th2, which are determined primarily by the presence or absence of IL-4 (15). In the absence of IL-4 and under the influence of IL-12, a differentiative set of responses leads to the production of Th1, which are cell-type subsets involved primarily in cellular immunity and which produce mainly IL-2 and IFN-γ. In the presence of IL-4, the Th0 differentiate into Th2 cells, which are involved in antibody production and which continue to produce IL-4 as well as IL-5, IL-6, IL-10, and IL-13, among others. The IFN-γ, in addition to its proliferative and stimulative functions on the cell types already described above, also exerts a negative inhibitory effect on the actions of the Th2 subset inhibiting antibody production.

Allergic Inflammation and IgE Production

Following interaction of antigen with macrophages, production of IL-1 and IFN-α is seen, and in the presence of IL-12 proceeds to a set of cellular differentiative events involved in cellular immunity as described previously (Figure 3). In the presence of IL-4, the stimulated Th2 subset exerts its effects on B-cell differentiative activity. Of importance in this respect is that the actions of various interleukins are seen at different stages of B-cell development. For example, IL-4 exerts its stimulatory effect primarily on resting B cells, IL-5 on activated B cells, and IL-6 on terminally differentiated B cells with the ultimate production of IgE. Moreover, the most recently identified IL-13 has been shown to share similar functions of IL-4, e. g., induction of Ig heavy-chain gene switching. The inhibitory effects of IFN-γ on differentiation are shown schematically in this illustration. In addition, other cytokines exert an effect on the cascade, including the stimulatory effects of IL-5 on eosinophil differentiation and IL-3 on mucosal mast cell differentiation.

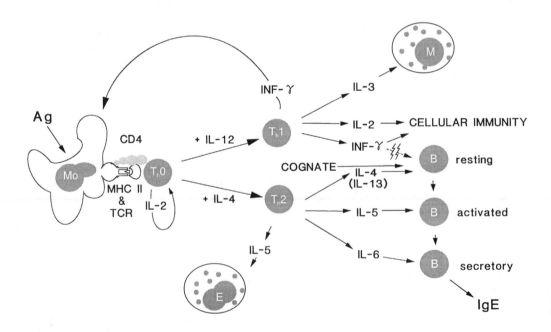

Figure 3. Cytokine cascade: Allergic inflammation and IgE production.

Clinical Relevance of the Cytokines to Human Allergic Diseases

From what has been described, it is now possible to illustrate some of the applications of this knowledge concerning cytokines to the treatment of allergic diseases (20). Spontaneous IgE synthesis by peripheral blood mononuclear cells (PBMC) of allergic atopic patients has been demonstrated *in vitro* (21–23); this can be enhanced by IL-4 and suppressed by IFN-γ or IFN-α (12). Further, elevated serum concentrations of IL-4 have also been detected in children with allergic diseases (24). In addition, profound defects of IFN-γ production by PBMCs from atopic dermatitis (AD) and hyper-IgE syndrome (HIES) patients have been observed (25–28). Collectively, these data suggest that the alterations of the above-mentioned IgE regulatory mechanisms may be involved in the pathogenesis of human diseases characterized by the hyper-production of IgE. As a direct result of these observations, there have been several clinical trials using IFN-α or IFN-γ to treat patients with AD or HIES which have yielded variable and sometime conflicting results. IFN-γ, for example, has been shown to have beneficial effects on severe AD and HIES (20), though most of the patients demonstrated a recurrence of disease once treatment was discontinued. Similarly, IFN-α has been shown to have a beneficial therapeutic effect in one patient with HIES, but failed to show clinical efficacy in two other patients with AD. Of particular interest was the demonstration that IFN-γ not only has the ability to increase the expression of IFN-α receptors, but also has multiple synergistic effects with IFN-α or IFN-β in antiviral, antiproliferative, and antitumor activities as well as potential natural killer (NK) cell function (29–30). These pleiomorphic effects of the combined or sequential uses of IFN-γ and IFN-α as demonstrated *in vivo* in the experimental animal and humans has shown great promise and has prompted us to explore this mode of treatment in several patients with allergic diseases.

Clinical Cases – Subjects and Treatment Regimen

A total of four patients with severe AD were studied; the clinical characteristics are summarized in Table 3. Prior to their entry into the study, each subject (or the parents) was explained the nature of the investigation, and informed consent was obtained.

- Patient no. 1 is a 22-year-old white man with severe AD since childhood which only partially responded to systemic steroids. Certain foods (i.e., corn and peanut) aggravated the AD. His serum IgE was 3300 IU/mL, and the severity score was 14/15, which involved 90% of the total body surface. IFN-γ ($0.05\,mg/m^2$) was given thrice weekly for 4 weeks, the dosing frequency being increased to every day for another 8 weeks when the medication was changed to IFN-α ($3 \times 10^6\,U/m^2$) thrice weekly for 20 weeks.
- Patient no. 2 is a 2-year-old white male with severe AD with normal IgE levels (1.2 IU/mL). At 6 months of age, he was diagnosed with asthma, which was controlled by daily β-agonist syrup (albuterol). His AD did not respond to potent topical steroids and intensive skin-care methods. The AD severity score was 12/15 and involved 70% of the body surface. A dosage of IFN-γ, $0.05\,mg/m^2$, was given subcutaneously three times a week for 4 weeks, and the dose was increased to $0.1\,mg/m^2$ for another 2 weeks, at which time the medication was changed to IFN-α ($0.5 \times 10^6\,U/m^2$) thrice weekly for another 20 weeks.

Table 3. Clinical characteristics of the patients.

Patient no.	Age (years)	Sex	Diagnosis	Duration of disease (years)	Serum IgE (IU/ml)	Severity score
1	22	M	AD	15	3300	14/15
2	2	M	AD	1.5	1.2	12/15
3	5	M	HIES	3	21000	11/15
4	12	F	AD	11	3601	13/15

Table 4. Results of treatment.

Patient no.	Treatment		Serum IgE (IU/ml)		Severity score (0–15)	
	IFN-γ	IFN-α	Pre	Post	Pre	Post
1	+	+	3300	2393	14	3
2	+	+	1.2	–	12	0
3	+	–	21000	8500	11	3
4	+	+	3601	3368*	13	3

* determined after 1 week of IFN-γ

- Patient no. 3 is a 5-year-old black male who was diagnosed with HIES (recurrent bacterial pneumonia/empyema, multiple staphylococcal skin infections, candidal septicemia, and chronic eczematous dermatitis). His highest serum IgE concentration was 21,000 IU/mL. IFN-γ, 0.05 mg/m^2, was given thrice weekly for 20 weeks.
- Patient no. 4 is a 12-year-old Asian female with severe AD since childhood with sensitivities to multiple foods (crab, shrimp, cod, peanuts, wheat, and egg) found to aggravate the AD. She had required several courses of systemic steroids to control the eczema and was also receiving oral sodium cromolyn, 100 mg qid. The serum IgE was 3601 IU/mL, and the severity score was 13/15, which involved 50% of the total body surface. A dosage of IFN-γ, 0.05 mg/m^2 was given subcutaneously daily for 7 days followed by IFN-α (3.0 × 10^6 U/m^2) thrice weekly for 4 weeks.

Results

The results of treatment are shown in Table 4.
- Patient no. 1 improved with the starting dose (0.05 mg/m^2, thrice weekly) of IFN-γ in the first 4 weeks (severity score decreased from 14 to 9). Subsequent to the increased dosing frequency (daily injection), the lesions continued to improve and reached a plateau at the 12th week (severity score 6), at which time the medication was changed to IFN-α. By the end of 32 weeks (20 weeks of IFN-α), the severity score was 3. The requirements for local skin care, i.e., lubricants and steroids, were lowered together with a diminished rate of school absenteeism.
- Patient no. 2 had dramatic improvement in the first 3 weeks after IFN-γ treatment. The disease activity, however, flared up at the 4th week.

Despite increased dosage of IFN-γ (0.1 mg/m^2), the lesions worsened almost to the pretreatment state. After 6 weeks of treatment, IFN-γ was discontinued and IFN-α was begun. With the relative low dose of IFN-α 0.5 × 10^6 U/m^2 thrice weekly, the lesion severity score decreased from 14 to 5 and the surface area involvement diminished from 70% to 10% at the 16th week. Further, the lesions completely resolved by the 26th week, at which time the medication was discontinued. At the most recent follow-up visit (6 months after treatment) he remains disease-free.
- Patient no. 3 received IFN-γ, 0.05 mg/m^2, thrice weekly for 20 weeks. The serum IgE decreased from 21,000 IU/mL to 8,500 IU/mL, and severity score decreased from 11 to 3. He continues to remain well on this IFN-γ treatment schedule.
- Patient no. 4 had a severe flare up of the eczema during the first week of IFN-γ therapy followed by rapid clearing of the inflammatory lesions during the 4 weeks of IFN-α therapy. Over the first week the serum IgE decreased from 3401 UI/mL to 3368 IU/mL upon the completion of interferon treatment. Over the next months, *Staphylococcus aureus* was cultured from facial skin lesions, which contributed to an exacerbation of the facial erythema. Following treatment with tetracycline 1000 mg bid over a course of 10 days and an increase of the oral sodium cromoglycate to 400 mg qid, a dramatic clearing of the skin lesions occurred, the severity score falling from 13 to 3. She has not required systemic or local steroids to date.

The reported adverse reactions by these patients are flu-like symptoms including transient headache, malaise, and myalgia. One or two doses of acetaminophen usually alleviate these symptoms. There is no laboratory abnormality detected.

Discussion

The results of these studies support the potential therapeutic effects of the interferons for patients with severe atopic dermatitis (20). Further, the results suggest that different dose schedules may be crucial in obtaining optimal therapeutic effects. In the present study, the sequential use of IFN-γ followed by IFN-α appeared to offer therapeutic value. This may possibly be due to the induction of IFN-α receptors by IFN-γ or to the synergistic effect of this combination of cytokines.

Several recent studies have provided some additional exciting knowledge suggesting the use of other cytokines in the treatment of allergic diseases. Zurawski et al. (14) describe a Tyr → Asp IL-4 mutant which binds to the IL-4 receptor but loses the function of cellular activation; they indicated that this mutant IL-4 can block the effects of IgE-mediated disease. The effects of this receptor-antagonist may provide the most effective mode of inhibition of IgE synthesis in allergic patients. There is also evidence suggesting that IL-4 and IL-13 receptors share similarities, so that the use of this mutant may also antagonize IL-13 activities. Similarly, IL-12, which is known to stimulate natural killer cells, a major source of IFN-γ, could also be yet another interleukin useful in the treatment of allergic diseases (13). Further studies involving other interleukins in patients with allergic disease are clearly indicated.

Address for correspondence:

Joseph A Bellanti
Georgetown University Medical Center
3800 Reservoir Road, N. W.
Washington, D. C. 20007
USA

References

1. Jabara HH, Ackerman SJ, Vercell D, et al. Induction of interleukin-4 dependent IgE synthesis and interleukin-5 dependent eosinophil differentiation by supernatant of a human helper T cell clone. *J Clin Immunol* 1988; 8:437.

2. Pene J, Rousset F, Briere F, et al. IgE production by normal human lymphocytes is induced by interleukin 4 and suppressed by interferon γ and α and prostaglandin E₂. *Proc Natl Acad Sci* 1988; 85:6880.

3. Del Prete GF, Maggi E, Parronchi P, et al. IL-4 is an essential factor for the IgE synthesis induced *in vitro* by human T cell clones and their supernatant. *J Immunol* 1988; 140:4193.

4. Snapper CM, Paul WE. Interferon-γ and B cell stimulatory factor-1 reciprocally regulate Ig isotype production. *Science* 1987; 236:944.

5. Heinzel FP, Sadick MD, Holaday BUJ, et al. Reciprocal expression of interferon γ on interleukin 4 during the resolution or progression of murine leishmaniasis. *J Exp Med* 1989; 169:59.

6. Coffman RL, Seymour BW, Lebman DA, et al. The role of helper T cell products in mouse B cell differentiation and isotype regulation. *Immunol Rev* 1988; 102:5.

7. Pene J, Rousset F, Briere F, et al. Interleukin-5 enhances interleukin-4 induced IgE production by normal human B cells: The role of soluble CD23 antigen. *Eur J Immunol* 1988; 18:929.

8. Vercelli D, Jabara HH, Arai K-I, et al. Endogenous interleukin 6 plays an obligatory role in interleukin 4-dependent human IgE synthesis. *Eur J Immunol* 1989; 19:1419.

9. Romagnani S, Del Prete G, Maggi E, et al. Role of interleukins in induction and regulation of human IgE synthesis. *Clin Immunol Immunopathol* 1989; 50:S13.

10. Coffman RL, Carty J. A T cell activity that enhances polyclonal IgE production and its inhibition by interferon-γ. *J Immunol* 1986; 136:949.

11. Finkelmann FD, Katona IM, Mosmann TR, et al. IFN-γ regulates the isotypes of Ig secreted during *in vivo* humoral immune responses. *J Immunol* 1988; 140:1022.

12. Rousset F, Robert J, Andary M, et al. Shifts in interleukin-4 and interferon-γ production by T cells of patients with elevated serum IgE levels and the modulatory effects of these lymphokines on spontaneous IgE synthesis. *J Allergy Clin Immunol* 1991; 87:58.

13. Trinchieri G. Interleukin-12 and its role in the generation of Th1 cells. *Immunology Today* 1993; 14:335.

14. Zurawski G, De Vries JE. Interleukin 13, an interleukin 4-like cytokine that acts on monocytes and B cells, but not on T cells. *Immunology Today* 1994; 15:19.

15. Seder RA, Paul WE, Davis MM, et al. The presence of interleukin-4 during *in vitro* priming determines the lymphokine-producing potential of CD4⁺-T cells from T cell receptor transgenic mice. *J Exp Med* 1992; 176:1091.

16. Bellanti JA, Kadlec JV, Escobar-Gutierrez A. Cytokines and the immune response. *Ped Clin N Am* 1994; 41: 597.

17. Lebman DA, Coffman RL. Interleukin 4 causes

isotype switching to IgE in T cell stimulated clonal B cell cultures. *J Exp Med* 1988; 168:853.

18. Geha RS. Regulation of IgE synthesis in humans. *J Allergy Clin Immunol* 1992; 90:143.

19. Vercelli D, Jabara HH, Arai K-I, et al. Induction of human IgE synthesis requires interleukin 4 and T/B cell interactions involving the T cell receptor/CD3 complex and MHC class II antigens. *J Exp Med* 1989; 169:1295.

20. Pung Y-H, Vetro SW, Bellanti JA. Use of interferons in atopic (IgE-mediated) diseases. *Ann Allergy* 1993; 71:2234.

21. Fiser PM, Buckley RH. Human IgE biosynthesis *in vitro*: Studies with atopic and normal blood mononuclear cells and subpopulations. *J Immunol* 1979; 123:1788.

22. Tijo AH, Hull WM, Gleich GJ. Production of human immunoglobulin E antibody *in vitro*. *J Immunol* 1979; 122:2131.

23. Buckley RH, Becker WG. Abnormalities in the regulation of human IgE synthesis. *Immunol Rev* 1978; 41:288.

24. Matsumoto T, Miike T, Yamaguchi K, et al. Serum levels of soluble IL-2 receptor, IL-4 and IgE-binding factors in childhood allergic diseases. *Clin Exp Immunol* 1991; 85:288.

25. Reinhold U, Pawelec G, Wehrmann W, et al. Immunoglobulin E and immunoglobulin G subclass distribution in vivo and relationship to *in vitro* generation of interferon-γ and neopterin in patients with severe atopic dermatitis. *Int Arch Allergy Appl Immunol* 1988; 87:120.

26. Reinhold U, Wehrmann W, Kukel S, et al. Evidence that defective interferon-γ production in atopic dermatitis patients is due to intrinsic abnormalities. *Clin Exp Immunol* 1990; 79:374.

27. Wierenga EA, Snoek MA, De Groot C, et al. Evidence for compartmentalization of functional subsets of CD4$^+$ T lymphocytes in atopic patients. *J Immunol* 1990; 144:4651.

28. Del Prete G, Tiri A, Maggi E, et al. Defective in vitro production of γ interferon and tumor necrosis factor-α by circulating T cells from patients with hyper-immunoglobulin E syndrome. *J Clin Invest* 1989; 84:1830.

29. Hannigan GE, Fish EN, Williams BR. Modulation of human interferon alpha receptor expression by human interferon γ. *J Biol Chemistry* 1984; 259:8084.

30. Weigent DA, Langford MP, Fleischmann WR, et al. Potentiation of lymphocytes natural killing by mixtures of α or β interferon with recombinant γ interferon. *Infect Immun* 1983; 40:35.

Cytokine and Cytokine Antagonists in the Therapy of Allergic Diseases

Steven Gillis*

Keywords: Allergy, IL-1 receptor, therapy

To date 15 interleukins (IL) have been identified. Many of these have naturally occurring soluble receptors (R). Allergic individuals have increased levels of IL-1. Treatment of allergies with recombinant IL-1R indicates that it can control the inflammatory response in a localized fashion resulting in a reduced allergen-induced late-phase reaction. This might lead to a new, safe and efficacious form of treatment for atopic patients.

The term interleukin (IL) refers to any one of a number of soluble molecules that function as potent mediators of cell growth and differentiation, inflammation, and immune responses. To date, fifteen distinct IL proteins have been identified and their cDNAs isolated. Of these, the pleiotropic IL-1α and IL-1β are known to induce thymocyte proliferation, activation of T and B lymphocytes, fibroblast proliferation, and protein secretion from hepatocytes. As with many cytokines, localized or systemic overproduction can lead to a variety of less desirable responses; with IL-1 these include septic shock, graft rejection, fever, inflammation, and bone resorption (1).

This wide variety of IL-1 specific responses exists as a result of a complex interactions between three IL-1 related molecules that interact with two distinct IL-1 receptors (IL-1Rs). The activities of IL-1α and IL-1β appear to completely overlap *in vitro*, and both cytokines bind with high affinity to the two IL-1Rs. In addition to the agonist forms of IL-1, a naturally occurring related molecule exists that binds to the IL-1Rs but does not signal. This IL-1 receptor antagonist (IL-1ra) is believed to act *in vivo* as a negative regulator of IL-1 activity (2, 3).

The IL-1Rs are referred to as the type I, or 80 kDa IL-1R (4), and the type II, or 60 kDa IL-1R (5). The type II IL-1R has three immunoglobulin (Ig)-like domains in its extracellular portion, a carboxy-proximal transmembrane region, and a short cytoplasmic domain. Although this receptor binds both IL-1α and IL-1β with high affinity, recent studies have indicated that it does not appear to signal in response to IL-1 binding. The type II IL-1R is shed rapidly from the surface of cells in response to certain stimuli, suggesting that this molecule may function *in vivo* as a naturally occurring antagonist of IL-1 activity (6, 7). The type I IL-1R also has three Ig-like domains in its extracellular portion, followed by a transmembrane domain and a long, 213-amino-acid cytoplasmic domain. This receptor appears to be responsible for all biological responses to both forms of IL-1 (7).

Numerous cytokines have been shown to have naturally occurring soluble forms of their receptors. These soluble receptors result from either alternative splicing, as in the case of the IL-4R, IL-7R, and GM-CSFR, or from proteolytic cleavage as with the IL-2R, IFNR-γ, and TNFR. The identification of such soluble cytokine receptors does not however, provide direct evidence that they function *in vivo* to modulate the effects of their respective cytokines. Perhaps the most compelling evidence for the use of soluble cytokine receptors as antagonists of cytokine activity comes from studies that have identified naturally occurring soluble cytokine receptors which are encoded within the genomes of several mammalian viruses. These soluble viral receptors include a TNFR homologue, an IFNR-γ homologue, and an IL-1R homologue (8). The poxvirus-encoded IL-1R homologue is the product of the B15R gene and, like both forms of cloned IL-1R, it contains three Ig-like domains. In parallel studies, two groups have shown that a recombinant form of this viral IL-1R can bind IL-1 with high affinity. Importantly, these groups also showed that mutant viruses in which this B15R gene product was specifically deleted were at-

*   Immunex Research and Development Corporation, Seattle, WA, USA.

tenuated compared to control viruses in an *in vivo* mouse model. This altered virus virulence provides direct evidence that a soluble IL-1R can function as IL-1 antagonists *in vivo* and suggests that the viral acquisition of such soluble cytokine receptors reflects an evolutionary advantage to the use of this form of antagonist (9, 10).

Previous work has shown that allergic individuals exhibit increased levels of IL-1 in the skin, lung, and nasal passages (11, 12). Together with its well known role in inflammation, these data suggest an important role for IL-1 in the exacerbation of allergic responses. The study described below examined the ability of a soluble form of the IL-1R to ameliorate the inflammatory response in atopic individuals.

The soluble IL-1R used in this study was a recombinant truncated form of the type I IL-1R, which was expressed as a soluble protein by the removal of the transmembrane and cytoplasmic domains. This recombinant IL-1R (rIL-1R) has been shown to bind IL-1α and IL-1β with an affinity identical to that of its membrane counterpart (13).

The investigation was a double-blind, randomized, placebo-controlled study which allowed evaluation of both rIL-1R safety (administering escalating doses of rIL-1R), and efficacy (measuring areas of induration, erythema, itching, and histopathology of affected areas) in atopic subjects (14). During the first portion of the study, 15 patients were tested for their response to timothy grass, dust mites, cat dander, alder, or orchard grass pollen allergens by intradermal (id) administration along the lower back. One allergen which elicited a strong response was selected per patient and titrated by intradermal injection on the upper back using serial 10-fold dilutions. The concentration of allergen necessary to elicit a 15–20 mm wheal was chosen as the endpoint titer. One to three weeks following determination of this endpoint, patients were tested for pre-existing antibodies to the rIL-1R. Serum samples were taken before and two weeks after the subcutaneous (subq) administration of the dose of rIL-1R which was equal to that scheduled to be given during the second part of the study. All patient sera throughout the study were negative for antibodies to the rIL-1R as measured by ELISA.

During the second portion of the trial, patients were administered id and in duplicate an amount of allergen equal to twice the concentration of the endpoint titer on each forearm. Patients received either the rIL-1R or a saline placebo directly under each allergen injection. Three individuals each received 1 µg, 10 µg, 25 µg, 50 µg, or 100 µg of rIL-1R in one forearm and the placebo in the opposite forearm. Each site was examined for induration and erythema at 10, 20, 30, or 40 min post injection, and again at 2, 4, 6, 8, 24, and 48 h post injection. Reactions occurring 2 h or more after allergen challenge were considered indicative of a late phase reaction.

The results of the measurements of both erythema and induration in this portion of the study were similar. Significant reduction in both measurements at all time points was noted at the site of allergen injection on the forearms of those individuals who had received either 1 µg or 10 µg of rIL-1R compared to the forearm which had received the placebo. At the higher doses of IL-1R administration, significant reduction in both measurements was seen compared to the response elicited by injection of the allergen alone; however, the diminished allergic response was not confined to the forearm which had received the rIL-1R, but was also seen in the forearm which had received the placebo. This response strongly suggested that the rIL-1R functioned in controlling the inflammatory response in a localized fashion and had also functioned systemically, diminishing the allergic reaction in the opposing arm as well.

To confirm this hypothesis, each patient simultaneously received a dose of allergen equal to the endpoint titer in two separate locations on the lower back, followed by an amount of rIL-1R equal to the amount administered on the forearm, but given in two separate locations away from the site of allergen inoculation. The protocol was specifically designed to examine whether rIL-1R could work in a systemic fashion. Erythema and induration measurements were taken in a manner analogous to that described for patient forearm inoculations. Consistent with the observations made in the forearms of patients who received the higher doses of rIL-1R, patients receiving 30 µg or more of the rIL-1R on the back showed significant reduction in induration and erythema at both sites of allergen inoculation.

Data on itching and discomfort gathered from all patient groups also showed that the administration of rIL-1R significantly decreased the irritation at the sites of allergen injection, consistent with the above described reduction in inflammation.

The results of this trial demonstrate that the administration of rIL-1R reduced allergen-induced late-phase reactions at a level similar to that seen for glucocorticoids. Subsequent challenge of the patients in this study with allergen several weeks after the completion of the trial suggested that the effects of rIL-1R were not permanent; therefore, additional studies will be necessary to address the question of long-term efficacy and route of administrations. Nonetheless, this trial clearly indicates that the rIL-1R functions as an effective antagonist of IL-1 activity *in vivo* and that it may provide a safe and efficacious form of treatment in an atopic patient population.

Address for correspondence:

Steven Gillis
Immunex Research and Development Corp.
51 University Street
Seattle, WA 98101
USA

References

1. Dinarello CA. Role of interleukin-1 in infectious diseases. *Immunol Rev* 1992; 127:119.

2. Dripps DJ, Brandhuber BJ, Thompson RC, Eisenberg SP. Interleukin-1 (IL-1) receptor antagonist binds to the 80-kDa IL-1 receptor but does not initiate IL-1 signal transduction. *J Biol Chem* 1991; 266:10331.

3. Hannum CH, Wilcox CJ, Arend WP, Joslin FG, Dripps DJ, Heimdal PL, Armes LG, Sommer A, Eisenberg SP, Thompson RC. Interleukin-1 receptor antagonist activity of a human interleukin-1 inhibitor. *Nature* 1990; 343:336.

4. Sims JE, March CJ, Cosman D, Widmer MB, MacDonald HR, McMahan CJ, Grubin CE, Wignall JM, Call SM, Friend D, Alpert AR, Gillis SR, Urdal DL, Dower SK. cDNA expression cloning of the IL-1 receptor, a member of the immunoglobulin superfamily. *Science* 1988; 241:585.

5. McMahan CJ, Slack JL, Mosley B, Cosman D, Lupton SD, Brunton LL, Grubin CE, Wignall JM, Jenkins NA, Brannan CI, Copeland NG, Huebner K, Croce CM, Cannizzaro LA, Benjamin D, Dower SK, Spriggs MK, Sims JE. A novel IL-1 receptor, cloned from B cells by mammalian expression, is expressed in many cell types. *EMBO J* 1991; 10:2821.

6. Colotta F, Re F, Muzio M, Bertini R, Polentarutti N, Sironi M, Giri JG, Dower SK, Sims JE, Mantovani A. Interleukin-1 type II receptor: A decoy target for IL-1 that is regulated by IL-4. *Science* 1993; 261:472.

7. Sims JE, Gayle MA, Slack JL, Alderson MR, Bird TA, Giri JG, Colotta F, Re F, Mantovani A, Shanebeck K, Grabstein KH, Dower SK. Interleukin 1 signaling occurs exclusively via the type I receptor. *Proc Natl Acad Sci USA* 1993; 90:6155.

8. Spriggs MK. Molecular strategies in the evolution of the virus-host interaction (cytokine and cytokine receptor genes 'captured' by viruses). *Curr Opin Immunol* 1994, in press.

9. Spriggs MK, Hruby DE, Maliszewski CR, Pickup DJ, Sims JE, Buller RML, VanSlyke J. Vaccinia and cowpox viruses encode a novel secreted interleukin-1-binding protein. *Cell* 1992; 71:145.

10. Alcamí A, Smith GL. A soluble receptor for interleukin-1β encoded by Vaccinia virus: A novel mechanism of virus modulation of the host response to infection. *Cell* 1992; 71:153.

11. Bochner BS, Charlesworth EN, Lichtenstein LM, Derse CP, Gillis S, Dinarello CA, Schleimer RP. Interleukin-1 is released at sites of human cutaneous allergic reactions. *J Allergy Clin Immunol* 1990; 86:830.

12. Sim TC, Alam R, Hilsmeier KA, Grant JA. Detection of inflammatory cytokines in nasal secretions (NS) of allergic subjects following antigen challenge. *J Allergy Clin Immunol* 1992; 89:287.

13. Sims JE, Acres RB, Grubin CE, McMahan CJ, Wignall JM, March CJ, Dower SK. Cloning of the interleukin-1 receptor from human T-cells. *Proc Natl Acad Sci USA* 1989; 86:8946.

14. Mullarkey MF, Leiferman KM, Peters MS, Caro I, Roux ER, Hanna RK, Rubin AS, Jacobs CA. Human cutaneous allergic late-phase response is inhibited by soluble IL-1 receptor. *J Immunol* 1994; 152:2033.

Gene Therapy for Immune Deficiency Disorders

Gay M Crooks*, Kenneth I Weinberg*, Robertson Parkman*, Carl Lenarsky*, R Michael Blaese**,
Donald B Kohn*

Keywords: Gene therapy, immune deficiency disorders, severe combined immune deficiency,
adenosine deaminase deficiency, umbilical cord blood

The congenital immunodeficiency syndromes, specifically adenosine deaminase (ADA) deficient severe combined immune deficiency (SCID), have been a major focus of the preclinical and clinical development of human gene therapy. In general terms, the technical issues of gene transfer and gene expression are similar for the immunodeficiency syndromes as for the entire field of gene therapy. Specific technical issues of gene expression vary depending on the pathogenesis of the particular genetic abnormality. Currently, the most widely used method of gene transfer is with retroviral vectors. Target cells for gene insertion in the congenital immune deficiencies may be either the hematopoietic stem cell (HSC), lymphoid progenitors or mature effector cells. Currently, gene transfer efficiency is low (1–5%) into HSC and T lymphocytes using retroviral vectors. The first clinical case of the correction of a genetic deficiency using gene therapy was in a patient with ADA deficiency in 1990. Currently, of the approximately 70 clinical gene therapy and gene marking protocols approved internationally, four groups are studying ADA deficiency as the target disease. These clinical protocols have used the following cell targets for retroviral vector mediated gene transfer: peripheral blood T lymphocytes, or CD34+ cells isolated from the peripheral blood, bone marrow or umbilical cord blood. The patients have all tolerated the gene therapy without toxicity. In all cases, T lymphocytes containing the vector cDNA have been detected in the peripheral blood. Assessment of the effect of the gene therapy on immune reconstitution will be more accurate when concurrent enzyme replacement therapy with PEG-ADA is withdrawn.

There are currently approximately 70 gene therapy and gene marking protocols approved for clinical investigation around the world, more than 60 of which originate in the USA (1). A variety of congenital and acquired diseases are targets for these protocols. Congenital immune deficiency disorders, specifically severe combined immune deficiency (SCID), occupy a central role in the history and ongoing development of human gene therapy. The first human gene therapy trial in the world was performed in two children with adenosine deaminase deficient SCID (2).

A number of congenital immune deficiencies are potentially amenable to gene therapy. These include various forms of SCID, leukocyte adhesion defects, X-linked agammaglobulinemia, X-linked immunodeficiency with hyper-IgM, chronic granulomatous disease, and Wiskott-Aldrich syndrome. Currently, the mainstay of treatment for most children with these life-threatening conditions is supportive, relying on reducing the risk of infection with isolation and intravenous immunoglobulin and early use of antibiotics. Preclinical studies for gene therapy are underway for a number of the congenital immune deficiencies for which the genetic abnormality has been discovered. However, SCID and specifically ADA deficiency have led the way in the development of gene therapy.

SCID comprises a group of disorders with a variety of genetic defects, all of which result in absence of T and B lymphocyte function. The forms of SCID for which the genetic defects have been established and which are therefore potentially amenable to gene therapy are listed in Table 1.

The optimal therapy for SCID is a bone marrow transplant from a histocompatible sibling (3). For the approximately 75% of children who do not have a sibling donor, a haploidentical T cell depleted bone marrow transplant or a matched unrelated bone marrow transplant are possible alternatives. However, the morbidity and mortality associated

*   Division of Research Immunology/Bone Marrow Transplantation, Children's Hospital Los Angeles, Departments
     of Pediatrics and Microbiology, University of Southern California School of Medicine, Los Angeles, CA, USA.
** National Institutes of Health, Bethesda, MD, USA.

Table 1. Congenital immune deficiencies potentially amenable to gene therapy.

1. SCID
   ADA deficiency
   PNP deficiency
   X linked (γ_c deficiency)
   MHC defects or Bare lymphocyte syndrome
     (includes C11TA deficiency)
   ZAP-70 (Zeta-associated protein, CD8 deficiency)
   CD3γ deficiency
   IL-2 deficiency (gene unknown but some may be
     NF-AT abnormalities)
2. Leukocyte adhesion defect
3. X-linked agammaglobulinemia
4. X-linked immunodeficiency with hyper-IgM
5. Chronic granulomatous disease

with pretransplant chemotherapy, graft-versus-host disease, and prolonged immune dysfunction post-transplant are high in nonsibling allogeneic transplants (3, 4). Thus, for the majority of children with SCID who lack a histocompatible donor, gene therapy offers the possibility for curative treatment avoiding the substantial risks of haploidentical and unrelated bone marrow transplantation.

Technical Issues for Gene Therapy

The major technical issues in designing gene therapy for any disease can be broadly considered under two interrelated headings: gene transfer and gene expression. Under gene transfer the following questions must be answered: (1) how is the gene to be transferred, (2) into which type of cell is the gene to be inserted, and (3) what percentage of target cells need to be transduced? In relation to gene expression: (1) which cells need to express the gene, (2) what level of expression is required, (3) is overexpression likely to be toxic, and (4) is inducible expression required? Each of these questions are interrelated and dependent on the pathogenesis of the specific disease being treated.

Gene Transfer

At present, genetically modified retroviruses are the most widely used vectors for gene therapy as they produce stable integration of therapeutic genes

and are relatively nontoxic to human cells. However, target cells must be actively cycling for gene transfer to occur via retroviral vectors. As hematopoietic stems cells (HSC) are predominantly in a quiescent (noncycling) state, conditions must be found to induce proliferation and hence gene transfer into (transduction of) these target cells. Attempts to improve transduction of progenitor cells have mostly relied on stimulation of bone marrow with hematopoietic growth factors. The mechanism by which cytokines improve transduction efficiency is not well understood, although it appears to be at least partially by inducing cell cycling (5).

In most types of congenital immune deficiency, only the cells of the immune system are affected. Thus, transfer of the therapeutic gene may be targeted to the pluripotent HSC, the long-lived lineage committed progenitor cells or the mature effector cells. Transduction efficiency of both HSC and mature T lymphocytes is only 1–5% with current technology (6, 7).

Gene Expression

Approaches to the issues of gene expression depend very much on which particular genetic abnormality is being targeted. Gene expression needs to be quantitatively sufficient in the cells primarily affected by the disease process. Overexpression of certain genes may be toxic. Table 2 shows the normal pattern of expression of some of the genes affected in forms of SCID. For certain genes normal expression is nonspecific and constitutive, e.g., ADA. In others, expression is much more complex, restricted to specific cell types and/or induced by activation or receptor ligand interactions, e.g., IL-2 deficiency. Clearly, the more specific and complex the regulation of the gene the more technically difficult it will be to devise gene therapy for the disease state.

Table 2. Patterns of expression of genes causing SCID.

Disease	Pattern of expression
ADA	non-specific
X-SCID	all hematopoietic lineages??
ZAP-70	thymocytes, T lymphocytes
MHC deficiency	B cells, monocytes
(C11TA)	inducible in all lineages?
CD3γ	T lymphocytes
IL-2 deficiency	T lymphocytes
	inducible by TCR engagement

In some forms of SCID, expression of the normal gene may confer a selective advantage for transduced cells over cells which remain defective. Examples of such diseases are ADA deficiency, X-linked SCID, ZAP-70 (CD8 deficiency), and possible CD3 γ deficiency. This advantage may cause an increase in the proportion of corrected cells with time, allowing an initially low transduction efficiency to ultimately result in sufficient expression for clinical benefit.

ADA Deficiency

In many ways, ADA deficiency provides an ideal disease model for gene therapy. ADA deficiency is the most common autosomal recessive form of SCID. In the absence of ADA, deoxyadenosine metabolites accumulate and result in severe derangements of purine metabolism. ADA is expressed in all cells, but the deficiency of the enzyme appears to affect only lymphoid cells with reduction in cell viability and function and abnormal differentiation. Therapeutic gene transfer of the ADA gene can therefore theoretically be targeted to hematopoietic stem cells or to mature T lymphocytes.

T lymphocytes can be repeatedly isolated from peripheral blood and expanded ex vivo with IL-2 and a comitogen (8). However, the expanded mature T cells have only a limited repertoire of responsiveness and an unknown life span in vivo. The level of transduction of T cells with retroviral vectors is relatively low (1–5%). In severely lymphopenic patients, T cells are not available for transduction.

Transduction of HSC with the normal ADA gene should result in permanent and multi-lineage correction of the defect, avoiding the need for repeated leukapheresis, transductions and infusions. However, the efficiency of transduction of the HSC is only 1–5% with retroviral vectors (6, 7). Despite the low level of transduction into both HSC and T cells, lymphocytes expressing the normal gene may have a survival advantage over their abnormal counterparts, theoretically resulting in therapeutic benefit with time.

As with other forms of SCID, the treatment of choice for ADA is a histocompatible bone marrow transplant from a sibling. In the absence of a sibling match, T cell depleted haplo-identical or matched unrelated bone marrow transplants are alternatives

with the associated problems already mentioned. Enzyme replacement therapy with polyethylene glycol-modified ADA (PEG-ADA) is available by intramuscular injection once or twice weekly, and results in improvement of immune function in the majority of patients. However, treatment is not curative and so must be continued life-long, with significant potential issues of compliance and financial cost. One year of PEG-ADA therapy costs approximately $100,000 and the cost increases as the patient grows. In approximately 30–40% of patients the response to PEG-ADA is partial (9). Thus, for the majority of patients who lack a sibling BMT donor, therapy for ADA deficiency is currently imperfect.

In 1990, the first human gene therapy was performed at the National Institutes of Health in Bethesda, Maryland, in two patients with ADA deficiency (2). In this protocol, serial monthly leukapheresis was performed to collect peripheral blood mononuclear cells which were stimulated ex vivo with IL-2 and anti-CD3 antibody and then transduced with the LASN retroviral vector. Following 10 days of ex vivo expansion, the transduced cells were transfused back into the patients each month. The first patient, who had shown only a partial response to PEG-ADA prior to gene therapy, has had a progressive increase of T lymphocyte numbers, with significant improvement of her immune function (development of isohemagglutinins, cytotoxic T cells specific for influenza and delayed type hypersensitivity skin tests responses). Over her 2 years of treatment, her leukocyte ADA level increased to 25% of normal and 30–50% of her circulating T lymphocytes contained vector. One year after her last infusion of transduced cells, the presence of functional T lymphocytes with the ADA cDNA has been demonstrated. This implies that functional peripheral T lymphocytes can persist for at least 1 year. The second patient treated on this protocol had only 0.1–1% of her circulating T cells transduced. In 1993, she was treated by transduced G-CSF mobilized peripheral blood CD34+ cells using a different retroviral vector. Six months since her therapy, PCR of her peripheral blood leukocytes has failed to detect the second vector.

In 1992, Claudio Bordignon in Milan, Italy, performed gene therapy on two ADA deficient children by infusing transduced CD34+ cells from the bone marrow with peripheral blood T cells transduced with a different ADA containing vector (10). The relative contribution of lymphocytes derived from the bone marrow stem cells and the peripheral blood T cells will be studied in this protocol. Results to date show approximately 1% of bone marrow CFU-GM (by G418 resistance) and 1% of peripheral T cells transduced.

ADA gene therapy using CD34[+] bone marrow cells has also been performed by Dinko Valerio et al. in the Netherlands (11). Three ADA deficient children have been treated. The vector was detected by PCR in the peripheral blood for the first few months after treatment and in the bone marrow of one child six months after treatment. However, the vector in the peripheral blood is not detectable at 6 months (the latest follow-up).

In May and June of 1993, in collaboration with Michael Blaese of the NIH, Donald Kohn and his colleagues at Children's Hospital Los Angeles treated three newborn infants with ADA deficiency using CD34[+] cells isolated from autologous cord blood (12). The cord blood cells were transduced with the LASN vector in the presence of IL-3, IL-6 and Steel factor. Following transduction, on day 4 of post-natal life, the cells were infused back into the patients. No immune suppressive or myeloablative therapy was given. The infants were commenced on PEG-ADA therapy on day 4 and kept in protective isolation until their immune function was satisfactory. All three patients remain clinically well and continue on PEG-ADA therapy at home. Follow-up to 12 months shows the persistence of the vector ADA gene in 1/10,000 to 1/1,000 of the peripheral blood mononuclear cells.

In each of these clinical protocols, the gene therapy has been tolerated without toxicity and myeloablation and immune suppression have been avoided. The concurrent treatment with PEG-ADA in all patients complicates the interpretation of the results somewhat, by reducing the role of selective advantage of transduced cells and providing an alternative reason for the immune reconstitution seen in these patients. As PEG-ADA therapy is withdrawn, the efficacy of the gene therapy will be able to be assessed more fully.

Address for correspondence:

Gay M Crooks
Division of Research Immunology/
Bone Marrow Transplantation
Children's Hospital Los Angeles
Mailstop #62
4650 Sunset Boulevard
Los Angeles, California 90027
USA

References

1. Human gene marker/Therapy clinical protocols. *Hum Gene Ther* 1994; 5:553.

2. Culver KW, Anderson WF, Blaese RM. Lymphocyte gene therapy. *Hum Gene Ther* 1991; 2:107.

3. Parkman R. The application of bone marrow transplantation to the treatment of genetic diseases. *Science* 1986; 232:1373.

4. Moen RC, Horowitz SD, Sondel PM, Borcherding WR, Trigg ME, Billing R, Hong R. Immunologic reconstitution after haploidentical bone marrow transplantation for immune deficiency disorders: treatment of bone marrow cells with monoclonal antibody CT-2 and complement. *Blood* 1987; 70:664.

5. Nolta JA, Kohn DB. Comparison of the effects of growth factors on retroviral vector-mediated gene transfer and the proliferative status of human hematopoietic progenitor cells.*Hum Gene Ther* 1990; 1:257.

6. Brenner MK, Rill DR, Holladay MS, Hislop HE, Moen RC, Buschle M, Krance RA, Santana VM, Anderson WF, Ihle JN. Gene marking to determine whether autologous marrow infusion restores long-term haemopoiesis in cancer patients. *Lancet* 1993; 342:1134.

7. Dunbar CE, OShaughnessy JA, Cottler-Fox M, Carter CS, Doren S, Cowan KH, Leitman SF, Wilson W, Young NS, Nienhuis AW. Transplantation of retrovirally-marked CD34[+] bone marrow and peripheral blood cells in patients with multiple myeloma or breast cancer. *Blood* 1993; 82 (Suppl 1):854 a.

8. Culver K, Cornetta K, Morgan R, Morecki S, Aebersold P, Kasid A, Lotze M, Rosenberg SA, Anderson WF, Blaese RM. Lymphocytes as cellular vehicles for gene therapy in mouse and man. *Proc Natl Acad Sci USA* 1991; 88:3155.

9. Hershfield MS, Chaffee S. PEG-enzyme replacement therapy in adenosine deaminase deficiency. In Desnick RJ (Ed) *Treatment of genetic diseases*. New York: Churchill-Livingston, 1991, p. 169.

10. Ferrari G, Rossini S, Nobili N, Maggioni D, Garofalo A, Giavazzi R, Mavilio F, Bordignon C. Transfer of the ADA gene into human ADA-deficient T lymphocytes reconstitutes specific immune functions. *Blood* 1992; 80:1120.

11. Hoogerbrugge PM, van Beusechem V, Valerio D, Moseley A, Harvey M, Fischer A, Debree M, Gaspar B, Morgan G, Levinsky R. Gene therapy of 3 children with adenosine deaminase deficiency. *Blood* 1993; 82 (Suppl 1):315 a.

12. Kohn DB, Weinberg KI, Parkman R, Lenarsky C, Crooks GM, Shaw K, Hanley ME, Lawrence K, Annett G, Brooks JS, Wara D, Elder M, Bowen T, Herschfield MS, Berenson RI, Moen, RC, Mullen CA, Blaese RM. *Blood* 1993; 82 (Suppl 1):315 a.

289

Tipping the Th1/Th2 Balance: An Approach to the Immunotherapy of Autoimmune and Allergic Diseases

Luciano Adorini*

Keywords: Insulin-dependent diabetes mellitus, IL-12, immunosuppression

A powerful new paradigm has recently emerged in immunology: the Th1/Th2 dichotomy. Th1 cells are characterized by secretion of interferon-γ (IFN-γ), and Th2 cells selectively produce IL-4 and IL-5. The subdivision of T cells into Th1 and Th2 subsets can be oversimplified to suggest that most organ-specific autoimmune diseases are Th1-mediated, whereas immediate-type hypersensitivities are Th2-mediated. Although clinical situations are certainly more complex, this paradigm offers the possibility to design straightforward experiments probing the role of Th1 and Th2 cells in immunoregulation and in the pathogenesis of immunological diseases. In addition, tipping the Th1/Th2 balance may offer novel approaches for immunointervention in autoimmune diseases and allergies.

Th1/Th2 Cells: The Current Paradigm for Immunoregulation

Based on the repertoire of lymphokine production, both mouse (1) and human (2) CD4$^+$ T cells can be subdivided into two subsets, Th1 and Th2. Th1 cells are characterized by secretion of interferon-γ (IFN-γ) and IL-2, and they promote cell-mediated immunity appropriate for eliminating intracellular pathogens. Conversely, Th2 cells selectively produce IL-4 and IL-5, and are involved in the development of humoral immunity protecting against extracellular pathogens. The generation of Th1 and Th2 subsets depends on the cytokines present during the initial phase of the immune response, a major role being played by IL-12 and IL-4, respectively (3, 4).

Th1 and Th2 cells not only protect against pathogens, they are also involved in the pathogenesis of immunological disorders. Th2 cells have a prominent role in immediate-type hypersensitivity, as IL-4 is the critical stimulus inducing switch to IgE antibody production (5). Th1-derived the proinflammatory cytokines, such as IFN-γ, IFN-α, and TNF-α, are involved in induction of autoimmune diseases (6, 7). Their role in autoimmunity is clearly illustrated by mice transgenic for cytokine genes. Transgenic mice expressing genes encoding IFN-γ (8) or IFN-α (9) under the control of the insulin promoter develop insulitis and diabetes. Similarly, mice transgenic for TNF-α develop severe rheumatoid arthritis, which is completely prevented by treatment from birth with anti-TNF-α antibody (10). In contrast, selective expression of TNF-α in pancreatic β cells leads to insulitis but not to diabetes (11), indicating the complexity of effector and regulatory mechanisms involved in insulin dependent diabetes mellitus (IDDM) induction. This is further emphasized by the observation that islet-specific production of IL-10 accelerates IDDM in genetically susceptible non obese diabetic (NOD) mice, suggesting that, in this case, β-cell destruction may also involve Th2-cell-mediated events (12).

Each Th cell subset inhibits its counterpart, and this is actually the driving force polarizing CD4$^+$ T cells toward either the Th1 or Th2 phenotype. IFN-γ directly inhibits proliferation of Th2 but not of Th1 cells (13), whereas IL-4 and IL-10 downregulate class II expression by monocytes, reducing their antigen-presenting capacity and inhibiting lymphokine production by Th1 clones (14). In addition, IL-4 (15) and possibly also IL-13 (16) suppress the development of Th1 cells through downregulation of IL-12 production by monocytes. Conversely, IFN-α inhibits development of Th2 cells. This reciprocal regulation indicates a role for

*   Roche Milano Ricerche, Milan, Italy.

Th2-derived lymphokines in inhibition of autoimmune diseases, as suggested by the reduced IDDM incidence following IL-4 administration to NOD mice (17). Evidence for Th2 cells regulating the onset of IDDM is further suggested by their capacity to inhibit the spontaneous onset of diabetes in rats (18).

We recently tested the role of IL-12 in the spontaneous development of IDDM in NOD mice, an autoimmune disease considered to be primarily mediated by Th1-type CD4+ T cells (S. Trembleau, et al., *J Exp Med*, in press). Administration of recombinant mouse IL-12 induces rapid onset of IDDM in NOD, but not in BALB/c mice. Activation of pancreas-infiltrating T cells from IL-12-injected NOD mice by insolubilized anti-TCR induces enhanced secretion of IFN-γ and low levels of IL-4 production, consistent with induction of Th1 cells. Histologically, IL-12 administration induces massive infiltration of lymphoid cells, mostly T cells, in the pancreatic islets of NOD mice. Therefore, IL-12 accelerates IDDM in genetically susceptible NOD mice, which correlates with increased Th1 cytokine production. These results hold implications for the pathogenesis, and possibly for the therapy, of IDDM and of other Th1-cell-mediated autoimmune diseases. In particular, it will be interesting to ascertain whether administration of IL-12 antagonists (25) interfere with IDDM development.

Th1-type cells appear to be involved not only in experimental but also in human-organ-specific autoimmune diseases. CD4+ T-cell clones isolated from lymphocytic infiltrates of Hashimoto's thyroiditis or Graves' disease exibit a clear-cut Th1 phenotype (19). In addition, most T-cell clones derived from peripheral blood or cerebrospinal fluid of multiple sclerosis patients show a Th1 lymphokine profile (20). The situation is less clear in systemic autoimmune disorders: A prevalent Th0/Th1 phenotype was found among clones derived from rheumatoid arthritis or Sjögren's syndrome patients, whereas a Th0/Th2 profile predominated among clones derived from systemic lupus patients (21).

Undoubtedly, selective inhibition of Th1 or Th2 cells, or deviation of Th1/Th2 cell development toward the opposing phenotype will represent an important strategy for induction of a relatively selective immunosuppression potentially applicable to the treatment of human autoimmune and allergic diseases.

Cytokines and Cytokine Antagonists

Cytokines, soluble molecules transmitting information among cells, are essential components of the immune response, and an imbalance of the cytokine network plays an important role in disease states like autoimmunity and allergy.

Elucidation of the structure and function of individual cytokines, as well as their selective production by Th1 and Th2 CD4+ T cells, has identified novel strategies for selective immunosuppression. Several approaches can be used to inhibit a given cytokine: the cytokine itself can be neutralized by specific monoclonal antibodies or by soluble cytokine receptors, whereas the cytokine receptor can be inhibited by monoclonal antibodies or by receptor antagonists competing with the ligand for the receptor binding site.

Recently, clinical trials have been performed targeting the proinflammatory cytokines IL-1 and TNF-α in patients with rheumatoid arthritis. Results of anti-TNF-α therapies are very promising. Animal studies have clearly documented the important role of TNF-α in rheumatoid arthritis. Mice transgenic for the human TNF-α gene produce high levels of this cytokine and develop arthritis beginning at 4 weeks of age (10). The disease is mediated by the transgenic molecule, as demonstrated by the prevention of arthritis following administration of monoclonal antibodies to human TNF-α. In addition, in a type-II collagen arthritis model, administration of anti-mouse TNF-α even after disease onset significantly reduced inflammation and tissue destruction (22). Based on these results, chimeric anti-TNF-α monoclonal antibody was administered to rheumatoid arthritis patients (23). Treatment with anti-TNF-α was safe and well tolerated, and led to significant clinical and laboratory improvements. Remissions lasted about 3 months, on the average, but reinjection of anti-TNF-α antibody induced a significant antiglobulin response in most patients, reducing considerably the efficacy of the treatment. An alternative approach, using the soluble TNF receptor p55 chain fused to the constant region of human IgG1 heavy chain (sTNFR-IgG1), has been demonstrated to be about 10-fold more effective than anti-TNF-α antibody at neutralizing the activity of endogenous TNF, as assessed in a model of murine listeriosis (24). This fusion protein appears to achieve the same clinical effects as anti-TNF-α antibody administration, but without induction of neutralizing antibodies.

These results demonstrate the efficacy of cytokine-specific treatments in inflammatory disease states, though even more promising are immunosuppressive strategies selectively targeting Th1- or Th2-type T cells. In particular, antagonists of IL-12 and IL-4 offer the possibility to selectively manipulate Th1 and Th2 cell induction, with great potential for the treatment of autoimmune diseases and allergies, respectively.

Tolerance Induction in Th1 Cells

Besides immunointervention based on the inhibition of Th1-promoting cytokines, Th1 cells can be physically eliminated or functionally inactivated by tolerance induction. The most obvious way to induce tolerance is to administer antigen in tolerogenic form. Tolerance induction by intravenous antigen administration takes place in the periphery, since it can be established in athymic mice, and it appears to be mediated more frequently by clonal anergy (26, 27) rather than by clonal deletion (28).

Induction of peripheral tolerance by administration of autoantigens has a beneficial effect in several autoimmune models. EAE can be ameliorated by inducing T cell anergy to synthetic peptides corresponding to the immunodominant epitopes of MBP (29). In this case, tolerance induction by MBP peptides at EAE onset, 10 days after administration of MBP, blocked the progression and decreased the severity of EAE. These results clearly demonstrate that selective immunotherapy by administration of autoantigenic peptides can be effective in acute experimental autoimmune diseases. However, amplification and broadening of the autoimmune response to other epitopes of the same autoantigen appears to occur in chronic diseases (30), suggesting that induction of immunosuppression by immunodominant peptides alone (31) may not be effective. This problem could be circumvented by tolerance induction to the entire autoantigenic protein, as demonstrated by induction of tolerance to glutamic acid decarboxylase, a putative autoantigen in IDDM, able to prevent diabetes development in NOD mice (32, 33). In addition, repeated intravenous administration of large amounts of

soluble myelin basic protein (MBP) could delete peripheral autoreactive T cells, and thereby improve the course of EAE (34).

Interestingly, tolerance induction by parenteral administration of soluble antigen affects primarily Th1-type cells, whereas the activity of Th2 cells can even be enhanced (35). This may suggest that tolerance induction by parenteral administration of soluble antigen may be effective in treating autoimmune but not allergic diseases. A critical point for the applicability of this approach is the possibility of inducing specific unresponsiveness in antigen-primed individuals.

We tested induction of peripheral T-cell tolerance by administration to mice of proteins or synthetic peptides in soluble form. Hen egg-white lysozyme (HEL), delivered continuously over a 10-day period by an osmotic minipump implanted subcutaneously, efficiently and specifically prevents the subsequent priming of T cells by the injection of HEL emulsified in adjuvant. Similar results can be obtained by administration of soluble HEL peptides (Guéry et al., manuscript in preparation).

T cells specific for dominant or subdominant HEL epitopes can be tolerized equally well. The set of overlapping HEL peptides used defines in mice of $H-2_k$ haplotype three dominant epitopes, included in HEL sequences 1–18, 46–61, and 107–129, and a subdominant one corresponding to the sequence 25–43 (36). The administration of soluble HEL very effectively inhibits T-cell responses to both dominant and subdominant HEL epitopes. This result is quite interesting, since one point of debate is the dominance of autoantigenic peptides presented by class II molecules associated with autoimmune disease susceptibility. Acccording to one theory, autoreactive pathogenic T-cell clones could recognize cryptic determinants and for this reason have escaped thymic deletion during negative selection (37). The opposite view considers autoantigenic peptides as dominant and therefore highly antigenic. Their antigenic potential can be expressed when events such as molecular mimicry (38) or regulatory imbalances (39) lead to a breakdown of tolerance. Our results, which demonstrate effective inhibition of T-cell responses induced by dominant and subdominant antigenic epitopes, would indicate that induction of peripheral T cell tolerance may in either case be capable of interfering with the activation of autoreactive T cells.

Th1 cells, which produce IL-2 and IFN-γ, preferentially induce synthesis of antibodies expressing the IgG2a isotype. Conversely, Th2 cells, producing IL-4, IL-5 and IL-10, mainly elicit antibody responses of IgG1 and IgE isotype and cause B-cell proliferation and differentiation (40). As documented by *in vivo* inhibition of anti-HEL antibody responses of IgG2a – but not IgG1 isotype – tolerance induction effectively prevents the helper function of Th1-, but not Th2-type cells. Our protocol of tolerance induction very efficiently inhibits (about a 100-fold decrease) IgG2a/IgG2b isotypes, whereas anti-HEL antibodies of IgG1 isotype show only a 5-fold reduction. These results indicate that Th1- but not Th2-type helper cells are inhibited by tolerance induction – consistent with the observation that antigen-specific unresponsiveness induced by pretreatment with aqueous antigen selectively tolerizes Th1-like cells (35, 41). Since Th1-type cells are the pathogenic cells in most organ-specific autoimmune diseases (7, 21), tolerance induction of this T-cell subset may interfere with the course of disease. Conversely, human CD4+ T-cell clones specific to allergenic and helmintic antigens exhibit Th2-like lymphokine production profile (2); in these cases tolerance induction may not affect pathogenic T cells.

The addition of IL-2 to cultures from tolerant mice only partially restores T cell responsiveness, indicating both anergy and deletion of T cells as possible mechanisms of tolerance induction. Mixing experiments have failed to demonstrate induction of suppressor T cells in tolerant mice. Moreover, tolerance induced in normal BALB/c and in BALB/c mice with a disrupted β2 microglobulin gene is indistinguishable, further excluding a role of CD8+ suppressor T cells in this tolerance protocol. Tolerance is long-lasting, and it is still active 5 months after administration of antigen in tolerogenic form. Interestingly, tolerance, rather than a secondary response, is induced by continuous peptide administration to protein antigen-primed mice, suggesting the possible applicability of this form of tolerance induction to selective immunosuppression of established autoimmune diseases. However, protein antigen administration to antigen-primed mice can inhibit T-cell responses, though under the conditions we have so far tested it invariably results in induction of a secondary antibody response. This indicates that the establishment of tolerance at the B-cell level by parenteral administration of soluble intact proteins to primed mice is difficult, if at all possible.

Prospects for Therapy

Selective immunosuppression can be induced by a variety of approaches and mediated by several different mechanisms. They could be grouped into two broad categories: approaches selectively directed at autoreactive T cells by targeting the MHC/antigenic peptide/TCR complex, and less selective approaches targeting a substantial fraction of T cells, including the pathogenic ones.

The first category represents, in principle, the most effective and selective form of immunosuppression. Induction of autoantigen-specific immunosuppression requires, obviously, knowledge of the autoantigens. At present, they are poorly defined in most autoimmune situations, though progress is expected in their identification and characterization. Once the inciting autoantigen has been identified, selective immunosuppression of T cells recognizing it could be induced by exploiting one or more of the mechanisms controlling peripheral tolerance. It is too early to judge how realistic the prospects are for clinical applicability of autoantigen-based immunosuppression, but the problems surfacing represent major challenges for pharmacological development.

In the second category of approaches, very heterogeneous indeed, some strategies have been clinically tested more thoroughly. Among them, some look extremely promising, for example, sTNFR-IgG in rheumatoid arthritis. It is likely that the next generation of immunosuppressive drugs will include several cytokine antagonists, particularly those able to inhibit, directly or indirectly, the development and function of Th1 or Th2 T cells.

Address for correspondence:

Luciano Adorini, MD
Roche Milano Ricerche
Via Olgettina, 58
I-20132 Milano
Italy

References

1. Mosmann TR, Cherwinski H, Bond MW, Giedlin MA, Coffmann RL. Two types of murine helper T cell clone. I. Definition according to profile of lym-

phokine activities and secreted proteins. *J Immunol* 1986; 136:2348.

2. Del Prete G, De Carli M, Mastromauro C, Biagiotti R, Macchia D, Falagiani P, Ricci M, Romagnani S. Purified protein derivative of mycobacterium tuberculosis and escretory-secretory antigen(s) of *Toxocara canis* expand *in vitro* human T cells with stable and opposite (type 1 T helper or type 2 T helper) profile of cytokine production. *J Clin Invest* 1991; 88:346.

3. Trinchieri G. Interleukin-12 and its role in the generation of Th1 cells. *Immunol Today* 1993; 14:335.

4. Paul WE, Seder RA. Lymphocytes responses and cytokines. *Cell* 1994; 76:241.

5. Finkelman FD, Katona IM, Urban JJ, Snapper CM, Ohara J, Paul WE. Suppression of *in vivo* polyclonal IgE responses by monoclonal antibody to the lymphokine B-cell stimulatory factor 1. *Proc Natl Acad Sci USA* 1986; 83:9675.

6. Powrie F, Coffmann RL. Cytokine regulation of T cell function: Potential for therapeutic intervention. *Immunol Today* 1993; 14:270.

7. O'Garra A, Murphy K. T-cell subsets in autoimmunity. *Curr Op Immunol* 1993; 5:880.

8. Sarvetnick N, Liggitt D, Pitts SL, Hansen SE, Stewart TA. Insulin-dependent diabetes mellitus induced in transgenic mice by ectopic expression of class II MHC and interferon-γ. *Cell* 1988; 52:773.

9. Stewart TA, Hultgren B, Huang X, Pitts-Meek S, Hully J, Maclachian NJ. Induction of type I diabetes by interferon-α in transgenic mice. *Science* 1993; 260:1942.

10. Keffer J, Probert L, Cazlaris H, Georgopulos S, Kaslaris E, Kioussis D, Kollias G. Transgenic mice expressing human tumor necrosis factor – a predictive genetic model of arthritis. *EMBO J* 1991; 13:4025.

11. Picarella DE, Kratz A, Li C-B, Ruddle NH, Flavell RA. Transgenic tumor necrosis factor (TNF)-α production in pancreatic islets leads to insulitis, not diabetes. *J Immunol* 1993; 150:4136.

12. Wogensen L, Myung-Shik L, Sarvetnick N. Production of interleukin 10 by islet cells accelerates immune-mediated destruction of β cells in nonobese diabetic mice. *J Exp Med* 1994; 179:1379.

13. Gajewski TF, Fitch FW. Anti-proliferative effect of IFN-γ in immune regulation. I. IFN-γ inhibits the proliferation of Th2 but not Th1 murine helper T lymphocyte clones. *J Immunol* 1988; 140:4245.

14. Moore K, O'Garra A, De Waal Malefyt R, Vieira P, Mosmann TR. Interleukin-10. *Annu Rev Immunol* 1993; 11:165.

15. Hsieh C-S, Macatonia SE, Tripp CS, Wolf SF, O'-Garra A, Murphy KM. Development of Th1 CD4+ T cells through IL-12 produced by *Listeria*-induced macrophages. *Science* 1993; 260:547.

16. Zurawski G, de Vries JE. Interleukin 13, an interleukin 4-like cytokine that acts on monocytes and B cells, but not on T cells. *Immunol Today* 1994; 15:19.

17. Rapoport MJ, Jaramillo A, Zipris D, Lazarus AH, Serreze DV, Leiter EH, Cyopick P, Danska JS, Delovitch TL. Interleukin 4 reverses T cell proliferative unresponsiveness and prevents the onset of diabetes in nonobese diabetic mice. *J Exp Med* 1993; 178:87.

18. Fowell D, Mason D. Evidence that the T cell repertoire of normal rats contains cells with the potential to cause diabetes. Characterization of of the CD4+ T cell subset that inhibits this autoimmune potential. *J Exp Med* 1993; 177:627.

19. De Carli M, D'Elios M, Mariotti S, Marcocci C, Pinchera A, Ricci M, Romagnani S, Del Prete GF. Cytolytic T cells with Th1-like cytokine profile predominate in retroorbital lymphocytic infiltrates of Graves' ophthalmopathy. *J Clin Endocrin Metab* 1993; 77:1120.

20. Brod SA, Benjamin D, Hafler DA. Restricted T cell expression of IL-2, IFN-γ mRNA in human inflammatory disease. *J Immunol* 1991; 147:810.

21. Romagnani S. Lymphokine production by human T cells in disease states. *Annu Rev Immunol* 1994; 12:227.

22. Williams RO, Feldmann M, Maini RN. Anti-tumor necrosis factor ameliorates joint disease in murine collagen-induced arthritis. *Proc Natl Acad Sci USA* 1992; 89:9784.

23. Elliott MJ, Maini RN, Feldmann M, Long-Fox A, Charles P, Katsikis P, Brennan FM, Walker J, Bijl H, Ghrayeb J, Woody JN. Treatment of rheumatoid arthritis with chimeric monoclonal antibodies to tumor necrosis factor α. *Arthritis Rheum* 1993; 36:1681.

24. Haak-Frendscho M, Marsters SA, Mordenti J, Brady S, Gillett NA, Chen SA, Ashkenazi A. Inhibition of TNF by a TNF receptor immunoadhesin. Comparison to an anti-TNF monoclonal antibody. *J Immunol* 1994; 152:1347.

25. Mattner F, Fischer S, Guckes S, Jin S, Kaulen H, Schmitt E, Rude E, Germann T. The interleukin-12 subunit p40 specifically inhibits effects of the interleukin-12 heterodimer. *Eur J Immunol* 1993; 23:2202.

26. Rammensee H-G, Kroschewski R, Frangoulis B. Clonal anergy induced in mature Vβ6+ T lymphocytes on immunizing Mls-1^b mice with Mls-1^a expressing cells. *Nature* 1989; 339:541.

27. Burkly LC, Lo D, Kanagawa R, Brinster L, Flavell RA. T cell tolerance by clonal anergy in transgenic mice with nonlymphoid expression of MHC class II I-E. *Nature* 1989; 342:564.

28. Webb S, Morris C, Sprent J. Extrathymic tolerance of mature T cells: Clonal elimination as a consequence of immunity. *Cell* 1990; 63:1249.

29. Gaur A, Wiers B, Liu A, Rothbard J, Fathman CG. Amelioration of autoimmune encephalomyelitis by myelin basic protein synthetic peptide-induced anergy. *Science* 1992; 258:1941.

30. Lehmann PV, Forsthuber T, Miller A, Sercarz EE. Spreading of T-cell autoimmunity to cryptic determinants of an autoantigen. *Nature* 1992; 358:155.

31. Clayton JP, Gammon GM, Ando DG, Kono DH, Hood L, Sercarz EE. Peptide-specific prevention of experimental allergic encephalomyelitis. Neonatal tolerance induced to the dominant T cell determinant of myelin basic protein. *J Exp Med* 1989; 169:1681.

32. Kaufman DL, Clare-Salzler M, Tian J, Forsthuber T, Ting GSP, Robinson P, Atkinson MA, Sercarz EE, Tobin AJ, Lehmann PV. Spontaneous loss of T-cell tolerance to glutamic acid decarboxylase in murine insulin-dependent diabetes. *Nature* 1993; 366:69.

33. Tisch R, Yang X-D, Singer SM, Liblau RS, Fugger L, McDevitt HO. Immune response to glutamic acid decarboxylase correlates with insulitis in non-obese diabetic mice. *Nature* 1993; 366:72.

34. Critchfield JM, Racke MK, Zuniga-Pflucker JC, Cannella B, Raine CS, Goverman J, Lenardo MJ. T cell deletion in high antigen dose therapy of autoimmune encephalomyelitis. *Science* 1994; 263:1139.

35. Burstein HJ, Shea CM, Abbas AK. Aqueous antigens induce *in vivo* tolerance selectively in IL-2- and IFN-γ-producing (Th1) cells. *J Immunol* 1992; 148:3687.

36. Adorini L, Appella E, Doria G, Nagy ZA. Mechanisms influencing the immunodominance of T cell determinants. *J Exp Med* 1988; 168:2091.

37. Gammon G, Sercarz E. How some T cells escape tolerance induction. *Nature* 1989; 342:183.

38. Oldstone MB. Molecular mimicry as a mechanism for the cause and a probe uncovering etiologic agent(s) of autoimmune diseases. *Curr Top Microbiol Immunol* 1989; 145:127.

39. Nepom GT. MHC class II molecules and autoimmunity. *Annu Rev Immunol* 1991; 9:493.

40. Mosmann TR, Coffman RL. Th1 and Th2 cells: Different patterns of lymphokine secretion lead to different functional properties. *Ann Rev Immunol* 1989; 7:145.

41. De Wit D, Van Mechelen M, Ryelandt M, Figueiredo AC, Abramowicz D, Goldman M, Bazin H, Urbain J, Leo O. The injection of deaggregated gamma globulins in adult mice induces antigen-specific unresponsiveness of T helper type 1 but not type 2 lymphocytes. *J Exp Med* 1992; 175:9.

Strategies for T-Cell Immunotherapy of Cancer

Cornelis JM Melief, W Martin Kast*

Keywords: Cytotoxic T lymphocyte, HLA system, tumor immunotherapy

In animal models anti-tumor effects have been obtained by vaccination with MHC class I binding peptides, inducing CD8$^+$ cytotoxic T lymphocyte (CTL) responses. While such vaccination can prevent the growth of subsequent tumor inocula, it cannot eradicate established tumor masses. Established tumor masses have been dealt with effectively in some models by adoptive transfer of cloned tumor-specific CTL in combination with interleukin-2 (IL-2). A prototype human papilloma virus type 16 peptide vaccine for cervical carcinoma patients has been developed. Similar vaccines are feasible for non-virally induced cancers such as malignant melanoma.

Introduction

In animal models involving both virus-induced and nonvirus induced tumors, the most powerful component of the immune system is the cytotoxic T lymphocyte (CTL) response directed against peptides presented by MHC class I molecules (reviewed in 1–4). The efficacy of CTL was proven by adoptive transfer of CD8$^+$ cytolytic T-cell clones. Adoptive transfer of CD4$^+$ noncytolytic T-cell clones was also shown to have strong anti-tumor potency in some models (1). The notion that T cells also have strong anti-tumor activity in human cancer has received strong support from the therapeutic activity of expanded tumor-infiltrating lymphocytes (TIL) in melanoma (6).

Below we discuss the relative merits and problems of T cell adoptive transfer and vaccination strategies in animal models and human cancer therapy.

T Cell Adoptive Transfer Versus Vaccination Strategies

Although cancer vaccination strategies based on modern immunological insights got under way only recently, it is likely that vaccination will never become an effective therapy for extensive established tumors in animal models (1–4). To which extent this also holds true in man remains to be seen, but impressive melomena regressions have been observed with uncloned TIL. Vaccination strategies must therefore be considered, especially in the form of adjuvant therapy following conventional cancer therapy to deal effectively with minimal residual disease. While adoptively transferred T cells, grown in large numbers prior to injection, are probably capable of dealing with a larger tumor burden, the growth and expansion of such tumor-specific T cells remains very laborious and costly at the present time and requires great skill. It is therefore not feasible to conduct adoptive T cell transfer therapy for large groups of patients. Vaccination on the other hand is intrinsically simple and inexpensive, once the appropriate vaccine components have been identified.

Tumor Eradication by Adoptive Transfer of T Cells

Murine tumors induced by such viruses as friend leukemia virus or human adenovirus type 5 (Ad5) can be eradicated by cloned CD8$^+$ CTL (1–4). These adoptively transferred CTL are most effective if combined with systemic interleukin-2 (IL-2) treatment, because most *in vitro* grown CD8$^+$ CTL clones do not produce sufficient IL-2 for autocrine expansion *in vivo* to sufficient numbers for effective therapy.

In the case of Ad5 induced tumors implanted in T cell deficient nude mice, large established tumors were eradicated within 14 days following adoptively transferred CTL directed against an E1a viral oncogene encoded peptide presented by the H-2 D^b MHC class I molecule (7, 8).

* Department of Immunohematology and Bloodbank, University Hospital Leiden, The Netherlands.

Nature of Antigens Detected by T Cells on Virus-Induced and Nonviral Tumors

Tumor antigens responsible for the generation of tumor-specific T cells against virus-induced tumors are encoded by viral genes (1, 7, 10). The actual antigens recognized by CD8+ CTL among TIL from melanoma patients are most likely directed against any one or a combination of recently defined melanoma-associated antigens that were found to be recognized by cloned CTL lines from melanoma patients. These include the antigens MAGE-1, tyrosinase, gp 100 and MART-1 (11–15). MAGE family antigens (MAGE-1, 2, and 3) are normally only expressed in the testis. Tyrosinase, gp 100, and MART-1 are melanocyte lineage-specific differentiation antigens, and are therefore also expressed in normal melanocytes. The HLA-binding peptides recognized by CTL against these antigens are encoded by the normal gene sequences; thus, these tumor-specific CTL are in essence autoreactive. Indeed, in patients with melanoma, skin depigmentation (vitiligo) is often associated with a favorable clinical course.

The Concept of Peptide Vaccination

Because MHC class I presented peptides are the key elements recognized by CD8+ CTL, and because few peptides are recognized by CTL in most virus infections, we argued that vaccination with such peptides should confer CTL mediated protection aginst virus-induced disease. We were indeed able to protect C57BL/6 mice against virulent Sendai virus-induced death by vaccination with the immunodominant CTL epitope (16, 17). Similar results were observed by Schulz et al. in the LCM virus system (18). In both cases the peptide was administered in incomplete Freund adjuvant (IFA).

Antitumor Effects by Vaccination with MHC Class I Binding Peptides

We set up a murine model for vaccination against human papilloma virus type 16 (HPV-16)-induced cervical carcinoma. To identify vaccine candidates we generated a set of 240 overlapping nonameric peptides derived from the sequence of the HPV-16

oncogenes E6 and E7. These peptides were tested for their ability to bind H-2 K^b and H-2 D^b MHC class I molecules. The high affinity H-2 D^b-binding peptide and the putative CTL epitope E7–49–57 (R A H Y N I V T F) emulsified in IFA was used for vaccination. Immunization with this peptide led to resistance against a subsequent challenge with HPV-16 transformed syngeneic tumor cells. Protection was associated with CTL memory (5).

Encouraged by these results, we identified peptides of HPV-16 E6 and E7 that bound with high affinity to the most frequent human HLA class I allele, HLA-A*0201, using a cellular binding assay (20), as well as peptides that bound to HLA-A*0201 and four other HLA-A alleles with a molecular binding assay (20). Two HLA-A*0201 binding peptides have been chosen for vaccination of patients with HPV-16 positive cervical carcinoma who have failed conventional therapy. The peptide vaccine also includes a synthetic helper peptide and an adjuvant resembling IFA, but of better defined composition (Montanide ISA 51, produced by Seppic). Vaccinations will be started in the autumn of 1994. If clinical peptide vaccination is effective, the issues of HLA polymorphism and HPV heterogeneity will have to be dealt with. Fortunately, the 5 HLA alleles (A*0101, A*0201, A*0301, A*1101, and A*2401) for which HPV binding peptides have been identified together occur in more than 95% of the Caucasian human population. Also, both HPV-16 and HPV-18 E6 and E7 peptides binding to these HLA molecules have been identified. These HPV types are associated with the great majority of human cervical carcinomas worldwide. Thus, a peptide cocktail vaccine is feasible, especially because the number of high affinity binding peptides for each HLA allele is limited (20).

Discussion

The results of vaccination with MHC class I binding peptides in animal models show that protective CTL responses can be induced against virulent virus infections and against virus induced tumors. A major advantage of such peptide vaccination is that protective CTL responses can be induced not only against immunodominant epitopes but also against subdominant epitopes. Subdominant peptides are peptides against which a T-cell response does not arise upon immunization with the intact native antigen (e. g., tumor cell or minor derived protein), but only following immunization with a predigested fragment containing the subdominant peptide or with the synthetic subdominant peptide (21).

Indeed, the protective CTL epitope in our murine HPV model is a subdominant one, because protective CTL against this epitope are only induced following vaccination with peptide in IFA but not after immunization with HPV transformed tumor cells (19), despite the fact that the tumor cells express this epitope. Apparently, on intact tumor cells the immunogenicity of this epitope is too low, possibly as a result of low expression. A similar phenomenon was observed by us in CTL against an epitope of Moloney leukemia virus (22). The advantages of peptide vaccination over conventional vaccination are listed in Table 1.

Table 1. Advantages of peptide vaccination for induction of CD8[+] CTL responses.

---

1. Omission of irrelevant material from vaccines.
2. Bypass of requirement for biosynthetic processing for entry of proteins into MHC class I molecules.
3. Induction of protective responses against otherwise silent peptides such as autologous peptides and non-dominant (subdominant) viral peptides. Thus, utilization of the full potential of the T-cell repertoire against target molecules of choice.

The strategy of peptide vaccination is not limited to virus-induced tumors, but can also be applied to other cancers. In the latter category of tumors, peptide vaccination may help to overcome natural tolerance or anergy towards self peptides of cancer-associated molecules (23–25).

If peptide vaccination by itself has insufficient therapeutic potency, combining peptide vaccination with *ex vivo* amplification of the induced CTL and combination of vaccination and/or adoptive transfer with systemic cytokine treatment (IL-2, IL-7) must be considered.

Address for correspondence:

Cornelius JM Melief
Rijnsburgerweg 10
2333 AA Leiden
The Netherlands

References

1. Greenberg PD. Adoptive T cell therapy of tumors: mechanisms operative in the recognition and elimination of tumor cells. *Adv Immunol* 1990; 49:281.

2. Melief CJM. Tumor eradication by adoptive transfer of cytotoxic T lymphocytes. *Adv Cancer Res* 1992; 58:143.

3. Melief CJM, Kast WM. Lessons from T cell responses to virus induced tumors for cancer eradication in general. *Cancer Surveys* 1992; 13:81.

4. Melief CJM, Kast WM. Potential immunogenicity of oncongene and tumor suppressor gene products. *Curr Opin Immunol* 1993; 5:709–713.

5. Feltkamp MCW, Smits HL, Vierboom MPM, Minnaar RP, De Jongh BM, Drijfhout JW, Ter Schegget J, Melief CJM, Kast WM. Vaccination with cytotoxic T lymphocyte epitope-containing peptide protects against a tumor induced by human papillomavirus type 16-transformed cells. *Eur J Immunol* 1993; 23:2242–2249.

6. Rosenberg SA, Packard BS, Hebersold PM, Solomon D, Topalian SL, Toy ST, Suinon P, Lotze MT, Yang JC, Serpp C, Simpson C, Carter C, Bock S, Schwarzentruber DJ, Wei JP, White DE. Use of tumor infiltrating lymphocytes and interleukin-2 in the immunotherapy of patients with metastatic melanoma: a preliminary report. *N Engl J Med* 1988; 319:1676.

7. Kast WM, Offringa R, Peters PJ, Voordouw AC, Meloen RH, Van der Eb A, Melief CJM. Eradication of adenovirus E1-induced tumors by E1A specific cytotoxic T lymphocytes. *Cell* 1989; 59:603–614.

8. Kast WM, Melief CJM. Fine peptide specificity of cytotoxic T lymphocytes directed against adenovirus-induced tumors and peptide-MHC binding. *Int J Cancer* 1991; 6:90–94.

9. Sijts AJAM, Ossendorp F, Mengedé EAM, Van den Elsen PJ, Melief CJM. Immunodominant mink cell focus-inducing murine leukemia virus (MuLV)-encoded CTL epitope, identified by its MHC class I-binding motif, explains MuLV-type specificity of MCF-directed cytotoxic T lymphocytes. *J Immunol* 152:106–116.

10. Tanaka Y, Anderson RW, Maloy WL, Tevethia SS. Localisation of an immunorecessive epitope on SV40 T antigen by H-2D[b]-restricted cytotoxic T-lymphocyte clones and a synthetic peptide. *Virology* 1989; 171:205.

11. Van der Bruggen P, Traversari C, Chomez P, Lurquin C, De Plaen E, Van den Eijnde B, Knuth A, Boon T. A gene encoding an antigen recognized by cytolytic T lymphocytes on a human melanoma. *Science* 1991; 254:1643.

12. Traversari C, Van der Bruggen P, Immanuel F, Luescher IF, Lurquin C, Chomez P, Van Pel A, De Plaen

E, Amar-Costesec A, Boon T. A nonapeptide encoded by human gene MAGE-1 is recognized on HLA-A1 by cytolytic T lymphocytes directed against tumor antigen MZ2-E. *J Exp Med* 1992; 176:1453.

13. Brichard V, Van Pel A, Wölfel Th, De Plaen E, Lethe B, Coulie P, Boon T. The tyrosinase gene codes for an antigen recognized by autologous cytolytic T lymphocytes on HLA-A2 melanomas. *J Exp Med* 1993; 178: 489.

14. Bakker ABH, Schreurs MWJ, De Boer AJ, Kawakami Y, Rosenberg SA, Adema GJ, Figdor CG. Melanocyte lineage-specific antigen gp 100 is recognized by melanoma-derived tumor-infiltrating lymphocytes. *J Exp. Med* 1994; 179:1005.

15. Kawakami Y, Eliyahu S, Delgado CH, Robbins P, Rivoitini L, Topalian SL, Miki T, Rosenberg SA. Cloning of the gene encoding a shared human melanoma antigen recognized by autologous T cells infiltrating into tumor. *Proc Natl Acad Sci USA* 1994; 91:3515.

16. Kast WM, Roux LM, Curren J, Blom HJJ, Voordouw AC, Meloen RH, Kolakovsky D, Melief CJM. Protection against lethal Sendai virus infection by *in vivo* priming of virus-specific cytotoxic T lymphocytes with a free synthetic peptide. *Proc Natl Acad Sci USA* 1991; 88:283–2287.

17. Kast WM, Brandt RMP, Melief CJM. Strict peptide length is not required for the induction of cytotoxic T lymphocyte-mediated antiviral protection by peptide vaccination. *Eur J Immunol* 1993; 23:1189–1192.

18. Schulz M, Zinkernagel RM, Hengartner H. Peptide-induced antiviral protection by cytotoxic T cells. *Proc Natl Acad Sci USA* 1991; 88:991.

19. Kast WM, Brandt RMP, Drijfhout JW, Melief CJM.

Human leukocyte antigen-A2.1 restricted candidate cytotoxic T lymphocyte epitopes of human papillomavirus type 16 E6 and E7 proteins identified by using the processing-defective human cell line T2. *J Immunother* 1993; 14:115–120.

20. Kast WM, Brandt RMP, Sidney J, Drijfhout JW, Kubo RT, Grey HM, Melief CJM, Sette A. The role of the HLA-A motifs in identification of potential CTL epitopes in human papillomavirus type 16 E6 and E7 proteins. *J Immunol* 1994; 152:3904–3912.

21. Sercarz EE, Lekmann PV, Ametani A, Benchou G, Miller A, Mondgil K. Dominance and crypticity of T cell antigenic determinants. *Ann Rev Immunol* 1993; 11:729.

22. Sijts AJAM, De Bruijn MHL, Ressing ME, Nieland JD, Mengede EAM, Boog CJP, Ossendorp F, Kast WM, Melief CJM. Idenfication of an H-2 K^b-presented Moloney MuLV CTL epitope that displays enhanced recognition in H-2D^b mutant bm 13 mice. *J Virol* 1994; 68:6038–6046.

23. Houbiers JGA, Nijman HW, Van der Burg SH, Drijfhout JW, Kenemans P, Van de Velde CJH, Brand A, Momburg F, Kast WM, Melief CJM. *In vitro* induction of human cytotoxic T lymphocytes responses against peptide of mutant and wild-type p53. *Eur J Immunol* 1993; 23:2072–2077.

24. Nijman HW, Van der Burg SH, Vierboom MPM, Houbiers JGA, Kast WM, Melief CJM. p53, a potential target for tumor-directed T cells. *Immunol Lett* 1994; 40:171–178.

25. Melief CJM, Kast WM. Potential immunogenicity of oncogene and tumor suppressor gene products. *Curr Opin Immunol* 1993; 5:709–713.

Allergic Inflammation and Asthma

Michael A Kaliner*

Keywords: Inflammation, vascular permeability, edema, epithelial lining fluid, airway hyperresponsiveness, mucus

Over the past decade, the concept that asthma is an inflammatory disease of the airways has been popularized. In this manuscript, the cardinal signs of inflammation and the evidence that they actually play a role in asthma are addressed. Vasodilation (redness) may participate in asthma, but only in restricted circumstances. Edema (vasopermeability) is thought to be quite important in acute and chronic airflow obstruction, and to be largely ignored therapeutically. It is suggested that increased vascular permeability with subsequent movement of fluid into the airway lumen is one of the important mechanisms leading to acute asthma deaths. Airway inflammation (the infiltration of inflammatory cells) and increased hyper-responsiveness (the airway equivalent to pain) are very important in asthma. Thus, the four cardinal signs of inflammation may be found in the asthmatic airway, and it is thought that they are indeed quite important in causing and propagating airflow obstruction. While we have reasonable medications to help reduce cellular infiltration and airway reactivity, we do not have any effective medications, other than steroids, to treat increased vascular permeability.

The cardinal signs of inflammation are redness, swelling, cellular inflammation and pain (or increased irritability). Over the past decade, since the late phase allergic reaction was recognized to be a sequelae of mast cell activation (1, 2), a great deal of attention has been directed at the role that airway inflammation plays in asthma. Support for inflammation occurring in asthma has been centered on models directed at cellular infiltration of the airway mucosa and movement of inflammatory cells into the epithelial lining fluid where they can be recovered by bronchoalveolar lavage (BAL). Substantial data has suggested that increased inflammation concomitantly increases airway reactivity, and that aiming therapy at the inflammation reduces airway responsiveness. However, relatively little interest has been shown toward airway edema and its role in asthma. In this review, data for each of the signs of inflammation, their pathogenesis, and roles in asthma will be briefly discussed. In the end, vascular permeability and its contribution to acute airflow obstruction as well as death from asthma will be underscored.

A working definition of asthma is as follows: A disease of reversible airflow obstruction manifested as wheezing and caused by various combinations of airway mucosal edema and inflammation, increased secretions, and smooth muscle contraction. Asthmatics exhibit airway hyper-reactivity, and the clinical course is quite variable (modified from reference 3). This definition stresses the four causes of airflow obstruction, as well as emphasizing the influence of airway hyperresponsiveness. Part of the intention of this review will be to integrate how inflammation participates in both airflow obstruction and airway hyperresponsiveness.

The four cardinal signs of inflammation are: edema (swelling), vasodilation (redness), cellular infiltration, and pain (increased airway responsiveness). In this review, each of these signs of inflammation will be reviewed in the context of asthma to determine if there is sufficient evidence to support its role in the disease. because the airways have no pain fibers, pain will be translated as increased airway responsiveness, accepting that this phenomena reflects increased sensory responses.

Airway Edema

In the classical description of the pathology of fatal bronchial asthma, Dunnill noted the presence of edema of the mucosa in 18 of 20 cases (4). The overlying mucosal denudation was attributed to the force of the mucosal edema, and the contribution of the plasma exudate to the excessive fluid in the

* Institute for Asthma and Allergy, Washington Hospital Center, Washington DC, USA.

bronchial lumen was discussed. The presence of large amounts of plasma proteins in the airway fluid has been confirmed many times (reviewed in 5), and was carefully documented in a recent study of broncho-lavage after allergen challenge (6). In the human nasal mucosa, a careful study of the dynamics of the formation of respiratory epithelial lining fluid was recently published (7) which documents that a mammoth movement of plasma-protein-rich fluid occurs within minutes of allergen exposure of allergic individuals. The microvascular permeability leading to the plasma exudate causes both mucosal edema and a marked increase in nasal secretions. There is speculation of the precise causes for the plasma protein exudation, but after allergen exposure mast cell mediators are the most likely cause (Table 1). However, mast cell mediator release also causes secondary reflexes, which might also participate in the microvascular per-

Table 1. Mediators thought to cause microvascular permeability in asthma.

Mast cell mediators:
    Histamine
    Bradykinin
    Leukotrienes
    Several prostaglandins
    Chymase
    Platelet-activating factor
    Reactive oxygen species
Neuropeptides:
    Substance P
    Neurokinin A
    Calcitonin gene-related peptide

meability. The capacity of histamine antagonists to effectively reduce the acute response to allergen suggests that histamine release is an important factor in nasal allergic reactions. There is, however, a contribution from reflex-stimulated submucosal glands, accounting for about 20% of the proteins secreted into nasal epithelial fluid.

In animal models, the process of microvascular permeability in the airways has been carefully studied and involves the following events: release of the vasoactive substance, development of intercellular openings between post-capillary venule endothelial cells, escape of plasma protein rich fluid into the tissues surrounding the venule, movement of water into the tissues and the formation of mucosal edema. In the conducting airways, the

responding post-capillary venules are part of an extensive plexus of sub-basement membrane vessels which probably act to warm and humidify inspired air. These vessels leak fluid into the area just deep to the basement membrane, which is precisely the area in which edema is found in asthmatic lungs. The edema may be cleared by two mechanisms: lymphatic clearance or epithelial secretion into the lumen. Lymphatic clearance undoubtedly contributes to the removal of the plasma exudation, but this process is slow and unproven. On the other hand, the process of paracellular transport of edema fluid between epithelial cells and into the bronchial or nasal lumen has been well documented. This process occurs within seconds of the formation of edema and may participate in the development of increased luminal fluid, which is a major factor in the airflow obstruction of asthma.

Thus, the evidence that airway edema plays an important role in asthma is based upon morphologic evidence of its presence, proof that plasma proteins are increased in luminal fluid, and an understanding of the processes involved in the dynamics of both microvascular permeability and the movement of the edema fluid into the lumen.

A protective role of this process in asthma has been suggested (8). The edema fluid that transverses the epithelium into the respiratory lining fluid would provide volume for increased mucociliary clearance, albumin to nonspecifically absorb proteins, IgG (and other plasma immunoglobulins) to interact with pathogens, inflammatory mediators (bradykinin, anaphylatoxins) to amplify the reaction, and enzyme inhibitors to limit the tissue destruction induced by pathogenic products. It seems more likely however that the process itself may be a useful primitive host defense mechanism. But in asthma, the edema and increased lining fluid are certain to be detrimental, contributing to airflow obstruction and the increased secretions thought to actually be responsible for death in many severe asthmatics. The admixture of plasma proteins with mucus and dead and dying cells must contribute to the increased viscosity of secretions.

Vasodilation

Inflammatory responses always initiate concomitant hyperemia due to vasodilation. This response can be seen in the skin or nasal mucosa after applying inflammatory mediators. Several mediators which cause increased blood flow also cause increased vascular permeability (PAF, bradykinin, leukotrienes, histamine), while other primarily increase blood flow (PGE, VIP, CGRP). Addition of agents which increase blood flow to those causing vascular permeability potentiates the permeability (reviewed in 9). However, increased vasodilation by itself does not lead to increased vascular permeability (10). Thus, increasing the blood flow through the mucosa does not by itself lead to plasma protein exudation, but in the presence of vasoactive amines, will potentiate the action of the amines.

Inflammation (Infiltration of Inflammatory Cells)

The association of asthma with airway inflammation has been recognized since the first recognition of eosinophils in the airways and sputum of asthmatics was noted. The classical descriptions of asthma pathology note the presence of eosinophils and neutrophils both in the lamina propria and airway lumen of asthmatics (11). However, the understanding of the potential contribution of inflammatory events in asthma took a giant leap forward with the use of bronchoalveolar lavage and bronchial biopsy of mild, ambulatory asthmatics.

The presence of eosinophils in the bronchial wall, in the absence of diseases associated with hypereosinophilia, is pathognomonic of asthma. Some reputable investigators now describe asthma as "chronic eosinophilic bronchitis" (12). Biopsies of mild asthmatics have confirmed the presence of eosinophils in the mucosa, often found beneath the basement membrane and in the epithelium (reviewed in 13). Not only are eosinophils present, but their granule derived proteins may be found in both the tissue and in BAL.

Another consistent finding is the presence of activated mucosal mast cells in the airways, along with an increased number of mast cells. The relationship between mast cell degranulation and severe asthma was noted many years ago (reviewed in 11). The finding of increased mast cell mediators in BAL confirms the presence of ongoing mast cell activation even in apparently healthy asthmatics (reviewed in 13).

Lymphocytes also appear to be increased in asthma, with increased numbers having been noted both in the epithelium and in the lamina propria (14). These lymphocytes have been noted to express the cell surface marker for IL-2, suggesting that they have been activated (15). It has been suggested that these activated lymphocytes might be producing cytokines of the Th2 subtype which might participate in the airway hyper-reactivity and cellular infiltration in asthma.

Other changes which have been noted by biopsy include a thickening of the basement membrane due to the deposition of collagen and fibronectin. Myofibroblasts along the basement membrane are increased in conjunction with this thickening and may be responsible (16). Mucous gland and goblet cell hyperplasia are also constant features.

Pain or Increased Irritability

The airways of asthmatics express increased irritability in response to diverse nonspecific stimuli. As the airways have few pain fibers, this increased reactivity is taken to be the equivalent of the pain noted with cutaneous inflammation. The underlying causes for bronchial hyperresponsiveness have not been identified with precision, although many contributing factors have been suggested (17, 18). While the underlying hyperresponsiveness seen in all asthmatic patients is unexplained, increases in hyperresponsiveness in relationship to allergen challenge, natural allergy exposure, late phase allergic reactions, viral infections, exposure to noxious fumes, inhalation of chemical sensitizers, and a variety of other stimuli have been documented. One of the features of these diverse provocations which all lead to airway reactivity is the development of cellular infiltrates. Precisely how mast cell activation, eosinophil infiltration, lymphocyte activation, and the other events which are associated with increased reactivity actually cause the change is not clear. One recent study in a monkey model of asthma suggested that mast cell activation and elaboration of tumor necrosis factor led to the generation of adhesion molecules which then facilitated eosinophil infiltration and the generation of increased airway reactivity. Pretreatment with antibodies directed at TNF prevented the response (19). Compelling arguments, however, can also be raised for the role of neutral endopeptidase, increased or decreased amounts of neuropeptides, and specific actions of mediators derived from mast cells, lymphocytes or eosinophils.

Conclusions

The cardinal features of inflammation are present in asthma, and are important in the disease. Cellular infiltration and activation participates in the airflow obstruction as well as increasing airway reactivity. Edema is a major contributor to airflow obstruction and leads to increased airway fluid, which is often the cause of death in acute asthma. Vasodilation is part of asthma, and has been suggested as an important part of exercise induced asthma. Therapy aimed at reducing inflammation in asthma will become increasingly important, not only to reduce airflow obstruction but also to reduce airway reactivity. Currently there is a great deal of attention being directed at reducing the cellular infiltration in asthma, particularly the eosinophilia. In the future, therapy aimed at reducing airway edema may also be available, and will likely produce important new therapeutic advantages.

Address for correspondence:

Michael A Kaliner
Medical Director
Institute for Asthma and Allergy
Washington Hospital Center
Washington DC 20010
USA

References

1. Tannenbaum S, Oertel H, Henderson W, Kaliner M. The biologic activity of mast cell granules. I. Elicitation of inflammatory responses in rat skin. *J Immunol* 1980; 125:325.

2. Lemanske RF, Kaliner M. Mast cell-dependent late phase reactions. *Clin Immunol Rev* 1982; 1:547.

3. Kaliner M, Eggleston P, Mathews K. Rhinitis and asthma. *JAMA* 1987; 258:2851.

4. Dunnill MS, The pathology of asthma, with special reference to changes in the bronchial mucosa. *J Clin Pathol* 1960; 13:27–33.

5. Perrson CGA. Plasma exudation and asthma. *Lung* 1988; 166:1.

6. Fick RB, Metzger WJ, Richerson HB, Zavala DC, Moseley PL, Schoderbek WE, Hunninghake GW. Increased bronchovascular permeability after allergen exposure in sensitive asthmatics. *J Clin Invest* 1987; 63:1147.

7. Raphael GD, Igarashi Y, White MV, Kaliner MA. The pathophysiology of rhinitis. V. Sources of protein in allergen-induced nasal secretions. *J Allergy Clin Immunol* 1991; 88:33.

8. Perrson CGA, Erejefalt I, Alkner U, Baumgarten C, Greiff L, Gustafsson B, Luts A, Pipkorn U, Sundler F, Svensson C, Wollmer P. Plasma exudation as a first line respiratory mucosal defense. *Clin Exp Allergy* 1991; 21:17.

9. Cheung KF, Rodgers DF, Barnes PJ, Evans TW. The role of increased airway microvascular permeability and plasma exudation in asthma. *Eur Respir J* 1990; 3:329.

10. Mullol J, Raphael GD, Lundgren JD, Baraniuk JN, Merida M, Shelhamer JH, and Kaliner MA. Comparison of human nasal mucosal secretion *in vivo* and *in vitro*. *J Allergy Clin Immunol* 1992; 89:584.

11. Kaliner MA, Blennerhassett J, Austen KF. Bronchial asthma. In Meischer PA, Muller-Eberhard HJ (Eds) *Textbook of Immunopathology*. New York: Grune & Stratton, 1976, pp. 387.

12. Frigas E, Gleich GJ. The eosinophil and the pathophysiology of asthma. *J Allergy Clin Immunol* 1986; 77:527.

13. Djukanovic R, Roche WR, Wilson JW, Beasley CRW, Twentyman OP, Howarth PH, Holgate ST. Mucosal inflammation in asthma. *Am Rev Resp Dis* 1990; 142:434.

14. Jeffery PK, Wardlaw AJ, Nelson FC, Collins JV, Kay AB. Bronchial biopsies in asthma. An ultrastructural, quantitative study and correlation with hyperreactivity. *Am Rev Resp Dis* 1989; 140:1745.

15. Azzawi M, Bradley B, Jeffery PK, Frew AJ, Wardlaw AJ, Knowles G, Assoufi B, Collins JV, Durham S, Kay AB. Identification of activated T lymphocytes and eosinophils in bronchial biopsies in stable atopic asthma. *Am Rev Resp Dis* 1990; 142:1407.

16. Brewster CEP, Howarth PH, Djukanovic R, Wilson J, Holgate ST, Roche WR. Myofibroblasts and subepithelial fibrosis in bronchial asthma. *Am J Respir Cell Mol Biol* 1990; 3:507.

17. Boushey HA, Holtzman MJ, Sheller JR, Nadel JA. Bronchial hyperreactivity. *Am Rev Resp Dis* 1980; 121:389.

18. Barnes PJ. New concepts in the pathogenesis of bronchial hyperresponsiveness and asthma. *J Allergy Clin Immunol* 1989; 83:1013.

19. Wegner CD, Gundel RH, Reilly P, Haynes N, Letts LG, Rothlein R. Intercellular adhesion molecule-1 (ICAM-1) in the pathogenesis of asthma. *Science* 1990; 247:456.

Eosinophil Granule Proteins and Cytokines as Monitors of Asthma

Sohei Makino*, Shinji Motojima*, Takeshi Fukuda*, Ikuo Akutsu*, Seihi Takatsu**

Keywords: Bronchial asthma, eosinophil granule proteins, sputum, serum IL-5

Bronchial asthma is a chronic inflammatory disease of the airway accompanied by infiltration of eosinophils, T cells, and mast cells. Toxic granule proteins from eosinophils are thought to cause the damage of the bronchial epithelium and induce airway hyperresponsiveness. *In vitro* monitoring of this airway inflammation is necessary to control asthma.

Eosinophil cationic protein (ECP) was increased in the sputum of asthma patients and its level correlated with the damage to the bronchial epithelium as assessed by fallen bronchial epithelial cells in the sputum. ECP was increased in the serum of asthma patients, and its level was higher in symptomatic asthma than in remission.

IL-5 and GM-CSF are released from CD4+ T cells and activate eosinophils for tissue damage and survival. Sputum from asthma patients had eosinophil survival enhancing activity, and the main factors found were GM-CSF and IL-5. In serum of asthma patients, the level of IL-5 was increased; it was higher in patients with moderate symptoms than in those with mild symptoms.

These observations suggest that measurement of eosinophil granule proteins and eosinophil stimulating cytokines in serum and sputum would be useful to monitor the inflammation of the airway in asthma.

bronchial epithelium, which is thought to induce airway hyperresponsiveness (3).

The most abundant inflammatory cells in the airway in asthma are lymphocytes, and CD4+ T cells were significantly higher in patients with symptomatic asthma than in nonsymptomatic asthma patients and nonasthmatic controls (5).

Th2 cells produce eosinophil growth-stimulating cytokines, including IL-5, IL-3 and GM-CSF (5, 6). These cytokines also activate eosinophils for tissue damage and production of lipid mediators. Among these cytokines, IL-5 is the most potent and specific for eosinophil activation. IL-5 enhances the release of granule proteins from eosinophils and prolongs their survival (7, 8). In the sensitized guinea pig model of asthma, treatment with anti-IL-5 antibody significantly suppressed the infiltration of eosinophils after the allergen inhalation (9).

Before eosinophils infiltrate into the bronchial mucosa, eosinophils in the peripheral blood have to adhere to the endothelial cells in the airway and transmigrate into the bronchial mucosa. Activation of eosinophils by cytokines, especially IL-5, and of adhesion molecule expression on epithelial cells, are critical for eosinophil migration (10, 11).

Mechanisms of Asthma, Roles of Eosinophils and T Cells (1)

Bronchial asthma is a chronic inflammatory disease of the airway accompanied by the infiltration of eosinophils, T cells and mast cells. An eosinophil has approximately 200 specific granules, which contain major basic protein (MBP), eosinophil cationic protein (ECP), and eosinophil peroxidase (EPO) (2). These granule proteins are highly basic and toxic to tissues. They cause damage to the

Monitoring Asthma

Asthma is characterized by reversible narrowing, hyper-responsiveness, and inflammation, and atopy of the airways. Environmental allergen exposure induces inflammation of the airway, which causes airway inflammation. A variety of stimuli can cause reversible airway narrowing.

In order to control asthma symptoms, it is essential to have information on the present caliber, re-

---

* Department of Medicine and Clinical Immunology, School of Medicine, Dokkyo University, Tochigi, Japan.
** Department of Immunology, Insitute of Medical Science, Tokyo University, Tokyo, Japan.

sponsiveness, and inflammation of the airways. The airway narrowing can be assessed by measurement of peak expiratory flow or $FEV_{1.0}$ (12). Airway responsiveness is measured by PC_{20} to inhaled acetylcholine, histamine, or methacholine, and is related to the severity of asthma (13) and eosinophil infiltration in the airway (14). An increase in diurnal variation is associated with an increase in airway responsiveness (12). These physiologic changes are thought to be induced by airway inflammation (1, 14).

Monitoring of Airway Inflammation

Monitoring of airway inflammation includes direct examination of biopsy specimens from the bronchial mucosa and epithelium, and indirect study by bronchoalveolar lavage fluid (BALF), sputum, and peripheral blood.

Biopsy of the Bronchial Mucosa

Histological examination of the bronchial biopsy can show: the number of infiltrating inflammatory cells, including eosinophils, T cells, and mast cells; damage of the bronchial epithelium; mRNA expression; the content of inflammatory cytokines (e. g., IL-5, GM-CSF) in infiltrating cells; and expression of adhesion molecules on the cells in the bronchial mucosa.

The number of eosinophils correlates with the degree of the damage to the bronchial epithelium, which also correlates with the airway responsiveness as expressed by the PC_{20} to inhaled acetylcholine (4, 14). The number of lymphocytes and their CD25/CD4+ subset in the bronchial mucosa is correlated with the number of eosinophils (4, 5). These lymphocytes are mostly CD4+ helper T cells. mRNA for IL-5 was observed in these cells (6, 15). These observations suggest that examination of eosinophils, T cells, and their subsets, and of mRNA expression for inflammatory cytokines, could indicate the degree of inflammation of the airway and the severity of asthma.

The adhesion molecule ICAM-1 is expressed on the walls of blood vessels and bronchial epithelial cells (16, 17), and VCAM-1 is expressed on the walls of the blood vessels (18). The expression of these adhesion molecules is enhanced in symptomatic asthmatic patients as compared to non-symptomatic asthma patient. It appears that the examination of the bronchial mucosa biopsy can give the most definite information about the inflammation of the airway and the usage of anti-inflammatory agents in asthma, although the precise indications for this examination have not yet established.

Bronchoalveolar Lavage Fluid (BALF)

It is thought that BALF can provide another direct indication of airway inflammation. Increases in eosinophils, eosinophil granule proteins, T cells, and mRNA for cytokines, including IL-4 and IL-5, and fallen epithelial cells are observed in antigen-induced late-phase asthmatic responses and in patients with symptomatic asthma as compared to patients in remission (16, 19, 20).

Among several sets of adhesion molecules on eosinophils and vascular endothelial cells, VLA-4 and VCAM-1 binding is specific to eosinophils rather than neutrophils. IL-4 is a specific stimulant to the expression of VCAM-1 in the endothelial cells (21). VLA-4 is expressed on eosinophils but not on neutrophils (22–24).

In order to investigate this further, Fukushima and Fukuda carried out BAL and bronchial biopsy on atopic asthma patients, and examined whether the BALF level of IL-4 could be used to predict eosinophil infiltration and VCAM-1 expression in the bronchial mucosa.

The BALF level of IL-4 was significantly higher in atopic asthma than in nonasthmatic controls or nonatopic asthma. Asthma patients whose BALF IL-4 level was raised tended to have increased expression of VCAM-1 in the bronchial mucosa, which showed a significant correlation with the degree of eosinophil infiltration (18). These observations suggest that IL-4 upregulates the eosinophil-specific adhesion molecule VCAM-1 on the vascular endothelium, and may be one of the major factors for eosinophils in the bronchial mucosa of atopic asthmatics. Supporting this possibility, antibody against VLA-4 suppressed antigen-induced eosinophil infiltration and the late asthmatic response in a sensitized guinea pig asthma model (25). These observations show that BALF can be a good monitor for airway inflammation, except for the difficulty of obtaining it in routine clinical practice.

306

Sputum

Sputum is thought to give information on the inflammation of the airway surface from which the sputum originated. Eosinophil granule proteins in sputum can be used to predict the number and activation of eosinophils inside the airway channels and the resultant damage of the bronchial epithelium. Ohashi and others measured the percentage degranulation of eosinophil specific granules by electron microscopy, and found that the concentration of ECP in the sputum of patients who were admitted because of asthma exacerbation showed a significant correlation with eosinophil degranulation (26).

The sputum level of ECP is increased in asthma as compared to COPD, pneumonia, respiratory infection, and other nonrespiratory diseases: the mean levels of sputum ECP were 1905 (n = 24), 832 (n = 29), 794 (n = 15), 339 (n = 10) and 526 ng/ml (n = 17), respectively (27).

Creola Body in Sputum: Bronchial epithelium that is shed during asthma attacks is called a Creola body. The number and size of the Creola bodies is inversely correlated with bronchial responsiveness to inhaled acetylcholine (28). Similarly, the number and size of the Creola bodies were higher in patients who showed a rise in airway responsiveness after antigen inhalation challenge compared to patients who did not (29). The amount of Creola bodies increased during severe asthmatic attacks which needed hospital admission. The ECP content was higher in sputum which had increased amounts of Creola bodies (30), suggesting that increased infiltration of eosinophils can produce more desquamation of the bronchial mucosa and enhances airway responsiveness.

These observations suggest that measurement of sputum ECP can give information on the destruction of the bronchial epithelium and on the activation of eosinophils in sputum. BALF from asthma patients has eosinophil survival enhancing activities (31).

In order to examine this activity in sputum of asthmatic patients, Adachi and Motojima examined the eosinophil viability enhancing activity of an extract of sputum from asthmatic patients by using guinea pig peritoneal eosinophils as an indicator. The sputum extract from asthmatic patients had more eosinophil viability enhancing activity than that from nonasthmatic controls. In asthmatic patients, sputum extract obtained during exacerbations had more eosinophil viability enhancing activity than that obtained during remission, suggesting that sputum contains factors for eosinophil survival. This eosinophil survival enhancing effect showed significant correlations to the sputum content of eosinophil cationic protein and to the asthma symptom score, suggesting that the eosinophil viability enhancing factor stimulates eosinophil migration into the airway and contributes to asthmatic symptoms. Anti-GM-CSF and anti-IL-5 antibodies significantly suppressed this activity (32).

BODY-KERN = These observations show that desquamated bronchial epithelium, eosinophil granule proteins, and eosinophil survival activity or the amount of GM-CSF and IL-5 in sputum can be used to monitor airway inflammation in asthma, though the sources of these cytokines remain to decided (33, 34).

Peripheral Blood

Serum Level of ECP: The number of eosinophils and their hypodense population in the peripheral blood is increased in asthma. Hypodense eosinophils show increased degranulation, which may elevate the serum level of eosinophil granule proteins (7).

These observations suggest that serum levels of eosinophil granule protein may be related to inflammation of the airway. To examine this possibility, Motojima and others measured the serum level of ECP and found that it was significantly higher in asthma patients than in patients with COPD and normal subjects. The serum level of ECP was higher during exacerbation of asthma as compared to during remission (27, 33). These findings suggest that the serum level of ECP can be used for diagnosis of asthma and to predict the inflammation of the airway.

Serum Level of Il-5: IL-5 is a selective eosinophil activating cytokine (10), and its serum level was found to be higher in diseases with eosinophilia. T cells in the airway in asthma showed increased expression of mRNA for eosinophil-poietic cytokines, including IL-5 (5, 6).

In order to examine this further, Akutsu and others measured the serum level of IL-5 in asthmatic patients and normal subjects using ELISA (26). The serum level of IL-5 is significantly higher in asthmatics than in nonasthmatic control subjects. The asthma was defined as mild, moderate, and severe. The serum level of IL-5 was higher in moderate asthma than in mild asthma, showing that activation of eosinophils induced by eosinophil-poietic cytokines contributes to worsening of asthma. In fact, it has been reported that only eosinophils stimulated by IL-5 can adhere to the vascular endothelium (10). Oral corticosteroid suppressed the serum level of IL-5 in asthma, with an increase in the PC_{20} to methacholine, and expression of IL-4 and IL-5 (36).

These observations in peripheral blood suggest that the serum level of ECP and IL-5 could be used as *in vitro* monitors of airway inflammation, though apparently the extent of their relationship to the airway inflammation must be examined before they are used in clinical practice.

Address for correspondence:

Sohei Makino, MD
Department of Medicine and Clinical Immunology
Dokkyo University School of Medicine
Mibu, Tochigi 321–02
Japan

References

1. Makino S, Fukuda T, Motojima S, Yukawa T. Eosinophils in asthma, part 2. In Makino S, Fukuda T (Eds) *Eosinophils, Biological and clinical aspects*. Boca Raton: CRC Press, 1992, pp. 329–346.

2. Ackerman SJ. Characterization and functions of eosinophil granule proteins. In Makino S, Fukuda T (Eds) *Eosinophils, Biological and clinical aspects*. Boca Raton: CRC Press, 1992, pp. 33–74.

3. Motojima S. Tissue damage due to eosinophils in allergic reactions and parasitic infection. In Makino S, Fukuda T (Eds) *Eosinophils, Biological and clinical aspects*. Boca Raton: CRC Press, 1992, pp. 75–94.

4. Ohashi Y, Motojima S, Fukuda T, Makino S. Airway hyperresponsiveness, increased intracellular spaces of bronchial epithelium, and increased infiltration of eosinophils and lymphocytes in bronchial mucosa in asthma. *Am Rev Respir Dis* 1992; 145:1469–1476.

5. Fukuda T, Ando N, Numao T, Akutsu I, Nakajima H, Makino S, Lymphocyte subsets in bronchial mucosa of symptomatic and asymptomatic asthmatics. *J Allergy Clin Immunol* 1991; 87 (Suppl):302.

6. Bentley AM, Meng Q, Robinson DS, Hamid Q, Kay AB, Durham SR, Increase in activated T lymphocytes, eosinophils, and cytokine mRNA expression for interleukin-5 and granulocyte/macrophage colony stimulating factor in bronchial biopsies after allergen inhalation challenge in atopic asthmatics. *Am J Respir Cell Mol Biol* 1993; 8:35–42.

7. Fukuda T, Makino S. Heterogeneity and activation. In Makino S, Fukuda T (Eds) *Eosinophils, Biological and clinical aspects*. Boca Raton: CRC Press, 1992, pp. 155–170.

8. Wardlaw AJ, Kay AB. Interrelationship between T lymphocytes and eosinophils. In Makino S, Fukuda T (Eds) *Eosinophils, Biological and clinical aspects*. Boca Raton: CRC Press, 1992, pp. 261–272.

9. Akutsu I, Fukuda T, Takatsu K, Makino S. Anti-IL-5 antibody inhibits antigen-induced bronchial eosinophilia, late asthmatic response and increase of non-specific bronchial responsiveness in a guinea pig model of asthma. *Respir Crit Care Med* 1994; 149:A530.

10. Resnick MB, Weller PF. Mechanisms of eosinophil recruitment. *Am J Respir Cell Mol Biol* 1993; 8:349–353.

11. Walsh GM, Hartnell A, Wardlaw AJ. IL-5 enhances the *in vitro* adhesion of human eosinophils, but not neutrophils, in an leukocyte integrin (CD11/18)-dependent manner. *Immunology* 1990; 71:258–265.

12. Ryan G, Latimer KM, Dolovich J, Hargreave FE. Bronchial responsiveness to histamine: Relationship to diurnal variation of peak flow rate, improvement after bronchodilator, and airway caliber. *Thorax* 1982; 37:423–429.

13. Makino S, Ikemori R, Fukuda T, Motojima S, Namai S, Toda M, Yamai T, Yamada G, Yukawa T. Clinical evaluation of standard method of acetylcholine inhalation test in bronchial asthma. *Jpn J Allergy* 1984; 33:167–175.

14. Laitinen LA, Laitinen A, Haahtela T. A comparative study of the effects of an inhaled corticosteroid, budosenide, and a beta2-agonist, terbutalien, on airway inflammation in newly diagnosed asthma: A randomized, double-blind, parallel-group controlled trial. *J Allergy Clin Immunol* 1992; 90:32–42.

15. Fukuda T. Eosinophil infiltration in the airway and cytokines. *Jpn J Allergy* 1992; 41:982.

16. Fukuda T, Ando N, Makino S. Expression of ICAM-1 in bronchial mucosa and its relation to symptoms in asthma. *Jpn J Allergy* 1990; 39:1257.

17. Wegner CD, Gundel RH, Reiley P, Haynes N, Letts LG, Rothlein R. Intercellular adhesion molecule-1(ICAM-1) in the pathogenesis of asthma. *Science* 1990; 247:456–459.

18. Fukushima T, Fukuda T, Makino S. IL-4, VACM-1 expression and eosinophil accumulation in airway of asthmatics. *Allergy Clin Immunol News* 1994; 6 (Suppl 2):33.

19. Robinson DS, Hamid Q, Bentley AM, Yin S, Kay AB, Durham SR. Activation of CD4[+] T cells, in-

creased Th2-type cytokine mRNA expression, and eosinophil recruitment in bronchoalveolar lavage after allergen inhalation challenge in patients with atopic asthma. *J Allergy Clin Immunol* 1993; 92:313–324.

20. Adelroth E, Rosentall L, Johansson S-A, Linden M, Venge P. Inflammatory cells and eosinophilic activity in asthmatics investigated by bronchoalveolar lavage. The effects of antiasthmatic treatment with budosemide or terbutarine. *Am Rev Respir Dis* 1990; 142:91–99.

21. Moser R, Fehr J, Bruijnzeel PLB. IL-4 controls the selective endothelium-driven transmigration of eosinophils from allergic individuals. *J Immunol* 1992; 149:1432–1438.

22. Walsh GM, Mermod JJ, Hartell A, Kay AB, Wardlaw. Human eosinophil, but not neutrophil, adherence to Il-1-stimulated huamn umbirical vascular endothelial cells is alpha1, beta1(very late antigen-4) dependent. *J Immunol* 1991; 146:3419–3423.

23. Bochner BS, Luscinska FW, Gimgorne MA. Adhesion of human basophils, eosinophils, and neutrophils to interleukin-1 activated human vascular endothelial cells: Contribution of endothelial cell adhesion molecules. *J Exp Med* 1991; 173:1553–1563.

24. Fukuda T. Bronchial asthma and adhesion molecules (endothelial cells and eosinophils). In *Asthma '93*. Tokyo: Mejikaru-revyuu, 1993, pp. 45–54 (in Japanese).

25. Sagara H, Ra C, Matsuda H, Yagita H, Okumura K, Fukuda T, Makino S. A monoclonal antibody against VLA-4 inhibits eosinophil accumulation and late asthmatic response in a guinea pig model of asthma. *J Allergy Clin Immunol* 1994; 93:269.

26. Ohashi Y, Motojima S, Kushima A, Tateishi K, Fukuda T, Makino S. Eosinophil activation in acute asthma attacks evaluated by electronmicroscopic findings of eosinophils and the concentration of eosinophil cationic protein in sputum. *Jpn J Allergy* 1991; 40:1265–1301.

27. Motojima S, Akutsu I, Fukuda T, Makino S. Clinical significance of measuring levels of sputum and serum ECP and serum IL-5 in bronchial asthma. *Allergy* 1993; 48:98–106.

28. Motojima S, Kushima A, Ogata H, Tateishi K, Fukuda T, Makino S. Relationship between presence of Creola body and airway hyperresponsiveness in patients with bronchial asthma. *Jpn J Allergy* 1990; 39:377–383.

29. Kushima A, Motojima S, Yamai T, Makino S. The participation of epithelial desquamation in the increase of bronchial hyperresponsiveness after antigen challenge in patients with bronchial asthma. *Jpn J Allergy* 1990; 39:1581–1589.

30. Ogata H, Motojima S, Fukuda T, Makino S. Creola body and the eosinophil cationic protein in sputum in acute asthmatic attacks with respect to their clinical significance. *Jpn J Allergy* 1990; 39:1567–1575.

31. Ohnishi T, Kita H, Weller D, Sur S, Sedgwick JB, Calhoun WJ, Busse WW, Abrams JS, Gleich GJ. IL-5 is the predominant eosinophil-active cytokine in the antigen-induced pulmonary late-phase reaction. *Am Rev Respir Dis* 1993; 147:901–907

32. Adachi T, Motojima S, Hirata A, Fukuda T, Makino S. Eosinophil viability enhancing activity in sputum from patients with brochial asthma. *Allergy Clin Immunol News* 1994; Suppl 2.

33. Broide DH, Paine MM, Firestein GS. Eosinophils express interleukin 5 and granulocyte macrophage-colony-stimulating factor mRNA at sites of allergic inflammation. *J Clin Invest* 1992; 90:1414–1424.

34. Bradding P, Roberts JA, Britten KM, Montefort S, Djukanovic R, Meuller R, Heusser CH, Howarth PH, Holgate ST. Interleukin-4, -5 and -6 and tumor necrosis factor-alpha in normal and asthmatic airways: Evidence for the human mast cell as a source of these cytokines. *Am J Respir Cell Mol Biol* 1994; 10:471–480.

35. Numao T, Fukuda T, Hirata A, Sagara H, Majima K, Nakajima H, Akutsu I, Ando N, Makino S. Eosinophil cationic protein in patients with bronchial asthma. *Jpn J Allergy* 1991; 40:93–99.

36. Robinson D, Hamid Q, Ying S, Bentley A, Assoufi B, Durham SR, Kay AB. Prednisolone treatment in asthma is associated with modulation of bronchoalveolar lavage cell interleukin-4, interleukin-5, and interferon-A cytokine gene expression. *Am Rev Respir Dis* 1993; 148:401–406.

Treatment of Atopic Diseases With Glucocorticoids, Cyclosporin A, and FK506: Anti-Inflammatory Effects and Inhibition of IL-5 Gene Transcription

Hirokazu Okudaira*,**, Akio Mori*, Matsunobu Suko*, Koji Ito*, Takafumi Etoh**, Hidemi Nakagawa**, Nobuo Tsuruoka***

Keywords: Interleukin-5, cyclosporin A, FK506, NF-AT, AP-1

IL-5 was produced spontaneously *in vitro* by peripheral blood mononuclear cells (PBMC) of mite-sensitive atopic patients and markedly boosted upon challenge with specific allergen, while PBMC of healthy controls produced essentially no IL-5. Stimuli delivered by the combination of phorbol ester (PMA) and Ca^{2+} ionophore (IOM) induced marked IL-5 production by PBMC obtained from atopic and nonatopic asthmatics, suggesting that both protein kinase C and Ca^{2+} influx are required for IL-5 production. CD2- or CD4-bearing cell depletion almost completely removed IL-5-producing cells, while CD8-bearing cell depletion enriched them. These findings indicate that $CD4^+$ T cells are the principal source of IL-5 in PBMC. The capacity of PBMC of atopic asthmatics, nonatopic asthmatics, and healthy controls to produce IL-2, IL-4, IL-5, and IFN-γ was compared, and showed that cytokine-producing capacities other than that of IL-5 (IL-2, IL-4, IFN-γ) are not significantly different among the three groups. Dexamethasone (Dex), FK506, and cyclosporin A (CsA) suppressed IL-5 production *in vitro* in a dose-dependent manner. Clear dose-dependent suppression of IL-5 gene expression by FK506 was also observed. The results suggested that both activating protein 1 (AP-1) and nuclear factor of activated T cells (NF-AT) are essential for IL-5 gene expression. Treatment of asthmatic patients with inhaled glucocorticoid (beclomethasone dipropionate) ameliorated clinical symptoms, improved lung function, and markedly suppressed IL-5 production by PBMC, suggesting an essential role of IL-5 in the pathogenesis of bronchial asthma. Atopic dermatitis was markedly ameliorated with CsA and FK506, which inhibit IL-5 gene expression.

Specific Allergen Extract Induced IL-5 Production by PBMC of Atopic Asthmatics but Not of Healthy Controls

Peripheral blood mononuclear cells (PBMC) from house dust mite-sensitive atopic asthmatics and normal healthy controls were incubated with *Dermatophagoides farinae* (D.f.) mite extract for 6 days and the resulting supernatants were assayed for IL-5.

IL-5 was clearly produced by PBMC of mite-sensitive atopic patients upon challenge with specific allergen, while PBMC of healthy controls produced essentially no IL-5.

Both PKC Activation and Ca^{2+} Influx Are Required for IL-5 Production

It is known that stimulation through T cell receptors activates protein kinase C (PKC) and increases the cytoplasmic concentration of Ca^{2+}. Protein kinase C is directly activated by phorbol ester (PMA), and cytoplasmic Ca^{2+} concentration can be increased by Ca^{2+} ionophore (IOM). In the present study, stimuli delivered by a combination of optimal concentrations of PMA and IOM were used to mimic antigenic stimuli (1). PBMC of atopic and nonatopic asthmatics clearly produced IL-5 in response to

---

*   Department of Medicine and Physical Therapy, University of Tokyo, Japan.
**   Department of Dermatology, University of Tokyo, Japan.
*** Suntory Institute for Biomedical Research, Mishima, Osaka, Japan.

PMA and IOM. Significant IL-5 production by PBMC of atopic asthmatics was observed even without stimulation and was markedly boosted when both PMA and IOM were included in the culture. This result suggests that both PKC activation and Ca^{2+} influx are required for peripheral T cells to produce IL-5 maximally.

CD4^{+} T Cells in PBMC Produce IL-5

IL-5 has been reported to be produced not only by T cells, but also by mast cells, eosinophils, and other cells (2, 3). However, in the present study, CD2 or CD4 depletion almost completely abrogated IL-5 production, and CD8 depletion rather

enhanced it. IL-5 mRNA was detected in only the CD4^{+} population upon stimulation. These findings are in agreement with the report by Sewell et al. (4), and clearly indicate that CD4^{+} T cells are the principal source of IL-5 in PBMC.

Cytokine Production by PBMC from Atopic Asthmatics, Nonatopic Asthmatics, and Healthy Controls

PBMC obtained from asthmatics and control subjects were stimulated with PMA and IOM. After 24 h, supernatants were collected and assayed for IL-2, IL-4, IL-5, and IFN-γ. Results are shown in

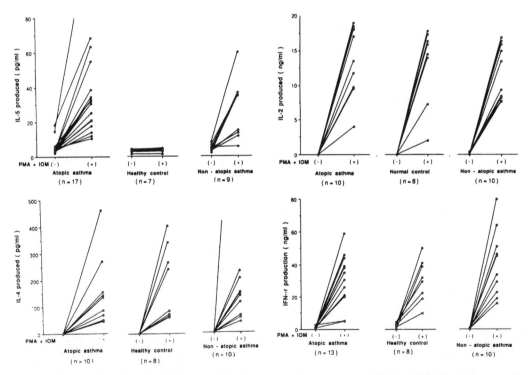

Figure 1. Comparison of IL-2, IL-4, IL-5, and IFN-γ production by PBMC obtained from atopic asthmatics, nonatopic asthmatics, and healthy controls. PBMC (2×10^{6}/ml) were stimulated with PMA (20 nM) and IOM (1 μM) for 24 h. Supernatants were assayed for IL-2, IL-4, IL-5, and IFN-γ by specific ELISA. The numbers of donors included in each study are shown in parentheses. IL-5 production was 37.6 ± 7.1, 3.6 ± 0.4, and 25.7 ± 5.5 pg/ml in atopic asthmatics, healthy controls, and nonatopic asthmatics, respectively. IL-2 production upon stimulation was 139.2 ± 16.0, 123.4 ±13.0, and 137.3 ± 18.1 ng/ml. IL-4 production upon stimulation was 146.0 41.2, 190.8 48.6, and 266.5 ± 117.2 pg/ml. IFN-γ production upon stimulation was 29.9 ± 4.4, 27.4 ± 2.0, and 28.7 ± 6.2 ng/ml. IL-5 production in atopic and nonatopic asthmatics was significantly greater than that in healthy controls (p < 0.05). No significant difference was observed among the three groups in the amounts of IL-2, IL-4, and IFN-γ produced.

Figure 1. No significant difference was observed among the three groups in the amounts of IL-2, IL-4, and IFN-γ produced. In contrast, significant IL-5 production was observed in atopic asthmatics and nonatopic asthmatics, but not in healthy controls. IL-5 production was 37.6 ± 7.1 pg/ml in atopic asthmatics, 25.7 ± 5.5 pg/ml in nonatopic asthmatics, and 3.6 ± 0.4 pg/ml in healthy controls. IL-5 production in atopic and nonatopic asthmatics was significantly greater than that in healthy controls (p < 0.05). This result indicates that T cells that produce IL-5 upon PMA and IOM stimulation exist in the peripheral blood of atopic and non-atopic asthmatics but not in that of healthy controls. The fact that the majority of PBMC of nonatopic asthmatics responded clearly to the stimuli of PMA and IOM to produce IL-5 suggests that so-called nonatopic asthmatics are actually hypersensitive at the level of T cells. Our recent study indicates that enhanced IL-5 production in asthmatics is the consequence of enhanced IL-5 gene transcription.

IL-5 Production Is Suppressed by FK506, CsA, and Dexamethasone

The above findings suggested an important role of IL-5 in the pathogenesis of atopic and nonatopic asthma and prompted us to investigate agents that can suppress IL-5 production. Glucocorticoids (GC) have been the most effective treatment for chronic asthma for a long time (5). Administration of GC in vivo suppresses eosinophilic inflammation and improves the symptoms of asthma. FK506 and cyclosporin A (CsA) are potent immunosuppressants used in organ transplantation (6). Their immunosuppressive action is suggested to be mediated by suppression of cytokine genes, including those for IL-2, IL-3, IL-4, IL-6, and GM-CSF (7). It is thus worthwhile to test their effects on IL-5, which may play an essential role in allergic inflammation.

Varying doses of FK506, CsA, and dexamethasone (Dex) were added simultaneously with PMA and IOM. All three agents inhibited IL-5 synthesis by PBMC obtained from atopic asthmatics. The viability of cells was not affected by any agents at the concentrations used.

As shown in Figure 2, FK506 clearly downregu-

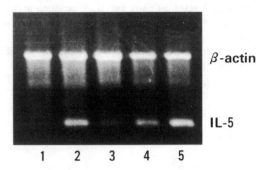

β-actin

IL-5

1   2   3   4   5

1. **no stimulation**
2. **PMA+IOM**
3. **PMA+IOM+FK506 1 μM**
4. **PMA+IOM+FK506 100nM**
5. **PMA+IOM+FK506 10nM**

Figure 2. FK506 suppressed IL-5 mRNA expression in activated PBMC. PBMC (2×10^6/ml) obtained from an atopic asthmatic patient were stimulated with PMA (20 nM) and IOM (1 μM) for 8 h. Cytoplasmic RNA was extracted, reverse transcribed, and amplified by PCR using IL-5 and β-actin primer sets.

lated IL-5 mRNA expressed in PBMC in a dose-dependent manner. β-Actin gene expression was not affected by FK506, thereby excluding the possibility of toxic effects of FK506 on the cells.

Possible Participation of NF-AT and AP-1 in IL-5 Gene Transcription

FK506 and CsA exert immunosuppressive effects through binding to their respective cellular ligands, FK-binding protein (FKBP) and cyclophilin (7). FK506-FKBP complex and CsA-cyclophilin complex inhibit the Ca^{2+}-calmodulin-dependent phosphatase, calcineurin, which is essential for a T cell-specific transcription factor, nuclear factor of activated T cells (NF-AT). This factor undergoes translocation into the nucleus for the initiation of IL-5 gene transcription (8). On the other hand, glucocorticoid and its receptor form a complex which competitively inhibits the activity of another transcription factor, activating protein-1 (AP-1), to bind to the enhancer element of cytokine genes (9,

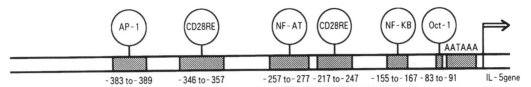

Figure 3. Presumed presence of transcription factor binding sites in human IL-5 promotor region.

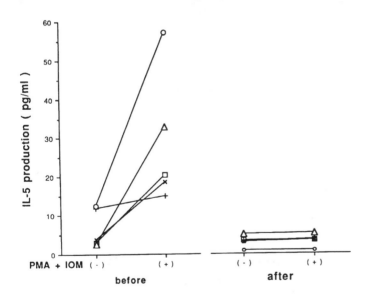

Figure 4. Treatment of atopic dermtitis with 1% FK506 ointment. Below: IL-5 production by atopic PBMC was suppressed by FK506 ointment.

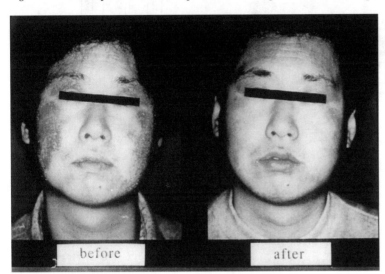

10). Both AP-1 and NF-AT are essential for IL-5 gene transcription (9). Although transcription factors and their binding elements for IL-5 await further elucidation in the future, we analyzed an approximately 500 bp segment upstream of the IL-5 transcription initiation site report by Tanabe et al. (11) using a computer system, GENETYX-CD (Ver. 16.0) (Software Development Co., Ltd.,

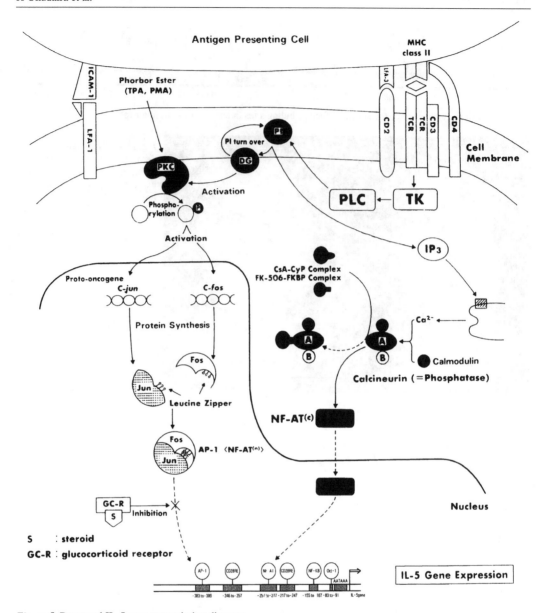

Figure 5. Presumed IL-5 gene transcription diagram.

Tokyo, Japan). We found possible AP-1 and NF-AT binding sites in the IL-5 promotor region, having more than 80% homology to the AP-1 and NF-AT binding sites identified in the IL-2 gene (12) (Figure 3). The effects of FK506, CsA, and Dex on IL-5 production suggest that the transcription factors NF-AT and AP-1 are both essential for the gene expression of IL-5 as well as IL-5.

Inhaled Corticosteroid Suppresses IL-5 Production by PBMC

Beclomethasone dipropionate (BDI) was administered with a metered dose inhaler to symptomatic asthmatic patients who had been treated with theo-

314

phylline and a β_2-stimulant. Marked improvement in both subjective symptoms and objective lung function tests was achieved in 2 weeks. PBMC obtained from the patients before and 2 weeks after the initiation of BDI were stimulated with PMA and IOM for 24 h. Supernatants were assayed for IL-2, IL-4, and IL-5. IL-2 and IL-4 production decreased about 50%, while IL-5 production decreased more than 90% after treatment. It is of great interest to find preferential suppression of IL-5 compared to other cytokines such as IL-2 and IL-4.

Treatment of Atopic Dermatitis with Agents that Inhibit IL-5 Gene Transcription

Accumulating evidence suggests that eosinophilic inflammation plays an important role in atopic dermatitis (13–15). If T cell-derived IL-5 is essential for the induction of eosinophilic inflammation, it is reasonable to use the agents which inhibit IL-5 gene transcription to treat atopic dermatitis. Clinical trials are in progress, and Figure 4 shows the preliminary data suggesting that the hypothesis is of value. Figure 4 shows that IL-5 production by PBMC is enhanced in atopic dermatitis patients and that the IL-5 production is downregulated after treatment with FK506 ointment.

Presumed processes from antigen presentation to IL-5 gene transcription are illustrated diagrammatically in Figure 5.

Address for correspondence:

Dr Hirokazu Okudaira
Department of Medicine and
Physical Therapy
Universitiy of Tokyo
7-3-1. Hongo, Bankyo-ku
Tokyo 113
Japan

References

1. Altman A, Mustelin T, Coggeshall KM. T lymphocyte activation: A biological model of signal transduction. *CRC Crit Rev Immunol* 1990; 10:347–391.

2. Plaut M, Pierce JH, Watson CJ, Hanley-Hyde J, Nordan RP, Paul WE. Mast cell lines produce lym-

phokines in response to cross-linkage of Fce RI or to calcium ionophores. *Nature* 1989; 339:64–67.

3. Broide DH, Paine MM, Firestein GS. Eosinophils express interleukin-5 and granulocyte macrophage-colony-stimulating factor mRNA at sites of allergic inflammation in asthmatics. *J Clin Invest* 1992; 90:1414–1424.

4. Sewell WA, Valentine JE, Cooley MA. Expression of interleukin-5 by the CD4+CD45R0+ subset of human T cells. *Growth Factors* 1992; 6:295–302.

5. Schleimer PR. Effects of glucocorticoids on inflammatory cells relevant to their therapeutic applications in asthma. *Am Rev Respir Dis* 1990; 141:S59–S60.

6. Schreiber SL, Crabtree GR. The mechanism of action of cyclosporin A and FK506. *Immunol Today* 1992; 13:136–142.

7. Sigal NH, Dumont FJ. Cyclosporin A, FK506 and rapamysin: Pharmacologic probes of lymphocyte signal transduction. *Annu Rev Immunol* 1992; 10:519–560.

8. Limaye AP, Abrams JS, Silver JE, Ottesen EA, Nutman TB. Regulation of parasite-induced eosinophilia: Selectively increased interleukin-5 production in helminth-infected patients. *J Exp Med* 1990; 172:399–402.

9. Vacca A, Felli MP, Farina AR, Martinotti S, Maroder M, Screpanti I, Meco D, Petrangeli E, Frati L, Gulino A. Glucocorticoid receptor-mediated suppression of the interleukin 2 gene expression through impairment of the cooperativity between nuclear factor of activated T cells and AP-1 enhancer elements. *J Exp Med* 1992; 175:637–646.

10. Weinberger C, Hollenberg SM, Ong ES, Harmon JM, Brower ST, Cidlowski J, Thompson EB, Rosenfeld NG, Evans RH. Identification of human glucocorticoid receptor complementary DNA clones by epitope selection. *Science* 1985; 228:740–742.

11. Tanabe T, Konishi M, Mizuta T, Noma T, Honjo T. Molecular cloning and structure of the human interleukin-5 gene. *J Biol Chem* 1987; 262:16580–16584.

12. Shaw JP, Utz PJ, Durand DB, Toole JJ, Emmel EA, Crabtree GR. Identification of a putative regulator of early T cell activation genes. *Science* 1988; 241:202–205.

13. Leiferman KM, Ackerman SJ, Sampson HA, et al. Dermal deposition of eosinophil-granule major basic protein in atopic dermatitis. Comparison with onchocerciasis. *N Engl J Med* 1985; 313:282–285.

14. Bruijnzeel PL, Bruijnzeel-Kooman CA. Skin eosinophilia in atopic dermatitis. *Allerg Immunol (Paris)* 1989; 21:224–227.

15. Paganelli R, Fanales-Belasio E, Carmini D, Scala E, Meglio P, Businco L, Aiuti F. Serum eosinophil cationic protein in patients with atopic dermatitis. *Int Arch Allergy Appl Immunol* 1991; 96:175–178.

Sensitization to Various Mite Species

Enrique Fernández-Caldas*, Leonardo Puerta**

Keywords: Mites, allergens, sensitization, asthma

The mites of the family Pyroglyphidae, *Dermatophagoides pteronyssinus* and *Dermatophagoides farinae*, are the main sources of house dust allergens and an important etiological factor in allergic respiratory diseases. Storage mites can also cause and exacerbate allergic respiratory diseases in exposed and sensitized individuals. A workshop on mite allergy and asthma applied the term "domestic mites" to the storage and house dust mite species that are found in house dust. The most common non-pyroglyphid domestic mites belong to the families Glycyphagidae (genera: *Blomia*, *Lepidoglyphus* and *Glycyphagus*), Acaridae (genera: *Tyrophagus*, *Acarus*, *Suidasia*, *Aleuroglyphus*), and Chortoglyphidae (genus: *Chortoglyphus*). There is an increasing interest in the allergenicity of these mites, since they have been found in house dust samples throughout the world and there is evidence that sensitization to their allergens is not limited to individuals with occupational exposure. Some investigators have found little or no cross-reactivity between *Dermatophagoides* spp. and storage mites, suggesting that this lack of cross-reactivity may imply important clinical consequences for individuals sensitized to their allergens. There is a high prevalence of sensitization to several nonpyroglyphid mites in subtropical and tropical regions. *Blomia tropicalis* is highly predominant in house dust and an important source of allergens.

Introduction

The mites of the family Pyroglyphidae, *Dermatophagoides pteronyssinus* and *D. farinae*, are the main sources of house dust allergens and an important etiological factor in allergic respiratory diseases (1, 2). The allergenicity of other species, such as *Blomia tropicalis*, *Tyrophagus putrescentiae*, *Aleuroglyphus ovatus*, *L. destructor*, *Acarus siro*, *Tyrophagus putrescentiae*, *Glycyphagus domesticus*, and *Chortoglyphus arcuatus*, previously known as storage mites, has also been demonstrat-

ed (3–8). These mites are commonly found in farming environments and in house dust in tropical and subtropical regions of the world. A workshop on mite allergy and asthma applied the term "domestic mites" to the storage and house dust mite species that are found in house dust (9).

It has been suggested that house dust mite allergy is involved in the increasing prevalence of allergic diseases (10–12). In recent years, significant advances have been made in the understanding of mite allergy and in the distribution of indoor allergens, including those from mite origin. While the allergenicity of the *Dermatophagoides* spp. has been extensively studied, extracts of *B. tropicalis* and other mite species only recently became available for research. This has allowed the study of the allergenic role of these species in urban and rural populations from different regions.

Mite Fauna in Tropical Environments

The pyroglyphid mites *D. pteronyssinus*, *D. farinae*, and *Euroglyphus maynei* and the glycyphagid mite, *B. tropicalis*, are the predominant mite species in the United States (13). Other species are also commonly described in house dust in regions with a temperate climates, but their total numbers tend to be small.

Studies conducted in tropical and subtropical regions have demonstrated that the composition of the house dust mite fauna is different from that in the United States and Europe. Studies in Brazil, Colombia, Costa Rica, Guatemala, and Venezuela have demonstrated that *B. tropicalis* is abundant and it has been detected in 16% to 96% of house dust samples in these regions (14–18). *B. tropicalis* and *D. pteronyssinus* are the most common mite

* University of South Florida College of Medicine, James A. Haley Veterans Hospital, Tampa, FL, USA.
** University of Cartagena College of Medicine, Cartagena, Colombia.

species in Cartagena, Colombia (16). In Barbados, *Blomia* spp. was the second most common mite in house dust along with *D. pteronyssinus* and *Cheyletus* spp. (19). The most important mite species in Mauritius, an island located in the tropical zone of the western Indian Ocean, seem to be *C. arcuatus, D. pteronyssinus, B. tropicalis, Tropilichus aframericanus, Hirstia domicola,* and *Euroglyphus maynei* (20). In São Paulo, Brazil, *B. tropicalis* is the most prevalent mite in house dust along with *D. pteronyssinus* (15). *B. tropicalis* has been described as the most numerous nonpyroglyphid house dust mite in Caracas, Venezuela and in Hong Kong, with occurrences of 96% and 75%, respectively (7, 14). In the United States, *B. tropicalis* has been found in subtropical cities such as New Orleans, (Louisiana), in Tampa and Delray Beach (Florida) and in San Diego (California) (13, 21). A scanning electron microscopy picture of *Blomia tropicalis* is shown in Figure 1.

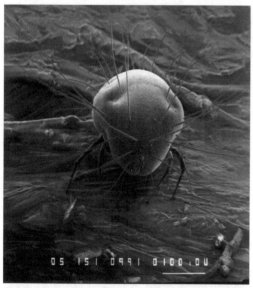

Figure 1. Rear view of *Blomia tropicalis* 150×. The small horizontal bar on the bottom represents 100 μm.

Cross-Reactivity Between Pyroglyphid and Non-pyroglyphid Mites

Miyamoto et al. suggested, by *in vitro* neutralization of skin sensitizing antibodies, that house dust and storage mites have common and species-spe-

cific antigens (8). It has been reported that *D. pteronyssinus* and *D. farinae* have two and four common antigens with *B. tropicalis*, respectively (22). In another study, Griffin et al. concluded that there is limited cross-reactivity among *Acarus siro, G. destructor,* and *D. pteronyssinus* and that these mites have common and species-specific allergenic determinants (23).

Minimal or no cross-reactivity between *Dermatophagoides* spp. and storage mites has been reported (5, 22–25). The major allergens from *Dermatophagoides* spp., Group I and Group II, are not present in *B. tropicalis* extracts (26). Nasal challenges with *B. tropicalis* extracts were performed in 12 subjects (4+ skin test positive to *B. tropicalis* and *Dermatophagoides* spp.) and 7 controls (skin test negative to *B. tropicalis* but positive to *Dermatophagoides* spp.) in Tampa, Florida. Ten of the 12 study subjects (83%) and none of the controls had a positive nasal challenge with *B. tropicalis* (p = 0.0024). A significant difference in inspiratory nasal airway resistance between both groups was achieved at a 1:1000 dilution (27). These results suggest that sensitization to *B. tropicalis* is species specific and should be considered of clinical significance in areas where this mite is endemic.

Bronchial provocation studies in farmers with positive RASTs to the storage mite *L. destructor* have also shown positive results (28). Since the cross-reactivity between *B. tropicalis* and *L. destructor* is high (5), sensitization to *L. destructor* in regions where this mite is not common could be due to cross-reactivity with *B. tropicalis* and vice versa (5, 16). However, the degree of specific IgE response to mite allergens also depends on the magnitude of exposure to a specific mite species present in the environment (29).

A high degree of cross-reactivity exists between *C. arcuatus* and *A. ovatus*. This could explain the high prevalence of sensitization to *C. arcuatus* and *A. ovatus* in regions where the latter mite is not common (16, 25).

The clinical significance of sensitization to cross-reacting allergens remains to be delineated.

Sensitization to Various Mite Species in Tropical Areas

Allergic asthma is common in tropical environments (30) and sensitization to multiple mite species is highly prevalent in these regions. Since pyroglyphid and nonpyroglyphid mites have minimal cross-reactivity, sensitization to nonpyroglyphid mites may be of clinical significance where these mites are abundant. Sensitization to *D. pteronyssinus*, *D. farinae*, *L. destructor*, *C. arcuatus*, *A. ovatus,* and *B. tropicalis* has been demonstrated by skin test and RAST in subjects with asthma and/or allergic rhinitis in Cartagena, Colombia (31, 32). The climatic conditions in this region offer a good environment for the growth of different mite species. The high prevalence of positive RASTs to various mites may be the result of the presence of multiple mite species in house dust. *B. tropicalis* is the most frequent sensitizer of asthmatic children in São Paulo, Brazil, and high levels of specific IgE to *B. tropicalis* have been detected in 20 mite allergic, asthmatic children in this city (26, 33).

Other investigators have described a high frequency of sensitizations to the storage mites *L. destructor*, *Tyrophagus putrescentiae*, *Acarus siro*, and *Gohieria fusca* in other areas of the world among *D. pteronyssinus*-sensitized subjects (34–36). These studies demonstrate that sensitization to storage mites is more common than expected and not only restricted to occupationally exposed individuals.

A study of 100 individuals with asthma and/or allergic rhinitis living in the subtropical Tampa Bay area of Florida revealed a prevalence of sensitization to the nonpyroglyphid mites *Acarus siro*, *A. ovatus*, *B. tropicalis*, *C. arcuatus*, *Glycyphagus domesticus*, *L. destructor,* and *T. putrescentiae* of between 32% and 69%; the prevalences of sensitization to *D. pteronyssinus* and *E. maynei* in this same population were 66% and 73%, respectively (37). Different IgE binding patterns were observed (Figure 2). Similar results have been observed elsewhere (31). While some patients respond primarily to the pyroglyphid mites (Figure 2 b), others respond to the majority of mite species in variable degree (Figure 2 a, c).

Iversen et al. reported a 27.5% prevalence of positive RASTs to storage mites in 326 asthmatic individuals with house dust mite allergy (38). In London, Luczynska et al. studied 196 individuals from an urban environment who were not occupationally exposed to storage mites. The authors found a 24% prevalence of elevated specific IgE to *D. pteronyssinus* and a 14% prevalence of positive RASTs to at least one of the storage mites tested (*Acarus siro*, *L. destructor* and *Tyrophagus longior*) (3).

The synergistic or additive effect of multiple

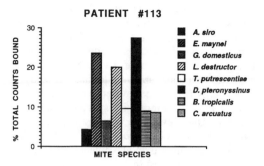

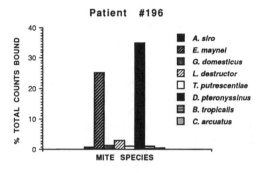

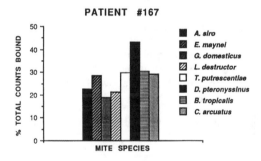

Figure 2. Different IgE binding patterns in three sera of asthmatic individuals from the Tampa Bay area of Florida.

mite sensitivities remains to be established. However, in a study on the clinical significance of the allergenic cross-reactivity of *E. maynei* and other nonpyroglyphid and pyroglyphid mite species, farmers with asthma alone or in combination with rhinitis were more frequently sensitized to storage mites and house dust mites than farmers with rhinitis alone (39). Sensitization to multiple domestic mites seems to be more common in allergic subjects with asthma than in patients with allergic rhinitis alone (6).

The prevalence of positive prick skin tests to the mite species *D. pteronyssinus, D. farinae, B. tropicalis, C. arcuatus, L. destructor* and *A. ovatus* was determined in 297 asthmatic adults and children living in seven cities of five Latin American countries in a collaborative international study on mite allergy (32). The prevalence of positive skin tests to the 6 different mite species is shown in Table 1. The prevalence of sensitization to the pyroglyphid mites *D. pteronyssinus* and *D. farinae* found in this study is in agreement with previous reports, which suggest that the prevalence of positive skin tests to pyroglyphid mite allergens among asthmatic individuals is in the range of 40–80% (2). The overall prevalence of sensitization to the four nonpyroglyphid mites (*A. ovatus, B. tropicalis, C. arcuatus,* and *L. destructor*) was lower in Bogotá and Mexico City than in the other geographical areas. These two cities accounted for the lowest rates of sensitization to these species (Bogotá for *A. ovatus* and México City for *B. tropicalis, C. arcuatus,* and *L. destructor*). These results are consistent with the fact that storage mites need higher humidity for survival than the *Dermatophagoides* spp. The highest degrees of sensitization were obtained in São Paulo and Caracas, both tropical cities.

There is evidence that sensitization to mite allergens may be less frequent in high altitude than in coastal environments in Europe (40, 41). Studies in patients living in high altitude areas in France have shown that in altitudes above 1000 and 1365 meters, mite growth and allergic sensitization to mite allergens is decreased (41, 42). However, the results of studies in Latin America in countries situated at a high elevation demonstrate that sensitization to mite allergens in asthmatic individuals, especially to *D. pteronyssinus* and *D. farinae*, is frequent in high altitude areas such as Bogotá and Mexico City; this two cities are situated over 2000 meters above the sea level. Studies in Colombia had previously demonstrated the presence of house dust mites in dust samples collected in dwellings of allergic individuals at high altitudes (43). Similar results have been obtained in Peru, where *D. pteronyssinus* was identified in dust samples collected at 3000 meters above the sea level (44).

Studies conducted in tropical and subtropical regions suggest that *D. pteronyssinus, B. tropicalis,* and *C. arcuatus* may be considered mites of clinical importance, due to the common occurrence of these species in house dust and the high prevalence of cutaneous and *in vitro* sensitivities. Extracts of these mites are warranted for a more accurate diagnosis and treatment of allergic respiratory diseases in these areas. *B. tropicalis* is a highly predominant mite species and an important source of mite allergens in tropical regions.

Acknowledgments

Leonardo Puerta is the recipient of an International Travel Grant from Colciencias.

Table 1. Positive skin tests (wheal ≥ 3 mm) to six mite species in 297 asthmatic patients.

Country	Ao	Bt	Ca	Df	Dp	Ld
Argentina						
Córdoba	43.3	58.3	55.0	53.3+	63.3	45.0
Santa Fe	39.4	57.5	42.4	66.6	72.7	40.7**
Brazil						
São Paulo	71.2*	93.7*	75.0	88.7	91.2*	76.2
Colombia						
Cartagena	57.1	71.4	64.3	75.0	60.7+	60.7
Bogotá	26.6+	56.6	36.6	66.6	70.0	40.0
Mexico						
Mexico City	40.0	46.6+	33.3+	73.3	73.3	30+
Venezuela						
Caracas	53.0	77.8	61.7	97.2*	75.5	64.7

* = highest prevalence; + = lowest prevalence; ** = 40.7% had a positive RAST

Address for correspondence:

Enrique Fernández-Caldas, Ph D
Division of Allergy and Immunology
C/o VA Hospital (VAR III D)
13,000 Bruce B. Downs Blvd.
Tampa, Florida 33612
USA

References

1. Voorhorst M, Spieksma FTH, Varekamp H. *House-dust atopy and the house-dust mite Dermatophagoides pteronyssinus.* Leiden: Staflus Scientific Publishing Company, 1969.

2. Platts-Mills TAE, Chapman MD. Dust mites: Immunology, allergic disease and environmental control. *J Allergy Clin Immunol* 1987; 80:755–765.

3. Luczynska CM, Griffin P, Davies RJ, Topping MD. Prevalence of specific IgE to storage mites (*A. siro, L. destructor* and *T. longior*) in an urban population and cross-reactivity with the house dust mite (*D. pteronyssinus*). *Clin Exp Allergy* 1990; 20:403–406.

4. Iversen M, Korsgaard J, Hallas T, Dahl R. Mite allergy and exposure to storage mites and house dust mites in farmers. *Clin Exp Allergy* 1990; 20:211–219.

5. Puerta L, Fernández-Caldas E, Caraballo LR, Lockey RF. Sensitization to *Blomia tropicalis* and *Lepidoglyphus destructor* in *Dermatophagoides* spp. allergic individuals. *J Allergy Clin Immunol* 1991; 88:943–950.

6. Silton RP, Fernández-Caldas, Trudeau WL, Lockey RF. Allergenicity of the mite *Aleuroglyphus ovatus*. *J Allergy Clin Immunol* 1991; 88:595–603.

7. Gabriel M, Cunnington AM, Allan WGL, Pickering CAC, Wraith DG. Mite allergy in Hong Kong. *Clin Allergy* 1982; 12:157–171.

8. Miyamoto T, Oshima S, Mizuno K, Sasa M, Ishizaki T. Cross-antigenicity among six species of dust mites and house dust antigens. *J Allergy* 1969; 44:228–238.

9. Dust mite allergens and asthma: Report of a second international workshop. *J Allergy Clin Immunol* 1992; 89(5):1046–1060.

10. Platts-Mills TAE, de Weck AL. Dust mite allergens and asthma-A world wide problem. *J Allergy Clin Immunol* 1989; 83:416–427.

11. Sears MR, Herbison GP, Holdaway MD, Hewitt D, Flannery EM, Silva PA. The relative risk of sensitivity to grass pollen, house dust mite and cat dander in the development of childhood asthma. *Clin Exp Allergy* 1989; 19:419–424.

12. Dowse GK, Turner KJ, Stewart GA, Alpers MP,

Woolcock AJ. The association between *Dermatophagoides* mites and the increasing prevalence of asthma in village communities within Papua New Guinea Highlands. *J Allergy Clin Immunol* 1985; 75:75–83.

13. Arlian L, Bernstein D, Bernstein IL, Friedman S, Grant A, Lieberman P, López M, Metzger J, Platts-Mills TAE, Schatz M, Spector S, Wasserman SI, Zeiger RS. Prevalence of dust mites in the homes of people with asthma living in eight different geographic areas of the United States. *J Allergy Clin Immunol* 1992; 90:292–300.

14. Hurtado I, Parini M. House dust mite in Caracas, Venezuela. *Ann Allergy* 1987; 59:128–130.

15. Neto J, Crocce J, Baggio D. Acaros da poeira domiciliar da cidae de São Paulo. Nota previa. *Rev Bras Alerg Imunopatol* 1980; 2:140–145.

16. Fernández-Caldas E, Puerta L, Mercado D, Lockey RF, Caraballo LR. Mite fauna, *Der p* I, *Der f* I and *Blomia tropicalis* allergen levels in a tropical environment. *Clin Exp Allergy* 1993; 23:292–297.

17 Vargas M V, Mairena H A. House dust mites from the metropolitan area of San José, Costa Rica. *Int J Acarol* 1991; 17(2):141–144.

18. García-Ibañez R, Fernández-Caldas E, García-Ramos E, Arango L, Lockey RF. Aeroallergen sensitivity in high altitude Guatemala City (abstract). *J Allergy Clin Immunol* 1991; 87(1):293.

19. Pearson RS, Cunnington AM. The importance of mites in house dust sensitivity in Barbadian asthmatics. *Clin Allergy* 1973; 3:299–306.

20. Guerin B, Levy DA, Lemao, Leynadier F, Baligadoo G, Fain A, Dry J. The house dust mite *Dermatophagoides pteronyssinus* is the most important allergen on the island of Maruritius. *Clin Exp Allergy* 1992; 22:533–539.

21. Fernández-Caldas E, Fox RW, Bucholtz GA, Trudeau WL, Ledford DK, Lockey RF. House dust mite allergy in Florida. Mite survey in households of mite-sensitive individuals in Tampa, Florida. *Allergy Proc* 1990; 11:263–267.

22. Arlian LG, Vyszenski-Moher DL, Fernández-Caldas E. Allergenicity of the mite, *Blomia tropicalis*. *J Allergy Clin Immunol* 1993; 91:1042–1050.

23. Griffin P, Ford AW, Alterman L, Thompson J, Parkinson C, Blainey AD, Davies RJ, Topping MD. Allergenic and antigenic relationship between three species of storage mite and the house dust mite, *Dermatophagoides pteronyssinus*. *J Allergy Clin Immunol* 1989; 84:108–117.

24. van Hage-Hamsten M, Johansson SG, Johansson E, Wiren A. Lack of allergenic cross-reactivity between storage mites and *Dermatophagoides pteronyssinus*. *Clin Allergy* 1987; 17:23–31.

25. Puerta L, Fernandez-Caldas E, Lockey R, Caraballo

L. Sensitization to to *Chortoglyphus arcuatus* and *Aleuroglyphus ovatus* in *Dermatophagoides Spp* allergic individuals. *Clin Exp Allergy* 1993; 23:117–123.

26. Arruda LK, Rizzo MC, Chapman MD, Fernández-Caldas E, Baggio D, Platts-Mills, Naspitz CK. Exposure and sensitization to dust mite allergens among asthmatic children in São Paulo, Brazil. *Cin Exp Allergy* 1991; 21:433–439.

27. Stanaland B, Fernández-Caldas E, Jacinto M, Trudeau WL, Lockey R. Positive nasal challenges with *Blomia tropicalis*. *J Allergy Clin Immunol* 1994; 93(2):217.

28. van Hagen-Hamsten M, Ihre E, Zetterstrom O, Johansson SGO. Bronchial provocation studies in farmers with positive RAST to the storage mite *Lepidoglyphus destructor*. *Allergy* 1988; 43:545–551.

29. van Hage-Hamsten M, Machado L, Barros MT, Johansson SGO. Immune Response to *Blomia kulagini* and *Dermatophagoides pteronyssinus* in Sweden and Brazil. *Int Arch Allergy Immunol* 1990; 91:186–191.

30. Caraballo LR, Cadavid A, Mendoza J. Prevalence of asthma in a tropical city of Colombia. *Ann Allergy* 1992; 68:525–529.

31. Puerta L, Fernández-Caldas E, Lockey RF, Caraballo LR. Mite allergy in the tropics: Sensitization to 6 domestic mite species in Cartagena, Colombia. *J Invest Allergol Clin Immunol* 1993; 3:198–204.

32. Fernández-Caldas E, Baena-Cagnani CE, López M, Patiño C, Neffen HE, Sánchez-Medina M, Caraballo L, Huerta López J, Malka S, Naspitz CK, Lockey RF. Cutaneous sensitivity to 6 mite species in asthmatic patients from 5 Latin American countries. *J Invest Allergol Clin Immunol* 1993; 3:245–249.

33. Rizzo MC, Arruda LK, Chapman MD, Fernadez-Caldas E, et al. IgG and IgE antibody responses to dust mite allergens among children with asthma in Brazil. *Ann Allergy* 1993; 71:152–158.

34. Ebner C, Feldner H, Ebner H and Kraft D. Sensitization to storage mites in house dust mite (*Dermatophagoides pteronyssinus*) allergic patients. Comparison of a rural and urban population. *Clin Exp Allergy* 1994; 24:347–352.

35. Berardino LD, Angrisano A, Gorli L, Cattaneo M, Lodi A. Allergy to house dust and storage mites in children: Epidemiologic observations. *Ann Allergy* 1987; 59:104–106.

36. Boner AL, Richelli C, Vallone G et al. Skin and serum reactivity to some storage mites in children sensitive to *Dermatophagoides pteronyssinus*. *Ann Allergy* 1989; 63:82–88.

37. Fernández-Caldas E, Trudeau WL, García-Ramos E, van Hage-Hamsten M, Johansson SGO, Lockey RF. Sensitization to house dust and storage mites in urban dwellers (abstract). *J Allergy Clin Immunol* 1991; 87(2):322.

38. Iversen M, Korsgaard J, Hallas T, Dahl R. Mite allergy and exposure to storage mites and house dust mites in farmers. *Clin Exp Allergy* 1990; 20:211–219.

39. van Hage-Hamsten M, Johansson SGO. Clinical significance and allergenic cross-reactivity of *Euroglyphus maynei* and other nonpyroglyphid and pyroglyphid mites. *J Allergy Clin Immunol* 1989; 83:581–589.

40. Spieksma FTM, Spieksma-Boezeman MIA. High altitude and house dust mites. *Br Med J* 1971; 1:82–84.

41. Vervloet D, Penaud A, Razzouk H, Senft M, Arnaud, A, Boutin C, Charpin J. Altitude and house dust mites. *J Allergy Clin Immunol* 1982; 69:290–296.

42. Charpin D, Birnbaum J, Haddi E, Genard G, Lanteaume A, Toumi M, Faraj F., Van der Brempt X, Vevloet D. Altitude and allergy to house dust mites: A pardigm of the influence of environmental exposure on allergic sensitization. *Am Rev Respir Dis* 1991; 143:983–986.

43. Acaros en Colombia y su relación con las alergias respiratorias. In Sánchez-Medina M, Fernández-Caldas E (Eds) Santafé de Bogotá: Editora Guadalupe Ltda, Colombia, 1994.

44. Cáceres I, Fain A. Notes on the mite fauna of the house dust of homes in Perú. *Bull Ann Soc R Belge d'Entomol* 1978; 114(10/12):301–303.

Mite Allergy in the Asia-Pacific Region

Pakit Vichyanond*

Keywords: House dust mites, allergy, asthma, Asia, Pacific

Allergy to house-dust mites (HDM) is extremely common among populations living in the Asia-Pacific region. Epidemiologic data from various countries in this region indicate that *Dermatophagoides pteronyssinus (Dp)* is the most prevalent species found, with *Dermatophagoides farinae (Df)* prevailing in certain areas, although variable counts in the same region have been demonstrated. *Blomia tropicalis (Bt)* are found exclusively in the Malaysia and Singapore areas. Infestations with house-dust mites are considered heavy in some areas, with counts amounting to thousands of mites per gram, and in other areas reaching tens of thousands mites per gram dust. In accordance with these counts, group I antigens have been determined to be in a moderate to high range, especially in countries near the equator. Sensitization rates in Asians to *Dermatophagoides (Ds)*, as determined by prick skin testing, are high (30–50%) compared to rates seen in caucasians (10–20%). Most asthmatic patients surveyed were sensitive to Ds. Since a large number of individuals with a high degree of mite sensitivity, who also resided in dwellings with high levels of antigens, do not develop clinical symptoms (of asthma and allergic rhinitis), international recommendations for group I antigens for the risk of sensitization (2 µg/gm) and for the development of disease (10 µg/gm) may have to be reexamined for populations who live in the Asia-Pacific region.

Introduction

The Asia-Pacific region is a dynamic area with economic growth in some parts reaching two-digit figures during the past few years. With its rapid industrial growth, life styles of people residing in these countries have changed dramatically. It is therefore inevitable that health problems, which in the past were mostly limited to infectious diseases, will switch over to those commonly encountered in more developed nations such as cancers and envi-

ronmental, allergic, and immunologic problems. Interests in allergic diseases have been well established in the region and existing data indicate that the incidences of allergic diathesis are on the rise, as is observed in other developed nations (1). Research to clarify this is in progress, as evident from efforts such as the formation of the Association of the Asia Pacific Societies of Allergy and Immunology, which held its first Congress in Bangkok in 1992 (the next Congress will be held in Taipei, ROC, in 1995). Allergy to house-dust mites is extremely common among people in this region. The symposium, "Mites in the Tropics", allows an opportunity to reexamine valuable information generated over the years from research laboratories in this region. Hopefully, this review will lead to a better understanding and definition of allergic problems related to house-dust mites in this area. Existing data obtained from Medline searches and from several collaborators within the region will be initially reviewed. Remaining questions will then be addressed and suggestions for future efforts to solve these problems will be finally attempted.

Japan

Japan has been at the forefront of research on mite allergy. Soon after the original work of Voorhost had been published, Miyamoto et al. established in 1968 that the antigens from house dust in Japan are also due to *Dermatophagoides* antigens (2). His earlier works mainly concentrated on Df (3), perhaps due to the work of his colleague, Oshima, who showed the dominance of Df in house dust from both Japan and Taiwan (4). Nevertheless, a later and wider-scale survey by the same group suggested that Dp was more prevalent all over the islands of Japan, and followed by storage mites,

---

* Department of Pediatrics, Faculty of Medicine, Siriraj Hospital, Mahidol University, Thailand.

Glycaphaginae privatus (2). This was in concordance with later studies by Kabasawa et al., who studied dusts from the homes of asthmatic children (5). The results indicated that *Dp* (53%) were twice as common as *Df* (23%). Average mite counts from these earlier Japanese studies pointed to heavy infestations, with counts varying from 518 (5) to 1054 mites/gm dust (2). Interestingly enough, *Blomia* species were the dominant species in dust from Taiwan (2). It was the study by Uchikoshi et al. which indicated that not only carpeted floor can host a large amount of mites, but that concrete floors, wooden floors, and tatami floors can contain a significant number of mites (6).

Up to 70% of patients with perennial allergy were sensitive to house dust allergens (7) and 34 of 35 asthmatic children were sensitive on skin prick tests to *Dp* extracts (5). It can therefore be concluded that dust mite antigens are among the most important allergens in Japan. Several Japanese children are extremely sensitive to these antigens on skin testing, as indicated by their large skin test reactions (up to 25 mm wheal and 45 mm flare was observed, (5)) and by their high RAST titers (8). As in caucasian populations, Shibasaki et al. later showed that specific IgE to mites (*Df*) correlated with the prevalence of asthma in children (8). In contrast to studies from New Zealand (9), a limited survey in asthmatic children by Takeda failed to show any correlation between either total IgE or specific IgE to *Df* and the degree of bronchial hyperresponsiveness (10). Since only 1/5 of children with high RAST titers were symptomatic with asthma, there is a suggestion that, at least in Japanese children, there must be factors other than specific IgE to mites that are important in the generation of the disease status (8).

Korea

Despite a lack of publications in the English language, plenty of reports relating to mite allergy are available in Korean (especially through the *Journal of the Korean Society of Allergology*). Results of these studies indicated high prevalences of positive skin prick tests to house dust mites (40–90%) in allergic individuals, both in children (11, 12) and in adults (13, 14). All studies except one (12) showed *Df* extracts to produce slightly higher positive rates than *Dp*. A large number of skin reac-

tivities to mites (30–40%) were noted in normal populations, both children (15) and adults (16). Studies of the mite fauna by several groups yielded conflicting data, with largest study suggesting *Dp* to be more prevalent than *Df* (17). Nevertheless, a more important study from Korea measuring group I antigens in Korean houses suggested that *Df* may be twice as prevalent as *Dp* (18). In this study, the mean group I antigen was only in a modest range (maximum on sofas, with a mean of 4.69 µg/g). Again, as in Malaysia (see below), some dusts from dry and smooth Korean floors ("Ondol") could contain large amounts of group I antigen (up to 10 µg/gm) (18).

China

As in Korea, several works regarding mite allergy in China are available, mostly in local medical journals. A good summary on mite allergy in China appeared in 1987 (19). It can be concluded that mean mite counts in China can be very high (1328 mites/gm dust), with *Dp* being predominant in the south, while *Df* is common in the northern part. Seasonal variation of asthma coincided with mite counts, with 2 peaks occurring in June and October (October > June) (19, 20) . Between 46% and 89% of asthmatics were sensitive to mite extracts. Mites were detected in the sputum of some patients with pulmonary symptoms, the significance of which is not completely known (21). Mass culturing of *Df* has been successful in Shanghai, and highly potent extracts have been produced for immunotherapy for at least the past 2 decades (20).

Taiwan, ROC

Despite an earlier work by Miyamoto which indicated *Blomia* as the predominant species in the Taipei area (2), a larger-scale survey conducted in the 1980s (1) implicated *Dp* as the major species of mites for this island (78.7%), while *Df* only accounted for a small number (6.2%). Using a standard method for counting, numbers of mites from homes of allergic patients and normal controls were found to be in a modest range (200–400 mites/g dust). There were no difference in the number of mites recovered from floors, carpets, couches, or mattresses. Furthermore, no difference in the number of mites from the homes of patients and controls was observed. There seemed to be a minor variation of mite count throughout the year in Taiwan, in contrast to the two peaks of asthma admissions (April to May and October to November). Mite density can not be predicted by the size of skin wheals to mite extracts since no differences in mite numbers were observed between houses of patients with larger vs. smaller wheals (14 mm cut off).

Using a larger-scale questionnaire survey and RAST to both *Dp* and *Df,* Tang et al. found the prevalence of positive RAST to *Dp* and/or *Df* to be 8.1%, with equal distribution between the two species (22). The prevalences of asthma, allergic rhinitis, and atopic eczema in this study were 4.3%, 9.4%, and 6.0%, respectively. The rates of positive RAST among those with asthma were the highest (52%), followed with those with rhinitis (28.7%) and atopic dermatitis (16.8%). Recent research in children with interesting results (including immunotherapy results) has been published. It was interesting that, besides *Der p I,* to which a large number of children in Taiwan reacted (70%), several (53%) reacted to a unique antigen, the gene of which has recently been cloned and described as *Der p VII* (23).

Hong Kong

Interest in mite allergy in Hong Kong began as early as in the 1970s, when Pickering and Gabriel reported a high incidence of skin reactivities to house-dust mites in patients with atopic asthma in Hong Kong (24). In 1982, a more thorough study on house-dust mites in Hong Kong was published (25). Dust was collected from modern resettlement flats in which Chinese asthmatics resided. Analysis of these samples revealed *Dp* to be the predominant species (51.8%) followed by *Euroglyphus maynei* (*Em*, 16%) and *Df* (13%). Surprisingly, *Blomia tropicalis (Bt)* was quite frequently recovered (10.6%), while other storage mites were relatively uncommon. This contrasted with dusts collected from London, where *Dp* were more common (73.5%) than *Df* (3.6%), and few storage mites were found. It was also established that quilts used in the winter time could be a major source of house dust mites.

In later study reported by Leung and Tseng, the prevalences of asthma, allergic rhinitis, and eczema in schoolchildren were determined by standard questionnaires to be of 7.2%, 21.9%, and 19.1%, respectively (26). Half of the respondents recruited for skin prick testing revealed high percentages (57%) to be atopic (positive SPT to one or more allergens). Among all allergens used, *Dp* was the most common allergen, eliciting the highest percent positive rate (96%), followed by cockroach mix (44.6%) and mold mix (40.6%). Only a handful of children were found to be allergic to pollen extracts, such as grass, trees, and weeds.

Thailand

The early results of an intradermal skin test survey performed in collaboration with the Japanese investigators in 1971 indicated that up to 76% of allergic patients in Thailand were sensitive to house-dust mite by intradermal testing (27). 53% of adult controls and 29% of pediatric controls also gave positive reactions. Later, larger-scale survey in asthmatic children confirmed this earlier contention (28). Moreover, as noted in this later study, sensitization to mites was not uncommonly observed in children less than 2 years of age. A survey of house dust mites from various provinces was reported as early as in 1972 (29). The number of mites in this study was astoundingly high, as some samples in Bangkok was reported to contain over 10,000 mites/g. Since skin prick test results in most of our patients were extremely large (wheal size could be up to 4 cm), we thus became interested in a dust-mite survey again in 1990. Surprisingly, in our initial survey in Bangkok (1990), we detected a much smaller number of mites per gram dust (mean = 23 mites/g). In our more extensive survey, we examined a larger number of dust samples from all over Thailand and found larger number of mites per gram dusts (92.2 mites/g), the majority of which were *Dp*, followed by *Df* (30). In addition, we measured group I antigens and found that while mite counts were relatively low, a large number of samples contained over 10 μg/g of group I antigen. Dust from the homes of allergic patients contained even higher amounts of group I antigens (31). Some samples in our ongoing studies contained group I antigen at up to 170 μg/gm dust! Our studies indicated that mites are ubiquitous in Thailand, and despite the numbers of mites not being large, antigens could be produced prolifically, perhaps due to the higher temperature range. In spite of the awareness of data from Singapore and Malaysia (see below), *Bt* was not commonly observed in any of our surveys.

Malaysia

Despite a relative lack of clinical work in the field of allergy from Malaysia (32), much basic research on the biology of mites has been accomplished by two dedicated acarologists in Kuala Lumpur (Drs. T.M. Ho and M. Nadchatram). From their extensive mite survey in the Peninsular Malaysia, it was apparent that among the many existing pyroglyphids, *Dp* was the most prevalent species encountered (33). Interestingly, the second most common species was *Bt*, followed by *Df and Em* (34). The degree of infestation was high, as counts per gram could reach 3500 mites/g in lower land (34). Common living quarters for the major socioeconomic class in the Southeast Asia, as described by these investigators in one of their later publications ("the houses were of single units with wooden walls and floors; the latter was raised and supported on timber pillars about a meter from the ground...usually without carpets but with some floor mats"), are quite different from those in developing countries (35) and several questions have been raised regarding to the ability of mites to survive in these milieus. From their studies, it was quite clear that mites in tropical areas such as Southeast Asia can survive fairly well on cement and wooden floors without any carpets or rugs (34, 35). Actually, wooden floors due to the presents of cracks and grooves are the densest sites for mite collection, followed by, surprisingly, cement floor, linoleum, and mattress (34). Cleaning such floors by sweeping and mopping with water did not influence the mite density (35). These findings are consistent with the experiences of many allergists within this region, that mite allergy is not limited to the affluent classes but also occurs in those of regular socioeconomic status who live in houses with bare floors. Mites in the tropics may adapt their metabolic activity to maturity (from egg stage to adult mites) faster in a higher temperature (> 25°C) than previously established temperature (at 25°C, (36)).

Singapore

House-dust mite, especially *Dp*, is the most common allergen that asthmatic Singaporians reacted to, both adults (69% (37)) and children (88% (38)). Interestingly, despite the abundance of plants and mold spores in the region, the majority of asthmatics in Singapore reacted to indoor allergen panels, indicating that Singaporians must have been spending a lot of time indoors.

The most interesting work on mite allergy from Southeast Asia perhaps came from theses by two graduate Singaporian students (39, 40), both of which have not yet been published in peer review journals. The first came from the work of Y.M. Neo of the National University of Singapore (in association with M. Nadchatram) (39). While trying to study the life cycle of *Austroglycyphagus malaysiensis*, Neo found that house-dust mites, which were present in all samples collected from homes in Singapore, were most often *Dp* (45%), followed very closely by, surprisingly, *Bt* (38%). It was also established that *Bt* were most commonly found in floor dusts (tiled>cement>carpet>linoleum), while *Dp* were commonly found on the sofa. The amounts of mites found at these two sites were phenomenal (sofa range 1229–33,833, floor range = 1105–30,000). Moreover, the degree of floor and sofa cleaning in this study did not influence the yield of these mites. Neo's findings confirmed the idea that bare floor could be the source of mites, and that merely removing carpet from rooms is not sufficient to remove of mites from these floors. Simultaneously, work by another graduate student, C.W. Ching, also from the National University of Singapore, confirmed that *Bt* was the dominant species found in mattress dusts, while *Dp* was more commonly found in dust from hotel samples (40), again suggesting that *Bt* could be more often associated with bare rather than carpeted floor. It is interesting that while *Bt* counts from Southeast Asia were highest in Singapore, followed by Malaysia, *Bt* was only occasionally found in dusts from Thailand.

Indonesia, the Philippines, and Other Countries

Limited dust mite surveys from the Philippines and Indonesia indicated that *Dp* are more commonly found (than *Df*) in these two countries (41, 42). Densities of *Dp* in Indonesia were reported to be low (between 20 and 104 mites/g, (41)), while those in the Philippines were higher (between 400 and 1000 mites/g (42)) Between 50% and 90% of asthmatics in these countries were sensitive to mite extracts. A field study in school children in Bali reported the prevalence of skin reactivity to be as high as 30% (41).

Limited numbers of patients were referred to the author's practice from Myanmar, Cambodia, and Vietnam for allergy evaluation. These patients exhibited large skin prick test reactions to *Dp* and *Df* extracts, leading the author to believe that, as in the rest of Southeast Asia, mites are the most important allergens for these countries as well.

Australia

This article would not live up to its title if it did not mention Australia, where numerous complex studies on mites have been carried out. In this limited review, two studies deserve particular mention. Although *Df* has been frequently described as rare in Australia, compared to *Dp*, both mites have been found to coexist at the same sites with varying frequencies and densities (43). Green et al. reported a mite survey from three different locations and found densities to vary from 10 to 440 mites/g (43). In a later survey performed at two different locations in New South Wales, Peat et al. reported *Der p I* to be as high as 83 µg/gm in Lismore (a more humid area), indicating a high degree of mite exposure in Australian children (44). Despite this, only 30% of Lismore children were found to be sensitive to mites. Surprisingly, no differences in the prevalences of atopy to mites or asthma (astoundingly high at 30%) were observed between humid area of Lismore and a dry area (Moree/Narrabri).

Special Remarks

Apparently, attempts by conscientious scientists and allergists from this region have confirmed that house-dust mites are among the most important allergens for people in the Asia-Pacific region. It was quite clear from the Japanese studies that a large proportion of individuals with mite sensitivity do not develop clinical allergic conditions. Limited surveys of mite antigens from these regions indicated that there is no correlation between mite counts and group I mite antigens. Moreover, people could live in dwellings with high antigen loads without developing any overt illnesses, indicating that international standards for group I antigens may not be entirely applicable to populations living in this region. Either mite exposure alone is not the most important factor leading to the development of clinical disease (particularly asthma), or people in this region with a long history of parasitic exposure have developed tolerance to high allergen loads. Which is the case is not entirely clear. Future research, both on the clinical effects and on the basic immune response to mites among those who live in the Asia-Pacific region, will be needed to answer these perplexing and unsolved mysteries.

Acknowledgments

I would like to acknowledge contributions from the followings collaborators without whom this work would not be entirely possible; Nat Malainual MS (NIH, Thailand), Martin D Chapman, PhD (Virginia, USA), Professors Chein-Soo Hong, MD and Hae Sim Park, MD (Yonsei University, Korea) Dr TS Wen (Shanghai University, China), F Cua-Lim, MD (the Philippines), Professors Drs PG Konthen, K Baratawidjaja and H. Sunduru (Indonesia), TM Ho, PhD (Malaysia), Chew Fook Tim and B W Lee, MD (Singapore), Drs Anne Woolcock and E Tovey (Australia) and R Tseng, MD (Hong Kong).

Address for correspondence:

Pakit Vichyanond, MD
Associate Professor of Pediatrics
Department of Pediatrics
Faculty of Medicine Siriraj Hospital
Bangkok 10700
Thailand

References

1. Chang Y, Hsieh K. The study of house dust mites in Taiwan. *Ann Allergy* 1989; 62:101–106.
2. Miyamoto T, Oshima S, Domae A, et al. Allergenic potency of different house dusts in relation to contained mites. *Ann Allergy* 1970; 28:405–412.

3. Miyamoto T, Oshima S, Ishizaki T, Sato S. Allergenic identity between the common floor mite (*Dermatophagoides farinae* Hughes, 1961) and house dust as a causative antigen in bronchial asthma. *J Allergy* 1968; 42:14.

4. Oshima S. Studies of the mite fauna in the house dust from Japan and Taiwan. *Jpn J Sanit Zool* 1970; 21:1.

5. Kabasawa Y, Ishii A, Murata H, Takaoka M. Clinical significance of the house dust mite (Dermatophagoides pteronyssinus) in asthmatic children in Japan. *Acta Allergol* 1976; 31:442–454.

6. Uchikoshi S, Kimura H, Nomura K, Chien C, Iida M, Miyake H. A study fo the ecology of house dust mite in dwelling houses. *Tokai J Esp Clin Med* 1982; 7(2):233–243.

7. Uchikoshi S, M O, Ohtsuka H. A statistical study of nasal allergy seen in past 10 years. *Oto Rhino Larygo Tokyo* 1981; 24:145–154.

8. Shibasaki M, Tajima K, Morikawa A, Mitsuhashi M, Sumazaki R, Tokuyama K. Relation between frequency of asthma and IgE antibody levels against *Dermatophagoides farinae* and total serum IgE levels in schoolchildren. *J Allergy Clin Immunol* 1988; 82:86–94.

9. Sears M, Burrow B, Flannery E, Herbison G, Hewitt C, Holdaway M. Relation between airway responsiveness and serum IgE in children with asthma and in apparently normal children. *N Engl J Med* 1991; 325:1067–1071.

10. Takeda K, Shibasaki M, Takita H. Relation between bronchial responsiveness to methacholine and levels of IgE antibody against *Dermatophagoides farinae* and serum IgE in asthmatic children. *Clin Exp Allergy* 1993; 23:450–454.

11. Lee K, Kim K. A study on the method of exclusion of unnecessary allergens from the vaccines for immunotherapy. *J Korean Soc Allergol* 1988; 8(2):150–164.

12. Seo H, Park Y, Chen M, Lee Y. Results of skin test, IgE in pediatric patients with respiratory allergies in Incheon and Kyung Ki area. *J Korean Soc Allergol* 1988; 8(3):271–278.

13. Kang S, Choi B, Moon H, Min K, Kim Y. The prevalence of skin reactions in patients with respiratory allergies. *J Korean Soc Alllergol* 1984; 4(1):49–56.

14. Yoon Y, Lee M, Park H, Park S, Hong C. The skin test reactivity and the level of the total IgE in the allergic patients. *J Korean Soc Allergol* 1989; 9(3):385–398.

15. Ahn Y, Choi E. The result of skin prick tests with 9 common areoallergens in Korea and RAST reactivity to D farinae in a community school children. *J Korean Soc Allergol* 1990; 10(3):213–225.

16. Choi G, Hoe Y, Kang Y, Kim H, Sim N. Skin prick test and RAST reactivity in nonallergic population. *J Korean Soc Allergol* 1989; 9(3):579–586.

17. Cho B. Mite ecology in Korean house dusts. *J Korean Soc Allergol* 1991; 11(1):1–8.

18. Hong C, Lee M. Measurement of group I allergens of house dust mites of Seoul and monthly variations of *Der f* I *J Korean Soc Allergol* 1992; 12(4):482–492.

19. Chien Y, Yang W, Xue Z, Massey D. House dust mite asthma in China: A review. *Ann Allergy* 1987; 59:147–148.

20. Wen T. Mite allergy in China. *Asian Pac J Allergy Immunol* 1992; 10(suppl, Nov 92):S423.

21. Wen T. Mites in sputum and allergy in China. *J Allergy Clin Immunol* 1993; 91(1, part 2):357 (abstr. #863).

22. Tang R, Tsai L, Hwang H, Hwang B, Wu K, Hung M. The prevalence of allergic disease and IgE antibodies to house dust mite in schoolchildren in Taiwan. *Clin Exp Allergy* 1990; 20:33–38.

23. Shen H, Chua K, Lin K, Hseih K, Thomas W. Molecular cloning and characterization of house dust mite allergen Der p VII. *J Allergy Clin Immunol* 1994; 93(1, part 2):205 (abstr. #254).

24. Pickering C, Gabriel M. The pattern of atopic asthma in the Chinese of Hong Kong. *Bull Hong Kong Med Ass* 1973; 25:95.

25. Gabriel M, Cunnington A, Allan WGL, Pickering C, Wraith A. Mite allergy in Hong Kong. *Clin Allergy* 1982;12:157–171.

26. Leung R, Tseng R. Allergic diseases in Hong Kong Schoolchildren. *Hong Kong Practitioner* 1993; 15:2409–2420.

27. Choovivathanavanich P, Oshima S, Miyamoto T, Kanthavichitra N, Suwanprateep P. Mite sensitivity studies on *Dermatophagoides farinae* and house-dust allergy in Thai subjects. *J Thai Med Assoc* 1971; 54:826–835.

28. Tuchinda M, Habanananda S, Vareennil J. Asthma in Thai children: A study of 2000 cases. *Ann Allergy* 1987; 59:207–211.

29. Wongsathuaythong S, Lakshana P. House-dust mite in Thailand. *J Thai Med Assoc* 1972; 1972(5):272–286.

30. Malainual N, Chairat P, Chapman M, Vichyanond P. House-dust mites distribution in Thailand. *J Allergy Clin Immunol* 1994; 93(1, part 2):254 (abstr. #549).

31. Vichyanond P, Malainual N, Chapman M. House dust-mites and the allergic Thai patients. *J Allergy Clin Allergy* 1994; 93(1, part 2):225 (abstr. #554).

32. Thomas V, Tan B, Rajapaksa A. *Dermatophagoides pteronyssinus* and house dust allergy in West Malaysia. *Ann Allergy* 1978; 40:114–116.

33. Ho T. Pyroglyphid mites found in house dust in Peninsular Malaysia. *Trop Biomed* 1986; 3:89–93.

34. Ho T, Nadchatram M. Distribution of *Dermatophagoides pteronyssinus* (Astigmata: Pyroglyphidae) in Cameron Highlands, Malaysia. *Trop Biomed* 1985; 2:54–58.

35. Ho T, Nadchatram M. Distribution of house dust mites in a new settlement scheme in Jengka, Pahang, Malaysia. *Trop Biomed* 1984; 1:49–53.

36. Ho T, Nadchatram M. Life-cycle and longevity of *Dermatophagoides pteronyssinus* (Troussart) (Acarina: Astigmata: Pyroglyphidae) in a tropical laboratory. *Trop Biomed* 1984; 1:159–162.

37. Tan W, Teoh P. An analysis of skin prick test reactions in asthmatics in Singapore. *Ann Allergy* 1979; 43:44–46.

38. Lee B, Teo J, Vellayappan K. Role of atopy in childhiid asthma. *J Singapore Ped Soc* 1989; 31:53–59.

39. Neo Y. The mite fauna of house dust in Singapore with laboratory studies on the life history of *Austroglycyphagus malaysinesis* Fain & Nadchatram. Thesis, National University of Singapore, 1983.

40. Ching C. House dust mites of mattresses in Singapore; Distribution and effect of bedkeeping hygiene. Thesis, National University of Singapore, 1983.

41. Woolcock A, Konthen P, Sedgwick C. Allergic status of children in an Indonesian village. *Asian Pac J Allergy Immunol* 1984; 2:7–12.

42. Cua-Lim F. House dust mites and respiratory allergy in Metro Manila. *Phil J Internal Med* 1990; 28:127–32.

43. Green W, Sedgwick C, Woolcock A, Leeder S, Stuckey M. House dust mites and skin tests in different australian localities. *Aust NZ J Med* 1986; 16:639–643.

44. Peat J, Tovey E, Mellis S, Woolcock A. Importance of house dust mites and alternaria allergens in childhood asthma: an epidemiological study in two climatic reions of Australia. *Clin Exp Allergy* 1993; 23:812–820.

Mite Allergen Exposure in Latin America

Carlos E Baena-Cagnani*, Cecilia M Patiño**

Keywords: Mite, allergens, exposure, Latin America, asthma

Many studies on mite allergy and asthma have been done in Latin American countries in the last 10 years. The current knowledge gained on this matter is summarized here. It strongly suggests that indoor environment control must be carried out in homes from asthmatic patients.

Indoor allergens are considered to play a major role in the etiology of allergic diseases, and their distribution is currently being better understood, particularly those from house dust mite origen (1).

In the last 25 years many studies have shown the proliferation of house dust mites in different parts of the world. A strong association between asthma and mite-allergen exposure has been firmly established, and the WHO expert panel report has called this association "... a worldwide problem." However, information provided on mite allergy in Latin America in this publication was scarce (2).

The first studies on mite allergy in the region were done during the 1970s; since then, the interest in house dust mites has increased in Latin America, and studies from Colombia (3), Argentina (4), Uruguay (5), Brazil (6), and Venezuela (7), among others, have been published.

A considerable body of information regarding house dust mite distribution, epidemiology, and allergen exposure in Latin America has been gained. Recently, a high prevalence of skin sensitivity to mite extracts among asthmatic patients has been shown.

Argentinian studies have demonstrated a significantly higher prevalence of mite sensitivity in both children and adults with asthma compared to the nonallergic population (8, 9).

A multinational survey was conducted in seven cities from five Latin America countries including Argentina, Brazil, Colombia, Mexico, and Venezuela. This study demonstrated that skin test sensitivity to different mite species is very common, ranging from 40% to *Aleuroglyphus ovatus (Ao)* in Mexico city to 97.2% to *Dermatophagoides farinae (Df)* in Caracas, Venezuela. Moreover, skin test positivities to other four species studied, *Dermatophagoides pteronyssinus (Dp)*, *Lepidoglyphus destructor (Ld)*, *Chortoglyphus arcuatus (Ca)* and *Blomia tropicalis (Bt)*, were also found in patients from all these cities (10).

Mite Fauna in Argentina and Other Latin American Countries

Studies on mite allergy have mainly focused on the the pyroglyphids *D. pteronyssinus* and *D. farinae*, which have been found in house dust samples in Argentina. In the last few years the mite fauna of house dust recovered from aspirates from pillows and mattresses has been analyzed.

A preliminary survey conducted in Córdoba, Argentina, showed a great variety of mite species in dust samples from pillows and mattresses. Together with *D. pteronyssinus* and *D. farinae* we identified *Euroglyphus maynei, Tarsonemus* spp., *Cheyletus* spp., *Oribatidae, Lepidoglyphus destructor*, and *Chortoglyphus arcuatus*. The mean concentration of mites was higher in pillows (358.5 mites/g of dust) than in mattresses (76.4 mites/g). The number of mites ranged from 20 to 720 mites per gram of dust, the mean values being above the critical levels for sensitization (11). The asthmatic children from this study lived in an environment with a hea mite allergen load (Table 1).

* Division of Allergology & Clinical Immunology, Department of Pediatrics, Hospital Infantil Municipal, Universidad Nacional de Córdoba, Argentina.
** Also: Department of Histology and Genetics, University of Córdoba.

Table 1. Mite fauna and mite count in dust samples from pillows and mattresses from Cordoba, Argentina.

Species	Pillows (n = 13)	Mattresses (n = 11)
D. pteronyssinus	8 (20–420)	2 (60)
D. farinae	8 (20–440)	5 (20–40)
E. maynei	4 (20–160)	1 (40)
Tarsonemus spp.	2 (80–740)	2 (120–320)
Cheylatus spp.	3 (20)	1 (40)
Oribatidae	2 (20–40)	1 (20)
Lepidoghyphus spp.	1 (20)	0
C. arcuatus	2 (20)	0
Mean mite count/g	358.5	76.4

Exposure to Mite Allergens in Argentina and Other Latin American Countries

The different mite species must be identified and counted in house dust samples since there is a great variety of them, formerly called "storage mites", now designated "domestic mites". Most of them have the capacity for sensitizing human beings and expressing species-specific allergens.

Together with mite identification, the mite allergen content is an important issue when the environment is studied. Despite the fact that mite numbers can be low, the levels of mite allergen can be high. The assesment of the allergen content in house dust samples is required for a successful evaluation of dwelling environments and complements mite counts and identification (23).

Argentinian studies have analyzed the allergen content in both pillows and mattresses but have emphasized the allergen content in pillows for two main reasons: (i) The patients breathe close to the pillows and not to the mattresses; (ii) at night there are no disturbances, so that the allergens come to "rest" on the floor and carpets.

A study has detected high levels of group I (G-I, *Der p* I + *Der f* I) allergens in both mattresses and pillows above 2 µg/g of dust (11). Another survey has analyzed the allergen concentration in wool and foam mattresses and pillows. The mean G-I allergen concentration was higher in wool pillows and mattresses (13.8 and 11.7 µg/g, respectively) than those of foam material (6.1 and 6.1 µg/g, respectively). Although the difference was not statisticaly significant, it was demostrated that pillows constitute an important allergen reservoir (24). An Argentinian study from Santa Fé also showed high levels of G-I mite allergens in dust samples from pillows and mattresses (6.7 and 4.3 µg/g, respectively) (25), emphazising the importance of pillows as a mite allergen nest.

Allergen exposure has been studied in other regions of Latin America such as São Paulo, Brazil. In 18 out of 20 houses studied it was possible to detect levels of *Der p* I greater than 10 µg/g of dust. The highest level of *Der p* I and group II allergens was found in bedding, followed by bedroom floor. This study also showed more than 200 RAST units/ml to *Blomia tropicalis* in 13 out of 20 sera (26).

Other reports from Latin American countries

We recently completed a study concerning mite fauna in 108 pillows and 107 mattresses (12). The same mite fauna profile reported in the preliminary study was found, levels lying above that recommended as critical to sensitize susceptible individuals.

Baggio and Croce in Brazil reviewed the mite fauna from 16 studies conducted in different Brazilian cities and found a great variety of mites including *Blomia* spp., *Pyroglyphidae* spp. and *Glyciphagus*, among others (13).

Another survey from Chile has studied the mite fauna in different regions of the country which has great variations in climatic conditions from north to south and from the coastal side to the Andes (14).

Studies from Cartagena, Colombia, have shown a very rich mite fauna. This tropical caribbean city has a mean annual temperature of 28°C and a relative humidity of 82%, both of which favor mite growth, including *Ca* and *Ao* ranging from 20 to 800 mites/g of dust samples (15). Allergic patients from this region have IgE levels against *Dp, Ao* and *Ca* (16) and *Bt* and *Ld* (17).

An earlier investigation from Colombia detected different mite species such as *Acarus siro, Tyrophagus putrescentiae*, and *Suidasia nesbitii* in Bogotá (18). This city is situated 2680 m above sea level, and interestingly, mites and mite allergens were found despite the city's altitude (19); this agrees with a study from Perú, at 3000 m above sea level (20), and contradicts European studies (21, 22). However, it must be considered that, despite the high altitude of Bogota, both the temperature and humidity are higher than in the European areas studied, thus providing better conditions for mite growth.

have discovered mite allergens in dust samples from Cartagena, Colombia (27); Curitiba, Brazil (28); and 5 Mexican cities (39).

Conclusions

Many studies on mite allergy and asthma have been done in Latin American countries in the last 10 years. The current knowledge gained on this matter is summarized in Table 2 and strongly suggests that indoor environment control must be done in homes from asthmatic patients.

Table 2. Insights gained on mite allergy from studies conducted in Latin American countries.

– The mite fauna is rich and variated
– Storage mites have capacity to induce skin test
  positivities and specific-serum IgE levels
– Mites are able to grow in the altitude
  as long as high temperatures and humidity exist
– Pillows are important reservoirs for mites
  and mite allergens

Address for correspondence:

Dr Carlos E Baena-Cagnani
Santa Rosa 381
(5000) Córdoba
Argentina

References

1. Fernández-Caldas E, Reed CE, Lokey RF. Distribution of indoor allergens. In Lockey RF, Buckantz SC (Eds) *Allergen immunotherapy*. New York: Marcel Dekker Inc, 1991, 69–101.

2. Platts-Mills TAE, de Weck AL. Dust mite allergens and asthma-A worldwide problem. Report of an international workshop. *J Allergy Clin Immunol* 1989; 83:416–427.

4. Asrilant M. Acaros domésticos y alergia al polvo de habitación. *Arch Arg Alergia Inmunol* 1972; 9:9–12.

5. Schuhl JF. Asma y alergia a ácaros en Montevideo. Estudio preliminar. *Allergol Immunopathol* 1977; 5:177–80.

6. Neto J, Croce J. Baggio D. Acaros da poeira domicilar da cidade de São Paulo. *Rev Bras Alergia Imunopathol* 1980; 2:140–5.

7. Hurtado I, Parini M. House dust mites in Caracas,

Venezuela. *Ann Allergy* 1987; 59:128–30.

8. Patiño CM, Baena-Cagnani CE, Fernández-Caldas E, Bustos GJ, Lockey RF. Skin sensitivity to 6 different mite species in asthmatic children. *J Allergy Clin Immunol* 1993; 91:498 a.

9. Baena-Cagnani CE, Neffen HE, Fernández-Caldas E, Patiño CM, Sánchez Guerra ME, Cuello MN, Bustos GJ. Sensibilidad cutánea a ácaros domésticos y de depósitos en niños y adultos asmáticos. *Arch Arg Alergia Inmunol* 1992; 23:66–71.

10. Fernández-Caldas E, Baena-Cagnani CE, López M, Patiño C, Neffen HE, Sánchez Medina M, Caraballo LR, Huerta López J, Malka S, Naspitz C, Lockey RF. Cutaneous sensitivity to six mite species in asthmatics patients from five Latin American countries. *J Invest Allergol Clin Immunol* 1993; 3:245–9.

11. Baena-Cagnani CE, Fernández-Caldas E, Patiño CM, Cuello MN, Bustos GJ, Lockey RF. In preparation.

12. Fernández-Caldas E, Patiño C, Cuello M, Lockey RF, Baena-Cagnani CE. Mite allergen levels and mite fauna in pillows and mattresses in Córdoba, Argentina. Accepted to the XV ICACI, 1994.

13. Baggio D, Croce J. Acaros contaminantes de ambientes e causadores de doenças alérgicas no homen. Unpublished.

14. Artigas JN, Casanueva ME. House dust mites from Chile (acari). *Guyana Zool* 1993; 47:5–104.

15. Fernández-Caldas E, Mercado D, Puerta L, Lockey RF, Caraballo LR. House dust mite sensitivity and mite fauna in the tropics. *J Allergy Clin Immunol* 1992; 89:257 a.

16. Puerta L, Fernández-Caldas E, Lockey RF, Caraballo LR. Sensitization to *Chortoglyphus arcuatus* and *Aleuroglyphus ovatus* in *Dermatophagoides* spp. allergic individuals. *Clin Exp Allergy* 1993; 23:117–23.

17. Puerta LLerena L, Fernández-Caldas E, Caraballo Gracia LR, Lockey RF. Sensitization to *Blomia tropicalis* and *Lepidoglyphus destructor* in *Dermatophagoides* spp. allergic individuals. *J Allergy Clin Immunol* 1991; 88:493–50.

18. Mulla MS, Sánchez Medina M, Charlet L. Faunistic and taxonomy of domestic acari in from house dust in Columbia. In Mulla MS, Sánchez Medina M (Eds) *Acaros en Colombia: Bionomía y distribución. Su importancia en la enfermedades alérgicas.* Bogotá: Editora Guadalupe, 1980.

19. Sánchez Medina M, Correa C. Controversial study of altitude mites and asthma. *J Allergy Clin Immunol* 1994; 93:254 a.

20. Cáceres I, Fain A. Notes of the mite fauna of the house dust of homes in Perú. *Bull Ann Soc R Belg d'Entomol* 1978; 114:301–3.

21. Vervloet D, Penaud A, Razzouk H, Senft M, Arnaud A, Boutin C, Charpin D. Altitude and house dust mites. *J Allergy Clin Immunol* 1982; 69:290.

22. Charpin D, Birnbaum J, Haddi E, Genard A, Lanteaume A, Toumi M, Faraj F, Van Der Brempt X, Vervloet D. Altitude and allergy to house dust mite. A paradigm of the influence of environmental exposure on allergic sensitization. *Am Rev Respir Dis* 1991; 143:983–6.

23. Luczynska CM, Arruda LK, Platts-Mills TAE, Miller JD, López M, Chapman MD. A two-site monoclonal antibody ELISA for the quantification of the major *Dermatophagoides* spp. allergens, *Der p* I and *Der f* I. *J Immunol Meth* 1989; 118:227–235.

24. Baena-Cagnani CE, Fernández-Caldas E, Patiño C, Swanson MC, Trudeau WL, Cuello M, Lockey RF. Comparison of mite allergen levels in pillows and mattresses. *J Allergy Clin Immunol* 1993; 91:352 a.

25. Predolini N, Sánchez Guerra M, Neffen H, Arlian LG, Fernández-Caldas E, Trudeau WL, Lockey RF. Sensitization to 7 domestic mites and mite allergen exposure in Argentina. *J Allergy Clin Immunol* 1993; 91:355 a.

26. Arruda LK, Rizzo MC, Chapman MD, Fernández-Caldas E, Baggio D, Platts-Mills TAE, Naspitz CK. Exposure and sensitization to dust mites allergens among asthmatic children in São Paulo, Brazil. *Clin Exp Allergy* 1991; 21:433–39.

27. Fernández-Caldas E, Puerta L, Lockey RF, Caraballo LR. Mite allergy in the tropics: Sensitization to six domestic mite species in Cartagena. *Clin Exp Allergy* 1993; 23:292–7.

28. Sugisawa S, Rosario NA, Baggio D, Suzuki M. Exposure to mites in public schools. *J Allergy Clin Immunol* 1994; 93:256 a.

29. González Velazco RN, Canseco González CP, Villareal Barrera G, González Díaz SN, Ulloa Portillo JC, Villa Michel ER, Salas Cepeda A, Rodríguez Pérez N, Swanson MC, Alvarado Valdés CA, Reed CE. Indoor dust allergens from 5 cities in Mexico. *J Allergy Clin Immunol* 1993; 91:352.

Environmental Control of Mite Allergy

Charles K Naspitz*, M Candida Rizzo*, L Karla Arruda**, E Fernandez-Caldas***, Dirceu Solé*, Martin D Chapman**, Thomas AE Platts-Mills**

Keywords: Domestic mites, *Dermatophagoides pteronyssinus*, *Blomia tropicalis*, asthma, endotoxins, acaricides, avoidance

There are several lines of evidence for a causal relationship between the quantity of domestic mite allergen and both sensitization and asthma. In areas with a tropical climate, domestic mites are completely dominant, mainly *D. pteronyssinus* and *Blomia tropicalis*. Mite allergen levels in houses in São Paulo are quite high, and the highest levels of *Der p* I were measured in bedding samples. The high levels of IgE and IgG antibodies to domestic mites observed point to the importance of environmental avoidance measures in the management of asthma. The possibility that the clinical manifestations of asthma could be modulated by endotoxin (ET) is also under investigation; levels of ET and the growth of gram-negative bacteria (GNB) in the bedroom of atopic and nonatopic children were measured monthly for one year. The correlation of these data with clinical symptoms and spirometry may help to validate the hypothesis that ET are able to potentiate inflammatory responses as an important factor in modulating asthma severity. GNB, the source of ET, probably are brought in from the streets on the shoes. To the instructions for reducing exposure to domestic mites, it may be necessary to add: remove shoes before entering the house or bedroom. Allergen avoidance should be seen as the primary anti-inflammatory treatment for asthma.

The association between hypersensitivity to inhalant allergens and childhood asthma has long been recognized. However, it has been increasingly appreciated that this response is limited to those children who develop an IgE antibody response. In some areas of the world, domestic mites of the genus *Dermatophagoides* are completely dominant, with up to 85% of asthmatic children having positive skin tests to mite allergens (1). In other areas, cat, dog, or cockroach allergens are also important. The evidence for a causal relationship has been well established by several studies that have shown a direct link between the quantity of domestic mite allergen exposure and both sensitization and asthma (1): there is a strong association between sensitization to indoor allergens and asthma (specific association); there is a dose response relationship between exposure to domestic mites allergens and sensitization; the nebulization of domestic mites or their specific allergens can induce bronchospasm, bronchial hyper-reactivity (BHR), and a characteristic inflammatory infiltrate; viral infections, ozone, passive smoking, etc., can induce the symptoms of asthma, but not the eosinophilic infiltrate; avoidance of domestic mites can both reduce asthma symptoms and decrease nonspecific BHR.

Several investigators have been working on the identification and definition of mite allergens. Two main groups, I and II, account for most of its allergenicity. The group I allergens are found in the fecal pellets, and the group II allergens are derived from both the mite bodies and feces. Group III allergens have also been described, as well as groups IV and V.

It has been proposed that exposure to > 2 µg of *Der p* I/g of dust is a risk factor for the development of mite sensitization and asthma, and exposure to > 10 µg/g of dust has been associated with an increased risk of acute exacerbations of asthma (2).

At this point, it is logical to conclude that the environmental control of mites, reducing the relevant allergens, might be considered the primary anti-inflammatory treatment for asthma; dramatic improvements have been achieved in almost all studies that have reduced exposure (1).

* Division of Allergy, Clinical Immunology and Rheumatology, Department of Pediatrics, Escola Paulista de Medicina, São Paulo, Brazil.
** Division of Allergy and Clinical Immunology, Department of Medicine, University of Virginia Health Sciences Center, Charlottesville, Virginia, USA.
*** Division of Allergy and Immunology, University of South Florida College of Medicine, Tampa, Florida, USA.

We studied 20 allergic asthmatic children aged 6–12 years, living in São Paulo, regarding their degree of sensitization to domestic mites and exposure to mite allergens in their homes (3). In 18 out of 20 houses, at least one dust sample was obtained which contained > 10 µg *Der p* I/g of dust. The highest levels of *D. pteronyssinus* allergens were measured in bedding samples. Mite allergen levels in Brazilian houses were as high as those reported to be associated with sensitization and acute attacks of asthma in other parts of the world. As *D. farinae* is rarely found in Brazil, *Der f* I was undetectable or found only at very low levels. Levels of IgE antibodies to *D. pteronyssinus* were > 200 RAST U/ml in 19 out of 20 children. IgE antibodies to the mite *Blomia tropicalis* were also measured, and levels > 200 RAST U/ml were observed in 13 out of 20 sera. The absence of group I allergens in *Blomia tropicalis* was confirmed by both monoclonal and polyclonal antibody-based immunoassays. The results suggested that *B. tropicalis* produced allergens that were distinct from the major *D. pteronyssinus* allergens. Immunoabsorption studies demonstrated that the bulk of the IgE antibody to *B. tropicalis* (64%) was to species-specific allergens and that 36% were cross-reactive with *D. pteronyssinus*. This finding implies

that management of children with asthma in São Paulo should include skin testing and possibly immunotherapy with *B. tropicalis*. Recently, we described the identification and partial nucleotide sequence of cDNA clones that express a *B. tropicalis* IgE binding protein. This protein, tentatively designated as *Blo t* 5, appears to be a major *B. tropicalis* antigen (4).

The aim of the next study (5) was to quantify indoor allergen levels and antibody responses to those allergens in a group of mite allergic asthmatic children (positive skin tests to *D. pteronyssinus*), and to compare both exposure and sensitization to a group of nonasthmatic nonatopic children (negative skin tests to *D. pteronyssinus*, *D. farinae*, and *B. tropicalis*) from the same area. In 16/20 and 17/20 houses of asthmatic and control children, respectively, at least one sample was obtained which contained > 10 µg *Der p* I/g of dust. Major allergens from domestic mites, cat and cockroach were measured in four sites from all 40 houses. The highest levels of *Der p* I were measured in bedding samples, followed by bedroom floor, TV room, and kitchen (Figure 1). Similar results were obtained for group II allergens. Serum IgE antibodies to *D. pteronyssinus* and *B. tropicalis* were > 200 RAST U/ml in 19/20 and in 16/20 asthmatic chil-

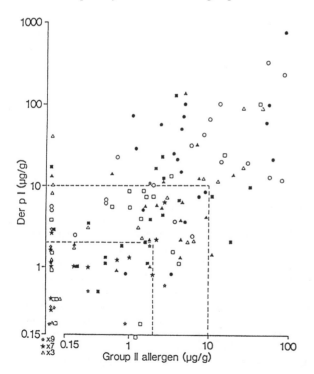

Figure 1. Levels of *Der p* I and group II allergens in 160 dust samples from houses of asthmatic patients (solid symbols) and controls (open symbols), collected from four sites of each subject's homes: bedding (●, ○); bedroom floor (■, ▢); TV room (▲, △); and kitchen (★, ☆). Dashed lines indicate 2 µg/g and 10 µg/g of dust, which have been proposed as threshold levels for sensitization and for development of acute symptoms of asthma in mite-allergic individuals, respectively.

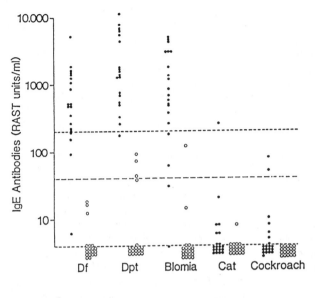

Figure 2. Measurements of IgE antibodies to *D. farinae* (Df), *D. pteronyssinus* (Dpt), *B. tropicalis* (Blomia), cat, and cockroach in sera from asthmatic children (●) and controls (○). The lower dashed line represents the detection level of the assay (4 RAST U/ml). The upper dashed lines represent 40 and 200 RAST U/ml, respectively.

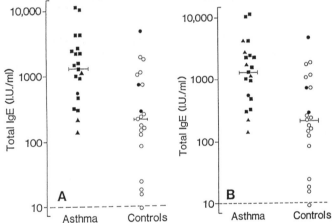

Figure 3. Total serum IgE levels in 20 patients with asthma and 20 controls. Sera were grouped according to the levels of IgE antibody, measured by RAST, to any of the five allergens studied (Figure 3A) or to the levels of IgE antibodies to *D. pteronyssinus* (Figure 3B) as follows:■ ≥ 800 U/ml; ▲ 200 to < 800 U/ml; ● 40 to < 200 U/ml; and ○ < 40 U/ml. The geometric mean values for the groups are shown by bars (GM for patients with asthma = 1318 IU/ml, GM for controls 212 IU/ml).

dren, respectively. In the control group, IgE antibodies to both mite species were < 40 RAST U/ml in most cases. IgE antibodies to cat and cockroach were undetectable or found in very low levels in most subjects (Figure 2). Total serum IgE was significantly higher in asthmatics and the highest levels of specific IgE were found in this group (Figure 3). IgG anti-*Der p* I and anti *Der f* I antibodies were detected in 17/20 asthmatics, as opposed to 3/20 controls (Figure 4). Although exposure to high levels of mite allergens was common in São Paulo, significant IgE and IgG antibody responses were detected only in children with asthma.

The high levels of IgE and IgG antibodies to domestic mites observed in all these studies stress the importance of environmental avoidance measures in the management of childhood asthma.

Although mites do not normally colonize humans, the scalp might be a potential source of mites, which could be deposited in the pillows. In some atopic and nonatopic children, we observed a variable number of different domestic mites in material obtained from the scalp using a handheld vacuum cleaner. Studies are in progress to determine the allergen levels and their eventual relationship to disease severity.

However, there is also another substance, endotoxin, composed of lipopolysaccharide (LPS)

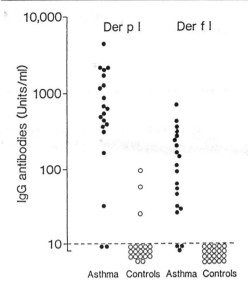

Figure 4. Quantitative measurements of IgG anti-Der p I and anti-Der f I antibodies in sera from patients with asthma (●) and controls (○), using antigen-binding RIA.

from the outer membrane of gram-negative bacteria (GNB). Endotoxins (ET) are very potent proinflammatory substances present in a variety of domestic and occupational dusts. Acute inhalation of 200 µg LPS induces a bronchial obstructive response in normal subjects; lower doses (20–40 µg) elicit a bronchial obstruction in subjects with asthma (6). The ET concentration and dust mite antigen content were determined in the houses of 28 adult asthmatics. There was no correlation between ET and mite concentrations. The asthma was more severe in the subjects exposed to higher ET concentrations. In conclusion, ET is present in the normal domestic environment and could have a deleterious effect on chronic asthma (7).

Based on these and other studies with ET, the possibility that the clinical manifestations of asthma could be modulated by ET was raised. To evaluate whether ET acts in synergy with specific domestic mite allergens, or whether it has its own actions on the asthma severity, we studied 10 asthmatic and 10 nonasthmatic patients (8–16 years old), from November 1992 to February 1994. *Der p* I, *Der f* I, and ET levels were measured in dust samples collected monthly from mattresses and floors in the 20 homes. To correlate the presence of ET with bacteria, bacterial growth was obtained from bedding, the bedroom floor, and indoor (ID)

and outdoor (OD) air samples. As there were (unexpectedly) more airborne gram-positive bacteria (ID, OD) and more GNB on the surfaces, we suspected that GNB were brought from the streets through the shoes. In fact, there was considerable growth of GNB when cultures were obtained from shoe soles. No significant correlation was observed between ET levels and GNB colony forming units (CFU). Overall, there was no correlation between ET and mite allergen levels, as was previously reported (7). RASTs to *B. tropicalis* and other mites are being analyzed, as well all the clinical data related to asthmatic symptoms, including AM and PM peak flowmeter values; all these data were collected daily, as were indoor and outdoor temperature and humidity. The correlation of all the data (ET and mite allergen levels, bacterial growth, clinical symptoms, spirometry and PFM readings) might help to validate the hypothesis that ET is able to potentiate inflammatory responses as an important factor in modulating asthma severity. It is important to stress that although all children in this study were submitted to the same load of ET and mite allergens, there were no symptoms in the control group, suggesting that in the absence of a genetic predisposition, ET by itself is not able to induce bronchial obstruction, as was reported in normal subjects after acute inhalations of ET (6).

Instructions for Reducing Exposure to Domestic Mites

Reducing the mite population is a difficult task. In an ideal case, one would remove the normal habitat of the mites and make what remains inhospitable for them. Methods to reduce the number of mites have mainly been developed in affluent countries, and very little is known about the influence of different types of housing on mite populations in partly affluent and nonaffluent countries. Education alone will not ensure compliance with domestic mite controls. Economic factors also influence the matter. Access to free or low cost mite-proof pillow and mattress covers may improve asthma care for poor children (8). Most attention should be directed to the patient's bedroom, although if possible the whole apartment or house should be treated. Mattresses, box springs, and pillows should be encased appropriately, not only to contain the allergen but also to deprive mites of an external source of humidity and food. Bed linen and blankets should be washed once a week in hot water (over 55°C) to ensure mite killing. Ideally, the carpet should be removed and replaced by vinyl or polished wooden floor boards. If it is impossible to remove the carpet, it can be completely covered by polyethylene sheeting, taped to the skirting board. Vacuum cleaning removes loose dust, but has no effect on the number of live mites in the carpet (the mites attach themselves to the fibers), and in fact some devices make large quantities of allergen airborne. Steam cleaning is inefficient at killing mites; they simply burrow deep into the carpet and are insulated from the heat. Curtains should be washable at 55°C. Children's soft toys can be a potent source of domestic mite allergen, and should be removed, washed in hot water, or deep frozen once a week. Furniture should not be fabric covered. Vinyl, leather, or plain wooden furniture is best. Reducing humidity may be important, since the concentration of domestic mites increases with increasing indoor humidity. Ambient humidity can be reduced with dehumidifiers or air conditioning. Room air cleaning devices include the high-efficiency particulate air unit, HEPA, a commonly used mechanical filter. The role of these devices is not defined (1)..

Acaricides (substances that kill mites via chemical action), including benzyl benzoate, pyrethoids, pirimiphos methyl, and liquid nitrogen, are being used, but have no proven effect at present. They can therefore not be recommended. Both benzyl benzoate (BB) and tannic acid (a 3% solution denatures domestic mite allergen) are very effective *in vitro*, although the difficulty of applying them so that they reach deep into the pile or padding of furniture or carpets reduces their effectiveness. The efficacy of acaricides is influenced by a variety of factors within each home and by the delivery systems, but these issues have not as yet been adequately addressed. Long-term exposure to acaricides requires rigorous safety and toxicity studies. Application of chemical acaricides to bedrooms where children have prolonged contact (via mattresses, pillows, carpets) is not recommended. In agricultural use, mites have developed resistance to acaricides. The available data do not justify the use of fungicides in the control of domestic mites (1, 7).

Recently, it was shown in a 12-month study involving 24 children aged 7–15 years, that a reduction in mite allergen exposure below a previously proposed threshold level of 2 µg/g of mattress dust could be achieved by the encasing procedure after as little as 14 days, whereas BB acaricide treatment appeared to be ineffective. More importantly, only in the encasing-regimen group was there a significant reduction in bronchial hyper-reactivity after 8 months of treatment (9).

Because of the possibility that a prejudicial association between GNB, ET, and domestic mites might be implicated in the severity of childhood asthma, removing shoes before entering the bedroom is a recommendation that may be added to the above instructions.

In conclusion, allergen avoidance should be seen as the primary anti-inflammatory treatment for asthma (1). Reducing allergen exposure allows a reduction in the amount of medication required. Allergen avoidance, however, requires a degree of effort and commitment from the parents of asthmatic children that has become alien in the treatment of asthma in an era when people are used to rapid bronchodilation treatment and short-term improvement. It also requires of the physician a considerable degree of conviction, explanation, encouragement, and persistence.

Address for correspondence:

Charles K Naspitz, MD
Rua Sergipe, 634 – 13 A
01243-000, São Paulo
Brazil.

References

1. Sporik R, Heymann PE, Fernandez-Caldas E, Platts-Mills TAE. Indoor allergens and asthma. In DG Tinkelman, CK Naspitz (Eds) *Childhood Asthma. Pathophysiology and Treatment.* New York: Marcel Dekker, 1993, pp 497–535.

2. Platts-Mills TAE, Thomas WR, Aalberse RC et al. Dust mite allergens and asthma: Report of a second international workshop. *J Allergy Clin Immunol* 1992; 89:1046–1060.

3. Arruda LK, Rizzo MC, Chapman MD, Fernandez-Caldas E, Baggio D, Platts-Mills TAE, Naspitz CK. Exposure and sensitization to dust mite allergens among asthmatic children in São Paulo, Brazil. *Clin Exp Allergy* 1991; 21:433–439.

4. Arruda LK, Fernandez-Caldas E, Naspitz CK, Montealegre F, Chapman MD. Molecular cloning of *Blomia tropicalis* allergen Blo t 5 and its sequence homology to *D. pteronyssinus* Der p 5. *J Allergy Clin Immunol* 1994; 93:205.

5. Rizzo MC, Arruda LK, Chapman MD, Fernandez-Caldas E, Baggio D, Platts-Mills TAE, Naspitz CK. IgG and IgE antibody responses to dust mite allergens among children with asthma in Brazil. *Ann Allergy* 1993; 71:152–158.

6. Michel O, Ginanni R, Le Bon B, Content J, Duchateau J, Serysels R. Inflammatory response to acute inhalation of endotoxin in asthmatic patients. *Am Rev Resp Dis* 1992; 146:352–357.

7. Michel O, Ginanni R, Duchateau J, Vertongen F, Le Bon B, Sergysels R. Domestic endotoxin exposure and clinical severity of asthma. *Clin Exp Allergy* 1991; 21:441–448.

8. Denson-Lino JM, Wilies-Jacobo LJ, Rosas A, O'-Connor RDO, Wilson NW. Effect of economic status on the use of house dust mite avoidance measures in asthmatic children. *Ann Allergy* 1993; 71:130–132.

9. Ehnert B, Lau-Schadendorf S, Weber A, Buetnner P, Schou C, Wahn U. Reducing domestic exposure to dust mite allergen reduces bronchial hyperreactivity in sensitive children with asthma. *J Allergy Clin Immunol* 1992; 90:135–138.

Index of Keywords*

A

acaricides 334
adenosine deaminase deficiency 286
adhesion molecules 13
adults 263
air pollution 83
airway hyperresponsiveness 301
airway responsiveness 63
allergen avoidance 126
allergen carrier 83
allergen-specific treatment 126
allergic diseases 161, 275
allergic rhinitis diary 160
allergotoxicology 83
allergy training programme 148
alveolar macrophages 1
antigen presentation 1, 215
anxiety 198
AP-1 310
Asia 323
asthma 13, 50, 55, 63, 90, 97, 104, 109, 119,
  126, 132, 156, 167, 174, 183, 194, 198, 208,
  251, 258, 305, 317, 323, 330, 334
asthma clinics 148
asthma diary 160
asthma management 203
asthmatic child 143
ATC/RCGP Asthma Diploma 148
atopic dermatitis (AD) 263, 275
atopic eczema 174
avoidance 334

B

B-cell epitope 220
basophils 19, 30, 268
Blomia tropicalis 334
bronchoconstriction 119
Btk 242
bullous pemphigoid 26

C

Ca^{2+} channel 113
calcium antagonists 113
cat 90
$CD8^+$ T cells 1
chemokines 30

children 97, 167
chloride channels 113
clinical efficacy 126
cockroach 90
coreceptor 69
corticosteroids 132
costimulation 69
cyclosporin A, 19, 132, 310
cytokine cascade 275
cytokines 26, 39, 50, 55, 275
cytotoxic T lymphocyte 296

D

dendritic cells 1
depression 198
Dermatophagoides pteronyssinus 334
diagnosis 226, 268
diagnostic procedures 268
documentation 152
domestic mites 334
double blind method 268
dyspnea 198

E

East Germany 174
edema 301
education 163
emotion 198
endotoxins 334
environment 97, 104
eosinophil granule proteins 305
eosinophils 13, 26, 30, 45, 55, 237, 251, 258
epidemiology 83, 174
epithelial lining fluid 301
epithelium 55
epitopes 215
European Community Respiratory Health
  Survey 172
exposure 330

F

families of asthmatic children 143
fatal asthma 189
fears 163
5-lipoxygenase 119
FK506 310

---

* This index was prepared on the basis of the keywords supplied by the authors. The page numbers refer to the first
  page of the chapter referring to the subject.